Handbook of Experimental Pharmacology

Volume 138

Springer
Berlin
Heidelberg
New York
Barcelona
Hong Kong
London
Milan
Paris
Singapore
Tokyo

Antiepileptic Drugs
Pharmacology and Therapeutics

Contributors

E. Ben-Menachem, R.G. Dickinson, F.E. Dreifuss, M.J. Eadie, N.B. Fountain, C.L. Harden, D. Heaney, W.D. Hooper, B. Jarrott, L.P. Johnson, C. Kilpatrick, H. Kutt, I.E. Leppik, R.H. Levy, W. Löscher, R.L. Macdonald, P.N. Patsalos, E. Perucca, J.W.A.S. Sander, S.C. Schachter, D. Schmidt, D.D. Shen, S. Shorvon, W.H. Theodore, F.J.E. Vajda, M.C. Walker, J.O. Willoughby

Editors

M.J. Eadie and F.J.E. Vajda

Springer

Professor Mervyn J. Eadie, AO, MD, PhD
University of Queensland
Department of Medicine
Royal Brisbane Hospital
Clinical Sciences Building
Herston, Qld. 4029
AUSTRALIA

Dr. Frank J.E. Vajda, M.D.
Australian Centre for Clinical Neuropharmacology
St. Vincent's Hospital
Fitzroy, Victoria 3065
AUSTRALIA

With 23 Figures and 42 Tables

ISBN 3-540-65374-0 Springer-Verlag Berlin Heidelberg New York

Library of Congress Cataloging-in-Publication Data
Antiepileptic drugs II / contributors, E. Ben-Menachem . . . [et al.]; editors, M.J. Eadie and F.J.E. Vajda.
p. cm. – (Handbook of experimental pharmacology; v. 138)
Includes bibliographical references and index.
ISBN 3-540-65374-0 (hardcover: alk. paper)
1. Anticonvulsants. 2. Epilepsy – Chemotherapy. I. Ben-Menachem, E. II. Eadie, Mervyn J. III. Vajda, F.J.E. (Frank J.E.) IV. Title: Antiepileptic drugs two. V. Title: Antiepileptic drugs 2. VI. Series.
[DNLM: 1. Anticonvulsants. 2. Epilepsy – drug therapy. W1 HA51L v. 138 1999 / QV 85 A6281 1999]
QP905.H3 vol. 138
[RM322]
615′.1 s – dc21
[616.8′53061]
DNLM/DLC
for Library of Congress 99-10225
CIP

Printed in Germany

Cover design: *design & production* GmbH, Heidelberg

Typesetting: Best-set Typesetter Ltd., Hong Kong

Production Editor: Angélique Gcouta

SPIN: 10568238 27/3020 – 5 4 3 2 1 0 – Printed on acid-free paper

Preface

In 1985, volume 74 of the Springer-Verlag *Handbook of Experimental Pharmacology*, under the editorship of H.-H. Frey and D. Janz, appeared. In this volume the then available data on the topic of *antiepileptic drugs* were collated and analysed. Over the intervening years knowledge in this area has grown progressively. More new antiepileptic drugs than the total number of agents that were in common use 15 years ago have in the interval either come on to the market or are about to do so. As well, further agents are at a fairly advanced stage of development, whilst the already established drugs have by and large held their places in clinical practice. Knowledge of epileptogenesis has advanced considerably. The mechanisms of action of antiepileptic drugs at the molecular level and in various animal models of epileptic seizures and of the epileptic state are much better understood than they were previously. As well, more information is available concerning the natural history of human epilepsy, and this knowledge is important in making optimal use of the various agents that are now available.

Therefore, it has seemed appropriate at this stage in the evolution of knowledge to produce a second volume dealing with Antiepileptic Drugs in the *Handbook of Experimental Pharmacology* series. The new volume has been written to supplement to the first volume rather than to supersede it, in an attempt to bring knowledge in the area to the level which applies at the present time in a field of therapeutics which is advancing steadily on several fronts and shows every sign of continuing to do so.

In attempting to produce such a volume, we are greatly indebted to colleagues in various countries who have been prepared to produce chapters dealing with particular topics in which their expertise is well recognised. We are most grateful to them all. The clarity of their writing, and their skill in communicating their knowledge, has greatly facilitated the preparation of this volume. In particular we would wish to pay tribute to the late Professor Fritz Dreifuss. He readily accepted our invitation to write his chapter (together with Dr. Fountain), and ensured that it was in our hands by the promised time, and yet only a few weeks later, sadly passed away. Thus Chap. 1 of this book may embody some of the last, if not the last, written work of one who made great contributions to the literature and practice of epileptology over many years and whose charm, expertise and generosity of spirit were so highly regarded internationally. We would also wish to acknowledge our gratitude to Mrs. Doris

Walker of Springer-Verlag, who patiently and good-naturedly co-ordinated the endeavour throughout, and to Emeritus Professor Gustav Born, who suggested it in the first place.

M.J. Eadie
Brisbane, Australia
F.J.E. Vajda
Melbourne, Australia

List of Contributors

BEN-MENACHEM, E., University of Göteborg, Department of Clinical Neuroscience, Section of Neurology, Sahlgren's Hospital, 413 45 Göteborg, Sweden

DICKINSON, R.G., Department of Medicine, University of Queensland, Royal Brisbane Hospital, Brisbane, Qld. 4029, Australia

DREIFUSS, F.E., Department of Neurology, Box 394, School of Medicine, University of Virginia Health Science Centre, Charlottesville, VA 22908, USA

EADIE, M.J., University of Queensland, Department of Medicine, Clinical Sciences Building, Royal Brisbane Hospital, Herston, Qld. 4029, Australia

FOUNTAIN, N.B., Department of Neurology, Box 394, School of Medicine, University of Virginia Health Science Centre, Charlottesville, VA 22908, USA

HARDEN, C.L., Cornell University Medical College and Comprehensive Epilepsy Center, New York Hospital-Cornell Medical Center, New York, NY 10021, USA

HEANEY, D., National Society for Epilepsy, Chalfont St. Peter, Gerrards Cross, Buckinghamshire SL9 ORJ, UK

HOOPER, W.D., University of Queensland Department of Medicine, Clinical Sciences Building, Royal Brisbane Hospital, Queensland 4029, Australia

JARROTT, B., Department of Pharmacology, Monash University, Clayton, Victoria, Australia 3168

JOHNSON, L.P., Division of Chemical Pathology, Royal Brisbane Hospital, Brisbane Queensland 4029, Australia

Kilpatrick, C., Melbourne Neuroscience Centre, Department of Neurology, The Royal Melbourne Hospital, Melbourne, Australia

Kutt, H., Cornell University Medical College and Comprehensive Epilepsy Center, New York Hospital-Cornell Medical Center, New York, NY 1002, USA

Leppik, I.E., MINCEP Epilepsy Care, University of Minnesota, 5775 Wayzata Blvd., Suite 255, Minneapolis, MN 55416, USA

Levy, R.H., Department of Pharmaceutics, University of Washington, Box 357610, H272 Health Sciences, Seattle, WA 98195, USA

Löscher, W., Department of Pharmacology, Toxicology and Pharmacy, School of Veterinary Medicine, Bünteweg, D-30559 Hannover, Germany

Macdonald, R.L., Departments of Neurology and Physiology, University of Michigan Medical Center, Neuroscience Lab Building, 1103 East Huron Street, Ann Arbor, MI 48104-1687, USA

Patsalos, P.N., Pharmacology and Therapeutics Unit, University Department of Clinical Neurology, Institute of Neurology, Queen Square, London WC1N 3BG, UK, and Chalfont Centre for Epilepsy, Chalfont St. Peter, Gerrards Cross, Buckinghamshire SL9 ORJ, UK

Perucca, E., Clinical Pharmacology Unit, Department of Internal Medicine and Therapeutics, University of Pavia, Piazza Botta 10, I-27100 Pavia, Italy

Sander, J.W.A.S., Epilepsy Research Group, Institute of Neurology, Queen Square, London WC1N 3BG, UK

Schachter, S.C., Clinical Research, Comprehensive Epilepsy Center, Department of Neurology, Beth Israel Deaconess Medical Center, KS-478, 330 Brookline Avenue, Boston, MA 02215, USA

Schmidt, D., Epilepsy Research Group, Goethestr. 5, D-14163 Berlin, Germany

Shen, D.D., Department of Pharmaceutics, University of Washington, Box 357610, H272 Health Sciences, Seattle, WA 98195, USA

Shorvon, S., The National Hospitals for Neurology and Neurosurgery, Epilepsy Research Group, Queen Square, London WC1N 3BG, UK

THEODORE, W.H., Clinical Epilepsy Section, NINDS, NIH, Bldg. 10, Room 5N-250, Bethesda, MD 20892-1408, USA

VAJDA, F.J.E., Australian Centre for Clinical Neuropharmacology, St. Vincent's Hospital, Fitzroy, Victoria 3065, Australia

WALKER, M.C., Epilepsy Research Group, Institute of Neurology, Queen Square, London WC1N 3BG, UK

WILLOUGHBY, J.O., Centre for Neuroscience and Department of Medicine, Flinders University, PO Box 2100, Adelaide, South Australia 5001, Australia

Contents

CHAPTER 2

Animal Models of Epilepsy and Epileptic Seizures

CHAPTER 3

Epileptogenesis: Electrophysiology

CHAPTER 4

Epileptogenesis: Biochemical Aspects

CHAPTER 5

Cellular Actions of Antiepileptic Drugs

CHAPTER 6

The Search for New Anticonvulsants

CHAPTER 10

Carbamazepine

R.G. DICKINSON, M.J. EADIE and F.J.E. VAJDA. With 1 Figure 267

CHAPTER 13

Valproate

CHAPTER 14

Vigabatrin

CHAPTER 18

Topiramate

CHAPTER 22

Anticonvulsant Combinations and Interactions

CHAPTER 1

Classification of Epileptic Seizures and the Epilepsies and Drugs of Choice for Their Treatment

F.E. DREIFUSS* and N.B. FOUNTAIN

A. Introduction

Since the beginning of the history of epileptology, the classification of the disorder has fascinated thoughtful people who were interested not only in describing individual seizures but also in enlarging the basis of fundamental knowledge by applying what was known of physiology and by inventing more advanced means of recording epileptic phenomena. Others proposed a classification, not of individual seizures, but of the conditions responsible for them. Thus Galen in the second century AD (TEMKIN 1971) postulated that epilepsy might be due to 'idiopathic causes', by which he meant that the underlying nidus of abnormality lay in the brain, but there also were 'symptomatic epilepsies' with their origin residing in the cardia of the stomach or elsewhere in the body.

Those early days constituted the philosophical era of speculation about the nature of the disease. TISSOT (1770) classified epileptic seizures but made a more specific contribution, elaborated by Bernard SACHS (1885), in speculating that epilepsy was an ongoing predisposing condition but that individual epileptic seizures are the expression of the epileptic process when triggered by a concatenation of circumstances which causes the seizure threshold to become exceeded. In this way he sought to answer the question of why a condition such as epilepsy, which is very long-standing, is manifested only on occasions by the symptom which brings the patient to the physician. There are many known precipitating factors for seizures, including flashing lights, the sound of certain music, eating, reading, playing mathematical games or electronic screen games, immersion in warm water and the presence of low blood glucose levels or hormonal imbalances. The underlying epileptic diathesis was felt to be either hereditary (idiopathic) or acquired (symptomatic). Subsequently one spoke of acute symptomatic and remote symptomatic epilepsies. Sigmund FREUD (1968) related childhood epileptic seizures to the major brain disturbances included under the heading of cerebral palsy.

The era of cerebral localization and pathology was characterized by the work of FRITSCH and HITZIG (1870) and FERRIER (1875), on which Hughlings JACKSON based many of his conclusions. This approach had less to do with the

* Professor Dreifuss died shortly after submission of this paper.

aetiology of epilepsy than it did with the classification of individual seizures according to their anatomical, physiological and pathological substrates. This type of endeavour was exploited by ASCROFT (1941) in studying head injury in World War I and by the clinical experience of PENFIELD, ERICKSON and JASPER. This type of detailed evaluation of individual epileptic seizures reached its zenith with the application of split-screen TV and EEG monitoring techniques.

The present period of study of the epilepsies includes the application of sophisticated physiological, neurochemical and pharmacological techniques to models of the epilepsies and the study of epilepsies in animal species. Investigations have ranged from the study of smaller and smaller units of structure, which have been analysed with techniques ranging from extracellular and intracellular recordings from individual cells derived from neuronal culture to integrated studies of whole animals involving all the structures of the intact nervous system. This work has led to the concept of kindling, as well as to a detailed study of neurotransmitters and their receptor binding sites. Furthermore, molecular biology has opened up the area of biochemical genetics, allowing more and more epileptic syndromes to be categorized.

The Commission on Classification of the International League Against Epilepsy has been challenged in its endeavours to classify both epileptic seizures and epileptic syndromes largely because of ignorance about the knowledge to be gained from a nosological approach, knowledge which in turn produces insights which lead to changes in the Classification as a part of a constantly evolving process. Moreover, classification is important from the point of view of achieving uniformity of terminology which permits the transmission of detailed information among individual researchers worldwide, thus leading to a poolability of data which is useful both for pharmacological and for genomic research. The study of individual seizures is essential in a surgical approach to their eradication by defining the symptomatogenic zone in the brain, though this region may be at a distance from the true site of ictogenic origin. Again, careful study will yield information concerning anatomico-functional correlations.

It appears that the individual epileptic seizure occurs when there is a change in the flux of ions across the charged nerve cell membrane leading to its discharge and the subsequent propagation of the derived impulse. Glutamate is the most common excitatory neurotransmitter and, when bound to α-amino-3-hydroxy-5-methyl-4-isoxazolepropionic acid (AMPA)-type receptors (the most common type of glutamate receptor), opens Na^+ channels to result in an excitatory postsynaptic potential (EPSP). When bound to the *N*-methyl-D-aspartate (NMDA)-type of glutamate receptor in the presence of an already depolarized membrane, glutamate opens Ca^{2+} channels, resulting in sustained depolarization which may further depolarize the cell in a self-perpetuating manner. Gamma amino-butyric acid (GABA) is the most common inhibitory neurotransmitter. It hyperpolarizes the cell membrane, causing inhibitory postsynaptic potentials (IPSPs), by opening Cl^- channels when it is bound to $GABA_A$ receptors and by opening K^+ channels by second messenger mechanisms when it is bound to $GABA_B$ receptors. Epileptiform discharges are ultimately expressed by augmentation of glutamate-mediated excitatory, or impairment of GABA-mediated inhibitory, mechanisms. The transmission and synchronization of the resulting discharge is largely contributed to by neuronal system instability at the hippocampus level, allowing discharge propagation and prolongation.

B. The International Classification of Epileptic Seizures

The International Classification of Epileptic Seizures (i.e. of the phenomenological aspect of epilepsy) was produced by the Commission on Classification and Terminology (1981) and is summarized in Table 1.

I. Partial Seizures

Partial seizures are those which begin locally, usually in six-layered isocortex. If they remain relatively confined to their area of origin for a length of time, the involved region imparts to the seizure its specific characteristics. Complex partial seizures occur when consciousness becomes impaired in partial seizures. It is then probable that the propagation of the seizure has occurred to brain regions, the integrity of which is essential to the maintenance of consciousness. Thus limbic system involvement usually results in a complex partial seizure. With impaired consciousness there are frequently aberrations of behaviour (automatisms). All partial seizures may generalize secondarily.

There has been much controversy as to what represents preservation of consciousness (Commission on Classification and Terminology 1981). The operational definition is preservation of awareness and/or responsiveness, though it is realized that full consciousness implies the appreciation of the totality of the experiential field. This is certainly difficult to test within the durations of individual seizures. While criticism of the practicality of recognizing the preservation of consciousness during seizures has some validity, the Classification has been used sufficiently long and in a sufficiently worldwide distribution to have gained acceptance. Also, better testing methods may ultimately solve some of the problems of assessing consciousness during seizures.

II. Generalized Seizures

The second main type of epileptic seizure is the generalized seizure, which is one in which both cerebral hemispheres are involved simultaneously and consciousness is usually impaired. The ictal EEGs generally show bilateral disturbances. The types of seizure here under consideration include absence seizures where there is an arrest of ongoing activities, a blank stare, frequently a brief upward rotation of the eyes and dilatation of the pupils. In addition there may be mild tonic components, eyelid myoclonus, increases or decreases

Table 1. International classification of epileptic seizures [adapted from Epilepsia (1981) 22:489–501]

I. Partial (focal, local) seizures

Partial seizures are those in which, in general, the first clinical and electroencephalographic changes indicate activation of a system of neurons limited to part of one cerebral hemisphere. A partial seizure is classified primarily on the basis of whether or not consciousness is impaired during the attack. When consciousness is not impaired, the seizure is classified as a simple partial seizure. When consciousness is impaired, the seizure is classified as a complex partial seizure. Impairment of consciousness may be the first clinical sign, or simple partial seizures may evolve into complex partial seizures. In patients with impaired consciousness, aberrations of behaviour (automatisms) may occur. A partial seizure may not terminate, but instead progress to a generalized motor seizure. Impaired consciousness is defined as the inability to respond normally to exogenous stimuli by virtue of altered awareness and/or responsiveness.

There is considerable evidence that simple partial seizures usually have unilateral hemispheric involvement and only rarely have bilateral hemisphere involvement; complex partial seizures, however, frequently have bilateral hemispheric involvement.

Partial seizures can be classified into the following three fundamental groups:

A. Simple partial seizures (consciousness not impaired)
  1. With motor symptoms
  2. With somatosensory or special sensory symptoms
  3. With autonomic symptoms
  4. With psychic symptoms

B. Complex partial seizures (with impairment of consciousness)
  1. Beginning as simple partial seizures and progressing to impairment of consciousness
     a) With no other features
     b) With features as in A. 1–4
     c) With automatisms
  2. With impairment of consciousness at the onset
     a) With no other features
     b) With features as in A. 1–4
     c) With automatisms

C. Partial seizures secondarily generalized

II. Generalized seizures (convulsive or nonconvulsive)

Generalized seizures are those in which the first clinical changes indicate initial involvement of both hemispheres. Consciousness may be impaired and this impairment may be the initial manifestation. Motor manifestations are bilateral. The ictal electroencephalographic patterns initially are bilateral, and presumably reflect a neuronal discharge which is widespread in both hemispheres.

A. 1. Absence seizures
   2. Atypical absence seizures

B. Myoclonic seizures

C. Clonic seizures

D. Tonic seizures

E. Tonic-clonic seizures

F. Atonic seizures

III. Unclassified epileptic seizures

Includes all seizures that cannot be classified because of inadequate or incomplete data and also some that defy classification in hitherto described categories. This includes some neonatal seizures, e.g. rhythmic eye movements, chewing, and swimming movements.

in postural tone or, if the seizure lasts a sufficient period of time, automatisms. Atypical absence seizures are frequently seen in the Lennox-Gastaut syndrome and are characterized by major changes in truncal tone, prolonged absence type behaviour with erratic myoclonic movements, drop attacks and occasionally generalized tonic-clonic convulsions. These may persist for a prolonged period of time.

Myoclonic seizures are sudden jerk-like contractions of the body or of its parts, even individual portions of muscles. While their origin is usually cortical, subcortical disturbances in Mollaret's triangle region are usually present. Tonic seizures are prolonged contractions of muscles leading to prolonged flexion or hyperextension of the trunk. These seizures may occur as isolated phenomena, as in the Lennox-Gastaut syndrome, or they may precede the clonic phase of tonic-clonic seizure activity. Tonic contractions usually represent the most severe form of seizures. It is during the tonic phase that fractures may result.

Atonic seizures are characterized by a sudden decrease of postural tone which may lead to drooping of the head, dropping of a limb or of objects held therein, or of the whole body. Occasionally a paroxysmal focal loss of muscle tone, as an epileptic phenomenon, is referred to as 'negative myoclonus'.

C. Classification of the Epilepsies and Epileptic Syndromes

This classification, described by the COMMISSION on CLASSIFICATION and TERMINOLOGY (1989), is summarized in Table 2. While the individual epileptic seizure is a symptom of the underlying condition causing it, the epilepsy or epileptic syndrome of which it is a manifestation is the primary aetiological entity. The diagnosis of the type of epilepsy that is present is based on the prognosis and such matters as the response to medication, the malignancy or the benignity of the condition, the presence or absence of other neurological abnormalities or of mental retardation and the presence or absence of interictal EEG abnormalities such as pathologically slow background rhythms.

The primary dichotomy within the Classification is determined by whether the epilepsy is idiopathic (genetic) or symptomatic. The secondary dichotomy depends on whether the seizures exhibited are partial seizures or generalized seizures. The following are some examples of the application of these classification principles.

I. Idiopathic Epilepsies

1. Idiopathic Epilepsies with Partial Seizures

The idiopathic epilepsies with partial seizures (NAYRAC and BEAUSSART 1958; LOMBROSO 1967; BEAUSSART 1972; LOISEAU and BEAUSSART 1973; BEAUMANOIR et al. 1974; HEIJBEL et al. 1975; GASTAUT 1982) include such conditions as benign Rolandic epilepsy or benign occipital epilepsy, frontal lobe epilepsy

Table 2. International classification of the epilepsies and epileptic syndromes [adapted from Epilepsia (1989) 30:389–399]

1 Localization-related (focal, local, partial) epilepsies and syndromes
- 1.1 Idiopathic (with age-related onset)
  At present, the following syndromes are established but more may be identified in the future:
  - Benign childhood epilepsy with centro-temporal spikes
  - Childhood epilepsy with occipital paroxysms
  - Primary reading epilepsy
- 1.2 Symptomatic
  This category comprises syndromes of individual variability and is mainly based on anatomical localization, clinical features, seizure types and aetiological factors (if known).
  - 1.2.1 Characterized by simple partial seizures with the characteristics of seizures:
    - Arising from frontal lobes
    - Arising from parietal lobes
    - Arising from temporal lobes
    - Arising from occipital lobes
    - Arising from multiple lobes
    - Locus of onset unknown
  - 1.2.2 Characterized by complex partial seizures, that is attacks with alteration of consciousness often with automatisms. Characterized by seizures:
    - Arising from frontal lobes
    - Arising from parietal lobes
    - Arising from temporal lobes
    - Arising from occipital lobes
    - Arising from multiple lobes
    - Locus of onset unknown
  - 1.2.3 Characterized by secondarily generalized seizures with seizures:
    - Arising from frontal lobes
    - Arising from parietal lobes
    - Arising from temporal lobes
    - Arising from occipital lobes
    - Arising from multiple lobes
    - Locus of onset unknown
- 1.3 Unknown as to whether the syndrome is idiopathic or symptomatic

2 Generalized epilepsies and syndromes
- 2.1 Idiopathic (with age-related onset – listed in order of age):
  - Benign neonatal familial convulsions
  - Benign neonatal convulsions
  - Benign myoclonic epilepsy in infancy
  - Childhood absence epilepsy (pyknolepsy)
  - Juvenile absence epilepsy
  - Juvenile myoclonic epilepsy (impulsive petit mal)
  - Epilepsy with grand mal (GTCS) seizures on awakening

  Other generalized idiopathic epilepsies, if they do not belong to one of the above syndromes can still be classified as generalized idiopathic epilepsies.
- 2.2 Cryptogenic or symptomatic (in order of age of onset)
  - West syndrome (infantile spasms, Blitz-Nick-Salaam Krampfe)
  - Lennox-Gastaut syndrome
  - Epilepsy with myoclonic-astatic seizures
  - Epilepsy with myoclonic absences

Table 2. *Continued*

2.3 Symptomatic
  2.3.1 Non-specific aetiology
    - Early myoclonic encephalopathy
  2.3.2 Specific syndromes
    - Epileptic seizures may complicate many disease states. Under this heading are included those diseases in which seizures are a presenting or predominant feature.

3 Epilepsies and syndromes undetermined whether focal or generalized
  3.1 With both generalized and focal seizures
    - Neonatal seizures
    - Severe myoclonic epilepsy in infancy
    - Epilepsy with continuous spike-waves during slow wave sleep
    - Acquired epileptic aphasia (Landau-Kleffner syndrome)
  3.2 Without unequivocal generalized or focal features
  All cases with generalized tonic-clonic seizures where clinical and EEG findings do not permit classification as clearly generalized or localization-related, as in many cases of sleep-grand mal.

4 Special syndromes
  4.1 Situation-related seizures (*Gelegenheitsanfalle*)
    - Febrile convulsions
    - Isolated seizures or isolated status epilepticus
    - Seizures occurring only when there is an acute metabolic or toxic event due to, for example, alcohol, drugs, eclampsia, non-ketotic hyperglycaemia, uraemia, etc.

with nocturnal seizures and benign temporal lobe epilepsy with prominent autonomic manifestations.

2. Idiopathic Epilepsies with Generalized Seizures

The idiopathic epilepsies with generalized seizures (Janz and Christian 1957; Currier et al. 1963; Livingston et al. 1965; Bjerre and Corelius 1968; Brown 1973; Penry et al. 1975; Tsuboi 1977; Asconape and Penry 1984; Delgado-Escueta and Enrile-Bascal 1984; Dravet et al. 1985a; Drury and Dreifuss 1985; Loiseau 1985; Wolf 1985; Dreifuss 1989) include many of the childhood epilepsy syndromes such as some forms of neonatal convulsions (most neonatal seizures are in fact partial by virtue of the immaturity of the developing brain). They also include benign myoclonic seizures of infancy, various syndromes associated with absence seizures including pyknoleptic petit mal, juvenile absence and juvenile myoclonic epilepsy. All have their characteristic clinical spectra and all are relatively easily controlled, lack other abnormalities of brain function and have normal interictal EEGs.

II. Symptomatic Epilepsies

1. Symptomatic Epilepsies with Partial Seizures

The causes of these epilepsies include typical traumatic, tumorous or vascular focal brain involvement. The nature of the seizures is dependent on the site of the lesion. In the case of complex partial seizures, the underlying lesions are frequently frontal or temporal. These epilepsies have a much poorer prognosis for remission or for control by medication than simple partial seizures due to a relatively static encephalopathy. The most terrifying symptomatic epilepsy with partial seizures is represented by epilepsia partialis continua (Rasmussen's syndrome), which is a childhood epileptic syndrome due to a rapidly progressive unilateral spreading condition with the development of hemiplegia, contralateral ventricular dilatation and dementia (RASMUSSEN et al. 1958). There is frequently histological evidence of focal encephalitis and there is some evidence of an immunological disturbance with antibody formation directed against the glutamate receptor (ROGERS et al. 1994).

2. Symptomatic Epilepsies with Generalized Seizures

These epilepsies are usually indicative of a severe underlying neurological disorder of developmental, biochemical or clastic aetiology. The underlying conditions include abnormal neural migrations, biochemical disorders (such as ceroid lipfuscinosis, Tay Sachs disease, sialidosis) or they may be on the basis of progressive myoclonic epilepsies such as Lafora disease, Baltic myoclonus, or mitochondrial abnormalities, such as mitochondrial encephalopathy with ragged red fibres or mitochondrial encephalopathy with lactic acidosis and strokes.

III. Epilepsies That Are Difficult to Categorize

Some epilepsies are difficult to categorize as to whether they are idiopathic, symptomatic or cryptogenic. By cryptogenic is meant an epilepsy which almost certainly is symptomatic by virtue of association with static encephalopathy or other neurology abnormality, but whose cause remains occult.

1. West's Syndrome

The epileptic syndromes that are difficult to categorize include West's syndrome (WEST 1841; JEAVONS and BOWER 1964; KELLAWAY et al. 1979; LOMBROSO 1983) in which the so-called idiopathic form, though demonstrating an interictal EEG hypsarrhythmia, may respond to ACTH or vigabatrin sufficiently well to abolish the EEG abnormality, terminate the seizures, and allow normal neural development. The seizures are massive spasms, either in flexion or extension, though the spasms may be incomplete. They frequently occur in clusters shortly after awakening. On the other hand, the majority of West's syndrome patients suffer significant intellectual retardation and many are found to have underlying structural abnormalities such as focal neuronal migration disorders, tuberous sclerosis or biochemical abnormalities such as non-ketotic hyperglycinaemia or phenylketonuria. Severe myoclonic epilepsy in infancy, similarly, is a rather severe form of probably cryptogenic or symptomatic epilepsy leading to abnormal neurological findings with apraxia and corticospinal tract signs (DRAVET et al. 1985b).

2. Lennox-Gastaut Syndrome

The Lennox-Gastaut syndrome (LENNOX and DAVIS 1949; GASTAUT et al. 1966; LENNOX 1966) is characterized by a severe encephalopathy with tonic extension spasms and atypical absence and episodic drop attacks as major features, as well as mental retardation and treatment intractability. It may be the end result of different aetiologies including West's syndrome, encephalitis or longstanding developmental defects. The outlook is uniformly dismal but seizures may improve gradually. Certain drugs such as felbamate or lamotrigine have relieved some aspects of the disorder.

3. Acquired Epileptic Aphasia (the Landau-Kleffner Syndrome)

This syndrome (LANDAU and KLEFFNER 1957) is a childhood disorder characterized by acquired aphasia, hemispheric or generalized spikes and spike and wave discharges. Many patients with this syndrome have psychomotor disturbances. They have a verbal auditory agnosia and reduction of spontaneous speech. The EEG frequently shows continuous spike-wave activity during slow wave sleep.

4. Epilepsy with Continuous Spike-Wave during Slow Wave Sleep

In this condition, nocturnal seizures are associated with continuous spike-wave activity during slow wave sleep (TASSINARI et al. 1985). The syndrome is virtually untreatable except that occasionally, as in the Landau-Kleffner syndrome, there may be a response to steroids. A neuropsychological disorder is frequent during the later phases of the disease.

D. Influence of Technological Advances on the Understanding of Semiology

Many idiopathic epilepsies have been found to have an underlying genetic basis. Rarely a month passes without new developments or the postulating of gene loci with putative sites responsible for the abnormal functions thought to contribute to the syndromes comprising the idiopathic epilepsies.

The following represent preliminary classificational data of the Commission on Genetics of the International League Against Epilepsy.

I. Singular Nuclear Gene Disorders

1. Without brain abnormalities, a category including, for example, such disorders as benign familial neonatal convulsions (20Q or 8Q) and familial frontal lobe seizures (20Q).

2. With brain abnormalities, a category including, for example, band heterotopias or X-linked lissencephaly (XQ22.3), paraventricular nodular heterotopia (XQ28), Unverricht-Lundborg disease (21), Lafora body disease (6Q) and ceroid lipofucscinosis (1Q,13, or 6P).

II. Complex Inheritance Disorders

1. Without brain abnormalities, a category including childhood absence epilepsy (?8Q) and juvenile myoclonic epilepsy (?6P,11, 15Q, 8Q), which seems a more heterogeneous condition than once thought.
2. With brain abnormalities, a category including, among the generalized seizures those with degenerative, infectious, tumorous and metabolic aetiologies and among the partial seizures those due to hippocampal scleroses, immunological disorders and trauma. So far, no specific gene defects have been defined in this group, but some of these disorders follow autosomal dominant or autosomal recessive inheritances, such as some neurocutaneous syndromes and various metabolic disorders. Specific chromosomal disorders associated with epilepsy include 4-P deletions, ring-chromosome 20, Down syndrome and the fragile-X syndrome.

It is clear that ultimately genetics will play a major role in epileptic syndrome identification and possibly in management because, wherever there is a gene anomaly there is a corresponding abnormal gene product, and this aberration may well be integrally associated with the clinical manifestation.

E. Drugs of Choice for Epileptic Seizures and the Epilepsies

The choice of antiepileptic drugs according to the specific seizure type under consideration or in keeping with the syndrome whose presenting symptom has precipitated therapeutic intervention, is a relatively recent possibility. The first rational treatment of epileptic seizures began with the introduction of bromides in 1857 (Locock), after which time it became quite apparent that effective therapy with these agents exacted a heavy cost in terms of toxicity. Newer drugs such as phenobarbitone tended to have less toxicity. The next advance came from the testing by Putnam and Merritt of hydantoins in the maximal electroshock animal model of convulsions. Subsequently all prospective antiepileptic drugs were tested for effectiveness and toxicity prior to their introduction, thus allowing at least a rough estimate of their tolerability and their efficacy from the outset (Putnam and Merritt 1937). In 1978, valproate was introduced and was thought to be effective by virtue of enhancing GABA actions in the nervous system, leading to a new avenue for the exploration of anticonvulsant agents. This was the first attempt at influencing excitatory or inhibitory neurotransmitter mechanisms and might be regarded as the beginning of the modern era of antiepileptic drug development. In general, the effectiveness of agents in enhancing neuronal inhibition or in antagonizing glutamate-mediated excitation was felt on theoretical grounds to augur well for antiepileptic drug development purposes. Furthermore, activation of the NMDA subtype of glutamate receptor allows an influx of Ca^{2+}, which may be cytotoxic. Evidence suggests that drugs such as felbamate, topiramate and lamotrigine may have an NMDA receptor blocking activity while phenytoin and carbamazepine predominantly tend to inhibit action potential propagation by blocking voltage gated Na^{+} channels. It is believed that most of these neurotransmitters affect the process of *ictogenesis*, i.e., the process which determines the production of seizures, from the nerve cell membrane. Though the process of *epileptogenesis* is not as well understood, it appears to result from anatomical changes in regions of the brain which have a relay-mobilizing and synchronizing function, e.g. the hippocampus. These changes can permanently render the organism considerably more vulnerable to an undue liability to seizures. The next stage in the development of antiepileptic drugs ideally should include seeking agents which will have an inhibitory effect on the process of epileptogenesis (Dreifuss 1994).

I. Drugs for Epileptic Seizures (Table 3)

1. Partial Seizures

At present a popular choice of medications for the management of partial seizures would include phenytoin, carbamazepine, valproate or phenobarbitone. In the case of complex partial seizures, carbamazepine is usually preferred but phenytoin and valproate are also used frequently. This type of seizure is frequently so recalcitrant, particularly in the presence of mesial temporal sclerosis, that other medications are frequently added to the initial drug used, and the option of surgery is frequently invoked.

Many other factors may influence the choice of antiepileptic drug, including whether the patient does not comply with treatment recommendations, in which case drugs which can be given less frequently than twice a day are preferred. Again, cosmetic considerations may sway the decision, as may the desire for pregnancy, which may incline the physician towards the use of phenytoin rather than valproate.

The newer antiepileptic drugs include gabapentin, lamotrigine, topiramate, and vigabatrin (the latter is not yet FDA approved in the United States). Felbamate is out of favour because of the hazard of its side effects, including aplastic anaemia and hepatic necrosis. Lamotrigine has become popular though its place in therapeutics has not yet been defined in partial seizures, nor has its place in monotherapy. Gabapentin is an almost ideal add-on medication because it is relatively free from side effects and interactions whilst, in simple partial seizures, its effectiveness is vitiated only by the need for a very high dose. Topiramate has similar attributes, but at high doses may cause cognitive side effects.

Table 3. Correlation between classification of epileptic seizures and drugs of choice for their treatment. The preferred agents are shown in italics

Seizure type	Drugs
Partial seizures	
Simple partial seizures	*Carbamazepine*, valproate, phenytoin, vigabatrin[a], (gabapentin, lamotrigine, topiramate)
Complex partial seizures	*Carbamazepine*, phenytoin, valproate, vigabatrin[a], primidone, (gabapentin, lamotrigine, topiramate)
Partial seizures, secondarily generalized	*Carbamazepine*, valproate, phenytoin, phenobarbitone, (gabapentin, lamotrigine, topiramate)
Generalized seizures	
Absence seizures	*Ethosuximide, valproate*
Myoclonic seizures	Valproate[b], clonazepam, lamotrigine[b], felbamate (but see side-effect profile), pyridoxine
Atonic seizures	Valproate[b], lamotrigine[b], felbamate (but see side-effect profile), corticosteroids
Tonic, clonic or tonic-clonic seizures	Valproate[b], carbamazepine, phenytoin, barbiturates

In parenthesis, FDA approval restricted to add-on medication.
[a] Not yet available in USA.
[b] Not yet FDA approved for this indication.

2. Generalized Seizures

In generalized seizures, valproic acid and its derivatives continue to be preferred. In the United States valproate is approved by the Food and Drug Administration for seizure types which include absence seizures, but most patients with generalized tonic-clonic seizures are also being afforded the benefit of this very effective drug. For treatment of seizures which are secondarily generalized, carbamazepine, phenytoin and valproate are popular.

On a worldwide basis, valproate is the most frequently used medication for absence seizures, though ethosuximide continues for some to be the drug of choice so long as tonic-clonic seizures are not a feature of the patient's epilepsy. The only reason that valproate is not uniformly preferred is that there continues to be some risk of hepatotoxicity in childhood age groups (BRYANT and DREIFUSS 1996). Some physicians therefore favour ethosuximide. In all other generalized seizure disorders valproate is regarded as the drug of choice, with benzodiazepines, particularly clonazepam, having a somewhat lesser place. Unfortunately clonazepam is associated with the development of tolerance which greatly reduces its desirability, and this to some extent is true also for clobazam, which is not available in the United States but which has a following in the United Kingdom and Canada. Lamotrigine may also be useful in treating generalized seizures.

Table 4. Classification of epilepsies correlated with their drugs of choice. The preferred agents are shown in italics

Epilepsy or epileptic syndrome	Drugs
Idiopathic epilepsies	
With partial seizures	*Carbamazepine*, valproate
With generalized seizures	
Childhood absence	*Ethosuximide, valproate*
Juvenile absence	*Valproate*
Juvenile myoclonic epilepsy	*Valproate*, phenytoin
Myoclonic absence	Valproate plus ethosuximide
Symptomatic epilepsies	
With partial seizures (lesional)	Carbamazepine, phenytoin, valproate, vigabatrin[a], (gabapentin, lamotrigine)
With generalized seizures	
West syndrome	*ACTH, prednisone*, valproate, (lamotrigine[b])
West syndrome in tuberous sclerosis	Vigabatrin[a], valproate[b]
Lennox-Gastaut syndrome	Felbamate (but see side-effect profile), valproate, clonazepam, (lamotrigine)
With known metabolic disorders	Pyridoxine, biotin, diets, steroids, benzodiazepines, as appropriate
Neonatal seizures	*Phenobarbitone* plus eliminate cause
Febrile convulsions	*Intermittent rectal diazepam,* long-term phenobarbitone (but note side-effect profile)
Reflex epilepsies	*Valproate*[b], benzodiazepines

In parenthesis, FDA approval restricted to use as add-on medication.
[a] Not yet available in USA.
[b] Not yet FDA approved for this indication.

II. Drugs for the Epilepsies (Table 4)

The management of the epilepsies and epileptic syndromes invokes elements which are more far-reaching than the treatment of individual seizure types and takes into consideration matters such as the natural history, prognosis, likelihood of a severe and progressive neurological ailment and the prospect of a benign self-limited condition whose individual elements may not require treatment. These issues which have to do with treating the patient rather than the seizure have been emphasized in recent years.

1. Idiopathic Epilepsies with Partial Seizures

These epilepsies, including the benign partial seizures of childhood, may or may not require medical intervention. If intervention is invoked it is a satisfying undertaking because most drugs useful in the treatment of partial seizures are effective and the disorder is usually self-limited.

2. Idiopathic Epilepsies with Generalized Seizures

Such epilepsies include childhood absence epilepsy, juvenile absence epilepsy, juvenile myoclonic epilepsy and primary generalized tonic-clonic convulsive epilepsy, usually nocturnal. The medications of choice include valproate and lamotrigine. The choice as to which drug should be used may depend upon collateral indications such as the patient's age, sex or intentions regarding pregnancy. In these various forms of epilepsy, apart from childhood absences, recurrence after discontinuation of medication is frequent so that medication is usually continued indefinitely.

3. Symptomatic Epilepsies with Localization-Related Seizures

These epilepsies are treated as described earlier under partial seizures. Heed should be paid to the syndrome of which the complex partial seizure is a part. If there is indication of a progressive tendency, of a crescendo, or of increasing number of seizures, or of the presence of mesial temporal sclerosis, early consideration should be given to surgical treatment. This should also be considered in patients with imaging evidence of malformations sufficiently localized to allow surgical removal.

4. Symptomatic Epilepsies with Generalized Seizures

Symptomatic epilepsies with generalized seizures come in two main varieties. The first includes diseases with named appellations which usually carry a very grim prognosis. Such diseases include ceroid lipofuscinosis, sialidosis, progressive myoclonic epilepsies, and malformations such as lissencephaly. These can be treated only symptomatically and palliatively.

The second group of conditions under this rubric include West's syndrome and the Lennox-Gastaut syndrome. West's syndrome is characterized by the occurrence of infantile spasms and on the EEG is frequently associated with hypsarrhythmia and a delay in neurological development. In some instances, early treatment with ACTH or prednisone or vigabatrin will result in immediate and significant improvement. In others, there will either be relapse or no improvement from the beginning. Valproate and vigabatrin have been used, as have been benzodiazepines. It has been found by Chiron et al. (1990) that infantile spasms due to tuberous sclerosis may respond successfully. Occasionally a PET scan or a high resolution MRI scan may reveal a focal malformation underlying the syndrome, and this may lead to a surgical approach.

The Lennox-Gastaut syndrome is one of the severest neurological handicaps of childhood. It is characterized by tonic axial seizures, drop attacks, atypical absence seizures and severe and progressive mental retardation. The syndrome is quite impervious to most modes of therapy. Felbamate showed some promise but is now rarely used because of the side effects referred to above, but continues to be tried as a measure of desperation, on occasions with some degree of success (Ritter et al. 1993). Lamotrigine may be of help in some of these cases, but the outlook remains poor.

Other causes of epileptic seizures include metabolic and electrolyte derangements which should be corrected, and deficiency disorders such as those involving pyridoxine, biotinidase and glucose, which should be corrected.

5. Febrile Convulsions

While febrile convulsions in infants are not always regarded as part of the problem of epilepsy, this matter is certainly sufficiently germane to warrant mention in a text on drugs involved in the management of epileptic seizures. Febrile convulsions raise the question of whether intermittent therapy, short-term prophylactic therapy or long-term therapy should be employed in their management. The consensus at the present time is that once the diagnosis of a simple febrile convulsive disorder has been made, intermittent rectal benzodiazepine therapy is at least one of the managements of choice and is preferable to long-term barbiturate management because of the considerably lesser behavioural disruption that it causes the child. Diazepam gel for rectal administration was recently approved in the United States for the treatment of clusters of seizures.

F. Conclusion

The choice of an antiepileptic drug for the management of a particular patient is thus seen to involve a number of possibilities, including not only the risk/benefit analysis for the particular seizure type but also, in a particular syndrome, with long- and short-range therapeutic goals abutting on personalities and lifestyles, involving most of a physician's medical and social responsibilities. The recent increase in the choice of an antiepileptic drug has also widened the economic issues to be considered in the decision as to whether drugs from one era, or from another, are used. The fashioning of a therapeutic plan, while far from perfect, is making it more possible to take care of a number of collateral problems while attempting to stop the patient's seizures.

References

Asconape J, Penry JK (1984) Some clinical and EEG aspects of benign juvenile myoclonic epilepsy. Epilepsia 25:108–114

Ascroft PB (1941) Traumatic epilepsy after gunshot wounds of the head. Brit Med J 1:739–744

Beaumanoir A, Ballist T, Varfis G et al. (1974) Benign epilepsy of childhood with rolandic spikes. Epilepsia 15:301–315

Beaussart M (1972) Benign epilepsy of children with rolandic (centro–temporal) paroxysmal foci. Epilepsia 13:795–811

Berkovic SF, Andermann F, Carpenter S et al. (1986) Progressive myoclonus epilepsies: specific cases and diagnosis. New Eng J Med 315:296–305

Bjerre I, Corelius E (1968) Benign familial neonatal convulsions. Acta Paediat Scand 57:557–561
Brown JK (1973) Convulsions in the newborn period. Develop Med Child Neurol 15:823–846
Bryant A, Dreifuss FE (1996) Valproic acid hepatic fatalities. III. U.S. experience since 1986. Neurology 46:465–469
Chiron C, Dulac O, Luna, D (1990) Vigabatrin in infantile spasms. Lancet 1:363–364
Commission on Classification and Terminology of the International League Against Epilepsy (1981) Proposal for revised clinical and electroencephalographic classification of epileptic seizures. Epilepsia 22:489–501
Commission on Classification and Terminology of the International League Against Epilepsy (1989) Proposal for revised classification of epilepsies and epileptic syndromes. Epilepsia 30:389–399
Currier RD, Kooi KA, Saidman LJ (1963) Prognosis of pure petit mal. A follow-up study. Neurology 13:959–967
Delgado-Escueta AV, Enrile-Bascal F (1984) Juvenile myoclonic epilepsy of Janz. Neurology 34:285–294
Dravet C, Bureau M, Roger J (1985a) Benign myoclonic epilepsy in infants. In: Roger J, Dravet C, Bureau M, Dreifuss FE, Wolf P (eds) Epileptic syndromes in infancy, childhood and adolescence. Libbey Eurotext, London, pp 51–57
Dravet C, Bureau M, Roger J (1985b) Severe myoclonic epilepsy in infants. In: Roger J, Dravet C, Bureau M, Dreifuss FE, Wolf P (eds) Epileptic syndromes in infancy, childhood and adolescence. Libbey Eurotext, London, pp. 58–67
Dreifuss FE (1989) Juvenile myoclonic epilepsy: characteristics of a primary generalized epilepsy. Epilepsia 30 [Suppl 4]:S1–S7
Dreifuss FE (1994) New antiepileptic drug development. Epilepsia 35 [Suppl 5]:S6-S9
Drury I, Dreifuss FE (1985) Pyknoleptic petit mal. Acta Neurol Scand 72:353–362
Ferrier D (1875) Experiments on the brain of monkeys. Proc Roy Soc Lond 23:409–430
Freud S (1968) Infantile cerebral paralysis. Translated by LA Russin. University of Miami Press, Floral Gables
Fritsch G, Hitzig E (1870) Uber die elektrische Erregbarkeit des Grosshirns. Arch Anat Physiol Wiss Med 37:300–332
Gastaut H (1982) A new type of epilepsy: benign partial epilepsy of childhood with occipital spike-waves. In: Advances in Epileptology, XIIIth Epilepsy International Symposium. Raven Press, New York, pp 18–25
Gastaut H, Roger J, Soularyrol R et al. (1996) Childhood epileptic encephalopathy with diffuse slow spike-waves (otherwise known as "Petit mal variant") or Lennox syndrome. Epilepsia 7:139–179
Heijbel J, Blom S, Rasmuson M (1975) Benign epilepsy of childhood with centrotemporal EEG foci: a genetic study. Epilepsia 16:285–293
Janz D, Christian W (1957) Impulsive-Petit mal. Dtsch Z Nervenheilkd 176:346–386
Jeavons PM, Bower BD (1964) Infantile spasms: a review of the literature and a study of 112 cases. Clinics in Developmental Medicine No 15, Heinemann Medical Books, London
Jeavons PM, Bower BD (1974) Infantile spasms. In: Vinken PJ, Bruyn GW (eds) Handbook of clinical neurology, Vol 15, North Holland, Amsterdam, pp. 219–234
Kellaway P, Hrachovy RA, Frost JD et al. (1979) Precise characteristics and quantification of infantile spasms. Ann Neurol 6:214–218
Landau WM, Kleffner FR (1957) Syndrome of acquired aphasia with convulsive disorder in children. Neurology 7:523–550
Lennox WG (1966) The slow-spike-wave EEG and its clinical correlates. In: Lennox WG (eds) Epilepsy and related disorders. Vol 1, Little Brown and Co, Boston, pp. 156–170
Lennox WG, Davis JP (1949) Clinical correlates of the fast and the slow spike and wave electroencephalogram. Trans Amer Neurol Assoc 74:194–197

Livingston S, Torres I, Pauli LL et al. (1965) Petit mal epilepsy. Results of a prolonged follow-up study of 117 patients. J Amer Med Assoc 194:113–118
Locock C (1857) Discussion of paper by E H Sieveking: Analysis of cases of epilepsy observed by the author. Lancet 1:527
Loiseau P (1985) Childhood absence epilepsy. In: Roger J, Dravet C, Bureau M, Dreifuss FE, Wolf P (eds) Epileptic syndromes in infancy, childhood and adolescence. Libbey Eurotext, London, pp. 106–120
Loiseau P, Beaussart M (1973) The seizures of benign childhood epilepsy with rolandic paroxysmal discharges. Epilepsia 14:381–389
Lombroso CT (1967) Sylvian seizures and midtemporal spike foci in children. Arch Neurol 17:52–59
Lombroso CT (1983) A prospective study of infantile spasms: clinical and therapeutic correlations. Epilepsia 24:135–158
Nayrac P, Beaussart M (1958) Les pointe-ondes prerolandique: expression EEG tres particuliere. Rev Neurol 99:201–206
Penry JK, Porter RJ, Dreifuss FE (1975) Simultaneous recording of absence seizures with videotape and electro-encephalography: a study of 374 seizures in 48 patients. Brain 98:427–440
Putnam TJ, Merritt HH (1937) Experimental determination of anticonvulsant properties of some phenyl derivatives. Science 85:525–526
Rasmussen TE, Olszewski J, Lloyd-Smith D (1958) Focal cortical seizures due to chronic localized encephalitides. Neurology 8:435–445
Ritter FJ, Leppik IE, Dreifuss FE et al. (1993) Felbamate in the treatment of Lennox-Gastaut syndrome. New Engl J Med 328:29–33
Rogers SW, Andrews PI, Gahring LC et al. (1994) Autoantibodies to glutamate receptor GluR3 in Rasmussen's encephalitis. Science 265:648–651
Sachs B (1895) A treatise on the nervous system of children for physicians and students. William Wood & Co, New York
Tassinari CA, Bureau M, Dravet C, Bernardina BD, Roger J (1985): Epilepsy with continuous spike and waves during slow sleep. In: Roger J, Dravet C, Bureau M, Dreifuss FE, Wolf P (eds) Epileptic syndromes in infancy, childhood and adolescence. Libbey Eurotext, London, pp. 194–204
Temkin O (1971) The falling sickness. A history of epilepsy from the Greeks to the beginnings of modern neurology. 2nd edn, John Hopkins Press, Baltimore
Tissot SA (1770) Traite de l'epilepsie faisant le tome troisieme du traite des nerfs et de leurs maladies. Didot, Paris
Tsuboi T (1977) Primary generalized epilepsy with sporadic myoclonias of myoclonic petit mal type. Theime, Stuttgart, pp. 19–35
West WJ (1841): On a peculiar form of infantile convulsions. Lancet 1:724–725
Wolf P (1985) Juvenile absence epilepsy. In: Roger J, Dravet C, Bureau M, Dreifuss FE, Wolf P (eds) Epileptic syndromes in infancy, childhood and adolescence. Libbey Eurotext, London, pp. 242–246

CHAPTER 2

Animal Models of Epilepsy and Epileptic Seizures

W. LÖSCHER

A. Introduction

In epilepsy research, animal models serve a variety of purposes. First, they are used in the search for new antiepileptic drugs. Second, once the anticonvulsant activity of a novel compound has been detected, animal models are used to evaluate the possible specific efficacies of the compound against different types of seizures or epilepsy. Third, animal models can be used to characterize the preclinical efficacy of novel compounds during chronic administration. Such chronic studies can serve different objectives, for instance, evaluation of whether drug efficacy changes during prolonged treatment, e.g. because of the development of tolerance, or examination of whether a drug exerts antiepileptogenic effects during prolonged administration, i.e. is a true antiepileptic drug. Fourth, animal models are employed to characterize the mechanism of action of old and new antiepileptic drugs. Fifth, certain models can be used to study mechanisms of drug resistance in epilepsy. Sixth, in view of the possibility that chronic brain dysfunction, such as epilepsy, might lead to altered sensitivity to drug adverse effects, models involving epileptic animals are useful to study whether epileptogenesis alters the adverse effect potential of a given drug. Seventh, animal models are needed for studies on the pathophysiology of epilepsies and epileptic seizures, e.g. the processes involved in epileptogenesis and ictogenesis (LOTHMAN 1996a).

Not all animal models of seizures and/or epilepsy can be used for all of the above described purposes. Furthermore, the intention of the experiment is essential for selection of a suitable animal model. For instance, simple seizure models such as the maximal electroshock seizure (MES) test, allowing testing of high numbers of compounds for anticonvulsant activity in a relatively short time, will be preferred to more complex models in screening approaches to anticonvulsant drug development. The use of animal models in the search for new anticonvulsants is dealt with in Chapter 6 of this volume. Nevertheless, in order to review the most important animal models currently used in epilepsy research, it will be necessary to characterize their pharmacological and predictive profile in terms of clinical types of seizures or epilepsy.

Most animal models used in epilepsy research are models of epileptic seizures rather than models of epilepsy. Since epilepsy is characterized by spontaneous recurrent seizures, a test such as the maximal electroshock seizure test, in which an acute seizure is electrically induced in a normal non-epileptic animal, cannot represent a model of epilepsy. On the other hand, there are true models of epilepsy, for instance animal mutants or transgenic animals with spontaneously recurrent seizures, which are obviously more closely related to human epilepsy than mere seizure models. Furthermore, epileptogenesis resulting in spontaneous recurrent seizures can be induced by chemical or electrical means. Unfortunately, many researchers do not differentiate between animal models of epilepsy and animal models of epileptic seizures, although the difference may be important in the interpretation of data obtained with such models. Of course, models of epilepsy, e.g. mutant animals with inherent epilepsy, can be used as models of seizures, e.g. in anticonvulsant drug potency studies, whereas a pure seizure model in a non-epileptic animal cannot be used as a model of chronic epilepsy.

An ideal animal model of epilepsy should fulfil the following requirements: (1) development of spontaneously occurring recurrent seizures; (2) seizure type(s) similar in clinical phenomenology to seizure types occurring in human epilepsies; (3) paroxysmal EEG alterations similar to EEG alterations occurring in the respective seizure types in humans; (4) a high seizure frequency to allow acute and chronic drug efficacy studies; (5) pharmacokinetics (particularly the rate of elimination) of antiepileptic drugs which allow the maintenance of effective drug levels during chronic treatment; (6) effective plasma (and brain) concentrations of antiepileptic drugs similar to those required for control of the relevant seizure types in epileptic patients. Although no model at present meets all these criteria, there are several so-called genetic animal models of epilepsy, i.e. species or strains of laboratory animals with "inborn" epilepsy, which resemble idiopathic epilepsy in humans more closely than any other experimental model (LÖSCHER 1984, 1992). However, out of practical reasons, the most commonly used animal models in anticonvulsant drug development are not models of chronic epilepsy but models of single epileptic seizures, in which seizures are induced in small laboratory animals (rats, mice) by simple chemical or electrical means.

Innumerable models of epilepsy and epileptic seizures have been described in the literature, so that it is not possible to review all these models in this chapter. In this respect, the interested reader is referred to previous reviews or volumes on this topic (PURPURA et al. 1972; KOELLA 1985; LÖSCHER and SCHMIDT 1988; FISHER 1989; ENGEL 1992). The various animal models can be assigned to different categories, e.g. models with spontaneously occurring seizures versus chemically or electrically induced seizures, models with recurrent seizures versus models with single seizures (i.e. chronic versus acute models), models with partial seizures versus models with generalized seizures, models with convulsive seizures versus models with non-convulsive seizures, screening models versus models for a more advanced phase of the screening procedure ("secondary screening"), mechanism-related models (i.e. with seizure induction by a known mechanism) versus models without a specific (or known) mechanism, and seizure threshold models versus models with (supra)maximal or suprathreshold induction of seizures.

One simple scheme of classification of experimental animal models of epilepsy and epileptic seizures is shown in Fig. 1. However, in a volume on antiepileptic drugs, it should be recognized that the clinical selection of an antiepileptic drug is based primarily on its efficacy for specific types of seizures and epilepsy (MATTSON 1995). Thus, for the purpose of preclinical drug evaluation, it may be more appropriate to classify the models on the basis of type of seizure or epilepsy. This should also allow a more precise interpretation of data from investigations into the mechanisms of any of these models and facilitate comparisons between experimental and clinical data. Therefore, in the present review, as far as applicable, the International Classification of Epilepsies and Epileptic Syndromes (COMMISSION 1989; DREIFUSS 1994) will be used to categorize animal models of epilepsy (Table 1). Similarly, animal models of seizures will be categorized with respect to seizure type (Table 2), using the International Classification of Epileptic Seizures (COMMISSION 1981). As pointed out above, the review will not attempt to cover all available or described models, but will be restricted to the relatively few models in the respective categories which have been studied in enough detail to judge their usefulness for the different purposes in epilepsy research outlined at the beginning of this section.

B. Animal Models of Epilepsy

By definition, animal models of epilepsy comprise animals with spontaneously occurring recurrent seizures. Furthermore, epileptic animals in which seizures occur not spontaneously but upon sensory stimulation, so called "reflex seizures" or "reflex epilepsy", will also be included in this section under the heading "Special Syndromes". In human epilepsy, only about 5% of epileptic patients get focal or generalized seizures in response to sensory stimulation (SCHMIDT 1993). About one-third of these patients with "reflex epilepsy" respond to photic stimulation. Seizures in photosensitive epilepsy are mostly of the absence type, whereas generalized tonic-clonic (grand mal), complex partial or simple partial seizures are less frequent (SCHMIDT 1993). Thus, the major drawback of all genetic animal models with reflex seizures is that this type of epilepsy is uncommon in humans. Furthermore, it should be noted that photomyoclonic seizures can occur in non-epileptic patients, which means that animals with photomyoclonic seizures are not necessarily models for epilepsy. The main advantage of genetic animals models with reflex seizures for anticonvulsant drug evaluation is that seizures can be easily and reproducibly evoked in these models without electrical or chemical means, and that the seizure types, at least in part, are similar in their clinical phenomenology to seizures occurring in human epilepsy.

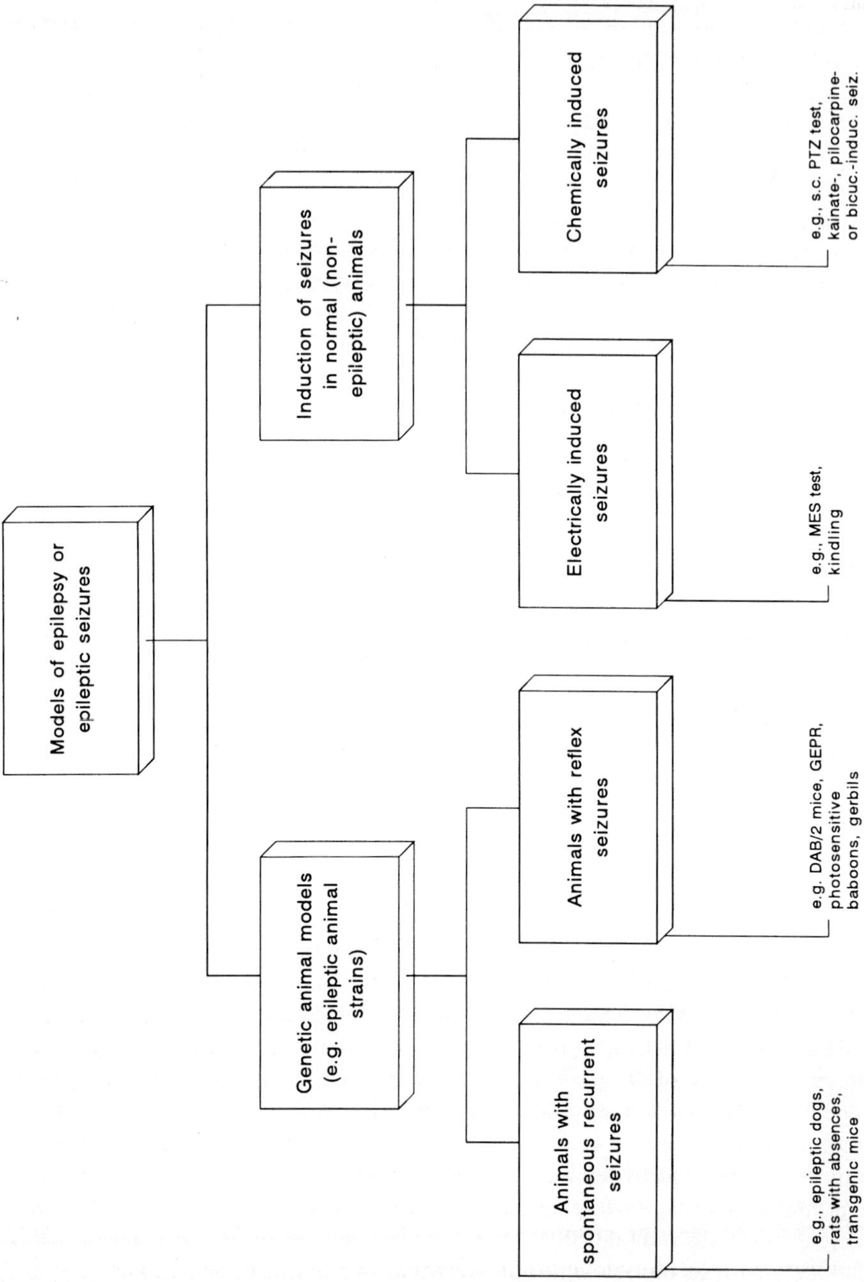

Fig. 1. Classification of experimental animal models of epilepsy and epileptic seizures

Table 1. International classification of epilepsies and epileptic syndromes in humans (COMMISSION 1989; DREIFUSS 1994) and proposed experimental animal models

Classification in humans	Potentially suitable animal models
1 Localization-related (focal, local, partial) epilepsies and syndromes	
1.1 Idiopathic	Dogs with localization-related epilepsy with age-related onset and no underlying cause other than a possible hereditary predisposition
1.2 Symptomatic	
Temporal lobe epilepsies	Amygdala or hippocampal kindling, kainate and pilocarpine models, local or topical application of metals, chemoconvulsants, or toxins
Frontal lobe epilepsies	Kindling or local application/injection of metals, chemoconvulsants, or toxins in respective areas
Parietal lobe epilepsies	As for frontal lobe
Occipital lobe epilepsies	As for frontal lobe
2 Generalized epilepsies and syndromes	
2.1 Idiopathic (primary), e.g. absence/myoclonic epilepsy	Lethargic mice, rat strains with spontaneous spike-wave discharges (e.g. GAERS)
Epilepsy with grand mal seizures	Double mutant rats (*zi/zi*, *tm/tm*) with spike-wave discharges and tonic seizures
2.2 Cryptogenic or symptomatic	
E.g. West syndrome, Lennox-Gastaut syndrome	No models as yet
3 Undetermined epilepsies	
3.1 With both generalized and focal seizures	*Tottering* mice with spike-wave discharges and focal seizures
4 Special syndromes e.g., reflex epilepsies	Epileptic gerbils, DBA/2 mice, genetically epilepsy prone rat, baboons, El mice

As in humans, an epilepsy in animal models is either idiopathic (and the epilepsy a primary epilepsy) or symptomatic (and the epilepsy a secondary epilepsy). Idiopathic or primary epilepsy is virtually synonymous with genetic epilepsy. The epilepsies occurring on the basis of structural disease or major identifiable metabolic derangements in the brain belong in the category of the symptomatic epilepsies (DREIFUSS 1994). In human epileptology, there is also the term "cryptogenic epilepsy", which is considered as a secondary epilepsy with unknown cause (DREIFUSS 1994), but this term will not be used for the animal models described in this review.

Based on the International Classification of Epilepsies and Epileptic Syndromes, four groups of epilepsies or epileptic syndromes are considered: (1) localization-related (focal, local, partial) epilepsies, (2) generalized epilepsies,

Table 2. International classification of epileptic seizures in humans (Commission 1981; Dreifuss 1994) and proposed experimental animal models

Classification in humans	Potentially suitable animal models
I. Partial (focal, local) seizures	
A. Simple partial seizures	Electrical induction of neocortical seizures via depth or screw electrodes
B. Complex partial seizures	Amygdala- or hippocampal-kindled seizures (stage 1 and 2); for other models see text
C. Partial seizures secondarily generalized	E.g. secondarily generalized (stage 4,5) kindled seizures
II. Generalized seizures	
A. Absence seizures	Lethargic mice, for other models see text
B. Myoclonic seizures	Pentylenetetrazole? (see text)
C. Clonic seizures	DBA/2 mice
D. Tonic seizures	MES, double mutant rats with spike-wave discharges and tonic seizures
E. Tonic-clonic seizures	MES, gerbils with 'major seizures', genetically epilepsy prone rat, epileptic dogs
F. Atonic seizures	
III. Unclassified epileptic seizures	

(3) undetermined epilepsies with both generalized and focal seizures or without unequivocal generalized or focal features, and (4) special syndromes, including reflex epilepsies (Commission 1989).

I. Localization-Related (Focal, Local, Partial) Epilepsies

This type of epilepsy is characterized by clinical or EEG evidence of local onset seizures, usually in a region of one cerebral hemisphere, which may spread to other parts of the brain during a seizure. More than half of all patients with this frequent type of epilepsy have both partial and secondarily generalized tonic-clonic seizures (Mattson 1995). Effective drugs for the treatment of partial epilepsies are carbamazepine, phenytoin, valproate, primidone, and phenobarbitone (Mattson 1995). Localization-related epilepsies are commonly symptomatic, but there are also some idiopathic types.

1. Idiopathic (Primary) Focal Epilepsies

According to the Classification Commission of the International League Against Epilepsy (ILAE), idiopathic localization-related epilepsies comprise benign childhood epilepsy with centrotemporal spikes, childhood epilepsy with occipital paroxysms, and primary reading epilepsy (Commission 1989). To our knowledge, no animal models have been described for these types of epilepsy. However, in dogs with idiopathic epilepsy, a localized onset of seizures is frequently seen, so that these animals will be described here. Genetic animal models of epilepsy with reflex seizures of focal onset will be described under the section "Special Syndromes".

a) Dogs with Idiopathic Localization-Related Epilepsy

Among domesticated animals, the dog is affected with epilepsy far more than any other species, making it a disease of considerable veterinary and comparative medical interest (Löscher 1984, 1992). Clinical and EEG observations strongly suggest that epilepsy in dogs approximates to the disease in man (Löscher et al. 1985). Thus, the prevalence of epilepsy in dogs is about 0.6% (with some variation between different breeds), which is quite similar to the value known for humans. Idiopathic epilepsy, as in humans, is more common than symptomatic epilepsy in dogs. A genetic background of most epilepsies in dogs is indicated not only by the absence of identifiable brain lesions but also by the differences in the prevalence of epilepsy among different breeds (Löscher et al. 1985). With respect to seizure types in epileptic dogs, generalized tonic-clonic seizures are by far the most common, but other types of seizures also occur, e.g. clonic, myoclonic, or tonic seizures, simple partial and complex partial seizures, and atypical seizures. Generalized tonic-clonic seizures in dogs are not only of the primary generalized type but often occur when focal seizures become secondarily generalized (Löscher 1986). The anticonvulsant pharmacology of the different types of epilepsies in dogs is similar to the situation in human epilepsy, although chronic administration of most antiepileptic drugs in dogs is hampered by their short elimination half-lives (Löscher 1986).

Although dogs with different types of idiopathic epilepsy would seem to provide an ideal model for epilepsy research, including research on localization-related idiopathic epilepsy, there are several drawbacks to this model. First, almost all studies on this species were done in dogs from private owners who are not willing to allow invasive experiments or to give away their animals for breeding purposes (Löscher 1997). Only a few studies on epilepsy in dogs have been performed in epileptic subgroups of dogs from beagle colonies (e.g. Edmonds et al. 1978). In this respect, the high prime and maintenance costs of dogs in the numbers necessary for selection and breeding of epileptic sublines limit the usefulness of this species for drug evaluation or pathophysiological studies. Furthermore, in contrast to genetic animal species with reflex seizures, or traditional electrically or chemically induced seizure models in normal animals, the naturally occurring seizures in dogs cannot be elicited at will by an investigator, which makes any scientific studies time-consuming, especially when the seizure frequency is low. Nevertheless, some groups, including our own, carry on studies with new drugs in epileptic dogs which are refractory to standard medications, but the primary goal of such studies is to help the animals and improve the current practice of epilepsy treatment in veterinary medicine rather than to obtain new information on drug resistance in general. One major drawback for chronic drug efficacy studies in epileptic dogs is that most new antiepileptics (and most of the clinically established antiepileptics) are so rapidly eliminated by dogs that it is not possible to maintain effective drug levels throughout the day using conventional drug preparations (LÖSCHER et al. 1985; LÖSCHER 1994). Indeed, the only drugs which allow maintenance of effective drug levels by one to three drug applications per day, and which are thus suited for chronic treatment of epilepsy in dogs, are phenobarbitone and primidone, the latter drug because of the accumulation of its active metabolite phenobarbitone (LÖSCHER et al. 1985; LÖSCHER 1994). Sustained-release formulations have been used to try to resolve the problem caused by the too rapid elimination of most antiepileptic drugs in dogs; however, sustained-release preparations developed for use in humans are not suitable for dogs because of the much shorter gastrointestinal retention time of such formulations (LÖSCHER 1981). More recently, the novel antiepileptic drug vigabatrin has been evaluated for control of epilepsy in dogs, because its mechanism of action (irreversible inhibition of GABA degradation) offers an effective treatment which should be independent of species differences in drug elimination. Vigabatrin proved to be effective in several epileptic dogs with phenobarbitone-resistant seizures, but at least in part vigabatrin had to be withdrawn because of the development of severe adverse effects such as haemolytic anaemia (SPECIALE et al. 1991).

2. Symptomatic (Secondary) Focal Epilepsies

According to the Classification Commission of the ILAE, symptomatic localization-related (focal, local, partial) epilepsies can be subdivided on the basis of the anatomical location of the epileptic focus into temporal lobe epilepsies, frontal lobe epilepsies, parietal lobe epilepsies, and occipital lobe epilepsies (DREIFUSS 1994). These types of epilepsy are the most common forms of chronic epilepsy in adults, and are often refractory to current antiepileptic drugs (LOISEAU 1986; LEPPIK 1992). Thus, animal models for these types of epilepsy are particularly important in the development of new antiepileptic drugs. However, models with partial seizures induced by electrical or chemical means (see Sect. C.I) may be more feasible in this respect than true models of symptomatic partial epilepsy with spontaneously recurring partial seizures.

The typical seizure types occurring in localization-related epilepsies are simple partial (i.e. without impaired consciousness) or complex-partial (i.e. with impaired consciousness) seizures, which both may evolve to secondarily generalized tonic-clonic seizures (DAM 1992). The majority (70%–85%) of complex partial seizures originate in the temporal lobes, while only about 10% are thought to originate from the frontal lobes (DAM 1992).

In patients, the localization-related symptomatic epilepsies may begin at any time of life, and have multiple aetiologies (MATTSON 1995). Among the most frequent causes are head trauma, vascular lesions, neoplasms, and infection. The majority of patients with temporal lobe epilepsy, the most common form of partial epilepsy, exhibit hippocampal sclerosis, and the seizures appear to originate within the sclerotic area. Often, the amygdala is also involved, explaining why most models of symptomatic localization-related epilepsy aim at the hippocampus or amygdala to produce seizures. Symptomatic focal epilepsy may occur as a chronic disease in dogs, e.g. in response to brain tumours (LÖSCHER et al. 1985), but because of the inherent problems of using such animals as preclinical models in epilepsy research (see Sect. B.I), they will not be further discussed here.

a) The Kindling Model of Temporal Lobe Epilepsy

The kindling phenomenon is a manifestation of the fact that "seizures beget seizures". Evidently through a kind of a positive feedback mechanism, a local epileptiform discharge, confined initially to a small focus or network, tends, if not "disturbed" (e.g. by treatment with antiepileptic drugs), to spread in space and severity. GODDARD et al. (1969) characterized this phenomenon in detail and in a systematic manner, which they came to refer to as "kindling". Animals chronically implanted with stimulation and recording electrodes in one structure of the limbic system or other brain areas (the amygdala being among the most responsive structures) develop seizures upon periodic electrical stimulation with an initially subconvulsive current. In rats stimulated in the amygdala, the initial stimulus often elicits focal paroxysmal activity (spikes, i.e. so-called "afterdischarges" in the EEG recorded from the amygdala) without overt clinical seizure activity. Subsequent stimulations induce the progressive development of seizures, generally evolving through the following stages: (1) immobility, facial clonus, eye closure, twitching of vibrissae, stereotyped sniffing, (2) head nodding, often accompanied by more severe facial clonus, (3) unilateral forelimb clonus, (4) rearing, often accompanied by bilateral forelimb clonus, and (5) continuous rearing and falling accompanied by secondarily generalized clonic seizures (RACINE 1972). All of these stages are associated with reduced responsiveness to sensory stimulation, in comparison to the normal waking state. The behaviour observed in stages 1 and 2 mimics that found in human complex partial (limbic or temporal lobe) seizures; the behaviour in the latter three stages would be consistent with complex partial seizures evolving to generalized motor seizures, the most devastating and difficult to treat form of epilepsy in adults (LOISEAU 1986). In addition to seizures becoming more severe during kindling acquisition, the paroxysmal EEG alterations (afterdischarges) associated with the clinical seizures increase in duration and amplitude. Furthermore, the electrical threshold for induction of afterdischarges in the focus significantly decreases during kindling development. Once the enhanced sensitivity (as evidenced by stage 5 seizures) has developed, the animal is said to be fully kindled. The increased convulsive sensitivity persists chronically after kindling has been established and thus appears to reflect permanent changes in brain function (SATO et al. 1990).

If kindling stimulations are continued, animals develop spontaneous seizures, demonstrating that kindling has resulted in epileptogenesis. The spontaneous seizures show the same characteristics as the electrically induced kindled seizures, and have been observed in kindled rats, baboons, cats, dogs, and other species (McNamara 1984). There is an ongoing controversy about whether kindling is also involved in humans, e.g. in post-traumatic epilepsy (e.g. Engel and Cahan 1986; Racine et al. 1989; Reynolds 1989; Adamec 1990; Sato et al. 1990).

Since its introduction in 1969, kindling has become the most widely used animal model of epilepsy, particularly because the mechanisms involved in kindling are thought to be relevant for epileptogenesis, including human epilepsy (Sato et al. 1990). Indeed, the kindling paradigm permits every possible facet of epilepsy research, ranging from membrane physiology involving brain slices to electroclinical phenomenology of spontaneously seizuring animals (Sato et al. 1990), so that the kindling model has provided us with a clearer insight into the nature of chronic epileptogenesis. An added advantage of the kindling model is that, in addition to increased seizure susceptibility, kindled animals exhibit lasting behavioural changes thought to be relevant for studies on psychosis in epilepsy (Sato et al. 1990; Trimble 1991). Most researchers use rats for the kindling model, but kindling can also be produced in other species, including primates (Sato et al. 1990).

In addition to classical kindling by focal electrical stimulation of sensitive brain sites, the term kindling is also used for repetitive bilateral transcorneal electrical stimulation ("corneal kindling") and for kindling induced by systemic administration of chemical convulsants such as pentylenetetrazol ("chemical kindling"). Repeated bilateral transcorneal stimulation of rats, e.g. with 8 mA, 60 Hz, for 4 s twice daily (White et al. 1995), induces kindling acquisition with seizures similar to those induced by conventional kindling through unilateral depth electrodes. This may indicate that the transcorneally applied electrical stimulus reaches the same brain circuits as the depth electrodes in limbic areas. However, the pharmacology of focally induced versus transcorneally induced kindled seizures may be different, for instance because a drug which affects the propagation of paroxysmal activity may be more effective in corneal kindling. Indeed, in a study in which the effect of standard anticonvulsants was compared in corneal-kindled and amygdala-kindled rats, phenytoin, carbamazepine and valproate were clearly more effective in corneal than in amygdala-kindled animals (Swinyard et al. 1993) so that in contrast to some statements in the literature (e.g. White et al. 1995), the pharmacology of the two models, and therefore their predictive character in terms of clinical drug efficacy, are different. Furthermore, corneal kindling with repeated transcorneal application of relatively high currents poses ethical problems in terms of animal welfare, whereas current application via a chronically implanted depth electrode in freely moving rats is not considered harmful for the animals.

In chemical kindling with systemic administration of pentylenetetrazol (SCHMIDT 1987; CRAIG and COLASANTI 1988), e.g. by intraperitoneal injection of 30 or 40 mg/kg every 2nd day in rats, some animals of a group may exhibit primary generalized convulsive seizures after the first or second injection, and most rats develop generalized clonic or tonic convulsions during subsequent pentylenetetrazole applications, indicating that this model represents a model of primary generalized seizures rather than localization-related focal seizures. In the following, the term kindling will be used only in its original sense, i.e. for focal (unilateral) electrical stimulation.

In view of the fact that most researchers use stimulation-induced seizures and not spontaneously occurring seizures in the kindling model as the endpoint for pharmacological studies, one may argue that kindling is a model of complex-partial seizures which become secondarily generalized rather than a model of localization-related (temporal lobe) epilepsy. However, in view of the kindling-associated phenomena, e.g. progressive increase in seizure severity and duration, a decrease in focal seizure threshold, a development of spontaneously recurrent seizures, and neuronal degeneration, kindling is certainly a model of chronic epilepsy which offers the advantage that seizures can be elicited at will. In this respect, the kindling model is similar to epileptic animals mutants with "reflex seizures", such as epileptic gerbils, which offer the advantage that both epileptogenesis and ictogenesis can be studied in the same model.

The pharmacological susceptibility of seizures in the kindling model and in human temporal lobe epilepsy is strikingly similar. Carbamazepine, phenobarbitone, and valproate block both the complex-partial and secondarily generalized seizure types in kindled rats (LÖSCHER and SCHMIDT 1988). Primidone is effective in this regard during chronic administration, due to slow accumulation of its active metabolite phenobarbitone. Phenytoin was long thought to exert only variable effects in kindled rats, but more recent reports showed that this major antiepileptic drug for the treatment of temporal lobe epilepsy in humans is also an effective drug in the kindling model, provided that certain technical factors are dealt with (MCNAMARA et al. 1989; RUNDFELDT et al. 1990; LOTHMAN et al. 1991). These factors include low or inconsistent absorption after intraperitoneal injection of basic solutions of phenytoin and the stimulus strength used for electrical induction of kindled seizures. If these factors are dealt with, phenytoin dose-dependently increases the threshold for induction of paroxysmal activity in the stimulated brain region (afterdischarge threshold), but does not decrease the severity or duration of secondarily generalized seizures at afterdischarge threshold current, indicating that phenytoin acts on seizure initiation in the focus but not on the propagation from the focus in this model (RUNDFELDT et al. 1990). Interestingly, when phenytoin's anticonvulsant activity was repeatedly tested in large groups of amygdala-kindled Wistar rats, subgroups with different sensitivities to phenytoin could be selected, another explanation for the variable effects of phenytoin in the kindling model reported previously (Löscher 1997). Three subgroups were characterized, i.e. phenytoin responders, phenytoin non-responders, and variable responders (Löscher and Rundfeldt 1991). While phenytoin responders always reacted to phenytoin with an anticonvulsant effect, i.e. an afterdischarge threshold increase, non-responders never showed such an effect, indicating that such non-responders might be an ideal model for studying mechanisms of drug resistance in epilepsy (Löscher 1997).

In addition to using fully kindled rats for drug potency studies, drugs can be administered during kindling acquisition in order to evaluate their antiepileptogenic efficacy. Interestingly, phenytoin and carbamazepine, which are used as drugs of first choice for the prevention of post-traumatic epilepsy, have not been found to be antiepileptogenic in the kindling model (Hernandez 1997). This result generally concurs with controlled clinical studies reporting that phenytoin or carbamazepine prophylaxis has no effect on the later development of epilepsy (Hernandez 1997).

Another interesting finding from the kindling model is that amygdala-kindled rats are much more sensitive to motor impairing and psychotomimetic adverse effects of certain drugs than age-matched non-kindled controls (Löscher and Hönack 1991, 1995). Thus, while *N*-methyl-D-aspartate (NMDA) antagonists proved ineffective in increasing the afterdischarge threshold or in affecting focal seizure activity in fully kindled rats, they induced much more marked adverse effects, including stereotyped behaviours, in kindled compared with non-kindled rats (Löscher and Hönack 1991). From this observation we concluded that epileptogenesis increases the adverse effect potential of certain anticonvulsant drugs (Löscher and Hönack 1991). In a subsequent study with a competitive NMDA antagonist in patients with partial epilepsy, no anticonvulsant effect was obtained, but patients showed marked adverse effects, including motor impairment and psychosis, that had not been observed with the drug in phase I studies in healthy volunteers (Sveinbjornsdottir et al. 1993). Interestingly, differences in anticonvulsant or adverse effects between epileptic and non-epileptic animals had previously been found also with other drugs in other epilepsy models. For instance, by comparing the anticonvulsant potency of an investigational drug on electrically induced seizures in non-epileptic and epileptic beagle dogs, Edmonds et al. (1978) found that epileptic and non-epileptic subjects did not respond similarly to anticonvulsant treatment, in that epileptic beagles were less sensitive to the anticonvulsant effect but more sensitive to the adverse effects of the test drug than non-epileptic dogs were. A similar finding in another species was reported by Laird et al. (1976), who showed that phenytoin, carbamazepine, and phenobarbitone all were 4 times more effective in blocking seizures in normal rats than in audiogenic-seizure susceptible epileptic rats. These data suggest that preclinical evaluation of an anticonvulsant *only* in non-epileptic animals may exaggerate its potential clinical usefulness. Furthermore, the data indicate that the chronic alterations in brain function induced by epileptogenesis may render the brain less susceptible to anticonvulsant drug effects, a suggestion which is substantiated by our recent findings with NMDA antagonists in the kindling model of temporal lobe epilepsy (Löscher and Hönack 1991).

b) The Kainate Model

Seizures induced by the excitotoxic glutamate analogue kainate are increasingly being used as a model of temporal lobe epilepsy (Sperk 1994). Kainate-induced seizures are associated with widespread brain damage, which is not seen in other models of temporal lobe epilepsy, such as the kindling model. Nevertheless, some of the convulsive behaviours seen after kainate injection in rats are remarkably similar to those observed in fully kindled rats (Sperk 1994), thus suggesting that the anatomical networks involved in seizure propagation may, at least in part, be similar (Löscher and Ebert 1996a). With respect to the susceptibility of kainate-induced seizures to systemic administration of standard antiepileptic drugs, benzodiazepines and trimethadione are the most effective, whereas phenytoin, carbamazepine, and valproate have no overt anticonvulsant action in this model (Sperk 1994). In other words, striking differences from the clinical efficacy of antiepileptic drugs in temporal lobe epilepsy exist, so that the predictive value, if any, of kainate seizures for the development of therapeutic strategies for temporal lobe epilepsy is difficult to ascertain.

Most researchers use the kainate model as a model of seizures rather than a model of epilepsy, because kainate is injected only once at a convulsant dose, and the acute seizures induced by this kainate injection are used as the endpoint for drug activity studies. However, this one injection of kainate can also result in spontaneous recurrent seizures, which may occur weeks after the termination of the initial drug-induced seizures, thus providing a true model of chronic epilepsy (Sperk 1994). These late spontaneous seizures are accompanied by shrinkage of the amygdala, and presumably originate in this area (Sperk 1994). The expression of spontaneous seizure activity as a late consequence of kainate-induced seizures has also been related to hippocampal damage and/or synaptic plasticity. This chronic state following kainate injection is the reason for discussing this model here, because the fact that administration of kainate may lead to spontaneous recurrent seizures might be useful in the search for mechanisms of chronic (temporal lobe) epilepsy. Furthermore, the model can be used in the search for drugs which block the development of chronic epilepsy, and the associated neurodegeneration.

c) The Pilocarpine Model

Seizures induced by the cholinergic (muscarinic) agonist, pilocarpine, have been proposed as an experimental model of intractable epilepsy with seizures resembling complex partial ("limbic") seizures that become secondarily generalized (Turski et al. 1989). This proposal was based, at least in part, on the lack of anticonvulsant effect of carbamazepine and phenytoin, drugs of first choice for the treatment of complex partial seizures in humans, against convulsions produced by pilocarpine (TURSKI et al. 1989). Effective anticonvulsants in this model comprised benzodiazepines, phenobarbitone, valproate and trimethadione, drugs which are normally not effective in patients with complex partial seizures resistant to phenytoin or carbamazepine (SCHMIDT 1993; MATTSON 1995). Thus, the predictive value of pilocarpine-induced seizures for developing "rational" therapeutic strategies for difficult-to-treat complex-partial seizures is uncertain. Furthermore, similar to the kainate model, seizures induced by injection of pilocarpine are certainly a model of seizures rather than a model of epilepsy. However, again similar to the kainate model, animals which survive the acute seizures induced by pilocarpine may develop late spontaneous seizures, i.e. develop chronic epilepsy. The first spontaneous seizure is usually observed 5–10 days after pilocarpine-induced status epilepticus (TURSKI et al. 1989). These seizures resemble stage 4/5 seizures of amygdala-kindled rats and continue to appear for several weeks following a status epilepticus. The spontaneous recurrent seizures observed in the pilocarpine model differ in their pharmacological susceptibility from the acute pilocarpine-induced seizures (LEITE and CAVALHEIRO 1995) and seem to be more comparable to human complex partial seizures in this respect (see Sect. C.I). An added advantage of the spontaneous seizures is that the mechanisms involved in the occurrence of spontaneous recurrent seizures might be relevant for studies on how chronic epilepsy develops. In this regard, however, it should be realized that pilocarpine, like kainate, induces widespread brain damage, involving regions that do not contain lesions in temporal lobe epilepsy.

d) *Chronic Epilepsy Following Status Epilepticus*

It is interesting to note that in both the pilocarpine and kainate models, spontaneous recurrent seizures, i.e. chronic epilepsy, have been observed in rats which survived the prolonged activity of acute convulsant-induced seizures, i.e. a status epilepticus (TURSKI et al. 1989; SPERK 1994). In addition to structural brain damage and enduring neurological deficits following status epilepticus, it has been suggested that status epilepticus can establish a chronic condition of active epilepsy in animal models and in humans (LOTHMAN and BERTRAM 1993). LOTHMAN and BERTRAM (1993) have proposed a two-step model: morphological brain injury in response to status epilepticus takes place first and this change, in turn, promotes seizures. This model was proposed as one way in which chronic active epilepsy, particularly of the often refractory temporal lobe type, can be established by a transient episode of status epilepticus (LOTHMAN and BERTRAM 1993). LOTHMAN et al. (1990) demonstrated that in rats spontaneous seizures not only developed following status epilepticus induced by convulsants such as kainate or pilocarpine but also after a period of continuous hippocampal electrical stimulation. This established an acute condition of self-sustaining status epilepticus which was followed by chronic neuropathological changes reminiscent of the hippocampal sclerosis encountered in many epileptic patients with temporal lobe epilepsy and, about 1 month following status epilepticus, recurrent spontaneous hippocampal seizures (LOTHMAN and BERTRAM 1993). Although this model may present an interesting approach to temporal lobe epilepsy, to our knowledge no pharmacological studies have been reported as yet. Furthermore, in humans the start of an epilepsy with status epilepticus is rather uncommon.

e) Spontaneous Focal Seizures Following Local Application of Metals, Chemical Convulsants or Toxins

Spontaneous recurrent seizures have also been observed in some models of focal epileptogenesis produced by local (commonly cortical) application of metals or metal salts, such as aluminium hydroxide, cobalt or iron, particularly when using monkeys as experimental animals (WARD 1972; KOELLA 1985; LÖSCHER and SCHMIDT 1988). Similarly, cortical or subcortical epileptogenic foci can be produced by the local application of various chemical convulsants or toxins (PRINCE 1972; KOELLA 1985; LÖSCHER and SCHMIDT 1988). However, most of these models have not been widely used in antiepileptic drug evaluation. Cobalt-induced focal seizures, which have been extensively characterized in pharmacological studies, seem to be more sensitive to antiepileptics used clinically for the treatment of absence seizures than to antiepileptics used for the treatment of focal seizures and generalized tonic-clonic seizures, and are thus apparently not a predictive model of localization-related epilepsies (CRAIG and COLASANTI 1992). In general, the topical use of convulsant metals or convulsant drugs is steadily decreasing in epilepsy research, possibly because of the development of more popular models for focal epilepsy, such as the kindling and kainate models. The same is true for the production of epileptogenic cortical foci in experimental animals by local freezing (LEWIN 1972; KOELLA 1985).

An interesting model of focal epilepsy has been obtained by injection of tetanus toxin into the rat neocortex or hippocampus (EMPSON et al. 1993). Within a day following focal injection of a small dose of tetanus toxin, spontaneous and stimulus-evoked paroxysmal discharges appeared in widespread regions of both hemispheres and these lasted for at least 9 months. An epileptic focus can also be produced by intrahippocampal injection of cholera toxin, but the resulting paroxysmal discharges are only transient (WILLIAMS et al. 1993). It should be noted that this approach of producing epileptic foci by toxins such as tetanus toxin is not new but had first been described several decades ago (KOELLA 1985).

II. Generalized Epilepsies

Generalized epilepsies are epileptic disorders with primarily generalized seizures, i.e. seizures in which the first clinical changes indicate initial involvement of both hemispheres, and in which ictal EEG patterns initially are bilateral (COMMISSION 1989). Most generalized epilepsies are idiopathic and usually begin in childhood, including types such as childhood absence epilepsy (pyknolepsy) or neonatal convulsions, whereas other types, such as juvenile myoclonic epilepsy (impulsive petit mal) or epilepsy with generalized tonic-clonic (grand mal) seizures, develop mostly in the 2nd decade of life (DREIFUSS 1994). Valproate is usually the drug of choice for the generalized idiopathic epilepsies (MATTSON 1995). Symptomatic or cryptogenic generalized epilepsies comprise epileptic syndromes such as the West syndrome (infantile spasms) and the Lennox-Gastaut syndrome, and epilepsy types such as epilepsy with myoclonic absences and myoclonic-astatic seizures (DREIFUSS 1994). To our knowledge, there are no animal models for such symptomatic or cryptogenic types of epilepsies or epileptic syndromes. Therefore, in the following, some models of generalized idiopathic epilepsy will be described. Only models with spontaneous recurrent seizures will be reviewed here, while models with reflex epilepsy will be considered under "Special Syndromes".

1. Animal Models of Idiopathic Primary Generalized Epilepsies

a) Epileptic Dogs

Epileptic dogs have been described above as a genetic animal model of epilepsy (Sect. B.I). Most generalized epilepsies in dogs occur in the absence of identifiable brain lesions, with an age-dependent onset between the 1st and 3rd year of life, and are commonly characterized by generalized tonic-clonic seizures, although other seizure types occur as well. Generalized tonic-clonic seizures in dogs with idiopathic epilepsy may be either primary or secondarily generalized. However, because of the described inherent disadvantages of epileptic dogs as an animal model of epilepsy, they will not be discussed further here.

b) Rats with Generalized Absence Epilepsy

Various mice and rat mutants with spontaneous non-convulsive patterns of epilepsy have been described (COENEN et al. 1992), but only a few have been used to characterize the basic mechanisms and pharmacological susceptibility of the syndromes. MARESCAUX and coworkers have selected a strain of Wistar rats in which 100% of the animals present recurrent generalized non-convulsive seizures characterized by bilateral and synchronous spike-wave discharges (7–11 cycles/s) accompanied by behavioural arrest, staring and sometimes twitching of the vibrissae (MARESCAUX et al. 1992). Based on its origin, this strain was termed the Genetic Absence Epilepsy Rat from Strasbourg (GAERS). A rat strain with similar electrographic and clinical features has been described by a Dutch group (COENEN et al. 1992). These two rat strains have been extremely helpful in elucidating pathophysiological, genetic, ontogenetic and pharmacological characteristics of non-convulsive epilepsy.

In both strains, drugs effective against absence or myoclonic seizures in humans (ethosuximide, trimethadione, valproate, benzodiazepines) suppress the spike-wave discharges, whereas drugs specific for convulsive or focal seizures (carbamazepine, phenytoin) or selective GABAmimetic drugs [$GABA_A$ receptor agonists such as muscimol and THIP (gaboxadol), GABA transaminase (GABA-T) inhibitors such as vigabatrin, GABA uptake inhibitors] increase the duration of spike-wave discharges (COENEN et al. 1992; MARESCAUX et al. 1992). Data on $GABA_A$ receptor antagonists such as bicuculline are controversial, showing either no effect (MARESCAUX et al. 1992) or an anticonvulsant effect on spike-wave discharges in the rat models (COENEN et al. 1992). The novel $GABA_B$ receptor antagonist CGP 35348 suppressed the spontaneous spike-wave discharges as well as the spike-wave discharges aggravated by concomitant injection of GABAmimetic drugs or γ-hydroxybutyrate, indicating the involvement of $GABA_B$-mediated neurotransmission in the development of spike-wave discharges in generalized non-convulsive epilepsy (MARESCAUX et al. 1992).

Whereas the above-described pharmacological findings with antiepileptic drugs in the rat model would be in line with the clinical efficacy of these drugs against absence epilepsy (MATTSON 1995), phenobarbitone was effective in blocking the seizures in GAERS, whereas this drug is ineffective in human absence epilepsy. More recent data from experiments with novel antiepileptic drugs substantiate that GAERS may be a model of myoclonic epilepsy rather than absence epilepsy (see Sect. C.II, below).

c) *The Lethargic (lh/lh) Mouse*

Lethargic (*lh/lh*) mice, a mutant mouse strain which functions as an animal model of idiopathic absence epilepsy, have spontaneous seizures that have behavioural and electrographic features and anticonvulsant sensitivity similar to those of human absence seizures (HOSFORD et al. 1992; HOSFORD and WANG 1997). Mice of different ages exhibit bilaterally synchronous electrographic bursts of 5- to 6-Hz spike-wave complexes which are accompanied by immobility and reduced responsiveness. The mean seizure frequency is about 130/h. Neurochemical and pharmacological experiments indicated that enhanced $GABA_B$ receptor-mediated transmission may underlie absence epilepsy in *lh/lh* mice (HOSFORD et al. 1992, 1995). Evaluation of clinically established antiepileptic drugs in the new model showed that the seizures were dose-dependently inhibited by ethosuximide, trimethadione, valproate, and clonazepam, whereas phenytoin and carbamazepine were ineffective (HOSFORD et al. 1992, 1995). Recently, HOSFORD and WANG (1997) demonstrated that the novel antiepileptic drug lamotrigine reduced the seizure frequency in *lh/lh* mice, while topiramate was without effect, and vigabatrin and tiagabine increased the seizure frequency, i.e. exerted proconvulsant activity. These interesting findings will be further discussed below in comparison with the findings from other models of absence seizures (Sect. C.II).

d) The Spontaneously Epileptic Double Mutant Rat

Spontaneously epileptc double mutant rats (*zi/zi*, *tm/tm*) that exhibit both absence-like seizures and tonic convulsions without external stimuli or when mildly stimulated by tapping or sound were obtained by mating the tremor heterozygous rat (*tm/+*) with the zitter homozygous rat (*zi/zi*) (SERIKAWA and YAMADA 1986). Absence-like seizures in the double mutant rat are characterized by immobility with fixed staring, without tremor or muscle twitches, being paralleled by 5–7 Hz spike-wave-like complexes in the cortical and hippocampal EEG (SASA et al. 1988). The non-convulsive seizures occur frequently, with 5–62 seizures observed in 15-min observation periods. Also, the rats exhibit generalized tonic convulsions with extension of all extremities, which occurred spontaneously between 68 and 128 times in an individual rat in a 12-h observation period (SASA et al. 1988). In addition, wild running and/or wild jumping is observed infrequently. Ethosuximide and trimethadione inhibited the absence-like seizures without affecting the tonic seizures (SASA et al. 1988). In contrast, phenytoin blocked the tonic but not the non-convulsive seizures. Phenobarbitone and valproate inhibited the number and total duration of both absence-like and tonic seizures in the mutant rats. These data demonstrate that the double mutant rat is an interesting model of generalized idiopathic epilepsy, combining both convulsive and non-convulsive seizures, thus allowing the evaluation of anticonvulsant activity against these different seizure types in the same model.

e) Transgenic or Knockout Mice

An alternative to animals with inborn epilepsy as a potential source of models of idiopathic generalized epilepsy may arise from the development of transgenic mice carrying epilepsy genes (ALLEN and WALSH 1996; NOEBELS 1996). Indeed, the ability to insert and delete genes in the nervous system provides a powerful strategy for generating new experimental models of epilepsy. These models are expected to reveal previously unknown cellular mechanisms of epileptogenesis, and may be used in new antiepileptic drug discovery (NOEBELS 1996). Furthermore, transgenic mice and knockout mice offer the possibility of selectively producing cellular or molecular abnormalities proposed to be involved in causing pharmaco-resistant epilepsy, thereby permitting an analysis of how critical these processes are (HEINEMANN et al. 1994). However, the various transgenic mice or mouse knockouts with seizures which have been produced so far are insufficiently characterized pharmacologically to allow conclusions about the usability of such animals in drug development for the treatment of specific types of epilepsy. Nevertheless, if the intractability of seizures has a genetic background, transgenic mice carrying the respective gene(s) could be ideal models for the development of more effective antiepileptic drugs.

III. Undetermined Epilepsies

In human epilepsy, this group comprises two subgroups, i.e. (1) epilepsies with both generalized and focal seizures, such as neonatal seizures, severe myoclonic epilepsy in infancy, and acquired epileptic aphasia, and (2) epilepsies without unequivocal generalized or focal features (COMMISSION 1989). To the writer's knowledge, only one animal model of epilepsy with both generalized and focal seizures has been described, i.e. the *tottering* mouse.

1. *Tottering* Mice

The homozygous *tottering* mouse (*tg*, autosomal recessive) is a presumed single-locus mutant, phenotypically characterized by spontaneous epileptic seizures (NOEBELS 1979). By 3–4 weeks of age, affected homozygotes can be recognized by a broad-based, ataxic gait. Spontaneous focal motor seizures are observed 1–3 days later and occur one or more times per day throughout the normal life span of the mutant. The initial stage of each episode begins with bilateral tonic flexor spasms in the hind legs. The second stage is marked by rapid, unilateral clonic jerks of the limbs, beginning in the hind leg and progressively spreading to affect both hind leg and fore leg simultaneously. In its final stage, the seizure terminates with prolonged clonic jerking of the forelimb alone. Generalized convulsions are never seen. In studies on *tottering* mice by FREY's group in Berlin, the focal motor seizures occurred irregularly a few times a day and 93% of the seizures lasted for 15 min or longer (LÖSCHER 1992). The focal seizures are not correlated with any reliable stereotyped EEG findings in surface electrocorticograms (NOEBELS and SIDMAN 1979). The focal motor seizures in *tottering* mice are not affected by ethosuximide and valproic acid but are potently suppressed by diazepam.

A second distinct seizure pattern in homozygous *tottering* mice is absence or myoclonic seizures associated with spike-wave discharges in the EEG. As early as day 32 postnatally, bilaterally synchronous 6–7/s spike-wave discharges appear as spontaneous bursts in electrocorticographic recordings (NOEBELS and SIDMAN 1979). These spike-wave bursts, 0.3–10 s in duration, occur hundreds of time per day and are in each case accompanied by a behavioural seizure, with arrest of movement, staring posture, twitching of the vibrissae, and single myoclonus jerks of the head or jaw. These seizures are present at least until 10 months of age. As shown by HELLER et al. (1983) in *tottering* mice with chronically implanted EEG electrodes, the spike-wave seizures can be dose-dependently blocked by ethosuximide, diazepam and phenobarbitone but not by phenytoin, which exacerbates the seizures at higher doses. These results thus demonstrate that in *tottering* mice the sensitivities to antiepileptic drugs of spike-wave absence seizures and of focal motor seizures differ. The model illustrates that – as in humans – animal mutants may combine different types of epileptic seizures. *Tottering* mice are not commonly used as a pharmacological model, but, like various other mouse mutants (SEYFRIED and

GLASER 1985; RISE et al. 1990; FRANKEL et al. 1994), their main use is in the evaluation of genetic and neuronal abnormalities involved in epilepsy (NOEBELS 1986; KOSTOPOULOS 1992).

IV. Special Syndromes

This group of epileptic syndromes includes epilepsies characterized by specific modes of seizure precipitation, i.e. the so-called "reflex epilepsies", which have already been discussed above (see Sect. B). Various species with reflex epilepsy have been reported in the literature, and several of these genetic epilepsy models are popular in epilepsy research, because they allow the induction of different types of epileptic seizures by simple non-invasive sensory stimuli.

a) Epileptic Gerbils

Reflex epilepsy in Mongolian gerbils (*Meriones unguiculatus)* occurs both in randomly bred and selectively bred colonies (LÖSCHER 1991). Seizures can be initiated by various precipitating environmental stimuli, e.g. a new environment, the onset of bright light, audiogenic stimuli, vigorous shaking of the cage, different handling procedures, or exposure of the animals to a blast of compressed air aimed at their backs (LÖSCHER 1991). By air blast stimulation, seizures could be evoked in more than 98% of randomly bred gerbils, so that no selective breeding procedures were needed to select seizure-susceptible animals (LÖSCHER 1991). The gerbils show an age-dependent onset and progression of seizures upon air blast stimulation with "minor" (facial myoclonic) seizures occurring at about 7–10 weeks of age and progression to "major" (generalized myoclonic and tonic-clonic) seizures occurring in most gerbils during subsequent stimulations, the maximum seizure severity being reached at about 7 months of age (LÖSCHER 1991). Epilepsy in gerbils usually does not remit and seizures can be evoked in most animals for their whole life span.

EEG studies in epileptic gerbils have suggested that the seizures might have a focal origin, beginning with localized spikes being recognized unilaterally in the parietal or occipital cortex, followed by the rapid spread of paroxysmal activity across the cortex and subcortical structures, involving areas of the limbic system (LOSKOTA and LOMAX 1975; SUZUKI and NAKAMOTO 1978). It has been suggested that the focal-onset ictal EEG paroxysms in parietal derivations might be related to the stimulus-bound nature of the seizures in epileptic gerbils (LOSKOTA and LOMAX 1975).

In pharmacological studies clonazepam, diazepam, valproic acid and ethosuximide were most potent against the minor seizures, whereas this type of seizure was resistant to phenytoin and could be only partially suppressed by carbamazepine (LÖSCHER 1991). Phenobarbitone was active against minor seizures but less so than against major ones. Major seizures were best suppressed by phenytoin, phenobarbitone, primidone, and carbamazepine as well as by diazepam and clonazepam. The benzodiazepines, however, were less potent against major seizures than against minor ones, which is consistent with clinical experience in humans (SCHMIDT 1993). Valproic acid was also less active against major seizures than it was against minor seizures, and ethosuximide protected against major seizures only at very high, sedative doses. Thus, it seems possible to differentiate in the gerbil between drugs clinically useful in humans against absence and myoclonic seizures (ethosuximide, valproic acid, benzodiazepines) and drugs particularly effective against generalized tonic-clonic seizures (phenytoin, phenobarbitone, primidone, carbamazepine), so that at least in terms of pharmacological sensitivity the epileptic gerbil is a model of generalized rather than of focal epilepsy.

However, because of a number of drawbacks (LÖSCHER 1992), this species is only rarely used in epilepsy research. First, although in gerbils seizures can be triggered by different external stimuli, usually handling or change in environment, most of these stimuli are poorly defined and not quantifiable. Second, following a seizure gerbils exhibit a refractory period that lasts for at least several days. Therefore, if a seizure is triggered without intention by handling during drug administration, evaluation of the drugs's effects is not possible. To overcome this problem, some investigators utilized inhalant anaesthetics during drug administration, further complicating the results because of possible pharmacological contamination by the anaesthetics. Third, familiarity with the experimental environment may lead to habituation of the stimulus that triggers the seizure. Fourth, pharmacological experiments in gerbils are time-consuming since, due to the long postictal refractoriness, the animals can be tested only once a week. Fifth, as in other rodent species the half-lives of common antiepileptic drugs in gerbils are much shorter than in man, which renders the maintenance of effective drug levels during chronic treatment difficult.

In spite of these drawbacks, the gerbil may be useful in improving the understanding of the neurophysiological and neurochemical mechanisms of seizure development. It offers the opportunity of studying the differential actions of anticonvulsants on young and adult animals and may thus prove valuable in the evaluation of anticonvulsant drugs used or usable in human epilepsy.

b) Audiogenic Seizure Susceptible Mice

Audiogenic seizures are violent generalized convulsions triggered by exposure to intense auditory stimulation in genetically susceptible strains of mice or rats (LÖSCHER 1992). Most studies on audiogenic seizure susceptible mice have been performed in the DAB/2 inbred strain of the house mouse (*Mus musculus*), which has been known since 1947 to be susceptible to sound-induced seizures (SEYFRIED 1979). Nearly 100% of the males and females of this strain undergo an age-dependent, often fatal, sequence of convulsions when initially exposed to a loud mixed-frequency sound (10-120 kHz, 90–120 dB), such as that of a doorbell. The seizures begin with a wild running phase, followed by clonic convulsions and a tonic extension, ending in respiratory arrest (in about 60%) or full recovery. Although the clonic seizures are normally used for the evaluation of anticonvulsant drug action, the wild running phase is probably the most important simple feature that distinguishes the syndrome from electroconvulsive seizures and most types of chemically induced seizures. The onset of audiogenic seizure susceptibility in DBA/2 mice generally occurs over a relatively short period of time (12–17 days of age). The age of peak susceptibility is between 19 and 24 days; thereafter, the susceptibility declines. By the time mice are adults (over 80 days old), they are completely resistant to auditory stimulation (Seyfried 1979).

Regarding evaluation of antiepileptic drugs in this model, all of the commonly used antiepileptic drugs protect against clonic seizures in DBA/2 mice (Chapman et al. 1984; Löscher 1992). Thus, in contrast to most other known models of epilepsy, sound-induced seizures in DBA/2 mice are not particularly sensitive to a specific clinical category of antiepileptic drugs. Besides antiepileptic drugs, various experimental anticonvulsants have proved active in audiogenic seizure susceptible mice. Among genetic animal models of epilepsy, DBA/2 mice with sound-induced seizures are at present certainly the most widely used model for anticonvulsant drug screening.

In conclusion, audiogenic seizure susceptible mice are useful as a sensitive gross screening model for potential anticonvulsant drugs. However, they do not discriminate between the different clinical categories of antiepileptic drugs, and thus they cannot predict antiepileptic activity against a specific type of epilepsy. In this respect, it should be noted that sound-induced seizures are uncommon in man (Bickford and Klass 1969) and thus the audiogenic seizure susceptible mouse is obviously not a model of a particular human convulsive disorder. On the other hand, it is unlikely that a potent anticonvulsant drug would be rejected by this model.

c) *Audiogenic Seizure Susceptible Rats*

Audiogenic seizures in selectively bred rats, such as the "genetically epilepsy prone rat" (GEPR), are first observed between 17 and 21 days of age, and, in contrast to audiogenic seizures in mice, the seizure susceptibility does not decline with age (Consroe et al. 1979). Sound-induced seizures in rats typically consist of the following sequence: a startle response, momentary quiescence, violent running, a tonic-clonic seizure, and postictal depression (Consroe et al. 1979). In contrast to audiogenic seizure susceptible mice, rats rarely die after the seizures. For anticonvulsant drug evaluation, the tonic-clonic component of the response pattern in the rats is commonly used.

Evaluation of common antiepileptic drugs in rats with sound-induced seizures (Consroe and Wolkin 1977; Consroe et al. 1979; Dailey and Jobe 1985) has shown that drugs which are effective against generalized tonic-clonic (grand mal) and partial seizures in humans, namely phenobarbitone, phenytoin, carbamazepine and clonazepam, are the most potent drugs in this model.

On the other hand, audiogenic seizures in rats are relatively insensitive to ethosuximide and valproate. Actually, ethosuximide failed to show a linear dose-response against audiogenic seizures, and even with high doses (600 mg/kg) no more than 60% of the animals could be protected (CONSROE and WOLKIN 1977). Determination of the protective index, i.e. the ratio between the median minimal neurotoxic dose (TD_{50}) in the rotarod test and the anticonvulsant ED_{50}, yielded high values for carbamazepine, phenytoin, clonazepam and phenobarbitone in audiogenic seizure susceptible rats, thus indicating a satisfactory margin of safety for these drugs (CONSROE and WOLKIN 1977; CONSROE et al. 1979). Considerably lower protective indices were found for trimethadione and valproic acid, and ethosuximide was protective only in neurotoxic doses.

These data demonstrate that the audiogenic seizure test in rats is similar to the maximal electroshock seizure test in rats or mice as regards the relative effectiveness of antiepileptic drugs. Although the maximal electroshock seizure test is the standard paradigm for identifying drugs with potential activity against generalized tonic-clonic seizures in man (see Sect. C.II), the audiogenic seizure susceptible rat seems to be a valuable alternative model in this respect, because it provides important pharmacogenetic, aetiological and pathophysiological information that is not readily apparent with the use of the more traditional electroshock seizure model.

The functional neuroanatomy of seizures in genetically epilepsy prone rats has been studied mainly with respect to the audiogenic seizure predisposition in these animals (FAINGOLD and NARIKOU 1992; JOBE et al. 1992; LÖSCHER and EBERT 1996a). The respective studies provided evidence for a role of the primary auditory pathway, particularly involving the inferior colliculus, in audiogenic seizure generation in the genetically epilepsy prone rat.

d) Epileptic Baboons with Photomyoclonic Seizures

A photomyoclonic syndrome in the baboon *Papio papio* was first reported by KILLAM et al. (1966). Since then, much work has been carried out elucidating the characteristics of this syndrome (NAQUET and MELDRUM 1972; KILLAM 1979). Myoclonic responses to intermittent photic stimulation (stroboscope at 25/s) occur in 60%–80% of adolescent baboons *P. papio* from the Casamance region of Senegal, whereas the seizure incidence is lower in *P. papio* from other areas. A minority (approximate 20%) of the animals show full tonic-clonic seizures. The clinical seizures are accompanied by paroxysmal discharges in the EEG, which usually consist of polyspikes or spikes and waves. The photosensitive responses, like the photoconvulsive response in humans, are age and sex dependent, being maximal in the adolescent female. The incidence of photosensitivity of other *Papio* species is generally less than 10%. Furthermore, in studies of other subhuman primates, the incidence of photosensitivity has been equally low (NAQUET and MELDRUM 1972). These data suggest that the photosensitivity is not a characteristic of genus or species but is a unique feature of *Papio* from the Casamance region. Photic stimulation is not the only effective provocative agent in *P. papio*, as hyperventilation, overexercise, the stress of capture, restraint, or heat and humidity can also induce seizures. Also, even in the absence of light, EEG paroxysms occur during sleep (KILLAM et al. 1967).

Photically induced seizures in *P. papio* begin with rapid, bilateral clonus of the eyelids and periocular musculature, followed by the spread of diffuse clonic twitching to the face and neck, often accompanied by more intense, isolated jerks of the head. The diffuse clonic twitching may be interrupted by isolated, or grouped clonic jerks involving the whole body, or tonic spasms of facial muscles, jaw opening, and grimaces. Finally, the entire body may become involved in violent clonic jerks with flexion of the head and upper body and tonic extension of the lower limbs. In some animals this is followed by marked generalized clonus. In the most severely epileptic animals, the generalized clonus gradually shifts to a tonic spasm and finally appears again in large clonic jerks which become more and more isolated. In the EEG, the onset of clinical seizures is accompanied by rapid spike, slower spike-wave, and slow polyspike-wave complexes (NAQUET and MELDRUM 1972).

The photomyoclonic response of *P.papio* has been suggested as a model for photomyoclonic seizures and myoclonic petit mal epilepsy in humans (NAQUET and MELDRUM 1972; KILLAM 1979). However, the sensitivity of this response to antiepileptic drugs is only in part similar to the human syndromes. Consistent with clinical experiences, valproic acid, phenobarbitone and benzodiazepines give complete protection against the myoclonic responses in baboons, whereas phenytoin and carbamazepine are only partially active. Plasma levels associated with protection are similar to human therapeutic levels for diazepam, clonazepam and phenobarbitone, whereas the level for valproic acid is higher than that necessary in humans. However, trimethadione, which is active against generalized myoclonic seizures in man, is only weakly active in baboons. Furthermore, ethosuximide and primidone were found to have little effect on the epileptic response in *P. papio*, although primidone is highly active against myoclonic seizures in humans (SCHMIDT 1993). Investigations with higher doses of ethosuximide showed that seizures in adult baboons could be reduced or abolished at 120–180 mg/kg, which produced blood levels up to 130 μg/ml. However, side effects were much greater than with equi-effective doses of phenobarbitone and benzodiazepines (RINNE et al. 1978). *P. papio* has also been used for chronic evaluation of antiepileptic drugs. During prolonged treatment, phenytoin was much more active than after single doses, while in the case of diazepam and clonazepam, tolerance to the anticonvulsant effect developed (STARK et al. 1970; KILLAM et al. 1973)

In conclusion, the baboon *Papio* offers a useful model of innate photomyoclonic seizures. Being the only subhuman primate model of idiopathic epilepsy, it offers special advantages for the study of age-related drug effects and chronic drug treatment, and has been used repeatedly in the evaluation of novel anticonvulsant drugs. However, with respect to the results with the antiepileptic drugs discussed above, the predictive value of this model for drugs effective against particular types of human epilepsy still requires clarification. Furthermore, in contrast to the kindling model (LÖSCHER and HÖNACK 1991), neither epileptic baboons nor audiogenic-seizure susceptible DBA/2 mice predicted the enhanced adverse effect potential of NMDA antagonists in epileptic patients (CHAPMAN et al. 1991), thus clearly restricting the validity of these models for the prediction of therapeutic indices of novel drugs.

e) El Mice

One of the few genetic animal models of reflex epilepsy with complex partial-like seizures is the El mouse (SEYFRIED and GLASER 1985; KING and LAMOTTE 1989). El mice exhibit seizures in response to vestibular stimulation (by repeated tosses into the air or by altering the equilibrium of the mice), which appear to originate in the hippocampus or other deep temporal lobe structures and then spread to other brain regions. The generalized tonic-clonic seizures which occur in these animals are preceded by excessive salivation and head, limb and chewing automatisms. EEG recordings indicate a localized onset of paroxysmal activity (SUZUKI and NAKAMOTO 1978). Thus, the seizures in El mice can best be classified as complex partial ones which become secondarily generalized. Accordingly, El seizures can be completely blocked by phenytoin and phenobarbitone (SEYFRIED and GLASER 1985). Despite these interesting features, the El mouse is not widely used in antiepileptic drug evaluation, but is employed primarily in the characterization of mechanisms underlying epileptogenesis and ictogenesis.

C. Animal Models of Epileptic Seizures

An epileptic seizure is a symptom of the condition which is responsible for it (DREIFUSS 1994). The present classification of epileptic seizures is based on the clinical seizure type and the ictal and interictal EEG expressions (COMMISSION 1981). Three groups of epileptic seizures are classified: (1) partial (focal, local) seizures, (2) generalized seizures (convulsive or non-convulsive), and (3) unclassified epileptic seizures (COMMISSION 1981). Partial, or focal, seizures have clinical or EEG evidence of local onset, usually in a region of one cerebral hemisphere, and may spread to other parts of the brain during a seizure. Generalized seizures have no evidence of a localized onset but essentially simultaneously involve all or large parts of both cerebral hemispheres from the beginning. Partial seizures are subclassified into three groups, i.e. simple partial seizures, complex partial seizures, and partial seizures secondarily generalizing to clonic and/or tonic seizures. Primary generalized seizures are subclassified mainly by the presence or absence of different patterns of convulsive movements. The major types of generalized seizures are absence, atypical absence, myoclonic, clonic, tonic, tonic-clonic, and atonic seizures (Mattson 1995). It should be noted that the term "petit mal" is not useful for the definition of experimental or clinical seizures, because it included historically a number of rather diverse epileptic syndromes with different anticonvulsant drug profiles (Löscher and Schmidt 1988). To allow a better interpretation of a model's predictive potency in terms of clinical seizure types, we have proposed that "petit mal" should be replaced by "absence" or – if applicable – "myoclonic" in experimental models.

Based on epidemiological data in European populations and in the United States (Gastaut et al. 1975; Hauser et al. 1993), the most frequent type of seizures in humans is complex partial seizures. Because these seizures are often resistant to current antiepileptic drugs (Leppik 1992), animal models of complex partial seizures are particularly important in the development of new treatment strategies (Löscher and Schmidt 1993, 1994).

I. Animal Models of Partial (Focal, Local) Seizures

As for other seizure types, two groups of models can be differentiated, models of epilepsy with focal seizures and non-epileptic animals in which acute (single) focal seizures are induced by electrical or chemical means.

1. Epileptic Animals with Focal Seizures

These models have been described above under the different categories of epilepsies and include genetic animal models, such as dogs with focal epilepsy and *tottering* mice, as well as models in which spontaneous recurrent focal seizures are induced by chemical (e.g. kainate, pilocarpine) or electrical means. Furthermore, because of the reasons discussed above, the kindling model should be included here. However, only a few researchers use the spontaneous recurrent seizures in these models for anticonvulsant drug evaluation, because such studies require chronic drug administration and 24-h recording of the animals. An example in this respect is the study of Leite and Cavalheiro (1995), who compared the efficacy of antiepileptic drugs in spontaneous seizures following pilocarpine-induced status epilepticus in rats. Phenobarbitone, carbamazepine, phenytoin, and high doses of valproate were effective against spontaneous complex partial-like seizures, while ethosuximide was inactive. The authors concluded that valid information can be obtained by using spontaneous seizures in the pilocarpine model for efficacy studies of drugs likely to be effective against complex partial seizures. However, because this is a time-consuming procedure, such a model should be reserved for more advanced stages of preclinical drug development.

An alternative to using spontaneous seizures in epileptic animals with focal seizures for drug evaluation is to induce seizures at will in such animals. An example in this respect is the kindling model. An overview of the anticonvulsant effect of old and new antiepileptic drugs against seizures induced

Table 3. Anticonvulsant effect of old and new antiepileptic drugs in animal models of temporal lobe epilepsy and against partial seizures in patients. For detailed data see LÖSCHER and SCHMIDT (1988, 1993, 1994), TURSKI et al. (1989), SPERK (1993), LEVY et al. (1995), DALBY and NIELSEN (1997), and text

Drug	Fully amygdala-kindled seizures in rats	Kainate-induced seizures in rats	Pilocarpine-induced seizures in rats	Partial seizures in patients
Old drugs				
Carbamazepine	+	NE	NE	+
Phenytoin	+	NE	NE	+
Phenobarbitone	+	+	+	+
Primidone	+[a]	?	?	+
Valproate	+	+	+	+
Benzodiazepines	+	+	+	+
Ethosuximide	NE	NE	NE	NE
Trimethadione	+	+	+	NE
New drugs				
Lamotrigine	+	?	?	+
Topiramate	+	?	?	+
Oxcarbazepine	?	?	?	+
Felbamate	+	?	+	+
Vigabatrin	+	+	?	+
Tiagabine	+	?	?	+
Gabapentin	+	NE	?	+
NMDA antagonists	NE[b]	+	+	NE

+, effective; +/–, inconsistent data; NE, not effective; ? no data available (or found).
[a] Only after chronic treatment because of accumulation of phenobarbitone.
[b] Some weak efficacy of some compounds against secondarily generalized seizures.

by focal electrical stimulation in fully kindled rats is shown in Table 3, together with the clinical efficacy of these drugs on focal seizures in patients. As shown by the data in this table, the kindling model provides clinically predictive data in terms of anticonvulsant efficacy against partial seizures. The only exception is trimethadione, which is effective in most models of convulsive seizures (see also Table 4), although most clinical studies suggest it has no broader spectrum of efficacy than non-convulsive (absence and myoclonic) seizures (see Table 5). A further advantage of the kindling model is that subgroups of animals which are refractory to most common antiepileptic drugs can be selected from large populations of amygdala-kindled rats, thus providing a model of pharmaco-resistant complex-partial seizures (LÖSCHER 1997). Because most kindled rats in such populations respond to antiepileptic drugs, responders and non-responders selected from the same model can be compared directly, which allows the study of the mechanisms involved in pharmaco-resistant epileptic seizures (LÖSCHER 1997).

Table 4. Anticonvulsant effect of old and new antiepileptic drugs against primary generalized convulsive (tonic and or tonic-clonic) seizures in animal models and patients. For detailed data see Löscher (1992), Löscher and Schmidt (1988, 1993, 1994), Levy et al. (1995), Dalby and Nielsen (1997), and text

Drug	MES test in mice or rats	Epileptic dogs	Double mutant rats (*zi/zi, tm/tm*)	Audiogenic DBA/2 mice	Audiogenic rats (GEPRs)	Epileptic gerbils	Generalized tonic-clonic seizures in patients
Old drugs							
Carbamazepine	+	NE[a]	?	?	+	+	+
Phenytoin	+	NE[a]	+	+	+	+	+
Phenobarbitone	+	+	+	+	+	+	+
Primidone	+	+	?	?	?	+	+
Valproate	+	NE[a]	+	+	+	+	+
Benzodiazepines	+	+[b]	?	+	+	+	+
Ethosuximide	NE	NE	NE	+	+/–	NE	NE
Trimethadione	+	?	NE	+	+	?	NE
New drugs							
Lamotrigine	+	?	?	+	+	?	+
Topiramate	+	?	?	?	?	?	+
Oxcarbazepine	+	?	?	?	?	?	?
Felbamate	+	?	?	?	?	?	+
Vigabatrin	NE	+	?	?	?	?	?
Tiagabine	NE	?	?	+	+	?	?
Gabapentin	+/–	?	?	+	?	+	?
NMDA antagonists	+	?	?	+	+	?	?

+, effective; +/–, inconsistent data; NE, not effective; ? no data available (or found).
[a] Only tested during chronic administration; half-life in dogs too short.
[b] Only effective after acute administration (status epilepticus); half-life too short for chronic administration.

Table 5. Anticonvulsant effect of old and new antiepileptic drugs against primary generalized non-convulsive (absence or myoclonic) seizures in animal models and patients. For detailed data see LÖSCHER (1992), LÖSCHER and SCHMIDT (1988, 1993, 1994); TURSKI et al. (1989), SPERK (1993), LEVY et al. (1995), DALBY and NIELSEN (1997), and text

Drug	s.c. PTZ test in mice or rats (seizures)	GHB model in rats	*Tottering* mice (SWD)	Double mutant rats (*zi/zi*, *tm/tm*) (SWD)	Rats with SWD (e.g. GAERS)	Lethargic mice (*lh/lh*)	Epileptic gerbils (minor seizures)	Baboons with photo-myoclonic seizures	Seizures in patients: Absence	Seizures in patients: Myoclonic
Old drugs										
Carbamazepine	NE	?	?	?	NE	NE	NE	+/–	NE	NE
Phenytoin	NE	NE	NE	NE	NE	NE	NE	+/–	NE	NE
Phenobarbitone	+	+	+	+	+	?	+	+	NE	+
Primidone	+	?	?	?	?	?	?	NE	NE	+
Valproate	+	+	?	+	+	+	+	+	+	+
Benzodiazepines	+	?	+	?	+	+	+	+	+	+
Ethosuximide	+	+	+	+	+	+	+	NE	+	+/–
Trimethadione	+	+	?	+	+	?	?	+/–	+	+
New drugs										
Lamotrigine	NE	?	?	?	NE	+	?	?	+	+
Topiramate	NE	?	?	?	?	NE	?	?	+/–	+
Oxcarbazepine	+/–	?	?	?	?	?	?	?	NE	NE
Felbamate	+	?	?	?	?	?	?	?	+/–	+
Vigabatrin	+	NE	?	?	NE	NE	?	+	NE	NE
Tiagabine	+	?	?	?	NE	NE	?	+	?	NE
Gabapentin	+/–	?	?	?	NE	?	?	NE	NE	NE
NMDA antagonists	+/–	?	?	?	+	?	?	+	?	?

+, effective; +/–, inconsistent data; NE, not effective; ? no data available (or found).

2. Focal Seizures Induced in Normal, Non-epileptic Animals

As discussed above, acute seizures in response to the systemic administration of kainate and pilocarpine in normal rats are increasingly being used as a model for focal seizures as occur in temporal lobe epilepsy, although the systemic administration of these convulsants induces bilateral paroxysmal activity in many brain regions and widespread brain damage in both hemispheres (Turski et al. 1989; Sperk 1994). Nevertheless, at least in part, the evoked seizures resemble the partial and secondarily generalized seizures in the kindling model, and the RACINE scale for kindled seizures is often used in a modified form for acute kainate- and pilocarpine-induced seizures. However, the pharmacology of the kindling model differs strikingly from that of the kainate and pilocarpine models. An overview of the anticonvulsant effect of old and new antiepileptic drugs in the kainate, pilocarpine and kindling models is shown in Table 3, together with the clinical efficacy of these drugs on focal seizures in patients. As shown by the data in this table, the only model in this category which provides clinically predictive data in terms of anticonvulsant efficacy is the kindling model, thus again demonstrating that seizures in epileptic animals may differ in their pharmacological sensitivity from seizures in non-epileptic animals, even when the seizure types are remarkably similar. A further potential disadvantage of using kainate and pilocarpine in anticonvulsant drug evaluation is the fact that these models are mechanism-related, i.e. seizures are induced by a specific mechanism – glutamate or acetylcholine receptor stimulation – so that drugs acting directly on these mechanisms will be particularly potent in these models. The inherent problems associated with mechanism-related models will be discussed below.

Besides kindling, i.e. repetitive focal electrical stimulation, acute focal stimulation can be used to produce localized afterdischarges as a model of focal seizures (Koella 1985). For example, Albright (1983) used this method to compare the effects of carbamazepine, clonazepam, and phenytoin on the focal seizure threshold (afterdischarge threshold) in the amygdala and cortex of rats. All three drugs were found effective in increasing the focal seizure threshold, with greater effects being produced in the cortex than in the amygdala. The author concluded that anticonvulsants may control partial attacks through their action on the focal seizure threshold. Interestingly, by comparing the effect of the same dose of phenytoin on the afterdischarge threshold before and after amygdala kindling, a loss of anticonvulsant activity was found after kindling, again demonstrating that epileptogenesis can markedly alter the sensitivity of seizures to anticonvulsant drug action (Löscher 1997).

An interesting novel model with focal electrical stimulation has recently been developed by Voskuyl et al. (1989, 1992). In this model, rats are implanted bilaterally with screw electrodes over the frontoparietal cortex and are then stimulated electrically by a ramp-shaped current which is stopped at the occurrence of the first sign of convulsive seizures, usually forelimb clonus. The seizure threshold thus determined has been termed "threshold for localized seizures" (TLS), which can be determined repeatedly in the same rat at short time intervals without a postictal seizure threshold increase (VOSKUYL et al. 1989, 1992), an advantage not shared by most other seizure models. Thus, this novel model allows the rapid evaluation of the anticonvulsant time course of a novel drug in individual rats. Even after large numbers of threshold for localized seizures determinations, there is no increase in the seizure severity or duration, i.e. no indication of kindling-like alterations. Pharmacological experiments showed that the threshold for localized seizures is elevated by valproate, phenobarbitone, and benzodiazepines, while carbamazepine, phenytoin and ethosuximide exerted only marginal effects (HOOGERKAMP et al. 1994). Thus, the predictive value of this model in terms of the clinical seizure type is unclear at present. Because of the bilateral current application, the direct cortical stimulation model may represent a model of a generalized convulsive seizure rather than a model of a focal seizure. Indeed, further increase of current above the threshold for localized seizures induced more severe and more generalized clonic activity (VOSKUYL et al. 1992). When this more generalized activity was used as the endpoint ("threshold for generalized seizures", TGS), valproate, phenytoin, carbamazepine, oxazepam, phenobarbitone, but not ethosuximide, were effective in increasing the seizure threshold (HOOGERKAMP et al. 1994), so that the pharmacological sensitivity of the threshold for generalized seizures resembles that for the maximal electroshock seizure test or maximal electroshock seizure threshold which will be discussed below. Our experiments have shown that a more anterior implantation of screw electrodes over the frontal neocortex produced seizures which resemble remarkably the motor seizures of frontal lobe epilepsy, both in terms of clinical and pharmacological characteristics (KRUPP and LÖSCHER 1998). Thus, this modified direct cortical stimulation model may be used as a new model of frontal lobe seizures.

Another strategy to produce acute (reactive) focal seizures is the topical or focal (unilateral) administration of convulsants, e.g. penicillin, bicuculline, picrotoxin, pentylenetetrazole, carbachol, kainate, and quinolinic acid (PRINCE 1972; KOELLA 1985; LÖSCHER and SCHMIDT 1988; ENGEL 1992). Based on the mechanism of action of these convulsants, they can be divided into compounds which block inhibition (e.g. penicillin, bicuculline, picrotoxin, pentylenetetrazole) and compounds that enhance excitation (e.g. carbachol, kainic acid, quinolinic acid), i.e. mechanisms thought to be important in ictogenesis of focal epileptic seizures (LOTHMAN 1996b). Such models are widely used in studies on the functional anatomy, networks, and neurochemical substrates involved in epilepsy and epileptic seizures (FAINGOLD and FROMM 1992; LÖSCHER and EBERT 1996a). One example is the focal unilateral injection of bicuculline into the anterior piriform cortex ("area tempestas") to study the role of the piriform cortex in the progression and generalization of the seizure discharge (LÖSCHER and EBERT 1996b).

II. Animal Models of Generalized Seizures

Again, models consisting of epileptic animals with generalized seizures, either occurring spontaneously or in response to sensory stimulation, should be distinguished from models in which generalized seizures are induced by chemical or electrical means in normal, non-epileptic animals. Although the seizure characteristics may be indistinguishable in these two types of models, seizures in an epileptic animal may differ in their pharmacological sensitivity from seizures in a non-epileptic animal. Furthermore, as discussed above, the therapeutic or protective index of an anticonvulsant drug, i.e. the ratio between its "neurotoxic" and anticonvulsant effect, may differ dramatically between epileptic and non-epileptic animals, even when the same seizure type is evaluated. Furthermore, the pharmacological sensitivity of primary generalized seizures may differ from that of secondary generalized seizures both experimentally and clinically (Löscher and Schmidt 1988); only models of primary generalized seizures will be described here.

1. Epileptic Animals with Primary Generalized Seizures

The most important models in this category are genetic animal models of epilepsy which have been described above (see Sect. B). Both models with spontaneously recurrent seizures and models with reflex epilepsy can be used as models of generalized seizures. These models can be further divided into models with generalized convulsive seizures and models with generalized non-convulsive seizures.

a) Genetic Animal Models of Epilepsy with Generalized Convulsive Seizures

These are epileptic dogs with generalized tonic-clonic seizures not preceded by focal seizures, generalized tonic seizures in the double mutant rat, baboons with photomyoclonic seizures or other types of generalized seizures, audiogenic seizure susceptible mice and rats, and gerbils with major (i.e. generalized tonic-clonic) seizures. An autosomal recessive mutation in the domestic fowl, resulting in tonic-clonic seizures in response to different sensory stimuli, has been described (Crawford 1969), but epileptic fowl are rarely used in epilepsy research. The most popular genetic animal models with generalized convulsive seizures are audiogenic seizure susceptible mice and rats. An overview of the pharmacological sensitivity of these models is given in Table 4.

b) Genetic Animal Models of Epilepsy with Generalized Non-convulsive Seizures

In this category are *tottering* mice with absence-like seizures, the double mutant rat with absence-like seizures, GAERS, young gerbils with minor seizures, and the lethargic (*lh/lh*) mouse. The effects of anticonvulsants in these models are compared in Table 5. As shown by these data, the only model which correctly predicts the anticonvulsant activity against absence seizures in patients is the *lh/lh* mouse, whereas all other models seem to be models of myoclonic rather than absence seizures (see also LÖSCHER and SCHMIDT 1988).

2. Primary Generalized Seizures Induced in Normal, Non-epileptic Animals

This group includes the most widely used models in antiepileptic drug development, because seizure induction is simple and the predictive value for detecting clinically effective anticonvulsant drugs is high. However, as will be outlined in the following, there are important exceptions in this respect, so that drug development strategies should not be based solely on models from this category (LÖSCHER and SCHMIDT 1988, 1993, 1994).

a) Models of Convulsive Seizures

The most widely used animal model in anticonvulsant drug screening is certainly the maximal electroshock seizure test (SWINYARD 1972). The endpoint in this test is tonic hind limb extension, and the test is thought to be a predictive model for generalized tonic-clonic seizures (KRALL et al. 1978b). Although this test appears so simple, there are a variety of technical, biological, and pharmacological factors which may affect the results obtained with this seizure model (LÖSCHER et al. 1991a). Normally, the test consists of the application of a suprathreshold 50- or 60-Hz electrical current (e.g. 50 mA in mice and 150 mA in rats) for 0.2 s via corneal electrodes, but the current application can also be performed via transauricular (or ear) and frontal electrodes. The location of current application is important, because some drugs are anticonvulsant after transcorneal but not after transauricular stimulus application (LÖSCHER et al. 1991a). This finding may be related to the origin of tonic seizures in the brain stem, because this brain region is preferentially activated when transauricular electrodes are used (BROWNING and NELSON 1985). Since the maximal electroshock seizure test has been proposed to indicate a drug's ability to prevent seizure spread (PIREDDA et al. 1985), tonic seizures induced by transcorneal electrodes may be more sensitive to inhibition of seizure spread than tonic seizures induced from transauricular or ear electrodes (LÖSCHER et al. 1991a).

A further important factor in the maximal electroshock seizure model is the current strength used. Inactivity of a drug in the supramaximal maximal electroshock seizure test, i.e. using a current far above the individual seizure threshold of the animals, does not necessarily mean that the drug is not effective against generalized tonic-clonic seizures in humans (LÖSCHER et al. 1991a). In this respect, determination of the threshold for maximal (tonic) electroconvulsions may have advantages (LÖSCHER and SCHMIDT 1988; LÖSCHER et al. 1991a; LÖSCHER and SCHMIDT 1993). Interestingly, a threshold tonic extension test has recently been added to the Antiepileptic Drug Development (ADD) Program of the National Institutes of Health (NIH), and is used for drugs which are inactive in the traditional identification tests comprising maximal electroshock seizures and subcutaneous pentylenetetrazole seizures (WHITE et al. 1995).

With respect to the predictive value of the maximal electroshock seizure test, based on retrospective comparisons of experimental and clinical data with commonly used antiepileptic drugs, it has been proposed that the maximal electroshock seizure test might not only detect drugs with activity against generalized tonic-clonic seizures, but also drugs effective against (complex) partial seizures (SWINYARD 1969; KRALL et al. 1978a,b). However, there are several more recently developed antiepileptic drugs, such as vigabatrin, which are effective against complex partial seizures in humans but are not capable of protecting animals against seizures in the traditional maximal electroshock seizure test (LÖSCHER and SCHMIDT 1988; see Table 4). Furthermore, there are some experimental anticonvulsants with a high potency in models of complex partial seizures, e.g. amygdala kindling, but no activity in the maximal electroshock seizure test (LÖSCHER and SCHMIDT 1988). Vice versa, both competitive and non-competitive NMDA antagonists are highly potent in the maximal electroshock seizure test, inactive in amygdala-kindled rats, and ineffective against complex partial seizures in humans (LÖSCHER and SCHMIDT 1994). Thus, although the maximal electroshock seizure test is probably the best validated of all seizure tests that predict drugs effective in generalized tonic-clonic seizures, it should not be used to predict drugs effective in partial seizures. Instead, animals models for partial seizures, such as amygdala-kindling, should be used for this purpose.

Another potential problem of the maximal electroshock seizure test is that electroconvulsive seizures are particularly sensitive to drugs blocking Na^+ channels (MELDRUM 1996). Thus, it is not surprising that almost all antiepileptic drugs that were initially detected by this test act, at least in part, via this mechanism (MELDRUM 1996). Seizure models which are also sensitive to other, potentially interesting mechanisms of anticonvulsant drug action against generalized convulsive seizures should be added to the early phase of screening or other drug development strategies.

Innumerable chemicals and drugs induce generalized convulsive seizures at toxic doses and several of these are used as tools in epilepsy research (KOELLA 1985; LÖSCHER and SCHMIDT 1988). Most of these chemoconvulsant models are characterized by generalized tonic-clonic convulsions, and either the clonic or the tonic seizure is taken as the endpoint. One of the most popular convulsants in this respect is pentylenetetrazole (Metrazol), which, however, is commonly used as a model of non-convulsive seizures and will be discussed below under that category. The main advantage of several chemical convulsants is their known mechanism of convulsant action, thus allowing study of the mechanisms of ictogenesis and the effect of anticonvulsant drugs on these mechanisms. Examples in this respect are GABA antagonists, such as bicuculline and picrotoxin, $glycine_A$ antagonists such as strychnine, and glutamate receptor agonists such as NMDA or *N*-methyl-D,L-aspartate (NMDLA). However, an anticonvulsant effect of a drug against seizures induced by a convulsant with a specific mechanism, e.g. bicuculline, does not necessarily mean that the anticonvulsant drug directly acts on this mechanism. For instance, phenobarbitone blocks almost all seizure types in almost all seizure models, so that the anticonvulsant effect in a given model does not allow a conclusion as to the mechanism of action of phenobarbitone. Another example illustrating the problem of using mechanism-related seizure models to elucidate the mechanism of action of anticonvulsant drugs stems from the NMDLA model, which is resistant to most standard antiepileptics, whereas – as was to be expected – NMDA receptor antagonists are effective, but so are GABAmimetic drugs (CZUCZWAR et al. 1985). Hence, a novel compound which acts as a GABAmimetic could be falsely interpreted as an NMDA antagonist in this model, thus delineating the inherent problem in drawing conclusions from using mechanism-related seizure models. Furthermore, a potent and selective anticonvulsant effect of a novel drug in a mechanism-related seizure model does not necessarily predict anticonvulsant efficacy in patients. For instance, NMDA antagonists are of course potent anticonvulsants against NMDA- or NMDLA-induced seizures; however, these drugs failed to be effective antiepileptic drugs in patients (LÖSCHER and SCHMIDT 1994). Interestingly, while the ADD program of the NIH previously used chemical convulsants (e.g. strychnine, picrotoxin, and bicuculline) to help elucidate differences in the mechanisms of action of the compounds (GLADDING et al. 1985), these have been replaced by more direct mechanistic studies, using electrophysiology and neurochemistry (WHITE et al. 1995).

b) Models of Absence or Myoclonic Seizures

The most widely used pharmacological model in this category is the subcutaneous pentylenetetrazole seizure threshold test in either mice or rats (SWINYARD 1949; SWINYARD et al. 1952). Indeed, most clinically effective antiepileptic drugs have been found either by their ability to block maximal electroshock seizure or pentylenetetrazole induced seizures, which was the reason for basing the initial drug detection of the ADD program of the NIH on these two seizure tests (KRALL et al. 1978a,b). In the subcutaneous pentylenetetrazole seizure threshold test, the convulsive dose inducing a clonic seizure of at least 5-s duration in 97% of the animals (CD_{97}) is injected and animals are observed for a postinjection period usually of 30 min for the occurrence of such a "threshold" seizure. The test is thought to be predictive of anticonvulsant drug activity against non-convulsive absence ("petit mal") seizures (WOODBURY 1972; KRALL et al. 1978a,b). However, this prediction was based almost solely on the efficacy of ethosuximide and trimethadione in this model (KRALL et al. 1978a). Experience with new antiepileptic drugs casts doubt on the predictive value of the subcutaneous pentylenetetrazole model (LÖSCHER and SCHMIDT 1988; HOSFORD and WANG 1997). Table 5 shows the anticonvulsant activity of various old and new antiepileptics in different models of absence and myoclonic seizures, including the subcutaneous pentylenetetrazole test, together with the clinical efficacy of the drugs against absence and myoclonic seizures. The data in this table clearly demonstrate that the pentylenetetrazole model is not a predictive test for absence seizures. Löscher and Schmidt (1988) have proposed that, based on the anticonvulsant effect of antiepileptics, it may represent a model of myoclonic seizures rather than absence seizures in man. Although pentylenetetrazole induces myoclonic seizures in addition to generalized clonic seizures at the doses commonly used in the subcutaneous pentylenetetrazole test, myoclonic seizures are rarely used as an endpoint in this model, but the pharmacological sensitivity of the pentylenetetrazole-induced clonic seizures is remarkably similar to the pharmacological sensitivity of myoclonic seizures occurring in human epilepsies (Table 5). In this respect, it should be considered that generalized myoclonic seizures in epilepsy are convulsive rather than non-convulsive, so that the term "non-convulsive" should not be used for all types of myoclonic seizures in animal models.

Interestingly, at much lower doses than those used for induction of clonic seizures by pentylenetetrazole, this convulsant produces electrographic and behavioural events more similar to generalized absence seizures (Snead 1992). However, this modified pentylenetetrazole model has not been used in epilepsy research to any significant extent, as yet.

Similarly to the maximal electroshock seizure test, various technical, biological and pharmacological factors may affect the results obtained with pentylenetetrazole induced seizures (Löscher et al. 1991b). One important factor in anticonvulsant drug evaluation is the drug's duration of action. Thus, a drug with a short duration of action in rodents may be missed in the subcutaneous pentylenetetrazole test because of the relatively long observation period following pentylenetetrazole (Löscher et al. 1991b). In this respect, the timed intravenous infusion of pentylenetetrazole might have advantages, because the anticonvulsant drug potency can be tested at the individual time of peak effect (Löscher and Schmidt 1988; Löscher et al. 1991b). A further factor which should be considered in the pentylenetetrazole and possibly other animal models is any seasonal differences in seizure susceptibility, even when laboratory animals are maintained under highly standardized conditions (Löscher and Fiedler 1996). In addition to season, circadian variation is an important factor in seizure models (Koella 1995) so that pharmacological studies in such models are strictly comparable only if performed at a similar time of the day.

Chemoconvulsant models that simulate the clinical features of non-convulsive absence/myoclonic epilepsy more closely than the conventional pentylenetetrazole model are the penicillin model of absence epilepsy in cats and the γ-hydroxybutyric acid (GHB) model in rats (Faingold and Fromm 1992; Snead 1992). Intramuscular injection of large doses of penicillin in cats produces a transient absence-like state with bilaterally synchronous 3/s spike-wave discharges in the EEG often accompanied by rhythmic motor movements, particularly of the eyelids, and behavioural arrest. Thalamic subnuclei are strongly implicated in generation of spike-wave activity in this model, based on electrical stimulation, lesion, and electrographic and neuronal recording studies. Interestingly, when given intramuscularly to rodents, penicillin does not consistently produce bilaterally synchronous spike-wave discharges similar to those seen in cats (SNEAD 1992). This restricts the use of the penicillin model, because cats are too expensive for large scale studies, such as drug screening.

In the γ-hydroxybutyrate model of absence seizures in rats, administration of γ-hydroxybutyric acid or its prodrug γ-butyrolactone (GBL) produces hypersynchronous spike-wave discharges (with 7–9 cycles/s) in the EEG which are associated with behavioural arrest, facial myoclonus and vibrissal twitching (SNEAD 1992). This γ-hydroxybutyrate induced syndrome is not restricted to rats but has also been induced in a similar manner in cats and monkeys. Interestingly, γ-hydroxybutyrate also occurs endogenously as a minor metabolite of GABA in the brain, and inhibition of γ-hydroxybutyrate synthesis and release by valproate has been implicated in the anticonvulsant mechanisms of this antiepileptic (LÖSCHER 1993). Using mapping of the EEG with bipolar depth recordings indicated that spike-wave discharges in the γ-hydroxybutyrate model in rats originate in the thalamus and cortex, whereas the hippocampus is not involved (SNEAD 1992). GABAmimetic drugs such as GABA agonists or GABA-T inhibitors exacerbate the γ-hydroxybutyrate induced syndrome in rats, and this has also been observed in other models of non-convulsive absence seizures as well as in humans with this type of epilepsy (SNEAD 1992). As discussed above, the mechanism of this proconvulsant effect of GABA on experimental and clinical generalized absence seizures may be enhanced $GABA_B$ receptor-mediated events. Again, based on data from pharmacological studies, LÖSCHER and SCHMIDT (1988) have suggested that the γ-hydroxybutyrate and most other models of non-convulsive epilepsy are models of epileptic myoclonic seizures (which are also associated with generalized spike-wave discharges in the EEG) rather than models of absence seizures. The only current exception to this proposal seems to be the *lh/lh* mouse (Table 5).

D. Conclusions

As mentioned in the "Introduction", the experimental models of epilepsy and epileptic seizures reviewed in this chapter are examples and are not meant to be comprehensive. Nevertheless, the great majority of animal models currently used in epilepsy research and antiepileptic drug development are included. For a more historical perspective, the interested reader is referred to previous reviews and volumes on this topic (STUMPF 1962; PURPURA et al. 1972; KRALL et al. 1978a; KOELLA 1985). All models have strengths and weaknesses and, as pointed out in the "Introduction", the choice of a model largely depends on the purpose of the experiment.

One problem in the preclinical use of animal models is the terminology used, because semantic inconsistencies contribute to controversy and confusion in the experimental literature, impairing communication between researchers (Löscher and Schmidt 1988; Engel 1992). As pointed out by Engel (1992), seizures should be referred to by their specific type, according to the International Classification of Epileptic Seizures, whenever possible. In the present review, an attempt was also made to refer to epilepsies and epileptic syndromes in animals as the specific types proposed by the ILAE, but – in contrast to seizures – for many types of epilepsy or epileptic syndromes no models exist as yet, and the clinical classification system applied in this review to animal models of epilepsies may be partially inadequate for this purpose. Nevertheless, the aim of this attempt was to improve communication and stimulate discussion between preclinical and clinical epileptologists. It is also important to recognize that the behaviour exhibited by certain mouse mutants and certain transgenic or knockout mice might represent non-epileptic disturbances (Engel 1992), which was the reason to limit this review to models with proven epilepsy or epileptic seizures.

Engel (1992) has recently proposed a somewhat different classification of experimental models of epilepsy and epileptic phenomena, including in vitro preparations, with four broad categories, i.e. (1) *presumed epileptic equivalents*, such as long-term and post-tetanic potentiation, and bursting neurons in vitro, which are not in themselves epileptic, but are believed to be valid models of specific neuronal events that underlie some aspects of epileptic seizures or disorders; (2) *acute experimentally induced seizure models*, which would be equivalent to reactive seizures in humans, but would not constitute epileptic conditions; this category would be consistent with the group of animal models of epileptic seizures in non-epileptic animals in the present review; (3) *chronic experimentally determined models*, which would be equivalent to symptomatic epilepsies in humans; and (4) *chronic genetically determined models*, which would be equivalent to idiopathic epilepsies in humans. There are many other possible classification systems (see, for instance, Fig. 1), but the ultimate goal of any system should be to minimize false interpretation of data obtained in a given model in terms of understanding the fundamental mechanisms of the human epilepsies or epileptic seizures for which the model stands. Furthermore, classification systems for animal models should aim at reducing false predictions in terms of anticonvulsant drug efficacy against specific types of epilepsy or epileptic seizures.

Acknowledgements. Critical discussions with Prof. Dieter Schmidt (Epilepsy Research Group, Berlin, Germany) during the preparation of the manuscript are gratefully acknowledged.

References

Adamec RE (1990) Does kindling model anything clinically relevant? Biol Psychiatry 27:249–279

Albright PS (1983) Effects of carbamazepine, clonazepam, and phenytoin on seizure threshold in amygdala and cortex. Exp Neurol 79:11–17

Allen KM, Walsh C (1996) Shaking down new epilepsy genes. Nature Med 2:516–518

Bickford RG, Klass DW (1969) Sensory precipitation and reflex mechanisms. In: Jasper HH, Ward AAJ, Pope A (eds) Basic mechanisms of the epilepsies. Little Brown, Boston, pp. 543–564

Browning RA, Nelson DK (1985) Variation in threshold and pattern of electroshock-induced seizures in rats depending on site of stimulation. Life Sci 37:2205–2211

Chapman AG, Croucher MJ, Meldrum BS (1984) Evaluation of anticonvulsant drugs in DBA/2 mice with sound-induced seizures. Arzneim-Forsch 34:1261–1270

Chapman AG, Graham JL, Patel S, Meldrum BS (1991) Anticonvulsant activity of two orally active competitive N-methyl-D-aspartate antagonists, CGP 37849 and CGP 39551, against sound-induced seizures in DBA/2 mice and photically induced myoclonus in *Papio papio*. Epilepsia 32:578–587

Coenen AML, Drinkenburg WHIM, Inoue M, van Luijtelaar ELJM (1992) Genetic models of absence epilepsy, with emphasis on the WAG/Rij strain of rats. Epilepsy Res 12:75–86

Commission on Classification and Terminology of the International League Against Epilepsy (1981) Proposal for revised clinical and electroencephalographic classification of epileptic seizures. Epilepsia 22:489–501

Commission on Classification and Terminology of the International League Against Epilepsy (1989) Proposal for revised classification of epilepsies and epileptic syndromes. Epilepsia 30:389–399

Consroe P, Wolkin A (1977) Cannabidinol – antiepileptic drug comparisons and interactions in experimentally induced seizures in rats. J Pharmacol Exp Ther 201:26–32

Consroe P, Piccione A, Chin L (1979) Audiogenic seizure susceptible rats. Fed Proc 38:2411–2416

Craig CR, Colasanti BK (1988) A study of pentylenetetrazol kindling in rats and mice. Pharmacol Biochem Behav 31:867–870

Craig CR, Colasanti BK (1992) Cobalt-induced focal seizures: neuronal networks and actions of antiepileptic drugs. In: Faingold CL, Fromm GH (eds) Drugs for control of epilepsy: actions on neuronal networks involved in seizure disorders. CRC Press, Boca Raton, pp. 125–142

Crawford RD (1969) A new mutant causing epileptic seizures in domestic fowl. Poultry Sci 48:1799

Czuczwar SJ, Frey H-H, Löscher W (1985) Antagonism of N-methyl-D,L-aspartic acid induced by antiepileptic drugs and other agents. Eur J Pharmacol 108:273–280

Dailey JW, Jobe PC (1985) Anticonvulsant drugs and the genetically epilepsy-prone rat. Fed Proc 44:2640–2644

Dalby NO, Nielsen EB (1997) Comparison of the preclinical anticonvulsant profiles of tiagabine, lamotrigine, gabapentin and vigabatrin. Epilepsy Res 28:63–72

Dam M (1992) Localization related epileptic syndromes. In: Trimble MR, Bolwig TG (eds) The temporal lobes and the limbic system. Wrightson Biomedical Publishing, Petersfield, pp. 115–128

Dreifuss FE (1994) The international classification of seizures and epilepsies: advantages. In: Wolf P (ed) Epileptic seizures and syndromes. Libbey, London, pp. 9–14

Edmonds HL Jr, Bellin SI, Mia Chen F-C, Hegreberg GA (1978) Anticonvulsant properties of rozipine in epileptic and nonepileptic beagle dogs. Epilepsia 19:139–146

Empson RM, Amitai Y, Jefferys JG, Gutnick MJ (1993) Injection of tetanus toxin into the neocortex elicits persistent epileptiform activity but only transient impairment of GABA release. Neuroscience 57:235–239

Engel JJ (1992) Experimental models of epilepsy: classification and relevance to human epileptic phenomena. In: Avanzini G, Engel JJ, Fariello R, Heinemann U (eds) Neurotransmitters in epilepsy. Elsevier, Amsterdam, pp. 9–20

Engel JJ, Cahan L (1986) Potential relevance of kindling to human partial epilepsy. In: Wada JA (ed) Kindling 3. Raven Press, New York, pp. 37–51

Faingold CL, Fromm GH (1992) Drugs for control of epilepsy: actions on neuronal networks involved in seizure disorders. CRC Press, Boca Raton
Faingold CL, Narikotu DK (1992) The genetically epilepsy-prone rat: neuronal networks and actions of amino acid neurotransmitters. In: Faingold CL, Fromm GH (eds) Drugs for control of epilepsy: actions on neuronal networks involved in seizure disorders. CRC Press, Boca Raton, pp. 277–308
Fisher RS (1989) Animal models of the epilepsies. Brain Res Rev 14:245–278
Frankel WN, Taylor BA, Noebels JL, Lutz CM (1994) Genetic epilepsy model derived from common inbred mouse strains. Genetics 138:481–489
Gastaut H, Gastaut JL, Geucalves CE, Silva CE, Fernandez Sanchez JL (1975) Relative frequency of different types of epilepsy: a study employing the classification of the international league against epilepsy. Epilepsia 16:457–467
Gladding GD, Kupferberg HJ, Swinyard EA (1985) Antiepileptic drug development program. In: Frey H-H, Janz D (eds) Antiepileptic drugs. Springer-Verlag, Berlin, pp. 341–350
Goddard GV, McIntyre DC, Leech CK (1969) A permanent change in brain function resulting from daily electrical stimulation. Exp Neurol 25:295–330
Hauser WA, Annegers JF, Kurland LT (1993) Incidence of epilepsy and unprovoked seizures in Rochester, Minnesota: 1935–1984. Epilepsia 34:453–468
Heinemann U, Draguhn A, Ficker E, Stabel J, Zhang CL (1994) Strategies for the development of drugs for pharmacoresistant epilepsies. Epilepsia 35 [Suppl 5]:S10–S21
Heller AH, Dichter MA, Sidman RL (1983) Anticonvulsant sensitivity of absence seizures in the *tottering* mutant mouse. Epilepsia 25:25–34
Hernandez TD (1997) Preventing post-traumatic epilepsy after brain injury: weighing the costs and benefits of anticonvulsant prophylaxis. Trends Neurosci 18:59–620
Hoogerkamp A, Vis PW, Danhof M, Voskuyl RA (1994) Characterization of the pharmacodynamics of several antiepileptic drugs in a direct cortical stimulation model of anticonvulsant effect in the rat. J Pharmacol Exp Ther 269:521–528
Hosford DA, Wang Y (1997) Utility of the lethargic (lh/lh) mouse model of absence seizures in predicting the effects of lamotrigine, vigabatrin, tiagabine, gabapentin, and topiramate against human absence seizures. Epilepsia 38:408–414
Hosford DA, Clark S, Cao Z, Wilson WAJ, Fu-hsiung L, Morrisett RA, Huin A (1992) The role of GABAB receptor activation in absence seizures of lethargic (*lh/lh*) mice. Science 257:398–401
Hosford DA, Wang Y, Liu CC, Snead OC (1995) Characterization of the antiabsence effects of SCH 50911, a GABAB antagonist, in the lethargic mouse, gamma-hydroxybutyrate, and pentylenetetrazole models. J Pharmacol Exp Ther 274:1399–1403
Hönack D, Löscher W (1995) Kindling increases the sensitivity of rats to adverse effects of certain antiepileptic drugs. Epilepsia 36:763–771
Jobe PC, Mishra PK, Dailey JW (1992) Genetically epilepsy-prone rats: actions of antiepileptic drugs and monoaminergic neurotransmitters. In: Faingold CL, Fromm GH (eds) Drugs for control of epilepsy: actions on neuronal networks involved in seizure disorders. CRC Press, Boca Raton, pp. 253–275
Killam EK (1979) Photomyoclonic seizures in the baboon. Fed Proc 38:2429–2433
Killam KF, Killam EK, Naquet RJ (1966) Mise en evidence chez certains singels d'un syndrome photomyoclonique. Can R Acad Sci 262:1010–1212
Killam KF, Killam EK, Naquet RJ (1967) An animal model of light sensitive epilepsy. Electroencephalogr Clin Neurophysiol 22:497–513
Killam EK, Matsuzaki M, Killam KF (1973) Effects of chronic administration of benzodiazepines on epileptic seizures and brain electrical activity in *Papio papio*. In: Garratini S, Mussini E, Randall LO (eds) Benzodiazepines. Raven Press, New York, pp. 443–460
King JT, LaMotte CC (1989) El mouse as a model of focal epilepsy: a review. Epilepsia 30:257–265

Koella WP (1985) Animal experimental methods in the study of antiepileptic drugs. In: Frey H-H, Janz D (eds) Antiepileptic drugs. Springer, Berlin, pp. 283–350
Kostopoulos GK (1992) The tottering mouse: a critical review of its usefulness in the study of the neuronal mechanisms underlying epilepsy. J Neural Transm 35 [Suppl]:21–36
Krall RL, Penry JK, Kupferberg HJ, Swinyard EA (1978a) Antiepileptic drug development: I. History and a program for progress. Epilepsia 19:393–408
Krall RL, Penry JK, White BG, Kupferberg HJ, Swinyard EA (1978b) Antiepileptic drug development: II. Anticonvulsant drug screening. Epilepsia 19:409–428
Krupp E, Löscher W (1998) Anticonvulsant drug effects in the direct cortical ramp-stimulation model in rats: comparison with conventional seizure models. J Pharmacol Exp Ther 285:1137–1149
Laird H, Consroe P, Straussner A (1976) Anticonvulsant drug comparisons in audiogenic and nonaudiogenic rats. Pharmacologist 18:136
Leite JP, Cavalheiro EA (1995) Effects of conventional antiepileptic drugs in a model of spontaneous recurrent seizures in rats. Epilepsy Res 20:93–104
Leppik IE (1992) Intractable epilepsy in adults. In: Theodore WH (ed) Surgical treatment of epilepsy. Elsevier, Amsterdam, pp. 7–11
Levy RH, Mattson RH, Meldrum BS (1995) Antiepileptic drugs. 4th edn, Raven Press, New York
Lewin E (1972) The production of epileptogenic cortical foci in experimental animals by freezing. In: Purpura DP, Penry JK, Tower D, Woodbury DM, Walter R (eds) Experimental models of epilepsy – A manual for the laboratory worker. Raven Press, New York, pp. 37–50
Loiseau P (1986) Intractable epilepsy: prognostic evaluation. In: Schmidt D, Morselli PL (eds) Intractable epilepsy: experimental and clinical aspects. Raven Press, New York, pp. 227–258
Löscher W (1981) Plasma levels of valproic acid and its metabolites during continued treatment in dogs. J Vet Pharmacol Ther 4:111–119
Löscher W (1984) Genetic animal models of epilepsy as a unique resource for the evaluation of anticonvulsant drugs. A review. Methods Findings Experiment Clin Pharmacol 6:531–547
Löscher W (1986) Experimental models for intractable epilepsy in nonprimate animal species. In: Schmidt D, Morselli PL (eds) Intractable epilepsy: experimental and clinical aspects. Raven Press, New York, pp. 25–37
Löscher W (1991) The epileptic gerbil. Neuronal networks and actions of antiepileptic drugs. In: Faingold CL, Fromm GH (eds) Drugs for control of epilepsy. CRC Press, Boca Raton, pp. 309–323
Löscher W (1992) Genetic animal models of epilepsy. In: Driscoll P (ed) Genetically defined animal models of neurobehavioral dysfunctions. Birkhäuser, Boston, pp. 111–135
Löscher W (1993) Effects of the antiepileptic drug valproate on metabolism and function of inhibitory and excitatory amino acids in the brain. Neurochem Res 18:485–502
Löscher W (1994) Neue Antiepileptika – ein Fortschritt für die Behandlung epileptischer Tiere? Kleintierpraxis 39:325–342
Löscher W (1997) Animal models of intractable epilepsy. Prog Neurobiol (in press)
Löscher W, Ebert U (1996) Basic mechanisms of seizure propagation: targets for rational drug design and rational polypharmacy. Epilepsy Res 11 [Suppl]:17–44
Löscher W, Fiedler M (1996) The role of technical, biological and pharmacological factors in the laboratory evaluation of anticonvulsant drugs. VI. Seasonal influences on maximal electroshock and pentylenetetrazol seizure thresholds. Epilepsy Res 25:3–10
Löscher W, Rundfeldt C (1991) Kindling as a model of drug-resistant partial epilepsy: selection of phenytoin-resistant and nonresistant rats. J Pharmacol Exp Ther 258:483–489

Löscher W, Hönack D (1991) Responses to NMDA receptor antagonists altered by epileptogenesis. Trends Pharmacol Sci 12:52
Löscher W, Schmidt D (1988) Which animal models should be used in the search for new antiepileptic drugs? A proposal based on experimental and clinical considerations. Epilepsy Res 2:145–181
Löscher W, Schmidt D (1993) New drugs for the treatment of epilepsy. Curr Opin Invest Drugs 2:1067–1095
Löscher W, Schmidt D (1994) Strategies in antiepileptic drug development: is rational drug design superior to random screening and structural variation? Epilepsy Res 17:95–134
Löscher W, Schwartz-Porsche D, Frey H-H, Schmidt D (1985) Evaluation of epileptic dogs as an animal model of human epilepsy. Arzneim-Forsch 35:82–87
Löscher W, Fassbender CP, Nolting B (1991a) The role of technical, biological and pharmacological factors in the laboratory evaluation of anticonvulsant drugs. II. Maximal electroshock seizure models. Epilepsy Res 8:79–94
Löscher W, Hönack D, Fassbender CP, Nolting B (1991b) The role of technical, biological and pharmacological factors in the laboratory evaluation of anticonvulsant drugs. III. Pentylenetetrazol seizure models. Epilepsy Res 8:171–189
Loskota WJ, Lomax P (1975) The Mongolian gerbil (*Meriones unguiculatus*) as a model for the study of the epilepsies: EEG records of seizures. Electroencephalogr Clin Neurophysiol 38:597–604
Lothman EW (1996a) Neurobiology as a basis for rational polypharmacy. Epilepsy Res [Suppl] 11:3–7
Lothman EW (1996b) Basis mechanisms of seizure spread. Epilepsy Res [Suppl] 11:9–16
Lothman EW, Bertram EH (1993) Epileptogenic effects of status epileptics. Epilepsia 34 [Suppl]:S59–S70
Lothman EW, Bertram EH, Kapur J, Stringer JL (1990) Recurrent spontaneous hippocampal seizures in the rat as a chronic sequela to limbic status epilepticus. Epilepsy Res 6:110–118
Lothman EW, Williamson JM, Van Landingham KE (1991) Intraperitoneal phenytoin suppresses kindled responses: effects on motor and electrographic seizures. Epilepsy Res 9:11–18
Marescaux C, Vergnes M, Depaulis A (1992) Genetic absence epilepsy in rats from Strasbourg – A review. J Neural Transm 35:37–69
Mattson RH (1995) Selection of antiepileptic drug therapy. In: Levy RH, Mattson RH, Meldrum BS (eds) Antiepileptic drugs. 4th edn, Raven Press, New York, pp. 123–136
McNamara JO (1984) Kindling: an animal model of complex partial epilepsy. Ann Neurol 16 [Suppl]:S72–S76
McNamara JO, Rigsbee LC, Butler LS, Shin C (1989) Intravenous phenytoin is an effective anticonvulsant in the kindling model. Ann Neurol 26:675–678
Meldrum B (1996) Action of established and novel anticonvulsant drugs on the basic mechanisms of epilepsy. Epilepsy Res 11 [Suppl]:67–78
Naquet R, Meldrum BS (1972) Photogenic seizures in baboon. In: Purpura DP, Penry JK, Tower D, Woodbury DM, Walter R (eds) Experimental models of epilepsy – A manual for the laboratory worker, Raven Press, New York, pp. 373–406
Noebels JL (1979) Analysis of inherited epilepsy using single locus mutations in mice. Fed Proc 38:2405–2410
Noebels JL (1986) Mutational analysis of inherited epilepsies. In: Delgado-Escueta AV, Ward AA, Woodbury DM, Porter RJ (eds) Basic mechanisms of epilepsies. Molecular and cellular approaches. Raven Press, New York, pp. 97–114
Noebels JL (1996) Using genes to create new models of epilepsy. Epilepsia 37 [Suppl 5]:2
Noebels JL, Sidman RL (1979) Inherited epilepsy: spike-wave and focal motor seizure in mutant mouse *tottering*. Science 204:1334–1336

Piredda SG, Woodhead JH, Swinyard EA (1985) Effect of stimulus intensity on the profile of anticonvulsant activity of phenytoin, ethosuximide, and valproate. J Pharmacol Exp Ther 232:741–745
Prince DA (1972) Topical convulsant drugs and metabolic antagonists. In: Purpura DP, Penry JK, Tower D, Woodbury DM, Walter R (eds) Experimental models of epilepsy – A manual for the laboratory worker. Raven Press, New York, pp. 51–84
Purpura DP, Penry JK, Tower D, Woodbury DM, Walter R (1972) Experimental models of epilepsy – A manual for the laboratory worker. Raven Press, New York
Racine RJ (1972) Modification of seizure activity by electrical stimulation: II. Motor seizure. Electroenceph Clin Neurophysiol 32:281–294
Racine RJ, Ivy GO, Milgram NW (1989) Kindling: clinical relevance and anatomical substrate. In: Bolwig TG, Trimble MR (eds) The clinical relevance of kindling. Wiley, Chichester, pp. 15–34
Reynolds EH (1989) The process of epilepsy: is kindling relevant? In Bolwig TG, Trimble MR (eds) The clinical relevance of kindling. Wiley, Chichester, pp. 149–160
Rinne SP, Bowyer JF, Barrows EB, Killam EK (1978) EEG effects of ethosuximide in *Papio papio*. Pharmacologist 20:161
Rise ML, Frankel WN, Coffin JM, Seyfried TN (1991) Genes for epilepsy mapped in the mouse. Science 253:669–673
Rundfeldt C, Hönack D, Löscher W (1990) Phenytoin potently increases the threshold for focal seizures in amygdala-kindled rats. Neuropharmacology 29:845–851
Sasa M, Ohno Y, Ujihara H, Fujita Y, Yoshimura M, Takaori S, Serikawa T, Yamada J (1988) Effects of antiepileptic drugs on absence-like and tonic seizures in the spontaneously epileptic rat, a double mutant rat. Epilepsia 29:505–513
Sato M, Racine RJ, McIntyre DC (1990) Kindling: basic mechanisms and clinical validity. Electroenceph Clin Neurophysiol 76:459–472
Schmidt J (1987) Changes in seizure susceptibility in rats following chronic administration of pentylenetetrazol. Biomed Biochem Acta 46:267–270
Schmidt D (1993) Epilepsien und epileptische Anfälle. Thieme Verlag, Stuttgart
Serikawa T, Yamada J (1986) Epileptic seizures in rats homozygous for two mutations, zitter and tremor. J Hered 77:441–444
Seyfried TN (1979) Audiogenic seizures in mice. Fed Proc 38:2399–2404
Seyfried TN, Glaser GH (1985) A review of mouse mutants as genetic models of epilepsy. Epilepsia 26:143–150
Snead OC (1992) Pharmacological models of generalized absence seizures in rodents. J Neural Transm 35 [Suppl]:7–19
Speciale J, Dayrell-Hart B, Steinberg SA (1991) Clinical evaluation of gamma-vinyl-gamma-aminobutyric acid for control of epilepsy in dogs. J Am Vet Med Assoc 198:995–1000
Sperk G (1994) Kainic acid seizures in the rat. Progr Neurobiol 42:1–32
Stark LG, Killam KF, Killam EK (1970) The anticonvulsant effects of phenobarbitone, diphenylhydantoin and two benzodiazepines in the baboon, *Papio papio*. J Pharmacol Exp Ther 173:125–132
Stumpf C (1962) Pharmakologische Methoden. In: Stumpf C, Petschke H (eds) Erzeugung von Krankheitszuständen durch das Experiment: Zentralnervensystem. Springer-Verlag, Berlin, pp. 1–105
Suzuki J, Nakamoto Y (1978) Sensory precipitation epilepsy focus in El mice and Mongolian gerbils. Folia Psychiat Neurol Jpn 32:349–350
Sveinsbjornsdottir S, Sander JWAS, Upton D, Thompson PJ, Patsalos PN, Hirt D, Emre M, Lowe D, Duncan JS (1993) The excitatory amino acid antagonist D-CPP-ene (SDZ EAA-494) in patients with epilepsy. Epilepsy Res 16:165–174
Swinyard EA (1949) Laboratory assay of clinically effective antiepileptic drugs. J Am Pharm Assoc 38:201–204
Swinyard EA (1969) Laboratory evaluation of antiepileptic drugs. Review of laboratory methods. Epilepsia 10:107–119

Swinyard EA (1972) Electrically induced convulsions. In: Purpura DP, Penry JK, Tower D, Woodbury DM, Walter R (eds) Experimental models of epilepsy – A manual for the laboratory worker. Raven Press, New York, pp. 433–458

Swinyard EA, Brown WC, Goodman LS (1952) Comparative assay of antiepileptic drugs in mice and rats. J Pharmacol Exp Ther 106:319–330

Swinyard EA, Wolf HH, White HS, Skeen GA, Stark LG, Albertson T, Pong SF, Drust EG (1993) Characterization of the anticonvulsant properties of F–721. Epilepsy Res 15:35–45

Trimble MR (1991) Epilepsy and behaviour. Epilepsy Res 10:71–79

Turski L, Ikonomidou C, Turski WA, Bortolotto ZA, Cavalheiro EA (1989) Review: Cholinergic mechanisms and epileptogenesis. The seizures induced by pilocarpine: a novel model of intractable epilepsy. Synapse 3:154–171

Voskuyl RA, Dingemanse J, Danhof M (1989) Determination of the threshold for convulsions by direct cortical stimulation. Epilepsy Res 3:120–129

Voskuyl RA, Hoogerkamp A, Danhof M (1992) Properties of the convulsive threshold determined by direct cortical stimulation in rats. Epilepsy Res 12:111–120

Ward AAJ (1972) Topical convulsant metals. In: Purpura DP, Penry JK, Tower D, Woodbury DM, Walter R (eds) Experimental models of epilepsy – A manual for the laboratory worker. Raven Press, New York, pp. 13–36

White HS, Woodhead JH, Franklin MR, Swinyard EA, Wolf HH (1995) Experimental selection, quantification, and evaluation of antiepileptic drugs. In: Levy RH, Mattson RH, Meldrum BS (eds) Antiepileptic drugs. 4th edn, Raven Press, New York, pp. 99–110

Williams SF, Colling SB, Whittington MA, Jefferys JG (1993) Epileptic focus induced by intrahippocampal cholera toxin in rat: time course and properties in vivo and in vitro. Epilepsy Res 16:137–146

Woodbury DM (1972) Applications to drug evaluations. In: Purpura DP, Penry JK, Tower D, Woodbury DM, Walter R (eds) Experimental models of epilepsy – A manual for the laboratory worker. Raven Press, New York, pp. 557–584

CHAPTER 3

Epileptogenesis: Electrophysiology

J.O. WILLOUGHBY

A. Introduction

It is now clear that a distinct epileptogenesis applies to each of the three common categories of clinical epilepsy, namely, partial, absence and primary generalized convulsive epilepsies. Partial epilepsy arises as a consequence of increased excitation within neurons close to a lesion. Absence epilepsy arises in relation to the remarkable effects of inhibition on a certain population of neurons. Primary generalized convulsive epilepsy, currently the least well understood, might be regarded as emerging out of neuronal synchronization. In this chapter, only the essentials pertaining to these three types of epileptogenic phenomena will be presented. There is a wealth of additional material that should be acknowledged; however, the few papers referenced herein do point to the larger literature. Expectably, many of the essentials arise from experimental work in animals, but the ideas are usually supported by some specific studies in humans.

In dealing with this complex subject, the essential information is contained predominantly in pathophysiology at two levels that cannot be separated. At the level of the single neuron, intrinsic or acquired neuronal characteristics alter neuronal behaviours that may lead, in association with other neurons, to promote abnormal neuronal discharges of different kinds. At the level of interconnected groups of neurons, abnormal neuronal discharges lead to altered function within the neurons themselves.

The term "generalized epilepsy" normally encompasses disorders characterized by attacks of absences, myoclonic jerks and major motor convulsions which sometimes occur in combination in the same individual. In contrast to focal epilepsy, generalized absence and generalized convulsive epilepsy occur in a macroscopically, and probably microscopically, normal brain. It is now clear that subtle changes in neuronal properties or in timing and/or synchronization are important in these particular epileptic disorders, even if the basic disturbances are currently elusive. Generalized epilepsies are common mono- or polygenic inherited disturbances (DELGADO-ESCUETA et al 1986). Their attacks are called generalized because, when the attacks have been studied using electroencephalography (EEG), a generalized electrical disturbance has been observed, that is, the electrographic disturbance occurs in all EEG leads over the entire cerebrum, apparently simultaneously. This contrasts with the

EEG of a partial seizure, in which the disturbance appears in EEG leads arising from a small area of brain, sometimes continuing for many seconds or minutes before more widespread, but frequently still localized discharges, or less often secondarily generalized discharges, occur.

B. Partial (Focal, or Lesional) Epilepsy

I. Overview

A most helpful starting point in understanding lesional epilepsy is to observe concurrently recorded electrical potentials from the surface EEG and from an intracellular micro-electrode within a neuron at an epileptic focus. Such recordings help to reveal important relationships between what can be seen in the EEG and what individual neurons are doing at the same time.

One of the features of the resting EEG between seizures is the appearance of single non-convulsive (interictal) electrical potentials, clinically referred to as interictal "spikes" and shown in Fig. 1. This single surface EEG event is actually associated with a burst of action potentials within the brain (MATSUMOTO and AJMONE-MARSAN 1964; CALVIN et al. 1968; CONNORS 1984) due to a special neuronal event in which there is a depolarization (excitation), superimposed on which there is a burst of action potentials (Fig. 1). This complex bursting phenomenon is known as a "depolarization shift" and the event is probably the characteristic feature of neurons in an epileptic focus. In addition, as shown in Fig 1, the neuronal correlate of the seizure process itself is a sustained depolarization and the generation of continuous high-frequency action potentials from neurons within the focus (AYALA et al 1973). Understanding the processes leading to depolarization shift development also assists in understanding some of the changes leading to a sustained seizure.

There are many processes that might result in cortical neurons near a focus acquiring the characteristic of discharging in depolarization shifts; these processes are best illustrated by reviewing what constitutes normal neuronal structure and function.

II. The Single Neuron: Normal Population

A schematic normal neuron is illustrated in Fig. 2. This cerebral cortical neuron has been chosen because the interconnectivity to be considered in the next section can most easily be illustrated for the cerebral cortex. Whether a neuron generates an action potential depends on a complex interaction involving the activity of excitatory and inhibitory inputs on its dendrites and cell body. Excitatory inputs normally synapse on the distal ends of dendrites, which are very long, and inhibitory inputs tend to be located on the cell body. Whether a neuron discharges depends on the integrated effect of all excitatory and inhibitory influences at the initial segment of the axon. If the overall depolarization (excitation) at this initial segment is sufficient, that is, it exceeds a depo-

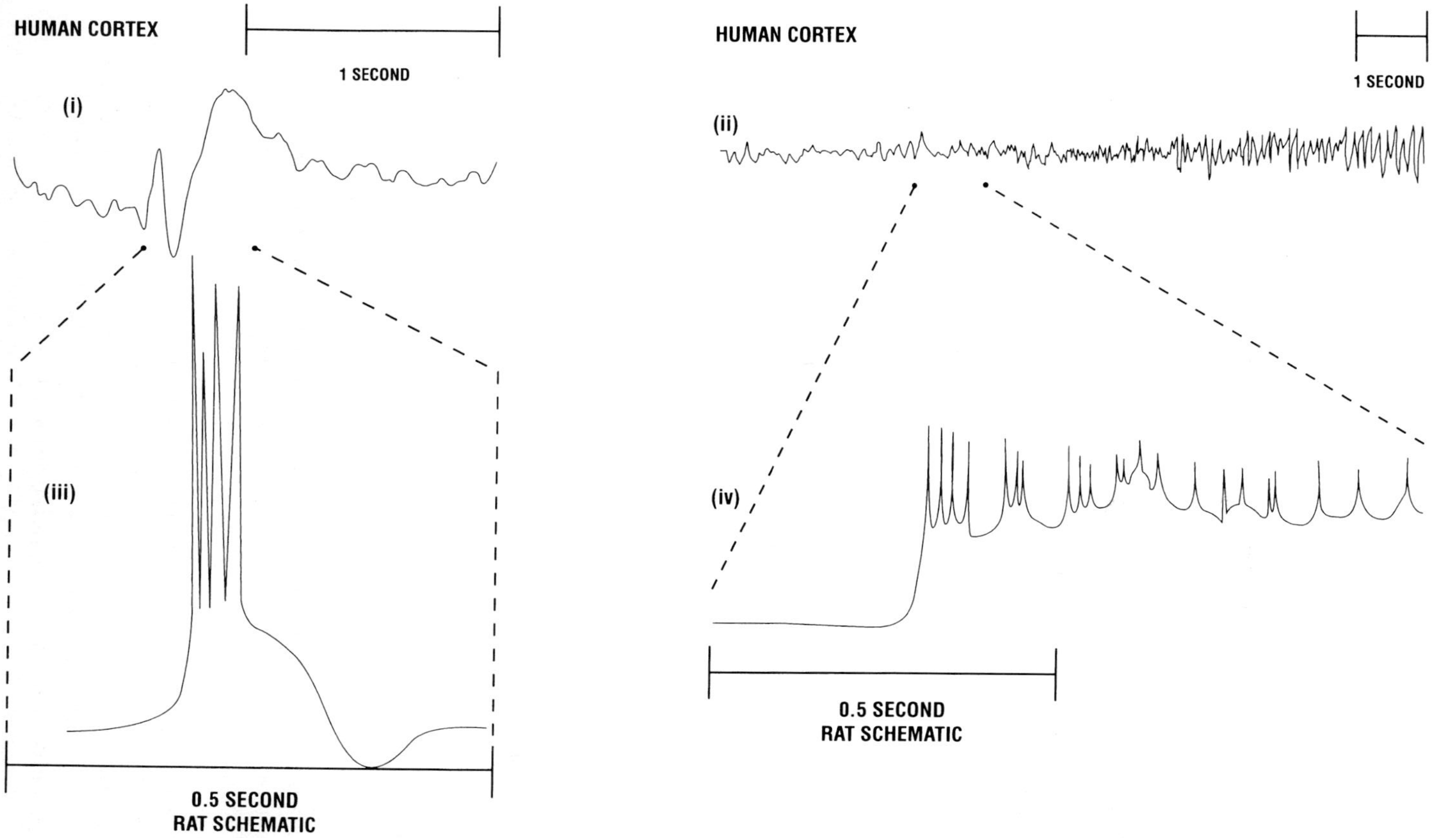

Fig. 1. Segments of EEG from clinical records showing *(i)* a typical interictal (non-convulsive) spike and *(ii)* the initiation of focal epilepsy. Below these segments is illustrated in schematic form in *(iii)*, intracellular events associated with the surface spike, the depolarization shift, and in *(iv)*, intracellular events associated with the initiation of the surface discharge. Figure modelled on representations from AYALA et al. (1973) and JEFFERYS (1993)

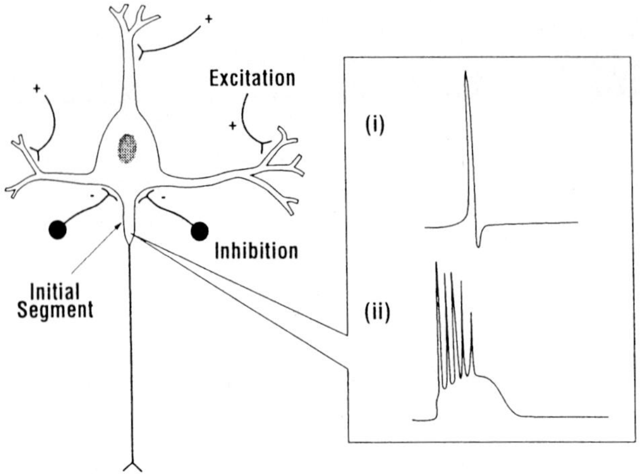

Fig. 2. Schematic pyramidal cortical neuron to indicate sites of excitatory and inhibitory inputs and the potentials recordable from the initial segment of the axon, *(i)* normally and *(ii)* after blockade of inhibitory inputs

larization threshold for the neuron, an action potential is generated which propagates along the axon to its synaptic terminals. Because the inhibitory inputs are very close to the initial segment of the axon, inhibitory synaptic activity has a potent effect at this site. Conversely, excitatory inputs are a relatively long distance from the initial segment and individually have less influence on the intracellular potential within it. During ongoing cerebral activity, the most frequent physiological outcome of the initial segment reaching the depolarization threshold is a single action potential.

Studies in which the properties of pyramidal neurons have been investigated in cultured brain slices show that the discharge behaviour of a pyramidal neuron can be changed remarkably by diminishing inhibitory activity, for example, by bathing the neuron in bicuculline, an antagonist of GABA at the GABAA receptor (SCHWARTZKROIN and PRINCE 1980). In this situation, instead of generating a single action potential, a burst of action potentials is generated in addition to a strongly sustained depolarization (excitation), mimicking the phenomenon referred to already – the depolarization shift (CONNORS 1984). The point of this observation is that neurons have an intrinsic capacity to exhibit a depolarization shift-like event as part of their normal repertoire of behaviours; indeed, a proportion of cerebral cortical and hippocampal neurons discharge in this fashion normally. The question then arises as to what biochemical or structural changes can be identified in neurons close to lesions associated with epilepsy that might increase the likelihood of more or all these neurons eventually firing with depolarization shifts?

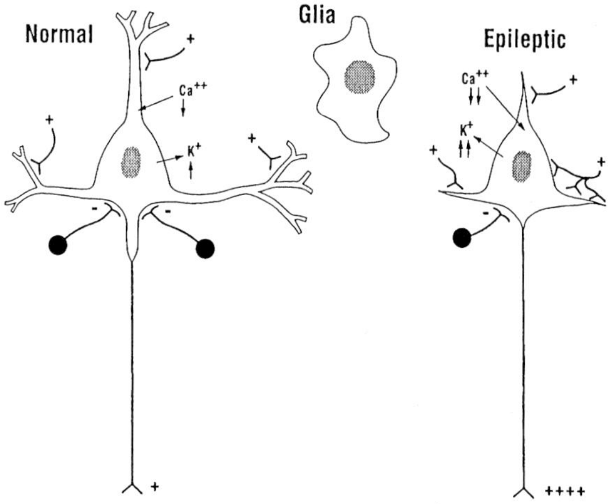

Fig. 3. Schematic normal pyramidal neuron and neuron within an epileptic focus to show structural and biochemical changes likely to be relevant in epileptogenesis, namely fewer inhibitory neurons, additional excitatory inputs, excitatory inputs closer to the initial segment, increased extracellular K^+ and reduced extracellular Ca^{2+}. Current evidence is that glia do not contribute to disturbances of the extracellular environment (HEINEMANN et al. 1986)

III. The Single Neuron: Epileptic Population

The potentially important changes are summarized in Fig. 3. One conceptually straightforward situation is that, in or near cerebral lesions, one would not normally expect a proportional loss of excitatory and inhibitory neurons, that is fewer, the same number, or more inhibitory neurons may be destroyed in comparison to the number of excitatory neurons lost (RIBAK et al. 1989). If the number of surviving inhibitory neurons is much reduced in comparison to the number of excitatory neurons, it is clear that surviving excitatory neurons could receive less inhibitory input (RIBAK et al. 1982; RIBAK 1986) and therefore be more readily excited to the threshold for action potential generation. Secondly, injurious processes may damage excitatory neurons without destroying them (PAUL and SCHEIBEL 1986; ISOKAWA 1997). As shown in the hippocampus from patients with temporal lobe epilepsy, one consequence of partial damage is that there are fewer dendritic processes and another is that surviving dendrites may have more excitatory inputs proximally as a result of regenerative sprouting of damaged excitatory inputs. Such sprouting has been demonstrated to occur, especially in hippocampus, and may lead to the establishment of additional inputs onto normal or injured neurons (MCKINNEY et al. 1997). Increased numbers of excitatory inputs and reduced numbers of inhibitory inputs have been shown in human temporal lobe neocortex in patients with temporal lobe epilepsy (MARCO and DEFILIPE 1997). If excitation occurs on the proximal dendrite, closer to the initial segment, the excitation will be more likely to cause neuronal activation.

There are other consequences of injury that may enhance excitation within small populations of neurons: normally close but separated neurons may come to have contiguous membranes, leading to direct excitatory field effects from an activated to adjacent quiescent neurons (JEFFERYS 1995), similar to the phenomenon of ephaptic transmission between demyelinated axons in multiple sclerosis. Furthermore, gap-junctions may exist between contiguous neurons in some circumstances (JEFFERYS 1995), thereby providing a very direct mechanism of excitation between neurons and one which might occur in pathological areas of brain, as suggested in one (NAUS et al. 1991) but not in another (ELISEVICH et al. 1997) recent report. There is evidence that gap junction coupling is increased in astrocytes from human chronic epileptic foci, a finding of possible relevance to enhancing focal synchrony (LEE et al. 1995). Although gliosis around lesions might also be expected to disturb control of the extracellular ionic environment and thus affect neuronal excitability, this has not been confirmed directly (HEINEMANN and DIETZEL 1984).

Thus, the net effect of the possible structural changes to the neurons near a pathological lesion may be such as to increase the overall ease with which neurons are brought to excitation and thereby increase the average firing rate of the population of neurons.

One consequence of increased neuronal firing rates is to intensify the activity-dependent changes in concentration of ions in the immediate environment of active neurons. Normally, these changes are rapidly corrected and include increases in K^+ released from neurons during the falling phase of each action potential, and falls in Ca^{2+} as it enters cells during the hyperpolarizing stage of each action potential (HEINEMANN et al. 1986). Increased firing rates may be such as to produce sustained changes in the ionic environment and these changes can directly increase neuronal membrane excitability (Fig. 2 – HEINEMANN et al. 1986; UEMATSU et al. 1990). Thus, morphological changes in conjunction with biochemical alterations significantly increase neuronal excitability such that, in response to the excitatory input from other neurons, neurons in the focus eventually produce depolarization shifts. On those occasions when there is sufficient coincident excitation, and inhibitory mechanisms are consequently rendered ineffective (BERMAN et al. 1992), sustained depolarizations (excitations) with sustained neuronal discharges occur.

IV. Connectivity

Some mechanisms of epileptogenesis acting at the neuronal level depend on excitation from an excitatory input, underscoring the importance of neuronal connectivity. Excitatory input to a cortical neuron arises mainly from other cortical neurons, much of it from local neurons on which the cortical neuron will have a reciprocal excitatory input (BERMAN et al. 1992). The main extrin-

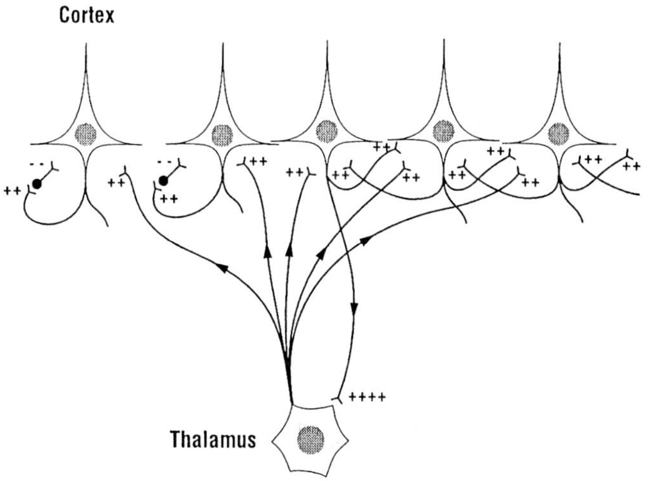

Fig. 4. Schematic to illustrate important excitatory connectivity of cortical neurons relevant to epileptogenesis. The inhibitory neurons are likely to be ineffectual in the presence of excitation in the form of synchronous or repetitive input

sic source of input to the cortex is from the thalamus; although it probably constitutes on the average less than 15% of the total inputs (BERMAN et al. 1992); again, the cortical neuron has a reciprocal excitatory relationship with thalamic neurons, i.e. there are cortico-thalamic neurons and also thalamo-cortical neurons which project back to the region of cortex from which they receive input (Fig. 4). The return projection to the cortex is not localized only to the neurons projecting to the thalamo-cortical neuron. Activation of the thalamo-cortical projection also results in excitation of cortical neurons near those from which each thalamic neuron receives an input. The effect of these reciprocal excitatory inputs is a powerful increase in excitation, both at the level of the epileptic focus and within the region of the thalamus to which it is connected. While inhibitory neurons within the cortex also receive collateral excitatory inputs from cortical neurons and from thalamic neurons, their influence is unlikely to be a significant factor once some excitation within the cortico-cortical and cortico-thalamic loops has been established because modelling studies have clearly demonstrated the ineffectiveness of inhibitory synaptic activity on neurons that receive several concurrent excitatory signals (BERMAN et al. 1992). An emerging property of neurons in this excited circuitry is the generation of depolarization shifts and sustained depolarizations (excitations) accompanying continuous discharges. When sufficient neurons are recruited into this process, clinical manifestations of the activity become apparent – the partial seizure.

The importance of the role of the cortex and the thalamus derived from animal experimental work has been reinforced by two positron emission tomographic (PET) studies in human, in which increased metabolism of the cortex and ipsilateral thalamus has been demonstrated during frequent or continuous partial epileptic seizures (HAJEK et al. 1991; DETRE et al. 1996).

V. Other Processes

Surprisingly, several situations have been described in experimental models of seizures (in hippocampal slices, including human slices) where GABA receptor activation is associated with neuronal discharges, usually where there has been considerable cellular micro-environmental change such as increased extracellular K^+ concentrations. In one situation, hyperpolarization (inhibition) mediated by GABA neurons with its associated rise in extracellular K^+ subsequently led to a synchronous depolarization (excitation) of groups of hippocampal neurons (AVOLI et al. 1994). In the other process, there was activation of terminals of excitatory neurons in the region of an epileptic focus. Here, extreme disturbances of the interstitial ionic environment that destabilize neuronal membranes and bring them close to firing threshold, also disturb membranes of nerve terminals innervating the epileptic focus (Fig. 5). Surprisingly, the process appears to be triggered by GABA receptor activation on nerve terminals (STASHEFF and WILSON 1992). It has been demonstrated indirectly by recording high frequency action potentials from thalamic neurons in circumstances when synaptic excitation has not occurred (NOEBELS and PRINCE 1978). Thus, the potentials arise at nerve terminals in the cortical focus and invade thalamo-cortical neurons and all their branches antidromically (Fig. 4). These project to and activate more widespread cortical regions and, because of very high frequency action potentials generated by the terminal excitation,

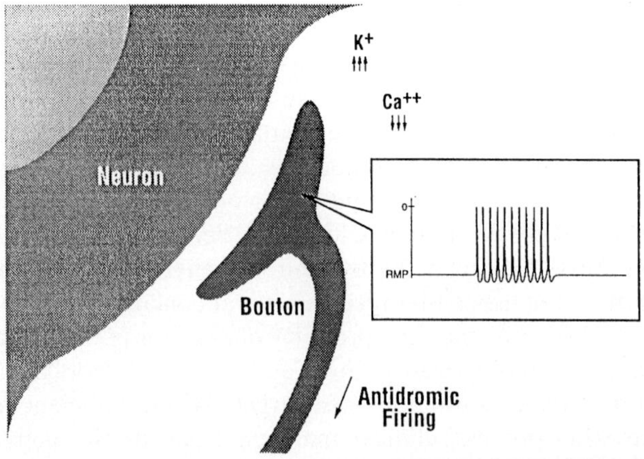

Fig. 5. Schematic to illustrate ectopic action potential generation within terminal boutons within an epileptic focus. Activation of GABA receptors appears to play a role in the initiation of these discharges (STASHEFF and WILSON (1992) (*RMP* resting membrane potential)

result in very much enhanced neurotransmitter release. The occurrence of this phenomenon at excitatory terminals throughout the cortex could constitute a very powerful and widespread synchronizing and excitatory stimulus, possibly relevant either to the first clinical manifestation of the focal discharge or to its becoming secondarily generalized.

Finally, genetic forms of apparently partial epilepsy are now recognized. For one, a molecular causal abnormality has been defined (STEINLEIN et al. 1995), but the disturbed mechanisms leading to the epilepsy remain to be elucidated.

C. Generalized Epilepsy: Absence Seizures

I. Overview

Human absence epilepsy is characterized behaviourally by a brief period of cessation of activity, associated electrographically with synchronous 3-Hz high voltage spike and wave activity over the entire cerebral cortex. Typically the affected individual is without a cerebral lesion and therefore it is not ethically feasible to implant electrodes to define the brain regions participating in the absence. Advances in a possible understanding of human non-convulsive generalized (absence) epilepsy have come from the examination of feline and rodent models of the condition. The rodent models in particular have an uncanny resemblance to the human disorder: there is a genetic tendency to spontaneous periods of behavioural inactivity for periods of seconds to a minute or so, accompanied by high-voltage spike and wave electrographic activity (VERGNES et al. 1986; COENEN and VAN LUIJTELAAR 1987; WILLOUGHBY and MACKENZIE 1992). Perhaps not surprisingly, however, the frequency of the discharges is different from that in the human (being at 7–9 Hz). In rodent models, the abnormal EEG discharge can be recorded from all cortical areas and from the thalamus, but not from other more primitive forebrain regions such as the hippocampus or amygdala (VERGNES et al. 1990). In the feline model too, it is the thalamus and cortex that have been demonstrated to generate 3 Hz spike and wave activity (KOSTOPOULOS et al. 1981a,b; MCLACHLAN et al. 1984).

The animal studies suggest that there are essentially four classes of neuron participating in discharge generation, two in the thalamus and two in the cortex (Fig. 6). The critical neurons for imposing synchronization are the GABA-synthesizing and -releasing inhibitory thalamic reticular neuron (SPREAFICO et al. 1991). These neurons project entirely within the thalamus (STERIADE et al. 1984) and inhibit thalamic neurons projecting to the cerebral cortex (thalamic projection neurons, also known as thalamo-cortical projection neurons). The second class of neurons are the thalamic projection neurons themselves, neurons that, for example, relay sensory activity to the cortex from the periphery (JONES 1991) or project pre-motor activity from the basal ganglia to the cortex. Figure 6 shows the connectivity of the thalamo-cortical projec-

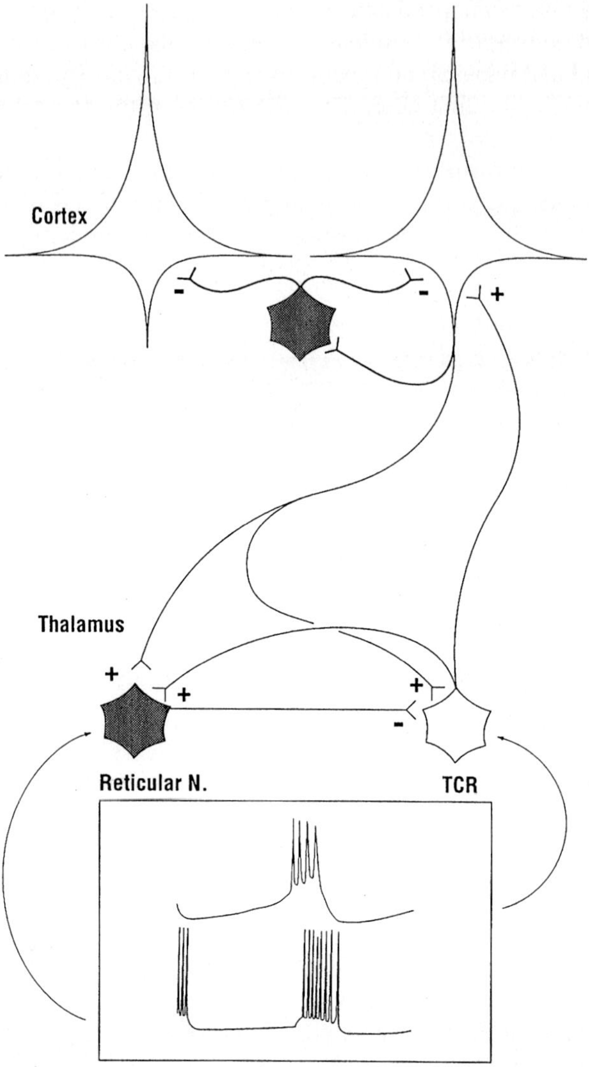

Fig. 6. Schematic to illustrate the neurons participating in the generation of absence epilepsy. The graphs illustrate intracellular potentials to show hyperpolarizations followed by calcium depolarizations with bursts of action potentials in thalamic neurons, with the thalamo-cortical neuron (*TCR*) reaching the threshold for discharge before the reticular thalamic neuron (*Reticular N.*). Figure modelled on representation in JEFFERYS (1993)

tion neurons with the cortical neurons (HERSCH and WHITE 1981), one of which projects back to the thalamus. Because the inhibitory thalamic reticular neurons innervate thalamic projection neurons broadly, the reticular neurons have a powerful inhibitory and synchronizing influence on thalamo-cortical projection neuron activity (CONTRERAS and STERIADE 1995). Also important are the reciprocal connections from cortex to thalamus and from thalamic projection neurons to thalamic reticular neurons, because these ensure excitation and reactivation of thalamic reticular neurons (CONTRERAS and STERIADE 1995).

II. Cortical Processes

As before, in considering the mechanisms of epileptogenesis it is helpful to start with the electrographic appearances. The cortical spike is caused by a synchronous volley of afferent excitation arising from the thalamus. The spike as recorded at the surface is a summation of electrical activity generated in the cortex, probably by a mixture of both thalamic projection neuron-induced cortical action potentials and by postsynaptic depolarizations (excitations) that do not quite cause action potentials (KOSTOPOULOS et al. 1981a,b). During the spike, excitatory and inhibitory neurons are activated. Because excitatory cortical neurons are reciprocally innervated by inhibitory neurons (Fig. 6), cortical activation is immediately followed by inhibition (hyperpolarization) of all cortical neurons, leading to a surface wave (KOSTOPOULOS et al. 1981a,b, 1983; KELLER and WHITE 1987). Another factor probably contributing to the prolonged cessation of cortical activity between spikes is simply a lack of excitatory input from the thalamus during this period, as demonstrated in another model of slow wave generation (CONTRERAS and STERIADE 1995), discussed below.

III. Thalamic Processes

It is the behaviour of the thalamic reticular and thalamic projection neurons that drives the cortically projected volley (STERIADE et al. 1990; LOPES DA SILVA 1991; SOLTESZ et al. 1991; CONTRERAS and STERIADE 1995). Both reticular and projection thalamic neurons have an interesting characteristic – in response to a lack of input, such as in states of low arousal with its associated reduced ascending cholinergic activation, the GABA-releasing inhibitory reticular neurons become more active and the thalamic projection neurons a little less depolarized (less activated). Eventually, as a consequence of reaching a sufficient state of hyperpolarization, a special class of Ca^{2+} channels, low threshold Ca^{2+} channels on the surface of thalamic neurons, becomes activated (more accurately, de-inactivated, in that they are again able to function, but only if there is sufficient depolarization of the neuronal membrane – SOLTESZ et al. 1991). From the state of hyperpolarization (inhibition), either of two mechanisms allows the neurons to progressively depolarize and reach a level of depolarization (excitation) at which the de-inactivated Ca^{2+} channels open. Via one mechanism, a class of ion channels that allows Na^+ and K^+ through the neuronal membrane also becomes activated by the hyperpolarization and permits slow Na^+ entry into the neurons, thereby gradually depolarizing the membrane (SOLTESZ et al. 1991). This process of slow depolarization (excitation) has similarities to cardiac pacemaker activity in the sino-atrial node. The second mechanism is the normal slow time-course of GABAB activated K^+ channels responsible for the sustained component of thalamic reticular neuron-mediated GABA-induced hyperpolarization (CRUNELLI and LERESCHE 1991). At a critical level of depolarization, the de-inactivated Ca^{2+} channels open, allowing Ca^{2+} entry into the neurons. The latter process results in a powerful depolarization (a more excitatory state) that exceeds the threshold for firing, and action potentials are generated (SOLTESZ et al. 1991). Furthermore, in thalamic neurons, the Ca^{2+} depolarization (excitation) frequently causes, not one action potential, but a burst of action potentials, to be generated. This burst of action potentials achieves two effects. Firstly, a volley of afferent impulses is projected from thalamo-cortical projection neurons to excite the cerebral cortex, thereby producing the surface EEG spike, and secondly, via collaterals back to thalamic reticular neurons, the volley also excites these reticular neurons to discharge. This reticular neuron discharge inhibits (hyperpolarizes) thalamic projection neurons and reticular neurons, thereby both terminating their discharges and again activating the pacemaker current and preparing the low threshold Ca^{2+} channels in thalamic neurons for later activation as described above. Because thalamic projection neurons have a low threshold Ca^{2+} channel that requires a lesser degree of depolarization to reach threshold than reticular neurons (HUGUENARD and PRINCE 1992), thalamic projection neurons, which are excitatory, reach their threshold for firing before reticular neurons, which are inhibitory. Thus alternating excitation and inhibition is established and rhythmic volleys from the thalamus reach the cerebral cortex.

IV. Human Studies

The recognition of the critical role of the special class of Ca^{2+} channels in pacemaking activity in the thalamus, the low threshold "T" type Ca^{2+} channels, provides corroboration that the processes observed in animal models reflect processes in human absence epilepsy, because it has now been shown that the clinically useful drug ethosuximide may be an antagonist of these Ca^{2+} currents (COULTER et al. 1990).

Functional imaging studies have also supported animal studies favouring a thalamo-cortical process in absence epilepsy. Human metabolic and blood flow studies examining changes from baseline and during hyperventilation-induced absence reveal increased cerebrocortical metabolism of glucose (ENGEL et al. 1985) and blood flow (PREVETT et al. 1995) as well as increased thalamic blood flow (PREVETT et al. 1995). There are no definitive disturbances interictally. These findings are of interest because they are consistent with the importance of the thalamus and cortex as proposed on the basis of the animal studies.

Possible primary pathogenetic mechanisms that have been proposed for absence epilepsy include increased cortical excitability (KOSTOPOULOS et al. 1981a,b; LUHMANN et al. 1995), thereby enhancing cerebral cortical responses to thalamic rhythmic activity and reciprocally affecting thalamic function, as well as disturbances of inhibition or of the low threshold Ca^{2+} currents in thalamic neurons. Disturbances in the latter have now been demonstrated in rat absence epilepsy in the reticular thalamic neurons (TSAKIRIDOU et al. 1995), but not in thalamic projection neurons (GUYON et al. 1993; TSAKIRIDOU et al. 1995). Specific abnormalities of Ca^{2+} currents have not yet been identified in humans. Enhanced cortical excitability has been demonstrated in human absence seizures, as judged by a reduction in the intensity of transcranial magnetic stimulation required to produce a contralateral limb motor response (REUTENS et al. 1993). In this study, there was a trend for individuals with myoclonic jerks and absences to have increased excitability compared to those with just absences. The results for patients with convulsive seizures were not presented. Transcranial magnetic stimulation probably causes motor neuronal activation by direct and transsynaptic actions (BURKE et al. 1993), so that a mechanism for the possibly increased cortical excitability as revealed in humans remains to be defined.

D. Generalized Epilepsy: Convulsive Seizures

I. Overview

Convulsive epilepsy in an apparently normal brain is a puzzle both in terms of the underlying brain state leading to the convulsion and the nature of the epileptic process itself – the state of knowledge has recently been summarized as: "in a somewhat mysterious manner, an epileptic event is generalized from the start" (NIEDERMEYER 1996). Human generalized convulsive epilepsy is characterized behaviourally by some combination of tonic and clonic convulsions and loss of consciousness. The clinical event is associated with an increasing strength of high frequency electrographical discharge over the entire cerebral cortex that gives way gradually to slow discharges of high voltage that progressively become even slower and eventually stop (GASTAUT and BROUGHTON 1972).

Typically, as in the case of absences, the affected individual is without a cerebral lesion and it is not ethically feasible to implant electrodes to define the brain regions participating in the seizure. There are only a few animal models of generalized convulsive epilepsy – evidence that many models exhibit synchronous bilateral EEG discharges with convulsions is unimpressive, although several baboon models do exhibit such a phenomenon (TICKU et al. 1992), but the process usually requires triggering by intermittent light stimulation (SILVA-BARRAT et al. 1986; MENINI et al. 1994; WADA 1994).

There are important clinical observations that point to some aspects of the pathophysiology of convulsive epilepsy in humans, as will be discussed below (Sect. D.V). However, the insight they provide can best be perceived after a consideration of the pathophysiological findings from studies in animals, because these animal models offer a deeper understanding of some of the processes likely to be occurring (BROWNING 1994; MENINI et al. 1994; WADA 1994). While these studies point to generalized convulsive epilepsies involving several types of motor convulsion arising from more than one neural substrate, the cortex and brain stem appear to interact in the generation of generalized tonic-clonic seizures (SILVA-BARRAT et al. 1986; MENINI et al. 1994; WADA 1994). Interestingly, it has been well demonstrated in rats that different motor convulsions are subserved by mechanisms with anatomical substrates which are sometimes situated in the brain stem, and sometimes in the forebrain and cerebral cortex (BURNHAM 1985; GALE 1992; BROWNING 1994).

II. Excessive Excitation or Impaired Inhibition

At present, the most widely held cellular hypotheses are that subjects with generalized convulsive epilepsy have a neuronal disturbance that lies somewhere on a spectrum between a reduction in the efficacy of inhibitory neuronal mechanisms and an increase in the efficacy of excitatory mechanisms. Certainly, animals (including humans) experience generalized convulsions after exposure to agents that block neuronal inhibition (JEFFERYS 1993; WILLOUGHBY et al. 1995) or cause neuronal excitation (LOTHMAN and COLLINS 1981; JEFFERYS 1993; CENDES et al. 1995; WILLOUGHBY et al. 1997).

One approach to generalized convulsive epilepsy, therefore, has been to study the seizure process in two pharmacological models in which the epileptogenic disturbance is well-defined. In one, a seizure is caused by widespread neuronal activation due to systemic administration of kainic acid, an excitatory amino-acid agonist at the kainate/a-amino-3-hydroxy-5-methyl-isoxazole-4-propionate (AMPA) receptor (YOUNG and FAGG 1990; WISDEN and SEEBURG 1993). In the other, a seizure is caused by a diffuse reduction in inhibition (by the systemic administration of picrotoxin, an antagonist at the g-aminobutyric acid $(GABA)_A$ receptor-gated Cl^- channel – GASS et al. 1992). This approach permits the study of convulsions induced by extremes of the spectrum of neuronal disturbances which possibly have an aetiological role in human generalized convulsive epilepsy.

III. Anatomical Distribution of Convulsions: Cortex and Hippocampus

To partially identify brain regions involved in a convulsion, immunohistochemistry for the presence of Fos protein can be used as a marker of neuronal activation. It is a method that provides anatomical definition with cellular resolution (DRAGUNOW and ROBERTSON 1987; MORGAN et al. 1987; SAGAR et al.

1988). Fos is the protein product of the c-*fos* gene, one of several immediate early genes that are activated in cells by different stimuli, including postsynaptic activation. By immunohistochemical staining for Fos, an image of brain regions and cell types that participate in the epileptic processes can be obtained. There are limitations to the technique: activated neurons may not always reveal Fos. With this caveat, after convulsions produced by both convulsants, Fos immunoreactivity is observed in all neurons in all laminae throughout the cerebral cortex without selectivity for specific laminae, cell classes or regions (Willoughby et al. 1995, 1997; Hiscock et al. 1996, 1998). In many seizures the hippocampus is also intensely involved. What is suggested by these anatomical studies is that the cortex and, in the excitation-induced form of epilepsy, the hippocampus are likely to be important participating structures, the hippocampus especially being of interest because it is not normally considered as relevant in human generalized convulsive epilepsy.

IV. Electrophysiological Distribution of Convulsions: Cortex and Brain Stem

It has recently become practicable to explore the distribution of seizure activity and the underlying preictal EEG states by analysing digitized records and using comprehensive mathematical/statistical methods. These methods permit the simultaneous analysis of both EEG frequencies and directions of propagation of rhythms between structures.

An examination of a wide range of frequencies (to over 100 Hz) in the hippocampus and cortex reveals different changes in the two pharmacological models referred to above. With excitation-induced epileptogenesis, there is a progressive development of more intense high frequency (above 30 Hz) rhythms out of the background state until non-convulsive discharges occur, during which stages low frequencies (below 20 Hz) also arise and increase in intensity. These non-convulsive discharges are presumptively a precondition to seizures. Eventually, a motor convulsion is manifested with only a small increase in very high frequency activity (above 100 Hz), without significant change in other frequencies in the cortical EEG (Fig. 7 – Medvedev et al. 1998). In inhibition-blocked seizures, there is doubtfully significant intensification of the background EEG at high frequencies (above 30 Hz) which precedes episodes of non-convulsive discharges associated with myoclonic jerks and, later, the convulsive EEG activity. The EEG in convulsive seizures induced by inhibition-blockade reveals the same changes evident with the non-convulsive discharges but at higher intensity, together with increased EEG frequencies at very high rates (above 100 Hz). The findings in both seizure types therefore point to the presence of intensified EEG rhythms in non-convulsive EEG discharges and qualitatively little change accompanying the convulsion. Because the cortical EEG is little different in non-convulsive discharges and convulsive discharges, the convulsive motor mechanism is possibly located elsewhere than in the cortex.

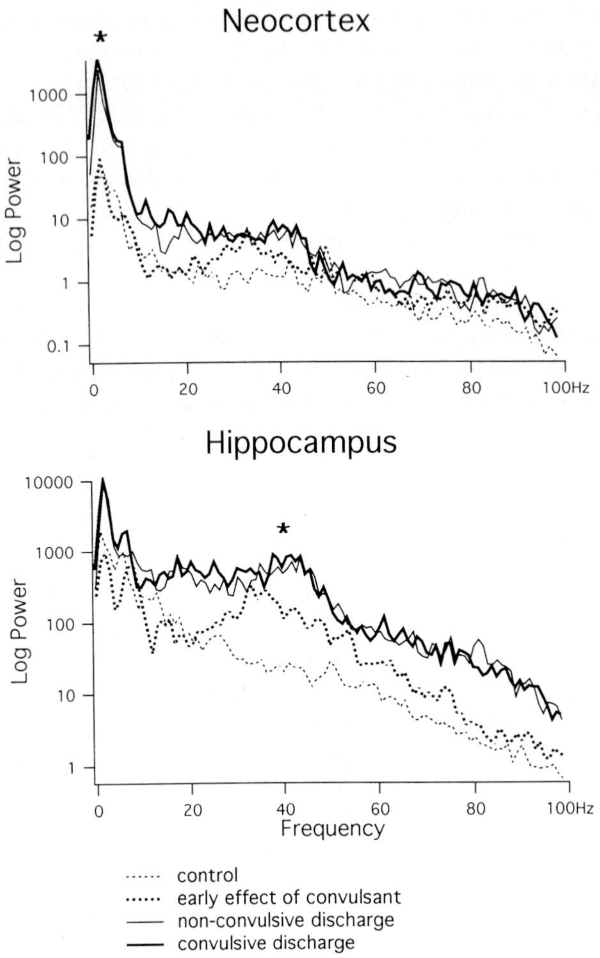

Fig. 7. Power spectra from cortex and hippocampus during excitation-induced epileptogenesis to show enhanced 40 Hz rhythms in background EEG, with further increases in power of frequencies up to at least 100 Hz in non-convulsive and convulsive discharges. The spectra from non-convulsive and convulsive discharges are little different, suggesting that the motor convulsion is mediated through the involvement of other structures than the cortex and hippocampus. *The asterisk* indicates much-enhanced frequencies in cortex and hippocampus. Note that the power is shown against a log scale, so that the increase in power of 40 Hz frequencies during discharges is approximately 100-fold, in comparison to approximately 10-fold increases in power of other frequencies. There is also an increase in power around 30–40 Hz caused by the convulsant, before any discharge occurs. (From Medvedev et al. 1998)

Of special interest from the EEG analysis studies of activation-induced convulsions is the observation (Fig. 7) of more large increases in the power of background rhythms in the 30–100 Hz frequency range, often the peak power increase being close to 40 Hz. The presence of intensified 40 Hz rhythms is especially notable because bursts of neuronal activity in rhythms of this frequency range have been proposed as integral to aspects of consciousness, to be discussed below (Sect. D.V). Furthermore, determination of the direction of flow of electrical signals through the brain during the non-convulsive discharges has shown that the frontal cortex leads fast frequencies in other regions after blockade of inhibition (MEDVEDEV et al. 1996) and that the hippocampus leads fast frequencies after the administration of excitatory convulsants (MEDVEDEV et al. 1998; MEDVEDEV and WILLOUGHBY 1998). The slow frequencies are more variable in origin, most often arising first in the frontal cortex, but later in the hippocampus or rarely in other cortical areas. Finally and importantly, during the convulsive discharges, the same brain regions have similar influences on EEG rhythms at different frequencies as they do during the non-convulsive discharges. Thus, impressive increases in the intensity of EEG frequencies occur during both non-convulsive and convulsive states and the rhythms in different regions may be driven by the same structures as those generating the non-convulsive discharges. This finding also suggests that these brain regions may not be subserving the convulsive component of the seizure.

Recording, stimulation and lesion studies suggest that brain stem (mesencephalic or pontine) structures mediate motor convulsions. For example, by using multi-unit recording techniques, high frequency rhythms in the mesencephalon and pontine nuclei have been identified in baboons which are the subject of photo-convulsive jerks or seizures (SILVA-BARRAT et al. 1986). The magnitude of the response as well as its critical timing (lying between the latencies to reach increased neuronal activity in visual and motor structures) both suggest an important mediation of the motor output by these pontine and mesencephalic structures. Lesions of brain stem regions in rats demonstrate an interference in the expression of generalized seizures initiated by various stimuli (BROWNING 1985, 1994). Finally, electrical stimulation of the brain stem can produce tonic seizure activity (BURNHAM 1985; GALE 1992; MATON et al. 1992), even in animals subjected to rostral midbrain transection. Thus, there is convincing evidence of the importance of brain stem structures in the expression of the motor convulsions in quite disparate models of generalized epilepsy, evidence that is likely to be relevant to understanding the process of generalized convulsions in humans.

V. Human Studies: Predisposing Brain Processes and a Synthesis

The existence of "40 Hz EEG oscillations" or oscillations, normal population discharges proposed to be the binding mechanism for coherent assemblies of cortical neurons in some forms of mental processing (ENGEL et al. 1992), makes it likely that the frequencies observed in the pharmacological epilepsy models are highly synchronized normal neuronal rhythmic bursting phenomena. In humans, there are many physiological situations or near physiological conditions that can provoke convulsions: photic stimulation, calculation, chess, reading, music, manipulating (RITACCIO 1994), some of which processes are known to evoke 40 Hz oscillations (ENGEL et al. 1992; DESMEDT and TOMBERG 1994; GEVINS et al. 1994; PULVERMULLER 1996).

Convulsions in response to such physiological stimuli might therefore be subserved by 40 Hz hyperresponsivity associated with the presence of that specific stimulus in prone individuals. Possibly also relevant in this context is the repeatedly confirmed observation in psychiatric wards that electrical stimulation of the frontal cortex during electroconvulsive therapy induces a convulsion lasting 1 min with a non-destructive 40–90 Hz stimulus lasting less than 1 s (SACKEIM et al. 1994). It may be asked how is it that benign stimuli produce such impressive, whole brain responses. Alternatively, perhaps, these provocations may simply indicate how easy it is for the normal brain to become synchronized and, therefore, convulsive.

Arousal also plays a triggering role especially in absences (INOUYE et al. 1990) and in convulsive epilepsy on awakening (NIEDERMEYER 1996). NIEDERMEYER (1996) has proposed that mildly arousing stimuli, insufficient to result in cortical desynchronization but enough to cause a cortical evoked potential in the setting of a mildly reduced state of cortical vigilance (drowsiness), lead to widespread cortical synchronization. As discussed by NEIDERMEYER, synchronization of cortical activity and suppression of fast activity occurs during states of drowsiness. Any excitatory stimulus applied at this stage of drowsiness is likely to meet a large population of neurons that is unstimulated and therefore ready to be activated, thus allowing the immediate initiation of regionally synchronized cortical activity that can propagate.

The following scheme of the pathophysiology of generalized convulsive epilepsy can therefore be proposed. The underlying disturbance, presumably a slight increase in neuronal excitability or reduction in neuronal inhibition, leads to an increased strength of normal neuronal activities including synchronization. As a consequence of increased synchronization of normal neuronal bursting, sometimes enhanced by physiological stimuli, there will be stronger activation and synchronization of cortical regions and thus more potent spread of the process, especially in the absence of competition from ongoing non-synchronized activity in cortical areas to be invaded. With progressively increasing cortical synchronization, activation of subcortical structures through descending projections might be the main event converting non-convulsive disturbances into a sustained tonic motor convulsion or allowing the emergence of clonic activity.

Acknowledgements. The author's work is supported by grants from the National Health and Medical Research Council, the Australian Brain Foundation, the Flinders Medical Centre Research Foundation and the Thyne-Reid Education Trust for Research in Epilepsy of the Royal Australasian College of Physicians. I thank my colleagues in the Epilepsy Laboratory and Centre for Neuroscience for many useful discussions.

References

Avoli M, Mattia D, Siniscalchi A, Perreault P, Tomaiuolo F (1994) Pharmacology and electrophysiology of a synchronous GABA-mediated potential in the human neocortex. Neuroscience 62:655–666
Ayala GF, Dichter MA, Gumnit RJ, Matsumoto H, Spencer WA (1973) Genesis of epileptic interictal spikes. 5. New knowledge of cortical feedback systems suggests a neurophysiological explanation of brief paroxysms. Brain Res 52:1–17
Berman NJ, Douglas RJ, Martin KAC (1992) Gaba-mediated inhibition in the neural networks of visual cortex. In: Mize RR, Marc RE, Sillito AM (eds) Progress in brain research, Vol 90, Elsevier, Amsterdam, pp. 443–476
Browning RA (1985) Role of the brain-stem reticular formation in tonic-clonic seizures: lesion and pharmacological studies. Fed Proc 44:2425–2431
Browning RA (1994) Anatomy of generalized convulsive seizures. In: Malafosse A, Genton P, Marescaux C, Broglin D, Bernasconi R (eds) Idiopathic generalized epilepsies: clinical, experimental and genetic aspects. John Libbey, London, pp. 399–413
Burke D, Hicks R, Gandevia SC, Stephen J, Woodforth I, Crawford M (1993) Direct comparison of corticospinal volleys in human subjects to transcranial magnetic and electrical stimulation. J Physiol 470:383–393
Burnham WM (1985) Core mechanisms in generalized convulsions. Fed Proc 44:2442–2445
Calvin WH, Sypert GW, Ward AA (1968) Structured timing patterns within bursts from epileptic neurons in undrugged monkey cortex. Exp Neurol 21:535–549
Cendes F, Andermann F, Carpenter S, Zatorre RJ, Cashman NR (1995) Temporal lobe epilepsy caused by domoic acid intoxication: evidence for glutamate receptor-mediated excitotoxicity in humans. Ann Neurol 37:123–126
Coenen AML, van Luijtelaar ELJM (1987) The WAG/Rij rat model for absence epilepsy: age and sex factors. Epilepsy Res 1:297–301
Connors WB (1984) Initiation of synchronized neuronal bursting in neocortex. Nature 310:23–29
Contreras D, Steriade M (1995) Cellular basis of EEG slow rhythms: a study of dynamic corticothalamic relationships. J Neurosci 15:604–622
Coulter DA, Huguenard JR, Prince DA (1990) Differential effects of petit mal anticonvulsants and convulsants on thalamic neurones: GABA current blockade. Br J Pharmacol 100:807–813
Crunelli V, Leresche N (1991) A role for GABA(B) receptors in excitation and inhibition of thalamocortical cells. Trends Neurosci 14:16–21
Delgado-Escueta AV, Ward Jr AA, Woodbury DM, Porter RJ (1986) New wave of research in the epilepsies. In: Delgado-Escueta AV, Ward Jr AA, Woodbury DM, Porter RJ (eds) Basic mechanisms of the epilepsies: molecular and cellular approaches. Raven Press, New York, pp. 3–55
Desmedt JE, Tomberg C (1994) Transient phase-locking of 40 Hz electrical oscillations in prefrontal and parietal human cortex reflects the process of conscious somatic perception. Neurosci Lett 168:126–129
Detre JA, Alsop DC, Aguirre GK, Sperling MR (1996) Coupling of cortical and thalamic ictal activity in human partial epilepsy: demonstration by functional magnetic response imaging. Epilepsia 37:657–661
Dragunow M, Robertson HA (1987) Generalized seizures induce c-fos protein(s) in mammalian neurons. Neurosci Lett 82:157–161
Elisevich K, Rempel SA, Smith BJ, Edvardsen K (1997) Hippocampal connexin 43 expression in human complex partial seizure disorder. Exp Neurol 145:154–164
Engel AK, Konig P, Kreiter AK, Schillen TB, Singer W (1992) Temporal coding in the visual cortex: new vistas on integration in the nervous system. Trends Neurosci 15:218–226

Engel JJ, Lubens P, Kuhl D, E, Phelps ME (1985) Local cerebral metabolic rate for glucose during petit mal absences. Ann Neurol 17:121–128
Gale K (1992) Subcortical structures and pathways involved in convulsive seizure generation. J Clin Neurophysiol 9:264–277
Gass P, Herdegen T, Bravos R, Keissling M (1992) Induction of immediate early gene encoded proteins in the rat hippocampus after bicuculline-induced seizures: differential expression of krox-24, fos and jun proteins. Neuroscience 48:315–324
Gastaut H, Broughton R (1972) Epileptic seizures: clinical features and pathophysiology. In: Gastaut H, Broughton R (eds) Epileptic seizures. Clinical and electrographic features, diagnosis and treatment. Thomas, Springfield, pp. 25–140
Gevins A, Cutillo B, Desmond J, Ward M, Bressler S, Barbero N, Laxer K (1994) Subdural grid recordings of distributed neocortical networks involved with somatosensory discrimination. Electroenceph clin Neurophysiol 92:282–290
Guyon A, Vergnes M, Leresche N (1993) Thalamic low threshold calcium current in a genetic model of absence epilepsy. Neuroreport 4:1231–1234
Hajek M, Antonini A, Leenders KL, Wieser HG (1991) Epilepsia partialis continua studied by PET. Epilepsy Res 9:44–48
Heinemann U, Dietzel I (1984) Extracellular potassium concentration in chronic alumina cream foci of cats. J Neurophysiol 52:421–434
Heinemann U, Konnerth A, Pumain R, Wadman WJ (1986) Extracellular calcium and potassium concentration changes in chronic epileptic brain tissue. Adv Neurol 44:641–661
Hersch SM, White EL (1981) Thalamocortical synapses with corticothalamic projection neurons in mouse SmI cortex: electron microscopic demonstration of a monosynaptic feedback loop. Neurosci Lett 24:207–210
Hiscock JJ, Mackenzie L, Willoughby JO (1996) Fos induction in subtypes of cerebrocortical neurons in rat after picrotoxin-induced seizures. Brain Res 738:301–312
Hiscock JJ, Mackenzie L, Willoughby JO (1998) Laminar distribution of Fos/calcium binding protein- and Fos/neurofilament protein-labelled neurons in rat motor and sensory cortex after picrotoxin-induced seizures. Exp Neurol (in press)
Huguenard JR, Prince DA (1992) A novel T-type current underlies prolonged Ca^{2+} dependent burst firing in GABAergic neurons of rat thalamic reticular nucleus. J Neurosci 12:3804–3817
Inouye T, Sakamoto H, Shinosaki K, Toi S, Ukai S (1990) Analysis of rapidly change in EEGs before generalized spike and wave complexes. Electroenceph clin Neurophysiol 76:205–221
Isokawa M (1997) Preservation of dendrites with the presence of reorganized mossy fiber collaterals in hippocampal dentate granule cells in patients with temporal lobe epilepsy. Brain Res 744:339–343
Jefferys JGR (1993) The pathophysiology of epilepsies. In: Laidlaw J, Richens A, Chadwick D (eds) A textbook of epilepsy. 4th edn Churchill Livingstone, London, pp. 241–276
Jefferys JGR (1995) Nonsynaptic modulation of neuronal activity in the brain: electric currents and extracellular ions. Physiological Reviews 75:689–723
Jones EG (1991) The anatomy of sensory relay functions in the thalamus. In: Holstege G (eds) Elsevier Science, pp. 29–52
Keller A, White EL (1987) Synaptic organization of GABAergic neurons in the mouse SmI cortex. J Comp Neurol 262:1–12
Kostopoulos G, Gloor P, Pellegrini A, Gotman J (1981a) A study of the transition from spindles to spike and wave discharge in feline generalized penicillin epilepsy: microphysiological features. Exp Neurol 72:55–77
Kostopoulos G, Gloor P, Pellegrini A, Siatitsas I (1981b) A study of the transition from spindles to spike and wave discharge in feline generalized penicillin epilepsy: EEG features. Exp Neurol 73:43–54

Kostopoulos G, Avoli M, Gloor P (1983) Participation of cortical recurrent inhibition in the genesis of spike and wave discharges in feline generalized penicillin epilepsy. Brain Res 267:101–112
Lee SH, Magge S, Spencer DD, Sontheimer H, Cornell-Bell AH (1995) Human epileptic astrocytes exhibit increased gap junction coupling. Glia 15:195–202
Lopes da Silva F (1991) Neural mechanisms underlying brain waves: from neural membranes to networks. Electroenceph clin Neurophysiol 79:81–93
Lothman EW, Collins RC (1981) Kainic acid induced limbic seizures: metabolic, behavioral, electroencephalographic and neuropathological correlates. Brain Res 218:299–318
Luhmann HT, Mittmann T, van-Luijtelaar G, Heinemann U (1995) Impairment of intracortical GABAergic inhibition in a rat model of absence epilepsy. Epilepsy Res 22:43–51
Marco P, DeFilipe J (1997) Altered synaptic circuitry in the human temporal neocortex removed from epileptic patients. Exp Brain Res 114:1–10
Maton B, Hirsch E, Vergnes M, Depaulis A, Marescaux C (1992) Dorsal tegmentum kindling in rats. Neurosci Lett 134:284–287
Matsumoto H, Ajmone-Marsan C (1964) Cortical cellular phenomena in experimental epilepsy: interictal manifestations. Exp Neurol 9:286–304
McKinney RA, Debanne D, Gahwiler BH, Thompson SM (1997) Lesion-induced axonal sprouting and hyperexcitability in the hippocampus in vitro: implications for the genesis of post-traumatic epilepsy. Nature Medicine 3:990–996
McLachlan RS, Gloor P, Avoli M (1984) Differential participation of some "specific" and "non-specific" thalamic nuclei in generalized spike and wave discharges of feline generalized penicillin epilepsy. Brain Res 307:277–287
Medvedev A, Willoughby JO (1998) Autoregressive analysis of the EEG in systemic kainic acid-induced epileptogenesis. Submitted
Medvedev A, Mackenzie L, Hiscock JJ, Willoughby JO (1996) Frontal cortex leads other brain structures in generalised spike-and-wave spindles and seizure spikes induced by picrotoxin. Electroenceph clin Neurophysiol 98:157–166
Medvedev A, Mackenzie L, Hiscock JJ, Willoughby JO (1998) Spectral analysis of the EEG in systemic kainic acid-induced epileptogenesis. Submitted
Menini C, Silva-Barrat C, Naquet R (1994) The epileptic and nonepileptic generalized myocolons of the *Papio papio* baboon. In: Malafosse A, Genton P, Marescaux C, Broglin D, Bernasconi R (eds) Idiopathic generalized epilepsies: clinical, experimental and genetic aspects. John Libbey, London, pp. 331–348
Morgan JI, Cohen DR, Hempstead JL, Curran T (1987) Mapping patterns of c-fos expression in the central nervous system after seizure. Science 237:192–197
Naus CC, Bechberger JF, Paul DL (1991) Gap junction gene expression in human seizure disorder. Exp Neurol 111:198–203
Niedermeyer E (1996) Primary (idiopathic) generalized epilepsy and underlying mechanisms. Clinical Electroencephalography 27:1–21
Noebels JL, Prince DA (1978) Development of focal seizures in cerebral cortex: role of axon terminal bursting. J Neurophysiol 41:1267–1281
Paul LA, Scheibel AB (1986) Structural substrates of epilepsy. In: Delgado-Escueta AV, Ward Jr AA, Woodbury DM, Porter RJ (eds) Basic mechanisms of the epilepsies. Molecular and cellular approaches. Raven Press, New York, pp. 775–786
Prevett MC, Duncan JS, Jones T, Fish DR, Brooks DJ (1995) Demonstration of thalamic activation during typical absence seizures using $H_2{}^{15}O$ and PET. Neurology 45:1396–1402
Pulvermuller F (1996) Hebb's concept of cell assemblies and the psychophysiology of word processing. Psychophysiology 33:317–333
Reutens DC, Berkovic SF, Macdonell RA, Bladin PF (1993) Magnetic stimulation of the brain in generalized epilepsy: reversal of cortical hyperexcitability by anticonvulsants. Ann Neurol 34:351–355

Ribak CE (1986) Contemporary methods in neurocytology and their application to the study of epilepsy. In: Delgado-Escueta AV, Ward Jr AA, Woodbury DM, Porter RJ (eds) Basic mechanisms of the epilepsies: molecular and cellular approaches pp. 739–764

Ribak CE, Bradburne RM, Harris AB (1982) A preferential loss of gabaergic, symmetric synapses in epileptic foci: a quantitative ultrastructural analysis of monkey neocortex. J Neurosci 2:1725–35

Ribak CE, Joubran C, Kesslak JP, Bakay RAE (1989) A selective decrease in the number of GABAergic somata occurs in pre-seizing monkeys with alumina gel granuloma. Epilepsy Res 4:126–138

Ritaccio AL (1994) Reflex seizures. In: Day LK (eds) Neurologic clinics. Saunders, Philadelphia, pp. 57–83

Sackeim HA, Long J, Luber B, Moeller JR, Prohovnik I, Devanand DP, Nobler MS (1994) Physical properties and qualifications of the ECT stimulus: I. Basic principles. Convulsive Therapy 10:93–123

Sagar SM, Sharp FR, Curran T (1988) Expression of c-fos protein in brain: metabolic mapping at the cellular level. Science 240:1328–1331

Schwartzkroin PA, Prince DA (1980) Changes in excitatory and inhibitory synaptic potentials leading to epileptogenic activity. Brain Res 183:61–76

Silva-Barrat C, Menini C, Bryere P, Naquet R (1986) Multiunitary activity analysis of cortical and subcortical structures in paroxysmal discharges and grandmal seizures in photosensitive baboons. Electroenceph clin Neurophysiol 64:455–468

Soltesz I, Lightowler S, Leresche N, Jassik-Gerschenfeld D, Pollard CE, Crunelli V (1991) Two inward currents and the transformation of low-frequency oscillations of rat and cat thalamo-cortical cells. J Physiol 441:175–197

Spreafico R, Battaglia G, Frassoni C. (1991) The reticular thalamic nucleus (RTN) of the rat: cytoarchitectural, golgi, immunocytochemical, and horseradish peroxidase study. J Comp Neurol 304:478–490

Stasheff SF, Wilson WA (1992) The genesis of seizures in vitro: axon terminal excitability. In: Engel JJ, Wasterlain C, Cavalheiro EA, Heinemann U, Avanzini G (eds) Molecular neurobiology of epilepsy. Elsevier, Amsterdam pp. 319–330

Steinlein OK, Mulley JC, Propping P, Wallace RH, Phillips HA, Sutherland GR, Scheffer IE, Berkovic SF (1995) A missense mutation in the neuronal nicotinic acetylcholine receptor alpha 4 subunit is associated with autosomal dominant nocturnal frontal lobe epilepsy. Nature Genetics 11:201–203

Steriade M, Parent A, Hada J (1984) Thalamic projections of nucleus reticularis thalami of cat: a study using retrograde transport of horseradish peroxidase and fluorescent tracers. J Comp Neurol 229:531–547

Steriade M, Gloor P, Llinas RR, Lopes da Silva FH, Mesulam M-M (1990) Basic mechanisms of cerebral rhythmic activities. Electroenceph clin Neurophysiol 76:481–508

Ticku MK, Lee JC, Murk S, Mhatre MC, Story JL, Kagan-Hallet K, Luther JS, MacCluer JW, Leland MM, Eidelberg E (1992) Inhibitory and excitatory amino acid receptors, c-fos expression, and calcium-binding proteins in the brain of baboons (papio hamadryas) that exibit "spontaneous" grand mal epilepsy. In: Engel JJ, Wasterlain C, Cavalheiro EA, Heinemann U, Avanzini G (eds) Molecular neurobiology of epilepsy. 9th edn, Elsevier, Amsterdam pp. 141–149

Tsakiridou E, Bertollini L, de-Curtis M, Avanzini G, Pape HC (1995) Selective increase in T-type calcium conductance of reticular thalamic neurons in a rat model of absence epilepsy. J Neurosci 15:3110–3117

Uematsu D, Araki N, Greenberg JH, Reivich M (1990) Alterations in cytosolic free calcium in the cat cortex during bicuculline-induced epilepsy. Brain Res Bull 24:285–288

Vergnes M, Marescaux C, Depaulis A, Micheletti G, Warter J (1986) Ontogeny of spontaneous petit mal-like seizures in wistar rats. Dev Brain Res 30:85–87

Vergnes M, Marescaux C, Depaulis A (1990) Mapping of spontaneous spike and wave discharges in Wistar rats with genetic generalized non-convulsive epilepsy. Brain Res 523:87–91

Wada JA (1994) Forebrain convulsive mechanisms examined in the primate model of generalized epilepsy: emphasis on the claustrum. In: Malafosse A, Genton P, Marescaux C, Broglin D, Bernasconi R (eds) Idiopathic generalized epilepsies: clinical, experimental and genetic aspects. John Libbey, London pp. 349–374

Willoughby JO, Mackenzie L (1992) Nonconvulsive electrocorticographic paroxysms (absence epilepsy) in rat strains. Lab Anim Sci 42:551–554

Willoughby JO, Mackenzie L, Medvedev A, Hiscock JJ (1995) Distribution of Fos-positive neurons in cortical and subcortical structures after picrotoxin-induced convulsions varies with seizure type. Brain Res 683:73–87

Willoughby JO, Mackenzie L, Medvedev A, Hiscock JJ (1997) Fos induction following systemic kainic acid: early expression in hippocampus and later widespread expression associated with seizure. Neuroscience 77:379–392

Wisden W, Seeburg PH (1993) A complex mosaic of high-affinity kainate receptors in rat brain. J Neurosci 13:3582–3598

Young AB, Fagg GE (1990) Excitatory amino acid receptors in the brain: membrane binding and receptor autoradiographic approaches. Trends Pharmacol Sci 11:126–132

CHAPTER 4

Epileptogenesis: Biochemical Aspects

B. Jarrott

A. Introduction

Epilepsies are defined as disorders of neuronal excitability characterized by periodic and unpredictable occurrences of seizures, while "seizures" are defined as transient changes of behaviour due to the disordered, synchronous, and rhythmic firing of populations of central nervous system neurons (McNamara 1994). These disorders of neuronal excitability can remain local or spread to other sites or engage all cortical regions simultaneously. Epileptogenesis could be defined as the molecular or cellular events producing the transient, disordered firing of a subpopulation of neurons in a key region of the brain, resulting in periodic seizures. A widely held view is that these seizures are caused by an abnormality in the major neurotransmitter systems of the brain such as excessive activity of the excitatory transmitters or impaired activity of the inhibitory transmitters, or a combination of both. However, the marked heterogeneity of syndromes (up to 50) diagnosed as epilepsy makes it most unlikely that there is a singular biochemical disorder that results in epileptogenesis. Furthermore, seizures set in motion a cascade of complex molecular and genomic changes, including changes in gene expression, sprouting of fibres, establishment of new synaptic contacts, alterations in expression of transmitters, modification of receptor expression, etc., that may contribute to the abnormally increased neuronal excitability and be responsible for a seizure-induced neuronal lesion. It is also recognized that epilepsy is an ongoing process in which repeated seizures may have an important impact on the brain and on the progression of the disorder. Thus it is essential that research should focus on understanding the biochemical basis of epileptogenesis since this should lead to the rational design of drugs both to prevent the development of epilepsy after insults such as head injury, brain tumours or febrile seizures, and also to minimize hyperexcitability at an existing epileptogenic focus which may be the result of a genetic disorder.

B. Methods for Studying Epileptogenesis

I. In Humans

1. Imaging Techniques

Technologies such as positron emission tomography and magnetic resonance imaging have had a dramatic impact on the evaluation for surgery of patients with intractable epilepsy and are now providing valuable insight into epileptogenesis through non-invasive, longitudinal studies (JACKSON and CONNELLY 1996; THEODORE 1996; KUZNIECKY 1997). Neurotransmitter receptors and transmitters such as γ-aminobutyric acid and glutamate can now be imaged with satisfactory resolution in epileptic patients and compared to controls (see Sect. C.I.2).

2. Neurophysiological Studies on Cortical Slices Maintained In Vitro

The increasing use of surgery to resect neocortical tissue containing the epileptogenic foci of patients whose seizures are resistant to pharmacological management, has provided a means for studying the neurophysiological, anatomical and neurochemical alterations in fresh human tissue. AVOLI and WILLIAMSON (1996) have comprehensively reviewed such published studies with human material. While the data are very interesting, these authors concluded that they have not yet revealed any definite cellular mechanism that may account for the expression of the epileptiform activity *in situ*. A major problem is access to control cortical slices from healthy subjects. Nevertheless such studies need to continue and to be guided by findings from studies of brain slices from animal models of epilepsy.

3. Microdialysis

The development of a combined microdialysis/depth electrode probe ('dialtrode') that can be stereotaxically implanted in the hippocampus of patients being investigated for their suitability for surgery has allowed chronic studies of transmitter efflux before, during and after seizures (DURING and SPENCER 1993) and has given insight into the biochemical basis of epileptogenesis (see Sects. C.I.1, C.I.2)

II. Animal Models

Animal models of epilepsy have played a key role for many years in both the screening and the development of potential anticonvulsant drugs and, more recently, in understanding the cellular and molecular basis of epileptogenesis (see also Chap. 2). The advantage of animal models is that adequate numbers of animals for meaningful statistical analysis can be obtained whilst invasive techniques, paying due regard to animal ethics principles, can give much more insight into the biochemical basis of epileptogenesis. Although over 50 different animal models have been reported that cover the multitude of types of epilepsy (FISHER 1989), this chapter deals primarily with the following 3 models:

1. Kindling

Kindling is an animal model of complex partial seizures (GODDARD et al. 1969), a common form of epilepsy in humans and one that is not well controlled by conventional anticonvulsant drugs. Kindling in rats is the process of repeated, intermittent (usually daily) application of subconvulsant electrical stimulation to the amygdala, normally with a depth electrode, which eventually induces generalized seizures after 15–30 applications. During the course of kindling, electrographic seizure activity is localized initially to the limbic areas but eventually spreads to other areas as seizures become generalized. The stages of kindling are classified behaviourally with stage 1 representing orofacial movements, stage 2 being head nodding, stage 3 forelimb clonus, stage 4 rearing and stage 5 rearing and falling (RACINE 1972). A rat is said to be fully kindled when stage 5 seizures are seen. This hyperexcitability is regarded as a permanent state that lasts the lifetime of the rat.

The kindling preparation of GODDARD et al. (1969) has been criticized as a model of human epilepsy because it relies on electrical stimulation to evoke a stage 5 seizure, whereas spontaneous seizures are a key feature of human epilepsy. However, it is not generally appreciated that if rats continue to be kindled after stage 5 has been reached, they will eventually develop spontaneous motor seizures (PINEL and ROVNER 1978), so that the widely held view that stage 5 represents the fully kindled state is mistaken. Nevertheless, the value of stopping kindling at stage 5, before spontaneous seizures occur, is that it is then possible to elicit a seizure when required, with electrical stimulation, and thus to separate the temporary biochemical changes due to the seizure itself from the biochemical changes due to the stage 5 kindled state many weeks after the last seizure.

2. Kainate Model

Kainic acid is a potent, long acting glutamate receptor agonist which, after systemic or intraventricular or intracerebral injection in rats, induces a syndrome similar to acute limbic status epilepticus and causes subsequent neuronal loss similar to that in temporal lobe epilepsy in humans (for a review, see SPERK 1994). This loss leads to a permanent decrease in seizure threshold similar to kindling, and kainate-treated rats months later become susceptible to spontaneous seizures. However, the neuronal loss after kainate is much greater than that with amygdaloid-kindling and it is difficult to determine whether the biochemical changes seen after kainate are due to the neuronal loss or to the epileptogenic state.

3. Genetic Strains

Genetic strains of mice, rats, fowl, gerbils and baboons have been used to study epileptogenesis as well as to screen for potential anticonvulsant drugs (see BUCHHALTER 1993; NOEBELS 1996). This approach will become more prominent and popular with the transgenic expression in mice of mutations in human epilepsy genes as they are identified.

III. Biochemical Techniques

The plethora of exciting techniques introduced over the last 10 years has shed new light on epileptogenesis. The cloning of receptors, enzymes, transporters, nerve growth factors, transcription factors and key structural proteins has allowed the application of techniques such as (a) *in situ* hybridization histochemical techniques to visualize the expression of these genes in brain sections, (b) generation of specific antibodies to localize the protein products of the genes by immunocytochemistry, (c) site-directed mutagenesis to determine the molecular mechanisms of the receptors, enzymes, transporters, growth factors, etc., (d) generation of transgenic rodents with null mutations to "knock-out" the actions of the cloned gene, and (e) synthesis of "anti-sense" oligonucleotides to inhibit the expression of the mRNA of the cloned gene. Other biochemical techniques such as high performance liquid chromatography and radioimmunoassays have permitted the measurement of transmitters in the extracellular space of brain nuclei after the stereotaxic implantation of microdialysis probes. The insights that such techniques have given into the biochemistry of epileptogenesis are detailed in Sects. C, D, and E of this chapter.

C. Role of Neurotransmitters in Epileptogenesis

I. Amino Acids

1. L-Glutamate

L-Glutamate and probably L-aspartate are the major excitatory amino acid transmitters in the brain and it has been long recognized that either excessive release of these excitatory amino acid transmitters or reduction in release of inhibitory transmitters leads rapidly to convulsions and death (CURTIS and JOHNSTON 1974).

a) Glutamate Release and Reuptake

In fully kindled amygdaloid rats, extracellular levels of glutamate and other amino acids have been measured after implantation of a microdialysis probe into the amygdala, both before and after an electrically stimulated seizure (KAURA et al. 1995). Basal levels of glutamate were elevated two- to threefold compared to sham-kindled rats, while a single electrical pulse resulted in a five- to sixfold increase in glutamate levels. On the other hand, basal GABA levels were significantly reduced by ~60%. It should be noted that the amino acid levels in the dialysate are the net result of release and reuptake by high affinity transporters and that therefore the maximum levels released may be much higher than the levels diffusing across the dialysis membrane. Nevertheless, the results for the basal release in kindled rats indicate a hyperactive state for glutamatergic release which could be due to impaired uptake, coupled with reduced release of GABA, a combination which could then initiate seizures.

A variation of this microdialysis technique has been applied to humans with complex partial epilepsy by DURING and SPENCER (1993) using a combination microdialysis/depth electrode ("dialtrode") implanted into each hippocampus. They found that the extracellular concentration of glutamate increased 1.5 min before, and for up to 16.5 min after, a seizure with a maximum rise of ~500% of basal release in the epileptogenic hippocampus, whereas in the non-epileptogenic hippocampus glutamate was increased only from 1.5 min before to 4.5 min after a seizure and then only by ~200%. On the other hand, when the dialysate was assayed for GABA, there was a significantly higher release from the non-epileptogenic hippocampus (~300%) only at 1.5 min after the seizure, compared with a ~100% value from the epileptogenic hippocampus. What was particularly significant and consistent in the six patients in this study was that: (a) the rise in glutamate preceded the EEG evidence of a seizure, which suggested that glutamate acted as a paracrine factor to produce a synchronized EEG population burst; (b) the delayed rise in GABA could indicate that it acted as a counter to the glutamate-induced excitation; (c) the lowered GABA response from the epileptogenic hippocampus suggests there may be altered release or reuptake of GABA at this site; and (d) the increased extracellular glutamate in the epileptogenic hippocampus, despite histological evidence of a loss of excitatory neurons, could be due to decreased glutamate uptake in this hippocampus.

More recently, Tanaka et al. (1997) have reported that transgenic mice homozygous to the null-mutation in the glutamate transporter gene, GLT-1, exhibit a 95% reduction in glutamate uptake into their cerebral cortex synaptosomes. Furthermore, electrophysiological experiments with hippocampal slices from these mice demonstrated that the peak concentration of synaptically released glutamate remained elevated in the synaptic cleft for longer periods than that recorded in slices from wild-type mice. Not only did these transgenic mice die prematurely but also they were observed to experience spontaneous seizures characterized by explosive running followed by a persistent opisthotonus posture and a Straub tail effect prior to dying a few minutes later. Postmortem examination ruled out haemorrhage, cardiovascular failure, ischaemia or major end-organ failure as the cause of death. Interestingly, histological examination of the brains of these homozygous mice aged 4–8 weeks revealed selective neuronal degeneration in the hippocampal CA_1 field in 7 out of 22 animals, which probably reflects individual differences in the occurrence of spontaneous seizures. These elegant studies emphasize the role of glutamate in causing excitotoxicity, as was first proposed by John Olney (see Rothman and Olney 1987). On the other hand, it does not necessarily mean that epileptogenesis is due to a failure of or deficiency in glutamate transporters; rather, that glutamate transporters play a key role in ensuring that the concentration of free glutamate in the synaptic cleft is kept low.

b) Glutamate Receptors

The receptors for the excitatory amino acids in brain have been divided into at least four broad subclasses based upon receptor sensitivity to synthetic agonists and antagonists: the three ionotropic subtypes: NMDA, AMPA and kainate receptors (NAKANISHI 1992; SOMMER and SEEBURG 1992) and the metabotropic G-protein linked receptors (SCHOEPP and JOHNSON 1993).

α) NMDA Receptors

These receptors are normally gated by Mg^{2+} in a voltage dependent manner and thus do not normally seem to be involved in low frequency synaptic transmission. If isolated rat brain slices are superfused with Mg^{2+}-free medium, this relieves the voltage-dependent block of the ion channel component of the NMDA receptor and leads to the appearance of spontaneous electrical paroxysmal events (HORNE et al. 1986). Similarly, if slices made from human epileptogenic neocortex removed during surgery for temporal lobe epilepsy are superfused with Mg^{2+}-free medium, seizure-like discharges are recorded that resemble the electrographic pattern associated with tonic-clonic seizures and which can be antagonized with an NMDA receptor antagonist (AVOLI et al. 1987). This indicates that NMDA receptors play a role in the genesis of prolonged epileptiform discharges.

Furthermore, after amygdala or hippocampal kindling in rats, the NMDA receptors in the dentate gyrus become actively involved in synaptic transmission (MODY and HEINEMANN 1987) as studied by intracellular recordings from granule cells. These authors concluded that this may underlie the long-lasting changes induced by kindling. More refined whole-cell patch clamp and cell-attached single channel recordings of granule cells acutely isolated from control and kindled rats by KÖHR et al. (1993) showed that kindling affects the mean open time of NMDA channels, and their sensitivity to intracellular adenosine triphosphate (ATP), but not their desensitization or single-channel conductance. These authors concluded that these alterations reflect a change in the molecular structure of NMDA channels and may underlie the maintenance of the epileptic state.

Biochemical studies on hippocampal slices from amygdaloid kindled rats also showed long-lasting enhanced responses to NMDA as measured by NMDA receptor-mediated inhibition of agonist-stimulated phosphoinositide hydrolysis (MORRISETT et al. 1989). This laboratory then demonstrated a selective and long-lasting (1 month) increased sensitivity to NMDA-evoked depolarizations in CA_3 pyramidal cells of the hippocampus of kindled rats (MARTIN et al. 1992). This was followed up by a complementary biochemical study (KRAUS et al. 1994). In this study, radioreceptor NMDA assays on microdissected regions (CA_1, CA_3 and fascia dentata) of the hippocampus of rats 28 days after the last kindled seizure showed a 2.8-fold increase in the Bmax (the maximum number of binding sites) only in the CA_3 region using ^{3}H-CPP but no change using ^{3}H-CGS 19755, another NMDA receptor antagonist. Furthermore, *in situ* hybridization histochemistry with riboprobes of NMDA receptor subunit genes (NMDAR1, NR2A, NR2B, NR2C, NR2D and GBP) were not altered by kindling. Thus KRAUS et al. (1994) concluded that a novel NMDA receptor subtype may be responsible for the increased sensitivity of

CA_3 neurons to NMDA in kindled rats. A similar result and conclusion was reached by PRATT et al. (1993), *viz.* that maintenance of enhanced seizure susceptibility in kindling is not due to altered expression of major NMDA receptor subunits, although a post-translational modification of the NMDA receptor would be an alternative possibility.

Pharmacological studies have also provided evidence that amygdaloid kindling in rats alters the susceptibility of NMDA receptors to their antagonists. Thus, the competitive NMDA receptor antagonists, CGP 37849 and CGP 39551, as well as the non-competitive antagonist, dizocilpine (MK-801), which were potent anticonvulsants against maximal electroshock seizures in naive rats, exerted only weak anticonvulsant effects in fully kindled rats and did not increase the focal seizure threshold (LÖSCHER and HÖNACK 1991). Furthermore, these NMDA receptor antagonists produced untoward, stereotypic behavioural responses in kindled rats that were not seen in non-kindled rats.

In human epileptic hippocampus slices after surgical resection, ISOKAWA and LEVESQUE (1991) used intracellular recordings of excitatory postsynaptic potentials to find an elevated NMDA response in dentate granule cells to perforant path stimulation. These authors suggested that activation of previously dormant NMDA receptors in pathologic neurons may be a mediator for epileptogenic synaptic transmission and associated neuronal degeneration.

β) AMPA/Kainate Receptors

Recent studies with the GluR3 subunit of the AMPA/kainate subclass of receptors have suggested that autoantibodies to this subunit could play a key role in the epileptogenesis which is characteristic of Rasmussen's encephalitis, a rare, progressive, catastrophic disease affecting previously normal children (ROGERS et al. 1994, 1996). A fortuitous observation was made that rabbits immunized with peptide sequences of GluR3, but not other glutamate receptor subunits, developed seizures and had early histopathological changes in the brain characteristic of Rasmussen's encephalitis. When these rabbit immunoglobulins were isolated and tested on isolated brain slices, rapid and reversible depolarizing responses were seen that could be blocked by the AMPA receptor antagonist, 6-cyano-7-nitroquinoxaline-2,3-dione (CNQX), but not the NMDA receptor antagonist, dizocilpine (TWYMAN et al. 1995). It was suggested that in Rasmussen's encephalitis, there may be a breakdown in the blood-brain barrier (as a result of injury or infection) which allows presentation of GluR3 antigen to the immune system for subsequent development of autoantibodies which then gain access to the brain and persistently activate the AMPA/kainate receptors on cortical or hippocampal neurons to cause epilepsy and/or excitotoxicity. This fits with clinical data showing some amelioration of seizures in affected children after plasma exchange, which suggests circulating GluR3 autoantibodies may have been removed (ANDREWS and MCNAMARA 1996). It also explains why hemispherectomy is effective, *viz.* that the affected cortex with its focal disruption of the blood-brain barrier that allowed access of the autoantibodies to the antigenic AMPA/kainate receptors is removed. Hopefully, a better understanding of this autoimmune disorder will lead to a less drastic treatment option.

Electrophysiological studies have shown that AMPA receptors in the open state gate only the entry of Na^+ and not Ca^{2+}. Molecular biology experiments have revealed that this selectivity is due to a key arginine residue at position 586 on the GluR2 receptor subunit. This is not gene encoded but is post-transcriptionally introduced by site-selective adenosine deamination. Brusa et al. (1995) have bred transgenic mice with an editing-deficient GluR2 allele that then express AMPA receptors with increased Ca^{2+} permeability. After 2 weeks postnatal development, these mice develop spontaneous and recurrent seizures and became progressively agitated with excessive jumping and running fits. All mice died by day 20 and postmortem analysis of their brains showed selective neuronal degeneration in the hippocampal CA_3 field with an absence of glial reaction. No other pathological features were seen. This experimental model of epilepsy raises the possibility that some human familial epilepsies could arise through aberrant expression of unedited GluR2 subunits in the hippocampus.

γ) Metabotropic Glutamate Receptors

It is now recognized that this is a family of G-protein coupled receptors (Schoepp and Johnson 1993) and that these receptors could play a role both in the development of the electrically kindled state in rats and also in the initiation of seizures in fully kindled rats (Attwell et al. 1995). This view is based on studies by these workers showing that the selective agonist, ACPD, when directly injected daily into the amygdala, inhibited the development of epileptogenesis beyond stage 2 (Racine's classification of electrical kindling), whereas rats injected with vehicle progressed to stage 5 (generalized seizure) over the same time period. On the other hand, in fully kindled rats, ACPD dose-dependently increased the generalized seizure threshold and decreased motor seizure duration after injections into the amygdala. Biochemical studies with cortical synaptosomes showed that ACPD was potent in inhibiting the depolarization-induced release of glutamate or aspartate via an action on presynaptic metabotropic receptors. These authors therefore suggested that glutamate-mediated excitation was a major influence in the development of kindling and the initiation of seizures in this rat model of complex partial seizures.

2. GABA

a) GABA Synthesis and Storage

γ-Aminobutyric acid (GABA) is the principal inhibitory neurotransmitter and exerts a hyperpolarizing action in all forebrain neurons. Neurons that store GABA can now be localized by immunohistochemistry with reasonable specificity in brain sections after fixation using polyclonal or monoclonal antibodies (SCHIFFMANN et al. 1988; LEHMANN et al. 1996). They can also be localized by staining with antiserum directed against glutamate decarboxylase, the enzyme that synthesizes GABA (SCHWARZER and SPERK 1995). These studies have shown that GABA is present in many interneurons or local circuit neurons in the central nervous system as well as in long projecting neurons such as striato-nigral, nigro-thalamic or cerebellar Purkinje-olivary neurons. More important, immunohistology studies have shown that other putative transmitter candidates such as neuropeptides are present in GABAergic neurons.

Ever since the discovery of the powerful inhibitory actions of GABA in the brain by Eugene Roberts in 1950, it has been postulated that epileptic seizures would result if GABAergic function was impaired (ROBERTS 1984). Similarly, LLOYD et al. (1985) reported significant decreases in glutamate decarboxylase activity, the enzyme that synthesizes GABA from glutamate, as well as reduced GABA binding, in resected samples of epileptogenic human cortex. However, subsequent studies with epileptogenic human hippocampus using immunohistochemical localization of glutamate decarboxylase showed that neurons containing this enzyme were relatively unaffected by the hippocampal sclerosis typical of temporal lobe epilepsy and even appeared to be resistant to the pathogenic mechanisms responsible for sclerosis and focal seizures (BABB et al. 1989). On the other hand, using the temporal cortex removed from patients with intractable temporal lobe epilepsy, MARCO et al. (1996) carried out a comprehensive immunohistochemical mapping study using antisera directed against (a) glutamate decarboxylase, (b) parvalbumin and (c) glial fibrillary acidic protein. They found multiple small regions with abnormal patterns of decreased immunostaining for glutamate decarboxylase and parvalbumin which were never seen in cortex from controls. The most conspicuous and common change was a loss of GABAergic chandelier interneurons which normally exert powerful regulation of impulse generation in cortical pyramidal neurons.

A novel, non-invasive technique, nuclear magnetic resonance spectroscopic editing, allows the serial measurement of GABA levels in regions of human brain such as the occipital lobe (PETROFF et al. 1996a). These workers compared GABA levels in the occipital cortex of patients with complex partial seizures with those in age-matched subjects without a history of seizures. The former group had levels that were 13% lower than the latter group. Interestingly, there were significant associations between low brain GABA levels in epileptic patients and recent seizures and, conversely, between high brain levels and patients whose seizures were well controlled. This exciting technique has also proved ideal for studying serial changes in brain GABA levels in epileptic patients treated with drugs such as vigabatrin (PETROFF et al. 1996b). The results with this imaging technique in conscious patients are consistent with the immunohistological data showing a loss of GABA interneurons in resected cortical tissue obtained by MARCO et al. (1996: see above). This raises the issue of whether delivery of exogenous GABA into brain areas would reduce or prevent epileptic seizures, by analogy with the strategy of elevating the dopamine levels in the striatum of parkinsonian patients whose dopaminergic neurons have become depleted below a threshold number. Preliminary studies with a polymer that releases GABA implanted bilaterally dorsal to the substantia nigra in amygdaloid-kindled rats, showed that seizures were suppressed significantly whilst the polymer was releasing GABA (KOKAIA et al. 1994). Unfortunately, the polymer was able to release sufficient GABA to have a marked anticonvulsant effect for only 2–3 days. Obviously, a much longer-acting polymer delivery technology needs to be developed before this approach could be considered for therapeutic trials.

b) *GABA Transporters*

Microdialysis probe studies in humans with temporal lobe epilepsy by DURING et al. (1995) have shed interesting light on the role of GABA in the hippocampus. A probe was implanted in both the epileptic hippocampus and the homotopic site of the contralateral hippocampus. Studies were carried out at least 7 days after implantation and a minimum of 24h after the last seizure. DURING et al. (1995) found that the basal GABA concentration was similar in dialysates from both probes but that high K^+ (56mM), Ca^{2+}-dependent release of GABA was significantly greater in the epileptogenic hippocampus than in the normal hippocampus (32-fold versus 14-fold respectively).On the other hand, the local perfusion with exogenous L-glutamate (5mM) induced a 4.6-fold increase in GABA in the dialysate from the non-epileptogenic hippocampus compared with a non-significant increase (1.7-fold) in the epileptogenic hippocampus. Parallel studies in amygdala-kindled rats gave similar results and further studies with these rats indicated both that glutamate-induced release was mediated by a GABA transporter and that this glutamate-impaired release of GABA after amydgaloid kindling was due to a decrease in the number of GABA-transporters in the hippocampus (DURING et al. 1995). These authors proposed that during periods of intense neural excitation, the release of GABA may be mediated in part by the GABA transporters (i.e. non-vesicular release) and that this diffusely increases inhibitory tone. The hypothesized loss of GABA transporters in human temporal lobe epilepsy would diminish this alternate release mechanism for GABA and thus neuronal hyperexcitability would predominate, leading to a seizure.

c) *GABA Receptors*

α) $GABA_A$ Receptors

$GABA_A$ receptors comprise a family of ligand-gated ion channels which consist of a heteropentameric protein that allows the passage of Cl^- into the neuron in the presence of GABA. The subunits are related but distinct as they are coded by different genes (OLSEN and TOBIN 1990; SMITH and OLSEN 1995).

Molecular biology studies have shown that there are at least six α subunits, 4 β, 4 γ, 1 δ and 2 ρ subunits, with splice variants of some as well. Thus, mathematically there are a large number (hundreds) of possible permutations for a pentameric subunit ion channel (SIGEL et al. 1990), and these could differ in sensitivity to modulators such as benzodiazepines or neurosteroids, although biochemical studies suggest there are 12–24 isoforms which are sufficiently abundant to have a physiological role.

Amygdaloid kindling in rats leads to a long-term decrease in neuronal sensitivity to applied GABA in dorsal raphe neurons which is still measurable 3 months after the last stage 5 seizure as recorded electrophysiologically (HERNANDEZ and GALLAGER 1992). While an obvious deduction would be that this may be due to altered expression of $GABA_A$ receptor subunits, a comprehensive analysis of the expression of 13 different $GABA_A$ subunits in rat brain sections by *in situ* hybridization histochemistry (KAMPHUIS et al. 1995) showed few long-term changes 1 month after the last seizure in fully kindled rats. Only a decrease in the long-splice $\gamma 2$ subunit was found in the pyramidal and granular neurons of the hippocampus although prominent enhanced changes in subunit expression were seen at the early stages of kindling acquisition. These authors suggested that the long-lasting impaired neuronal sensitivity to GABA might be due to modified receptor phosphorylation. This is a reasonable hypothesis given that *in vitro* biochemical studies have shown that protein kinase C is able to phosphorylate $GABA_A$ β and $\gamma 2$ subunits, and this results in a negative modulation of membrane currents in isolated cultured neurons (KRISHEK et al. 1994).

In the strain of the genetic absence epilepsy rat of Strasbourg (GAERS), the $\beta 2$ and $\beta 3$ $GABA_A$ subunits were reduced in frontal neocortex and anterior thalamic nuclei. This correlated with reduced binding of the benzodiazepine ligand, ^{3}H-flunitrazepam (SPREAFICO et al. 1993).

β) $GABA_B$ Receptors

$GABA_B$ receptors are located primarily on presynaptic GABA terminals in brain where they function as autoreceptors to decrease GABA release once the concentration of GABA builds up in the synaptic cleft. In contrast to the $GABA_A$ receptor, the $GABA_B$ receptor is a 7-transmembrane spanning protein that is coupled via a GTP-binding protein to a K^+ channel or adenylate cyclase, so that stimulation by GABA causes an increase in K^+ conductance and a hyperpolarizing response which reduces release of the transmitter. The typical $GABA_B$ receptor selective agonist is baclofen, while the most selective antagonists are phaclofen and CGP-353348.

Studies have shown that intracortical injections of baclofen in rats induces epileptogenic discharges, and phaclofen and CGP-355348 antagonize this action of baclofen (BRAILOWSKY et al. 1995). It is possible that the epileptogenic action of baclofen could be due to release of aspartate and activation of NMDA receptors in the hippocampus.

The inbred genetic mouse strain, lethargic (*lh/lh*), which has a single-locus defect on chromosome 2, exhibits spontaneous seizures that have behavioural and electrographic features of absence seizures in humans. Baclofen significantly increases seizure frequency in *lh/lh* mice but at the same dose in wild-type mice only causes sedation, which suggests that baclofen is not merely acting as a proconvulsant (HOSFORD et al. 1992). Furthermore, CGP-35348 produces a dose-dependent reduction in seizure frequency in *lh/lh* mice. Additionally, receptor binding assays show a significant increase (26%) in the density of $GABA_B$ receptors, but not in $GABA_A$- or NMDA-receptors, in neocortical membranes prepared from these mice, and also show synaptically evoked $GABA_B$ receptor-mediated inhibition of NMDA excitatory postsynaptic potentials in the CA_1 region of hippocampal slices from *lh/lh* mice. Autoradiographic localization of $GABA_B$ receptors in these mice brains also showed increased binding throughout the thalamic nuclei (HOSFORD 1995). This author also suggested that thalamic relay neurons are endowed with voltage-dependent T-type Ca^{2+} channels with the capacity to undergo burst-firing. After activation by GABA released by GABAergic inputs from tonically active nucleus reticularis thalami neurons, T-channels are quickly inactivated and they require lengthy hyperpolarization to remove their inactivation (a process called deinactivation). Thus, in this strain of mice, $GABA_B$ receptors play a role in the epileptogenesis of absence-like seizures, possibly by deinactivating T-type Ca^{2+} channels and triggering a synchronous burst firing of thalamic neurons.

II. Biogenic Amines

The biogenic amines, noradrenaline, dopamine, 5-hydroxytryptamine and acetylcholine, are now well accepted as neurotransmitters in the central nervous system. Pharmacological manipulation of levels of noradrenaline, 5-hydroxytryptamine and acetylcholine in the central nervous system influences seizure frequency or intensity. Thus it has been suggested that epileptogenesis may be due to altered aminergic neurotransmission in the central nervous system.

1. Noradrenaline

It is now established that noradrenergic mechanisms in the brain modulate and reduce epileptic discharges induced by a variety of chemical methods or by electrical kindling. In the case of amygdaloid kindling in rats, depletion of forebrain noradrenaline by reserpine markedly facilitates the rate of kindling development but, in contrast, depletion of noradrenaline after kindling has been established does not exacerbate kindled seizures (WESTERBERG et al. 1984). Pharmacological studies with selective adrenoceptor drugs have shown that the α_2-adrenoceptor agonist, clonidine, dose-dependently suppressed kindling development in rats while treatment with α_2-adrenoceptor antagonists (idazoxan, yohimbine) facilitated kindling development but neither type of drug modified seizures elicited in previously kindled rats (GELLMAN et al. 1987). Thus the exogenous α_2-adrenoceptor agonist, clonidine, and presumably the endogenous α_2-adrenoceptor agonist, noradrenaline, exert antiepileptogenic but not anticonvulsant actions in this animal model. On the other hand, the β-adrenoceptor antagonist propranolol significantly retarded the development of the fully kindled state in rats (KOKAIA et al. 1989a)

In particular, considerable evidence has shown that locus coeruleus noradrenergic neurons act to dampen epileptic activity in the brain (CHAUVEL and TROTTIER 1986). Pharmacological manipulation indicated that it was noradrenaline rather than dopamine that modulated seizure activity. In fully kindled rats with a microdialysis probe in the hippocampus, basal release of noradrenaline was reduced. This supports the hypothesis that attenuation of noradrenergic neurotransmission contributes to the kindling phenomenon (KOKAIA et al. 1989b). However, an electrically induced seizure gave a ~threefold rise in noradrenaline levels in the stimulated hippocampus within the first minute, which was similar to the response to seizures in non-kindled rats, suggesting that the noradrenergic pathways in the kindled hippocampus are still functional. Destruction of the noradrenergic forebrain neurons in rats using the chemical neurotoxin 6-hydroxydopamine markedly facilitates the rate of kindling to stage 5; conversely, bilateral implantation of locus coeruleus grafts into the hippocampus or piriform cortex of 6-hydroxydopamine-treated rats retards the development of kindling, an effect probably due to the noradrenergic neurons in the graft reinnervating the dorsal hippocampal formation (BARRY et al. 1989). Functional studies with intracerebral microdialysis probes in the hippocampus of 6-hydroxydopamine-treated rats after locus coeruleus grafts showed that there was a ~threefold increase in noradrenaline release during electrical kindling seizures, which was similar to the release in the hippocampus of control rats (KOKAIA et al. 1989b; BENGZON et al. 1990). Furthermore, the seizure-suppressant actions of intra-hippocampal locus coeruleus grafts were blocked by administration of the α_2-adrenoceptor antagonist idazoxan before each kindling stimulation. These results suggest that noradrenaline released from locus coeruleus grafts inhibits kindling via activation of α_2-adrenoceptors (BENGZON et al. 1990). Electrophysiological experiments (STANTON et al. 1989) on hippocampal slices from fully kindled rats showed that noradrenaline's normal action, which is to depolarize dentate gyrus granule cells, increase input resistance, firing and Ca^{2+} influx in response to repetitive stimulation and long-lasting potentiation of synaptic potentials, was markedly reduced. These reduced responses were probably due to down-regulation of both α_1- and β_1-adrenoceptors. It is interesting that a decrease in α_1-adrenoceptor binding sites was found in "actively spiking" temporal lobe tissue resected from epileptic patients (BRIERE et al. 1986).

JOBE et al. (1994) have reviewed the evidence for the role of noradrenergic neurotransmission in the seizure predisposition of genetically epilepsy-prone rats (GEPR). They concluded that a deficit in noradrenaline levels and turnover in the superior colliculus and/or ventrally adjacent regions acted as a determinant not only of seizure susceptibility but also of exaggerated seizure responsiveness and of deficient seizure thresholds in this rat strain. However, they cautioned that other neurotransmitter systems could also be involved in the predisposition to seizures.

2. 5-Hydroxytryptamine

In the case of the genetically epilepsy-prone rat (GEPR), sertraline, a highly selective and potent inhibitor of neuronal uptake of 5-hydroxytryptamine, produced a dose-dependent reduction in the intensity of audiogenic seizures and increased the extracellular levels of 5-hydroxytryptamine in the thalamus as assessed by microdialysis (YAN et al. 1995). This action countered the deficiencies in endogenous 5-hydroxytryptamine in the midbrain of these rats.

3. Acetylcholine

The basal forebrain cholinergic neurons have been implicated in the mechanisms of kindling since muscarinic antagonists (atropine) and atropine plus the nicotinic antagonist (mecamylamine) retard the development of amygdaloid kindling, while local injections of cholinergic agonists into the brain result in seizures. Furthermore, muscarinic cholinoceptors are downregulated during amygdaloid kindling, suggesting that there is increased acetylcholine release during kindling. On the other hand, destruction of cholinergic neurons in the hippocampus and neocortex markedly facilitates the initial stages of seizure development, but not the progression from focal to generalized seizures (KOKAIA et al. 1996).

Genetic Absence-Epilepsy Rats of Strasbourg (GAERS), which are derived from the Wistar rat strain, exhibit spontaneous bilateral and synchronous spike-and-wave discharges during quiet wakefulness but almost never during active behaviour and sleep. The frontoparietal cortex and relay nuclei of the ventrolateral part of the thalamus are critical in the generation of absence seizures (DANOBER et al. 1995). The activities of these structures are under the control of ascending cholinergic neurons originating in the nucleus basalis and the mesopontine cholinergic nuclei. Excitotoxic lesions of the nucleus basalis irreversibly suppressed absence seizures, presumably because of depletion of cortical cholinergic innervation producing a reduction of cortical excitability (DANOBER et al. 1994).

Biochemical studies of cholinergic markers (choline acetyltransferase and acetylcholinesterase) in human lateral temporal cortex removed to treat intractable epilepsy have shown modest increases (~25%) in areas of actively spiking cortex compared with non-spiking areas (KISH et al. 1988). These authors suggested that this represents sprouting of cholinergic nerve terminals in the spiking areas, but immunocytochemical evidence is required to confirm this hypothesis.

Autosomal dominant nocturnal frontal lobe epilepsy is a partial epilepsy which causes frequent, violent but brief seizures at night. STEINLEIN et al. (1995) have studied an Australian family with this disorder and found a missense mutation in the neuronal nicotinic acetylcholine receptor. This abnormality was in the $\alpha 4$ subunit, where a serine residue was replaced by a phenylalanine residue in the second transmembrane domain of this ionotropic receptor, resulting in impaired nicotinic cholinergic function. As cholinergic transmission is particularly active during sleep, impaired transmission in subjects with this mutation could be the molecular basis of their epileptogenesis.

III. Neuropeptides

It is now recognized that there are at least 40 diverse classes of peptides in the brain that are: (a) localized in subpopulations of neurons that contain the classical neurotransmitters such as glutamate, GABA, and biogenic amines, (b) processed in cell bodies from large protein precursors and packaged into vesicles for transport by axoplasmic flow to terminals, (c) preferentially released at high frequencies of nerve stimulation (>10 Hz), and (d) interact with specific receptors on postsynaptic neurons where they have potent depolarizing or hyperpolarizing effects (HÖKFELT 1991). These are the criteria that suggest a neurotransmitter function for these neuropeptides, although the general view is that these neuropeptides probably function as neuromodulators rather as primary transmitters since they do not appear to be released at low frequency nerve firing and nerve terminals have no mechanisms for conservation of neuropeptide stores such as active reuptake into the nerve terminal after transmitter release or local synthesis. These are essential mechanisms for conservation of the classical amino acid and biogenic amine transmitters. Another view of the role of neuropeptides in the brain is that they function as "volume" transmitters rather than as "point to point" transmitters across synapses, unlike the classical amino acid transmitters (AGNATI et al. 1995). This view is based on the fact that there is no mechanism for the rapid inactivation of some neuropeptides at the synaptic junction, unlike the situation for the classical transmitters; hence these neuropeptides are able to diffuse considerable distances from their point of release after high frequency stimulation, thereby interacting with their receptors on many other neurons (DUGGAN et al. 1990).

Many papers have now reported alterations in neuropeptides in the hippocampus and other limbic regions after experimental seizures in laboratory animals. It appears that these changes depend upon whether the seizures were induced either by conventional amygdaloid kindling or fast kindling or kainate injections or by status epilepticus methods. It is essential in these studies that the time courses be determined since many changes in peptide levels may simply be a consequence of a seizure rather than a key neurochemical component of epileptogenesis.

SCHWARZER et al. (1995, 1996) have recently reviewed the published literature on neuropeptide changes in limbic regions of rats after a variety of induced seizures (kainic acid, fast kindling and status epilepticus). It could be concluded that the key neuropeptides involved in epileptogenesis are the following: neuropeptide Y, somatostatin, cholecystokinin and dynorphin.

1. Neuropeptide Y

In the hippocampus of rats, neuropeptide Y is present in a subpopulation of hilar interneurons which also are immunoreactive for somatostatin and GABA. These neurons degenerate after kainate-induced seizures, whereas basket cells in the dentate gyrus which also stain for GABA and neuropeptide Y survive these seizures (SPERK et al. 1992). Interestingly, glutamatergic excitatory mossy fibres arising from the granule cells of the dentate gyrus do not contain neuropeptide Y constitutively, but express high levels of neuropeptide Y mRNA and immunoreactivity after kainate-induced seizures in rats (MARKSTEINER et al. 1990; SPERK et al. 1992) and in resected temporal lobes of epileptic patients (DE LANEROLLE et al. 1989).

In slices of hippocampus, exogenously applied neuropeptide Y inhibits potassium-stimulated release of glutamate (GREBER et al. 1994) and also reduces hippocampal epileptiform activity (COLMERS and BLEAKMAN 1994). In slices of hippocampus taken from electrically kindled rats, the release of neuropeptide Y was measured by a sensitive radioimmunoassay (RIZZI et al. 1993). With high potassium stimulation, there was enhanced release of neuropeptide Y from hippocampal slices from kindled rats compared with sham rats, but no difference in spontaneous efflux of the peptide. This enhanced release persisted for at least 1 month after kindling, which suggests that neuropeptide Y plays a role in the enduring changes in synaptic transmission found in kindled hippocampi.

In vivo studies have shown that, if neuropeptide Y is administered into the right lateral ventricle of rats in nanomole doses (1.5–6 nmol), it is very effective in blocking kainate-induced motor seizures as well as in strongly decreasing epileptiform EEG activity in limbic areas (WOLDBYE et al. 1997). It appears to exert this action through the Y_5 subtype of receptor. Conversely, neuropeptide Y gene "knock-out" mice, with undetectable brain levels of neuropeptide Y mRNA and immunoreactivity, exhibit mild seizures characterized by jerking of the head and body, forelimb clonus, tail erections and vocalizations particularly when placed on top of their cage. Also, these mice are more sensitive to pentylenetetrazole-induced seizures than wild-type or heterozygous littermates (ERICKSON et al. 1996). Thus there is a good case for regarding neuropeptide Y as an endogenous anticonvulsant (SPERK and HERZOG 1997).

2. Somatostatin

Somatostatin is present in hilar interneurons together with neuropeptide Y and GABA. There is an increased concentration of both peptides as measured by RIA and an increased projection to the outer molecular layer in the dorsal and ventral hippocampus as measured by immunocytochemistry, both at the proconvulsive stage 2 and after full kindling (SCHWARZER et al. 1996). It is believed that somatostatin released in these areas may serve to control granule and pyramidal cell excitability through a hyperpolarizing action and may have a tonic inhibitory action on kindling epileptogenesis since an infusion of an anti-somatostatin antibody into the dorsal hippocampus of rats undergoing kindling enhanced the rate of kindling (MONNO et al. 1993). In addition, injection of a peptidase-resistant somatostatin analogue had an anticonvulsant action against quinolinate-induced seizures in the hippocampus.

3. Cholecystokinin

Cholecystokinin has been reported to have anticonvulsant activity against electrically induced seizures in rats and increased cholecystokinin immunoreactivity was seen in the inner molecular layer of the dentate gyrus where the terminals form a dense plexus adjacent to the granule cells. These changes were more pronounced at stage 2 than at stage 5 of kindling (SCHWARZER et al. 1996). In the cortex of kindled rats, rapid but transient changes in preprocholecystokinin mRNA have been measured by *in situ* hybridization histochemistry, but these changes were associated with the acute seizure activity rather than the permanent kindling mechanism (BURAZIN and GUNDLACH 1996).

4. Dynorphin

The mossy fibre pathway from the dentate gyrus to the CA_3 pyramidal neurons contains both glutamate and the opioid peptide, dynorphin. High frequency stimulation, in addition to generating fast excitatory postsynaptic potentials due to release of glutamate, also generates a long-lasting inhibition of neighbouring mossy fibre synapses by a presynaptic action of released dynorphin achieved via activation of presynaptic$^+$ receptors (WEISSKOPF et al. 1993). The actions of endogenous dynorphin are slow and prolonged, reaching a peak within 2 min and lasting several minutes, and also result in a block of long-term potentiation (WAGNER et al. 1993) which is involved in both learning and kindling. Furthermore, intracerebral injection of dynorphin suppresses electrically kindled seizures (BONHAUS et al. 1987). However, neither endogenous dynorphin levels nor dynorphin mRNA are altered after kindling (ROSEN et al. 1992), which indicates that this opioid peptide is not involved in the permanent kindling state.

IV. Purines

The purine base, adenosine, and its nucleotide ATP, are present in high concentrations in brain and have potent electrophysiological effects (STONE 1981; EDWARDS and GIBB 1993). An interesting view is that ATP functions as a fast, excitatory transmitter across certain synapses in the CNS via stimulation of postsynaptic P_{2X}-purinoceptors, allowing influx of Ca^{2+}; however, the ATP is then rapidly catabolized to adenosine by ecto-ATPases at the synapse (EDWARDS 1996).This nascent adenosine could then act postsynaptically via P_1 purinoceptors to hyperpolarize the neuron by opening K^+ channels and even act presynaptically to inhibit release of transmitters including glutamate and GABA. In other words, ATP could act as a dual transmitter, causing brief excitation followed by inhibition, both pre- and postsynaptically due to its rapid breakdown to adenosine. Unfortunately, due to the lack of sufficiently sensitive histochemical techniques, the extent of ATP-releasing pathways in the brain is not known, nor is it known if adenosine is stored in vesicles in nerve terminals in the brain as a transmitter in its own right.

DRAGUNOW (1988) has comprehensively reviewed the literature on the putative role of adenosine in epilepsy, and the outcome strengthens his earlier, attractive hypothesis that adenosine is the brain's natural anticonvulsant, since synaptic inhibition is believed to play a critical role in limiting the size and duration of epileptic discharges. It is clear that adenosine and its synthetic analogues, as well as adenosine uptake inhibitors, are effective in decreasing epileptiform activity both *in vitro* and *in vivo* in models of seizures and that brain levels of adenosine increase within seconds following the onset of experimental seizures, a finding which could explain why seizures arrest spontaneously even in the absence of anticonvulsant drugs (DURING and SPENCER 1992). Interestingly, NAGY et al. (1990) reported that ecto-ATPase was about 30% reduced in human epileptic temporal cortex and anterior hippocampus compared to non-spiking human temporal tissue. This lessened amount of enzyme may reduce the extracellular concentration of adenosine in this area and thus delay the terminations of convulsions. On the other hand, there was enhanced ecto-ATPase activity in the posterior hippocampus which included the dentate gyrus and CA_3 field. The authors suggested that this was due to the presence of mossy fibres of the granule cells and represented a compensatory reaction of epileptic neurons. Thus, during seizure discharges, large amounts of ATP may be co-released with transmitters in the affected brain area. Increased ecto-ATPase activity would be necessary both to remove the excitatory transmitter and also to provide sufficient amounts of adenosine to depress the evoked release of transmitters.

A study of synthetic analogues of adenosine has demonstrated that compounds which are selective agonists for adenosine A_1 receptors, such as N^6-cyclohexyladenosine and N^6-cyclopentyladenosine, were most potent in preventing status epilepticus in a rat model involving continuous electrical stimulation of the hippocampus, whereas in another rat model of recurrent electrical stimulation of the hippocampus, the administration of adenosine A_1 receptor antagonists such as 8-cyclopentyl-1,3-dimethylxanthine precipitated status epilepticus (YOUNG and DRAGUNOW 1994). Interestingly, 6 days later, in this latter group of rats, as compared with vehicle-injected rats, there was a massive, bilateral loss of nerve cells in the CA_1 and CA_3 regions of the hippocampus. Conversely, in the rats that did not develop status epilepticus as a result of prior treatment with the adenosine A_1 receptor agonist, there was no loss of neurons. Since treatment with a selective adenosine A_2 receptor agonist had no effect in either stimulation paradigm, it was concluded that adenosine A_1 receptors play a key role in the anticonvulsant effects. Further support for a key role for the adenosine A_1 receptors comes from quantitative autoradiographic studies with the selective radioligand ^{3}H-cyclohexyladenosine in surgically excised neocortex from patients suffering from intractable temporal lobe epilepsy (ANGELATOU et al. 1993). These authors found that there was a significant (48%) increase in adenosine A_1 receptor binding in all six cortical layers from epileptic patients compared to control temporal lobe tissue. They concluded that there was a significant upregulation of these receptors which may constitute a protective mechanism against subsequent seizures by enhancing the depressant response of neocortical neurons to endogenous adenosine.

V. Nitric Oxide

Nitric oxide (NO) is a small, rapidly diffusible free radical that is generated enzymatically by a family of isoenzymes, nitric oxide synthase (NOS), from the amino acid L-arginine, the other product being citrulline (ZHANG and SNYDER 1995). Two isoforms of NOS have been found in the brain, an inducible, Ca^{2+}/calmodulin-dependent form and a constitutive form known as neuronal NOS which is coupled to the NMDA receptor (ZHANG and SNYDER 1995). Neurally released glutamate can stimulate both the NMDA receptor and neuronal NOS, resulting in generation of NO that then activates guanylate cyclase so that cyclic GMP is formed postsynaptically. NO may also act as a trans-synaptic retrograde messenger to modulate presynaptic release of glutamate and it has been suggested that it plays an important role in the hippocampus in long-term potentiation, a model of learning and memory (ZHANG and SNYDER 1995). The actions of NO are very short-lived with a half-life estimated to be ~10s. This makes it very difficult to quantitate the action of NO in the brain. However, as a free radical, NO can be spin-trapped with an iron diethyldithiocarbamate complex and measured *ex vivo* by cryogenic electron paramagnetic resonance spectroscopy in rat brain regions such as the hippocampus, striatum, and neocortex (MULSCH et al. 1994; OLESEN et al. 1997). It has been found that after kainate-induced seizures in rats, NO formation was increased sixfold within 30–60min in the amygdala/temporal cortex region and up to 12-fold, although more slowly, in the remaining cortex (MULSCH et al. 1994). Interestingly, pretreatment with either 7-nitroindazole, which is a specific inhibitor of neuronal NOS, or diazepam, resulted in a reduction in convulsions and NO formation. This led the authors to conclude that NO was a proconvulsant mediator in kainate-induced seizures.

The measurement of NOS mRNA expression by *in situ* hybridization histochemistry is a useful index of NOS activity in the brain. This technique has been used to study the effect of kindling on NOS. In the case of the fast kindling paradigm, ELMÉR et al. (1996) found that 2h after 40 rapidly recurring seizures evoked by hippocampal stimulation in rats, NOS mRNA expression had decreased by 56% in the dentate granule cell layer, whilst after 12–24h mRNA levels had increased by 420%, 105% and 1260% in the CA_1, CA_3 pyramidal cells and piriform cortex respectively. Gene expression returned to control levels after 7 days. It was concluded from these data that the presumed changes in NO production resulting from the altered mRNA levels resulted in a modulation of synaptic function during fast kindling and could also influence neuronal vulnerability after epileptic insults. Another marker of NOS in brain sections is the histochemical technique for NADPH diaphorase, which has been used to examine changes in NOS in rats that underwent amygdaloid kindling 1 month previously (AL-GHOUL et al. 1995). These authors found that there was increased staining in terminals in rat limbic regions, which is consistent with the above results from NOS mRNA *in situ* histochemistry.

Another useful approach to establish a neuronal role for NO in epileptogenesis is the use of pharmacological inhibitors of NOS such as N^G-nitro-L-arginine (NOLA) and N^G-nitro-L-arginine methyl ester (L-NAME). Unfortunately, the results reported in the literature for these inhibitors are conflicting, probably due to different modes of seizure induction as well as different doses and routes of administration. RUNFELDT et al. (1995) have resolved some of these discrepancies by using a refined model of the cortical seizure threshold in rats that allows the determination of the time course of anticonvulsant or proconvulsant drug effects in individual rats. They found that NOLA was the preferred NOS inhibitor. At intraperitoneal doses of 1–10mg/kg there was a significant increase in the seizure threshold, which was ~50% of the increase seen after use of the conventional anticonvulsant, valproate (200mg/kg, intraperitoneally), in this model. On the other hand, when the dose of NOLA was increased to 40mg/kg, a significant and long-lasting decrease in seizure threshold was seen. These authors concluded that a NOS inhibitor could be either anti- or pro-convulsant in this model, depending on the dose administered, and that the anticonvulsant effects suggest that NO may play a role as an endogenous anticonvulsant for NMDA-induced seizures.

D. Postsynaptic Effects

I. Role of Ca^{2+} Channels and Ca^{2+} Binding Proteins

The genetic mouse strain, known as the tottering (*tg*) mutant, has a single gene mutation on chromosome 8 which causes a delayed-onset, recessive neurological disorder resulting in ataxia, motor seizures, and behavioural seizures closely resembling petit mal epilepsy in humans (FLETCHER et al. 1996). EEG recordings are normal except during the frequent, spontaneous seizures, when generalized bilateral spike and wave discharges are recorded. A hyperinnervation of the central nervous system from locus coeruleus noradrenergic neurons was found as an early histopathological change (LEVITT and NOEBELS 1981). However, more recent investigations using a positional cloning strategy of the *tg* locus have revealed that the α_{1A} voltage-sensitive Ca^{2+} channel gene is mutated in *tg* mice (FLETCHER et al. 1996). The α_{1A} Ca^{2+} channel is a major component of the high threshold, voltage-sensitive P- and Q-type Ca^{2+} channels which play a role in excitatory transmission in the brain. The position and nature of the mutation suggested that pore function is altered in the *tg* strain, but it is not known whether this enhances or inhibits the function of the Ca^{2+} channel.

While it is now well established that sustained increases in intracellular Ca^{2+} are a key factor in initiating irreversible neuronal injury, it has been found that many neurons contain a variety of cytosolic calcium-binding proteins which either modulate or mediate the actions of Ca^{2+} (BAIMBRIDGE et al. 1992). Of particular importance are the proteins, calbindin-D28K and parvalbumin, which are found in separate subpopulations of neurons. For example, in the hippocampus, parvalbumin is present in a subset of fast-firing interneurons while calbindin-D28K is found specifically in the dentate granule cells and CA_1 pyramidal neurons. As the parvalbumin-containing neurons are more sensitive to kainate seizure-induced injury than calbindin-D28K positive neurons, this suggests that calbindin-D28K expression may have a protective function in conditions of prolonged excitation. During kindling, calbindin-D28K levels decline progressively from dentate granule cells until they are almost unmeasurable. Conversely, focal stimulation of the perforant pathway in rats for 6h led to a ~2.5-fold increase in expression of calbindin-D28K mRNA in the dentate granule cells of the hippocampus. This increase was maintained for ~6 h and returned to baseline after 12h (LOWENSTEIN et al. 1991). In a subsequent study in rats, LOWENSTEIN et al. (1994) reported seizures which occurred in rats for 4–6h after subcutaneous injections of kainic acid. They found a similar temporal pattern of calbindin-D28K mRNA expression to that which occurred with electrical stimulation of the perforant pathway. These authors concluded that changes in calbindin-D28K mRNA expression were part of a cellular response designed to protect the cell from calcium-mediated injury.

II. Immediate Early Genes

A substantial number of studies since 1987 have shown that neurotransmitter receptor stimulation can regulate gene expression which may, in turn, be involved in long-term alterations of neuronal behaviour achieved via synaptic plasticity. While the initial studies focussed on learning and memory as the behaviour that was changed, it soon became apparent that epileptic kindling also led to altered gene expression primarily in the hippocampus (DRAGUNOW and ROBERTSON 1987), a region which was known to regulate the development of kindling. At the same time, independent studies in rodents showed that injections of chemical convulsants such as pentylenetetrazole also resulted in rapid expression (within a few minutes) of proto-oncogenes c-*fos* and c-*jun* in the hippocampus and cortex and these substances persisted for half an hour (Morgan et al. 1987; Saffen et al. 1988). These two genes were referred to as cellular immediate early genes (IEGs) by analogy with the immediate early genes of viruses which are promptly transcribed upon infection of a cell by a virus. These cellular IEGs, c-*fos* and c-*jun*, encode for nuclear proteins that are known as the DNA-binding transcription factors Fos and Jun, respectively, which function as components of the mammalian transcription factor activator protein-1 (AP-1). Morgan and Curran (1989) coined the term "stimulus-transcription coupling" for this process in the brain following seizures. Further research showed that, in addition to Fos, several Fos-related peptides were induced by the chemical convulsants and these peptides also participated in the formation of AP-1 complexes, so that seizures elicited a stereotypic series of events that involved the staggered appearance and disappearance of proteins contributing to AP-1 complexes (Morgan and Curran 1991). It soon became obvious that the IEGs response was complex since these Fos-related peptides were expressed by several Fos-related genes called *fra*. The procedures for measuring the expression of IEGs were (a) Northern blots to quantitate specific mRNA in homogenates with radioactive cDNA or synthetic oligonucleotide probes, (b) *in situ* hybridization histochemistry to locate mRNA expression in brain sections with the same radioactive probes or (c) immunohistochemical stains with antisera raised against specific peptide sequences of Fos peptides. This latter technique, while simple and sensitive, had drawbacks due to problems with cross-reactivity with the several Fos-related peptides in brain sections.

While it was apparent that c-*fos* expression was an early step in the electrical kindling process, there was only a low level of constitutive expression of c-*fos* mRNA in the hippocampus of both fully kindled and naive rats (Shin et al 1990; Burazin and Gundlach 1996). This suggests that a permanent expression of Fos is not obligatory for the permanently kindled state in rats. Shin et al. (1990) also demonstrated that the electrophysiologically recorded "afterdischarge" in the hippocampus after pulse stimulation of the angular bundle of rats was obligatory for c-*fos* mRNA expression, but that a threshold of at least 30 s was required for c-*fos* expression. This represented an "all-or-none" relationship between afterdischarge and c-*fos* mRNA expression, rather than a linear or graded relationship (Shin et al. 1990).

It subsequently became apparent that, firstly, IEGs were part of a common cellular mechanism that modifies gene expression in response to alterations in the extracellular environment and, secondly, that different subsets of IEGs could be induced independently (Curran and Morgan 1995). Thus, in a rat model of status epilepticus which leads to selective neuronal loss in hippocampal subfields and the amygdala/piriform cortex after 3–6 days, Dragunow et al. (1993) found a massive bilateral induction of c-*jun* and a lesser induction of c-*fos* and *Jun* B in hippocampal pyramidal neurons with little or no induction in the dentate granule cells mirroring the sites of neuronal loss. These authors suggested that Jun may regulate the transcription of "suicide" genes that produce programmed cell death.

Not only did electrically induced seizures result in rapid expression of c-*fos* mRNA (Burazin and Gundlach 1996) in rat brain but also a single audiogenic seizure induced in the Wistar AS genetic strain of rats resulted in c-*fos* expression confined to the subcortical auditory nuclei in the brain stem. Interestingly, repeated daily audiogenic seizures (10–40) led to kindling and increased c-*fos* expression in forebrain areas such as the amygdaloid complex, piriform and perirhinal cortex and medial hypothalamus, which reflected the extent of propagation of EEG discharges after kindling (Simler et al. 1994).

The expression of IEGs is an attractive mechanism through which brief changes in electrical activity may produce long-lasting structural and functional changes achieved via alteration in gene expression. However, as these alterations in IEGs and their transcription factors appear to be transient (duration <2 h), they are not necessarily involved in the maintenance of changes in neural function such as kindling (Burazin and Gundlach 1996). Nevertheless, Fos expression is an essential component of kindling since the development of kindling was impaired if protein synthesis was blocked during the period of stimulation. This suggests that IEGs play a role in linking the transient kindling stimulus to the emergence of the permanent hyperexcitable state. But protein synthesis is not the sole factor leading to the permanent kindled state, since the degree of bursts of population action potentials in the dentate granule cells was also obligatory for c-*fos* expression in these neurons (Labiner et al. 1993).

While no one neurotransmitter can account for all instances of IEG expression in the brain, the NMDA-glutamate receptors appear to mediate most of the gene induction following seizures. This conclusion is based both on a close relationship between the distribution of Fos immunoreactivity induced by administration of pentylenetetrazole and the density of NMDA receptors (Morgan et al. 1987), and on the blockade of pentylenetetrazole-induced c-*fos* expression by the non-competitive NMDA channel antagonist dizocilpine (MK 801). Subsequent studies in cultured rat dentate gyrus neurons demonstrated that a sustained NMDA-induced increase in intracellular Ca^{2+} for several minutes was obligatory for the induction of c-*fos* mRNA, suggesting that Ca^{2+} is the second messenger coupling this receptor to c-*fos* induction. This interpretation helps explain why there is only a low constitutive expression of c-*fos* mRNA in normal brain, where sustained increases in Ca^{2+} concentration do not occur (Lerea et al. 1992). Dizocilpine caused a partial but not total block of the induction of c-*fos* mRNA by NMDA. Non-NMDA agonists also induced c-*fos* mRNA expression in dentate neurons, and this was blocked by nifedipine, suggesting that non-NMDA agonists depolarized the neurons, allowing Ca^{2+} to enter them through voltage-operated Ca^{2+} channels to induce c-*fos* mRNA expression (Lerea et al. 1992).

The recent development of transgenic mice and rats which express a gene comprising the promoter region of c-*fos* fused with *lac*Z (a bacterial reporter gene expressing β-galactosidase activity) allows c-*fos* expression to be monitored with single cell resolution by a simple and unambiguous histochemical method (SMEYNE et al. 1992; KASOF et al. 1995). This avoids the problem of variable cross-reactivity of Fos-related peptides with antisera raised against synthetic peptide sequences of Fos, which was inherent in the early immunohistochemical technique. These transgenic rodents have been used for a more precise comparison of the actions of the two different chemical convulsants, kainic acid and pentylenetetrazole. KASOF et al. (1995) found that kainic acid elicits seizures in the *c-fos-lacZ* rats after systemic injection, as does pentylenetetrazole, but the former elicits a massive and more sustained induction of c-*fos* in limbic structures whereas the latter induces c-*fos* equally well in both the limbic system and the cerebral cortex. The difference between the two chemicals is that kainic acid initially elicits a period of generalized seizures and c-*fos* expression, which is followed days later by degeneration of subpopulations of hippocampal neurons, whereas pentylenetetrazole elicits similar seizures and c-*fos* induction but does not lead to neuronal death. An advantage of this histochemical staining technique is that the β-galactosidase staining product was confined to the nucleus when c-*fos* was expressed, but the staining product appeared in the cytoplasm in neurons about to die.

The recent breeding of transgenic mice with a null mutation of the c-*fos* gene by gene targeting provides a new approach to define the role of c-*fos* in the structural and functional changes seen after kindling (WATANABE et al. 1996). In homozygous mice carrying the null mutation for c-*fos*, the development of kindling was impaired and seen as a delay in the onset of both electrophysiological and behavioural features. Also, in these mice, kindling-induced granule cell axon sprouting into the supragranular region of the dentate gyrus was attenuated, reflecting the formation of fewer mossy fibre terminals. WATANABE et al. (1996) suggested that this latter effect could be due to a reduction in the granule cells of seizure-induced transcriptional regulation of gene expression which normally encodes genes for neurotrophic factors, their receptors and axonal growth-associated proteins. In otherwise normal kindled mice, the expression of such genes would lead to induction of mossy fibre sprouting, but in the null mutation mice the absence of c-*fos* would limit the transcriptional activation of such growth-related genes. In the normal, kindled mice, mossy fibre sprouting innervates the granule cell dendrites, thereby forming a recurrent excitatory circuit that would promote the progressive intensification of evoked seizures in kindled animals.

E. Neurotrophins and Neurogenesis

Neurotrophins are a family of basic polypeptides (~120 amino acid residues) comprising nerve growth factor (NGF), brain-derived neurotrophic factor (BDNF), neurotrophin-3 (NT-3), neurotrophins-4/5 (NT-4/5) and glial derived neurotrophic factor (GDNF), which are believed to play a key role in regulating survival, proliferation, maturation and outgrowth of specific populations of neurons in the brain (LINDSAY et al. 1994; LINDVALL et al. 1994). It was first reported in 1989 that limbic seizures induced in rats by a unilateral lesion in the hilus of the dentate gyrus led to marked increases (~25-fold) in the mRNA that expresses NGF in the hippocampal dentate gyrus 4h after the onset of recurrent limbic seizures (GALL and ISACKSON 1989). Subsequently it was found that after rapid kindling of the ventral hippocampus of rats, BDNF mRNA and NGF mRNA, but not NT-3 mRNA, were elevated in the dentate gyrus, CA_1 region of the hippocampus and the piriform cortex after 1–4h and had returned to normal by 24h (ERNFORS et al. 1991).

The role of BDNF in the development of kindling has been examined further, using BDNF mutant mice (KOKAIA et al. 1995). While homozygous BDNF "knock-out" mice die within the 1st week after birth, heterozygotes (BDNF +/-) with one functional copy of the BDNF gene survive but with lower levels of BDNF mRNA in cortical and hippocampal neurons. Development of kindling is markedly suppressed in these mice, but the maintenance of kindling is unaffected. Interestingly, mossy fibre sprouting is augmented in the BDNF heterozygotes compared to wild-type mice, which argues against the idea that mossy fibre sprouting is responsible for the kindling phenomenon. Recently, similar experiments have also been carried out with NT-3 mutant mice (ELMÉR et al. 1997). Amygdala kindling was markedly retarded in mice heterozygous for a deletion of the NT-3 gene (NT-3 +/-), and this retardation was reflected as a dampening of the progression from focal to generalized seizures. These mice were also found to have a 30% reduction of basal NT-3 mRNA levels as determined by *in situ* hybridization histochemistry. It was concluded that endogenous NT-3 levels may influence the rate of epileptogenesis and that a link exists between NT-3 and BDNF gene regulation in dentate granular cells.

While the above studies have shown a dramatic but short-lived increased expression of the mRNAs for neurotrophins in the hippocampus after seizures, for technical reasons it has not been possible to demonstrate increased levels of their protein products. Nevertheless, it has been suggested that an increased level of neurotrophins could induce a cascade of gene changes for other proteins, leading to axonal sprouting and the establishment of new synaptic contacts which could play a key role in subsequent epileptogenesis (LINDVALL et al. 1994).

I. Mossy Fibre Sprouting in the Hippocampus

The hippocampus has a propensity to generate seizures and, within the hippocampal formation, the dentate gyrus is thought to play a pivotal role in epileptogenesis (WILLIAMSON et al. 1995). The hippocampal mossy fibre pathway originates in the granule cell bodies of the dentate gyrus and projects through the hilus to innervate CA_3 pyramidal cell dendrites. These neurons are regarded as glutamatergic (SORIANO and FROTSCHER 1994) and they receive direct synaptic input from the entorhinal cortex. However, a recent paper (SLOVITER et al. 1996) has radically challenged the accepted dogma that the dentate granule neurons are solely glutamatergic. These authors obtained convincing immunohistochemical evidence in rat, mouse and monkey brains that the mossy fibres of the dentate granule cells contain GABA-like immunoreactivity as well as glutamate decarboxylase, the enzyme synthesizing GABA from glutamate. Furthermore, electrical stimulation of the perforant pathway of rats for up to 24h, which reliably evoked population spikes and epileptoform discharges in the granule cells and CA_3 and CA_1 pyramidal cells, resulted in a reproducible induction of glutamate decarboxylase and GABA-like immunoreactivity in the contralateral hippocampal neurons that do not normally contain these markers. *In situ* hybridization histochemistry and biochemical assays confirmed the elevation of mRNA for glutamate decarboxylase in the dentate gyrus. These authors suggested that their ability to detect glutamate decarboxylase and GABA-like immunoreactivity in normal granule cells was due to greater methodological sensitivity. Their results suggest that dentate granule neurons contain two "fast-acting" amino acid neurotransmitters, one excitatory (glutamate) and one inhibitory (GABA), a situation which could lead to both excitatory and inhibitory postsynaptic effects. As well, they contain the neuropeptide dynorphin, which is believed to act presynaptically to inhibit afferent input into the hippocampus (WAGNER et al. 1993). Their finding that perforant pathway stimulation in rats induces GABA in additional granule cells suggests that spontaneous seizures in human temporal epilepsy may also induce granule cell glutamate decarboxylase and GABA levels above their basal values, thereby influencing the excitability of the hippocampal network in this form of epilepsy. An independent study by SCHWARZER and SPERK (1995) in rats after kainate-induced seizures showed that the constitutively glutamatergic mossy fibres expressed both the mRNA for glutamate decarboxylase and the enzyme after limbic seizures. These workers suggested that GABA could then be released from mossy fibres to provide an endogenous anticonvulsive mechanism to counteract seizure generation. While the results of SLOVITER et al. (1996) and SCHWARZER and SPERK (1995) challenge prevailing dogma, more research needs to establish both that GABA in mossy fibres is stored in vesicles and is released in response to depolarization, before accepting that these neurons can produce both excitatory and inhibitory postsynaptic actions.

Human temporal lobe epilepsy, which is difficult to manage with conventional anticonvulsant drugs, is frequently associated with a marked loss of hippocampal CA_1, CA_3 pyramidal cells, and hilar neurons, as well as glial proliferation, which is referred to as hippocampal sclerosis (PARENT and LOWENSTEIN 1997). Interestingly, dentate granule cells tend to be preserved relative to the other neurons. As the hippocampal sclerosis precedes the development of spontaneous seizures and as the surgical removal of the damaged portion of the hippocampus greatly reduces the incidence of seizures in a majority of patients (Falconer and Taylor 1968), it is believed that the degeneration facilitates the occurrence of seizures. Studies in laboratory animals have shown that repeated brief seizures evoked by kindling (Cavazos et al. 1994), or kainic acid-induced status epilepticus (Parent et al. 1997), induce progressive neuronal loss not only in the hippocampal formation, producing appearances that closely resemble hippocampal sclerosis, but also neuronal loss in other limbic areas. It is generally considered that glutamate excitotoxicity is the biochemical basis of the neuronal cell loss, particularly in the status epilepticus rat model (Sutula et al. 1992), and that therapeutic strategies to reduce excitotoxicity may reduce the occurrence of seizures in this type of epilepsy.

In addition to neuronal cell loss in the hippocampus in the seizure models in rats, the dentate granule cells that appear to be resistant to degeneration demonstrate sprouting of their mossy fibres and develop recurrent collaterals that form synapses in the dentate molecular layer (Parent and Lowenstein 1997). It has been suggested that this sprouting results either in recurrent excitatory circuits and subsequent hippocampal hyperexcitability or in an increased excitatory drive onto inhibitory interneurons in the inner molecular layer, thereby restoring recurrent inhibition. Recent studies with the rat pilocarpine model of status epilepticus (Parent et al. 1997) have demonstrated that prolonged seizure activity markedly increases neurogenesis in the dentate subgranular proliferative zone. Differentiation of these newly born granule cells with their axons projecting to both the CA_3 pyramidal cell region and the dentate inner molecular layer, rather than remodelling of mature granule cells, is the basis of the sprouting and the resultant epileptogenesis. Furthermore, intermittent perforant path stimulation of rats which produces hippocampal seizure activity without neuronal degeneration also stimulated neurogenesis in the dentate subgranular proliferative zone (Parent et al. 1997).

The reactive sprouting of mossy fibres also correlates with an increased expression in their neurons of origin of α-tubulin- and microtubule associated protein-mRNA whose protein products are essential cytoskeletal components of the "sprouts" back into the granule cell dendrites (Khrestchalisky et al. 1994). Interestingly, the mossy fibres do not "sprout" into the CA_3 field and it has been suggested that proliferating, tenascin-positive astrocytes impair axonal passage into the CA_3 field while non-proliferating, tenascin-negative astrocytes guide axonal outgrowth and synaptogenesis to the dentate gyrus (Represa et al. 1994).

Recent studies by Bengzon et al. (1997) have shown that even a single hippocampal kindling stimulation which produced focal epileptiform activity in the hippocampus with an afterdischarge lasting 82 ± 7 s, resulted in apoptotic death of neurons in the dentate gyrus 5 h later. Forty rapid kindling stimulations delivered at 5-min intervals resulted in a much higher number of neurons undergoing apoptotic death. Paradoxically, single and intermittent seizures also stimulated proliferation of both neurons and non-neuronal cells in the dentate gyrus. The authors concluded that both apoptotic death and proliferation of dentate gyrus neurons might constitute primary events in seizure-induced hippocampal pathology.

II. Neuronal Migration Disorders in the Cortex

Neuronal migration disorders are the result of disturbed brain development and are now recognized as a cause of some types of epilepsy (Brodtkorb et al. 1994). Magnetic resonance imaging can identify the abnormalities whose sites roughly correspond to the sites of focal epileptiform EEG activity. This facilitates surgical resection of these defects as a treatment option. Recently, it has been demonstrated that prenatal exposure of rats to methylazoxymethanol not only disrupts normal neuronal migration in the cortex and hippocampus but also results in epileptoform activity in hippocampal slices in the presence of moderately elevated (6 mM) K^+ levels (Baraban and Schwartzkroin 1995). This simple animal model shows great promise for studying epileptogenesis associated with neuronal migration disorders.

F. Conclusions

It is obvious that there is no simple biochemical defect that underlies epileptogenesis and it is likely that there are as many different biochemical disorders as there are different types of epilepsy. Molecular biology is making an important contribution to our understanding of epileptogenesis, if only to emphasize the molecular complexity of the components involved in chemical transmission in the central nervous system. Hopefully new techniques such as positional cloning of identified epilepsy genes will shed new light on epileptogenesis in the coming years and this will lead to new, rational therapies to manage these devastating neurological disorders.

References

Agnati LF, Zoli M, Strömberg I, Füxe K (1995) Intercellular communication in the brain: wiring versus volume transmission. Neuroscience 69:711–726

Al-Ghoul WM, Meeker RB, Greenwood RS (1995) Kindling induces a long-lasting increase in brain nitric oxide synthase activity. Neuroreport 6:457–460

Andrews PI, McNamara JO (1996) Rasmussen's encephalitis: an autoimmune disorder? Curr Opin Neurol 9:141–148

Angelatou F, Pagonopoulou O, Maraziotis T, Olivier A, Villemeure JG, Avoli M, Kostopoulos G (1993) Upregulation of A1 adenosine receptors in human temporal lobe epilepsy: a quantitative autoradiographic study. Neurosci Letts 163: 11–14

Attwell PJE, Kaura S, Sigla G, Bradford HF, Croucher MJ, Jane DE, Watkins JC (1995) Blockade of both epileptogenesis and glutamate release by (1S,3S)-ACPD, a presynaptic glutamate receptor agonist. Brain Res 698:155–162

Avoli M, Williamson A (1996) Functional and pharmacological properties of human neocortical neurons maintained in vitro. Prog Neurobiol 48:519–554

Avoli M, Pumain R, Olivier A (1987) Seizure-like discharges induced by lowering $[Mg^{2+}]_0$ in the human epileptogenic neocortex maintained in vitro. Brain Res 417:199–203

Babb TL, Pretorius JK, Kupfer WR, Crandall PH (1989) Glutamate decarboxylase-immunoreactive neurons are preserved in human epileptic hippocampus. J Neurosci 9:2562–2574

Baimbridge K, Celio M, Rogers J (1992) Calcium-binding proteins in the nervous system. Trends Neurosci 15:303–308

Baraban SC, Schwartzkroin PA (1995) Electrophysiology of CA_1 pyramidal neurons in an animal model of neuronal migration disorders: prenatal methylazoxymethanol treatment. Epilepsy Res 22:145–156

Barry DI, Kikvadze I, Brundin P, Bolwig TG, Björklund A, Lindvall O (1989) Grafts of fetal locus coeruleus neurons in rat amygdala-piriform cortex suppress seizure development in hippocampal kindling. Exp Neurol 106:125–132

Bengzon J, Brundin P, Kalen P, Kokaia M, Lindvall O (1991) Host regulation of noradrenaline release from grafts of seizure-suppressant locus coeruleus neurons. Exp Neurol 111:49–54

Bengzon J, Kokaia Z, Elmér E, Nanobashvilli A, Lindvall O (1997) Apoptosis and proliferation of dentate gyrus neurons after single and intermittent limbic seizures. Proc Natl Acad Sci USA 94:10432–10437

Bonhaus DW, Rigsbee CC, McNamara JO (1987) Intranigral dynorphin 1–13 suppresses kindled seizures by a naloxone insensitive mechanism. Brain Res 405:358–363

Brailowsky S, Montiel T, Meneses S, Di Scala G (1995) Effects of $GABA_B$ receptor antagonists on two models of focal epileptogenesis. Brain Res 702:126–132

Briere R, Sherwin AL, Robitaille Y, Olivier A, Quesney LF, Reader TA (1986) α_1-Adrenoceptors are decreased in human epileptic foci. Ann Neurol 19:26–30

Brodtkorb E, Torbergsen T, Nakken KO, Andersen K, Gimse R, Sjaastad O (1994) Epileptic seizures, arthrogryposis and migrational brain disorders: a syndrome? Acta Neurol Scand 90:232–240

Brusa R, Zimmerman F, Koh D-S, Feldmeyer D, Gass P, Seeburg PH, Sprengel R (1995) Early-onset epilepsy and postnatal lethality associated with an editing-deficient GluR-B allele in mice. Science 270:1677–1680

Buchhalter JR (1993) Animal models of inherited epilepsy. Epilepsia 34 [Suppl 3]:S31–S41

Burazin TCD, Gundlach AL (1996a) Rapid but transient increases in cholecystokinin mRNA in cerebral cortex following amygdaloid-kindled seizures in the rat. Neurosci Letts 209:65–68

Burazin TCD, Gundlach AL (1996b) Rapid and transient increases in cellular immediate early gene and neuropeptide mRNAs in cortical and limbic areas after amygdaloid kindling seizures in the rat. Epilepsy Res 26:281–293

Cavazos JE, Das I, Sutula TP (1994) Neuronal loss induced in limbic pathways by kindling: evidence for induction of hippocampal sclerosis by repeated brief seizures. J Neurosci 14:3106–3121

Chauvel P, Trottier S (1986) Role of noradrenergic ascending system in extinction of epileptic phenomena. In: Delgado-Escuetta AV, Ward AA, Woodbury DM, Porter RJ (eds) Basic mechanisms of the epilepsies: molecular and cellular approaches. Raven Press, New York (Advances in neurology, vol 44) pp. 475–487

Colmers WF, Bleakman D (1994) Effects of neuropeptide Y on the electrical properties of neurons. Trends Neurosci 17:373–379

Curran T, Morgan JI (1995) Fos: An immediate-early transcription factor in neurons. J Neurobiol 26:403–412

Curtis DA, Johnston GAR (1974) Amino acid transmitters in the mammalian central nervous system. Ergebn Physiol 69:97–188

Danober L, Vergnes M, Depaulis A, Marescaux C (1994) Nucleus basalis lesions suppress spike and wave discharges in rats with spontaneous absence-epilepsy. Neuroscience 59:531–539

Danober L, Depaulis A, Vergnes M, Marescaux C (1995) Mesopontine cholinergic control over generalized non-convulsive seizures in a genetic model of absence epilepsy in the rat. Neuroscience 69:1183–1193
De Lanerolle NC, Kim JH, Robbins RJ, Spencer DD (1989) Hippocampal interneuron loss and plasticity in human temporal lobe epilepsy. Brain Res 495:387–395
Dragunow M (1988) Purinergic mechanisms in epilepsy. Prog Neurobiol 31:85–108
Dragunow M, Robertson HA (1987) Kindling stimulation induces c-fos protein(s) in granule cells of the rat dentate gyrus. Nature 329:441–442
Dragunow M, Young D, Hughes P et al. (1993) Is c-Jun involved in nerve cell death following status epilepticus and hypoxic-ischaemic brain injury? Molecular Brain Res 18:347–352
Duggan AW, Hope PJ, Jarrott B, Schaible H-G, Fleetwood-Walker SM (1990) Release, spread, and persistence of immunoreactive neurokinin A in the dorsal horn of the cat following noxious cutaneous stimulation. Studies with antibody microprobes. Neuroscience 35:195–202
During MJ, Spencer DD (1993) Extracellular hippocampal glutamate and spontaneous seizure in the conscious human brain. Lancet 341:1607–1610
During MJ, Ryder KM, Spencer DD (1995) Hippocampal GABA transporter function in temporal-lobe epilepsy. Nature 376:174–177
Edwards FA (1996) Features of P2X receptor-mediated synapses in the rat brain: Why doesn't ATP kill the postsynaptic cell ? In: P2 purinoceptors: localization, function and transduction mechanisms. Wiley, Chichester. Ciba Foundation Symposium 198:278–289
Edwards FA, Gibb AJ (1993) ATP – a fast neurotransmitter. FEBS Letts 325:86–89
Elmér E, Alm P, Kokaia Z et al. (1996) Regulation of neuronal nitric oxide synthase mRNA levels in rat brain by seizure activity. NeuroReport 7:1335–1339
Elmér E, Kokaia M, Ernfors P, Ferencz I, Kokaia Z, Lindvall O (1997) Suppressed kindling epileptogenesis and perturbed BDNF and TrkB gene regulation in NT-3 mutant mice. Exp Neurol 145:93–103
Ernfors, P, Bengzon J, Kokaia Z, Persson H, Lindvall O (1991) Increased levels of messenger RNAs for neurotrophic factors in the brain during kindling epileptogenesis. Neuron 7:165–176
Falconer MA, Taylor DC (1968) Surgical treatment of drug-resistant epilepsy due to mesial temporal sclerosis. Arch Neurol 19:353–361
Fisher RS (1989) Animal models of the epilepsies. Brain Res Rev 14:245–278
Fletcher CF, Lutz CM, O'Sullivan TN et al. (1996) Absence epilepsy in tottering mutant mice is associated with calcium channel defects. Cell 87:607–617
Gall CM, Isackson PJ (1989) Limbic seizures increase neuronal production of messenger RNA for nerve growth factor. Science 245:758–761
Gellman RL, Kallianos JA, McNamara JO (1987) Alpha-2 receptors mediate an endogenous noradrenergic suppression of kindling development. J Pharmac Exp Ther 241:891–898
Goddard GV, McIntyre DC, Leech CK (1969) A permanent change in brain function resulting from daily electrical stimulation. Exp Neurol 25:295–330
Greber S, Schwarzer C, Sperk G (1994) Neuropeptide Y inhibits potassium-stimulated glutamate release through Y2 receptors in rat hippocampal slices in vitro. Brit J Pharmac 113:737–740
Hernandez TD, Gallager DW (1992) Development of long-term subsensitivity to GABA in dorsal raphe neurons of amygdala-kindled rats. Brain Res 582:221–225
Hökfelt T (1991) Neuropeptides in perspective. Neuron 7:867–879
Horne AL, Harrison NL, Turner JP, Simmonds MA (1986) Spontaneous paroxysmal activity induced by zero magnesium and bicuculline: suppression by NMDA antagonists and GABA mimetics. Eur J Pharmacol 122:231–238
Hosford DA (1995) Models of primary generalized epilepsy. Curr Opin Neurol 8:121–125

Hosford DA, Clark S, Cao Z, Wilson WA, Lin F, Morrisett RA, Huin A (1992) The role of $GABA_B$ receptor activation in absence seizures of lethargic (*lh/lh*) mice. Science 257:398–401

Isokawa M, Levesque MF (1991) Increased NMDA responses and dendritic degeneration in human epileptic hippocampal neurons in slices. Neurosci Letts 132:212–216

Jackson GD, Connelly A (1996) Magnetic resonance imaging and spectroscopy. Curr Opin Neurol 9:82–88

Jobe PC, Mishra PK, Browning RA, Wang C, Adams-Curtis LE, Ko KH, Dailey JW (1994) Noradrenergic abnormalities in the genetically epilepsy-prone rat. Brain Res Bull 35:493–504

Kamphuis W, De Rijk TC, Lopes da Silva FH (1995) Expression of $GABA_A$ receptor subunit mRNAs in hippocampal pyramidal and granular neurons in the kindling model of epileptogenesis: an in situ hybridization study. Mol Brain Res 31:33–47

Kasof GM, Mandelzys A, Maika SD, Hammer RE, Curran T, Morgan JI (1995) Kainic acid-induced neuronal death is associated with DNA damage and a unique immediate-early gene response in c-fos-lacZ transgenic rats. J Neurosci 15:4238–4249

Kaura S, Bradford HF, Young AMJ, Croucher MJ, Hughes PD (1995) The effect of amygdaloid kindling on the content and release of amino acids in vivo and in vitro from the amygdaloid complex: in vivo and in vitro studies. J Neurochem 65: 1240–1249

Khrestchalisky M, Ferhat L, Charton G, Bernard A, Pollard H, Represa A, Ben-Ari Y (1994) Molecular correlates between reactive and developmental plasticity in the rat hippocampus. J Neurobiol 26:426–436

Kish SJ, Olivier A, Dubeau F, Robitaille Y, Sherwin AL (1988) Increased activity of choline acetyltransferase and acetylcholinesterase in actively epileptic human cerebral cortex. Epilepsy Res 2:227–231

Köhr G, De Koninck Y, Mody I (1993) Properties of NMDA receptor channels in neurons acutely isolated from epileptic (kindled) rats. J Neurosci 13:3612–3627

Kokaia M, Bengzon J, Kalen P, Lindvall O (1989a) Noradrenergic mechanisms in hippocampal kindling with rapidly recurring seizures. Brain Res 491:398–402

Kokaia M, Kalen P, Bengzon J, Lindvall O (1989b) Noradrenaline and 5-hydroxytryptamine release in the hippocampus during seizures induced by hippocampal kindling stimulation: an in vivo microdialysis study. Neuroscience 32:647–656

Kokaia M, Aebischer P, Elmér E, Bengzon J, Kalen P, Kokaia Z, Lindvall O (1994) Seizure suppression in kindling epilepsy by intracerebral implants of GABA – but not by noradrenaline-releasing polymer matrices. Exp Brain Res 100:385–394

Kokaia M, Ernfors P, Kokaia Z, Elmér E, Jaenisch R, Lindvall O (1995) Suppressed epileptogenesis in BDNF mutant mice. Exper Neurol 133:215–224

Kokaia M, Ferencz I, Leanza G et al. (1996) Immunolesioning of basal forebrain cholinergic neurons facilitates hippocampal kindling and perturbs neurotropin messenger RNA regulation. Neuroscience 70:313–327

Kraus JE, Yeh G-C, Bonhaus DW, Nadler JV, McNamara JO (1994) Kindling induces the long-lasting expression of a novel population of NMDA receptors in hippocampal region CA_3. J Neurosci 14:4196–4206

Krishek BJ, Xie X, Blackstone C, Huganir RL, Moss SJ, Smart TG (1994) Regulation of $GABA_A$ receptor function by protein kinase C phosphorylation. Neuron 12:1081–1095

Kuzniecky R (1997) Magnetic resonance and functional magnetic imaging: tools for the study of human epilepsy. Curr Opin Neurol 10:88–91

Labiner DM, Butler LS, Cao Z, Hosford DA, Shin C, McNamara JO (1993) Induction of c-fos mRNA by kindled seizures: complex relationship with neuronal burst firing. J Neurosci 13:744–751

Lehmann H, Ebert U, Löscher W (1996) Immunocytochemical localization of GABA immunoreactivity in dentate granule cells of normal and kindled rats. Neurosci Letts 212:41–44
Lerea LS, McNamara JO (1993) Ionotropic glutamate receptor subtypes activate c-fos transcription by distinct calcium-requiring intracellular signaling pathways. Neuron 10:31–41
Lerea LS, Butler LS, McNamara JO (1992) NMDA and non-NMDA receptor mediated increase of c-fos mRNA in dentate gyrus neurons involves calcium influx via different routes. J Neurosci 12:2973–2981
Lindsay RM, Wiegand SJ, Altar A, DiStefano PS (1994) Neurotrophic factors: from molecule to man. Trends Neurosci 17:182–190
Lindvall O, Kokaia Z, Bengzon J, Elmér E, Kokaia M (1994) Neurotrophins and brain insults. Trends Neurosci 17:490–496
Lloyd KG, Bossi L, Morselli PL (1984) GABA hypothesis of human epilepsy: neurochemical evidence from surgically resected identified foci. In: Fariello RG (ed): Neurotransmitters, seizures, and epilepsy II. Raven Press, New York, pp. 285–293
Löscher W, Hönack D (1991) Anticonvulsant and behavioral effects of two novel competitive N-methyl-D-Aspartic acid receptor antagonists, CGP 37849 and CGP 39551, in the kindling model of epilepsy. Comparison with MK-801 and carbamazepine. J Pharmacol Exp Ther 256:432–440
Lowenstein DH, Miles M, Hatam F, McCabe T (1991) Up-regulation of calbindin-D28 K mRNA in the rat hippocampus following focal stimulation of the perforant path. Neuron 6:627–633
Lowenstein DH, Gwinn RP, Seren MS, Simon RP, McIntosh TK (1994) Increased expression of mRNA encoding calbindin-D28K, the glucose-regulated proteins, or the 72kDA heat-shock protein in three models of acute CNS injury. Mol Brain Res 22:299–308
Marco P, Sola RG, Pulido P, Alijarde MT, Sanchez A, Ramon y Cajal S, DeFelipe J (1996) Inhibitory neurons in the human epileptogenic temporal neocortex. Brain 119:1327–1347
Marksteiner J, Ortler M, Bellman R, Sperk G (1990) Neuropeptide Y biosynthesis is markedly induced in mossy fibres during temporal lobe epilepsy of the rat. Neurosci Letts 112:143–148
Martin D, McNamara JO, Nadler JV (1992) Kindling enhances sensitivity of CA_3 hippocampal pyramidal cells to NMDA. J Neurosci 12:1928–1935
McNamara JO (1994) Cellular and molecular basis of epilepsy. J Neurosci 14:3413–3425
Mody I, Heinrmann U (1987) NMDA receptors of dentate gyrus granule cells participate in synaptic transmission following kindling. Nature 326:701–704
Monna A, Rizzi M, Samanin R, Vezzani A (1993) Anti-somatostatin antibody enhances the rate of hippocampal kindling in rats. Brain Res 602:148–152
Morgan JI, Curran T (1989) Stimulus-transcription coupling in neurons: role of cellular immediate-early genes. Trends Neurosci 12:459–462
Morgan JI, Curran T (1991) Proto-oncogene transcription factors and epilepsy. Trends Pharmacol 12:343–349
Morgan JI, Cohen DR, Hempstead JL, Curran T (1987) Mapping patterns of c-fos expression in the central nervous system after seizure. Science 237:192–197
Morrisett RA, Chow C, Nadler JV, McNamara JO (1989) Biochemical evidence for enhanced sensitivity to N-methyl-D-aspartate in the hippocampal formation of kindled rats. Brain Res 496:25–28
Mulsch A, Busse R, Mordvintcev PI, Vanin AF, Nielsen EO, Scheel-Kruger J, Olesen S-P (1994) Nitric oxide promotes seizure activity in kainate-treated rats. NeuroReport 5:2325–2328
Nagy AK, Houser CR, Delgado-Escueta AV (1990) Synaptosomal ATPase activities in temporal cortex and hippocampal formation of humans with focal epilepsy. Brain Res 529:192–201

Nakanishi S (1992) Molecular diversity of glutamate receptors and implications for brain function. Science 258:597–603

Noebels JL (1996) Targeting epilepsy genes. Neuron 16:241–244

Olesen S-P, Moller A, Mordvintcev PI, Busse R, Mulsch A (1997) Regional measurements of NO formed in vivo during brain ischemia. Acta Neurol Scand 95:219–224

Olsen RW, Tobin AJ (1990) Molecular biology of $GABA_A$ receptors. FASEB J 4:1469–1480

Parent JM, Lowenstein DH (1997) Mossy fiber reorganization in the epileptic hippocampus. Curr Opin Neurol 10:103–109

Parent JM, Yu TW, Leibowitz RT, Geschwind DH, Sloviter RS, Lowenstein DH (1997) Dentate granule cell neurogenesis is increased by seizures and contributes to aberrant network reorganization in the adult rat hippocampus. J Neurosci 17:3727–3738

Petroff OAC, Rothman DL, Behar KL, Mattson RH (1996a) Low brain GABA level is associated with poor seizure control. Ann Neurol 40:908–911

Petroff OAC, Rothman DL, Behar KL, Mattson RH (1996b) Human brain GABA levels rise after initiation of vigabatrin therapy but fail to rise further with increasing dose. Neurology 46:1459–1463

Pinel JPJ, Rovner LI (1978) Electrode placement and kindling-induced experimental epilepsy. Exp Neurol 58:335–346

Pratt GD, Kokaia M, Bengzon J, Kokaia Z, Fritschy J-M, Möhler H, Lindvall O (1993) Differential regulation of N-methyl-D-aspartate receptor subunit messenger RNAs in kindling-induced epileptogenesis. Neuroscience 57:307–318

Racine RJ (1972) Modification of seizure activity by electrical stimulation: II. Motor seizure. Electroenceph Clin Neurophysiol 32:281–294

Represa A, Niquet J, Pollard H, Ben-Ari Y (1994) Cell death, gliosis, and synaptic remodeling in the hippocampus of epileptic rats. J Neurobiol 26:413–425

Rizzi M, Monno A, Samanin R, Sperk G, Vezzani A (1993) Electrical kindling of the hippocampus is associated with functional activation of neuropeptide Y-containing neurons. Eur J Neurosci 5:1534–1538

Roberts E (1984) GABA-related phenomena, models of nervous system function, and seizures. Ann Neurol 16 [Suppl]:S77–S89

Rogers SW, Andrews PI, Gahring LC et al. (1994) Autoantibodies to glutamate receptor GluR3 in Rasmussen's encephalitis. Science 265:648–651

Rogers SW, Twyman RE, Gahring LC (1996) The role of autoimmunity to glutamate receptors in neurological disease. Mol Medicine Today 3:76–81

Rosen JB, Cain CJ, Weiss SRB, Post RM (1992) Alterations in mRNA of enkephalin, dynorphin and thyrotropin releasing hormone during amygdala kindling: an in situ hybridization study. Mol Brain Res 15:247–255

Rothman SM, Olney JW (1987) Excitotoxicity and the NMDA receptor. Trends Neurosci 10:299–302

Rundfeldt C, Koch R, Richter A, Mevissen M, Gerecke U, Löscher W (1995) Dose-dependent anticonvulsant and proconvulsant effects of nitric oxide synthase inhibitors on seizure threshold in a cortical stimulation model in rats. Eur J Pharmac 274:73–81

Saffen DW, Cole AJ, Worley PF, Christy BA, Ryder K, Baraban JM (1988) Convulsant-induced increase in transcription factor messenger RNAs in rat brain. Proc Nat Acad Sci USA 85:7795–7799

Schiffmann S, Campistron G, Tugendhaft P, Brotchi J, Flament-Durand J, Geffard M, Vanderhaeghen J-J (1988) Immunocytochemical detection of GABAergic nerve cells in the human temporal cortex using a direct γ-aminobutyric acid antiserum. Brain Res 442:270–278

Schoepp DD, Johnson BG (1993) Pharmacology of metabotropic glutamate receptor inhibition of cyclic AMP formation in the adult rat hippocampus. Neurochem Int 22:277–283

Schwarzer C, Sperk G (1995) Hippocampal granule cells express glutamic acid decarboxylase-67 after limbic seizures in the rat. Neuroscience 69:705–709
Schwarzer C, Williamson JM, Lothman EW, Vezzani A, Sperk G (1995) Somatostatin, neuropeptide Y, neurokinin B and cholecystokinin immunoreactivity in two chronic models of temporal lobe epilepsy. Neuroscience 69:831–845
Schwarzer C, Sperk G, Samanin R, Rizzi M, Gariboldi M, Vezzani (1996) Neuropeptides-immunoreactivity and their mRNA expression in kindling: functional implications for limbic epileptogenesis. Brain Res Reviews 22:27–50
Shin C, McNamara JO, Morgan JI, Curran T, Cohen DR (1990) Induction of c-fos mRNA expression by afterdischarge in the hippocampus of naive and kindled rats. J Neurochem 55, 1050–1055
Sigel E, Baur R, Trube G, Möhler H, Malherbe P (1990) The effect of subunit composition of rat brain $GABA_A$ receptors on channel function. Neuron 5:703–711
Simler S, Hirsch E, Danober L, Motte J, Vergnes M, Marcscaux C (1994) C-fos expression after single and kindled audiogenic seizures in Wistar rats. Neurosci Letts 175:58–62
Sloviter RS, Dichter MA, Rachinsky TL, Dean E, Goodman JH, Sollas AL, Martin DL (1996) Basal expression and induction of glutamate decarboxylase and GABA in excitatory granule cells of the rat and monkey hippocampal dentate gyrus. J Comp Neurol 373:593–618
Smeyne RJ, Schilling K, Robertson L, Luk D, Oberdick J, Curran T, Morgan JI (1992) Fos-lacZ transgenic mice: mapping sites of gene induction in the central nervous system. Neuron 8:13–23
Smith GB, Olsen RW (1995) Functional domains of $GABA_A$ receptors. Trends Pharmacol 16:162–167
Sommer B, Seeburg PH (1992) Glutamate receptor channels: novel properties and new clones. Trends Pharmacol 13:291–296
Soriano E, Frotscher M (1994) Mossy cells of the rat fascia dentata are glutamate-immunoreactive. Hippocampus 4:65–70
Sperk G (1994) Kainic acid seizures in the rat. Prog Neurobiol 42:1–32
Sperk G, Herzog H (1997) Anticonvulsant action of neuropeptide Y. Nature Medicine 3:728–729
Sperk G, Marksteiner J, Gruber B, Bellman R, Mahata M, Ortler M (1992) Functional changes in neuropeptide Y and somatostatin containing neurons induced by limbic seizures in the rat. Neuroscience 50:831–846
Spreafico R, Mennini T, Danober L et al. (1993) $GABA_A$ receptor impairment in the GAERS: an immunocytochemical and receptor binding autoradiographic study. Epilepsy Res 15:229–238
Steinlein OK, Mulley JC, Propping P et al. (1995) A missense mutation in the neuronal nicotinic receptor $\alpha 4$ subunit is associated with autosomal dominant nocturnal frontal lobe epilepsy. Nature Genetics 11:201–203
Stone TW (1981) Physiological roles for adenosine and adenosine 5'-triphosphate in the nervous system. Neuroscience 6:523–555
Sutula T, Cavazos J, Golarai G (1992) Alterations of long-lasting structural and functional effects of kainic acid in the hippocampus by brief treatment with phenobarbital. J Neurosci 12:4173–4187
Tanaka K, Watase K, Manabe T et al. (1997) Epilepsy and exacerbation of brain injury in mice lacking the glutamate transporter GLT-1. Science 276:1699–1702
Theodore WH (1996) Positron emission tomography and single photon emission computed tomography. Curr Opin Neurol 9:89–92
Twyman RE, Gahring LC, Spiess J, Rogers SW (1995) Glutamate receptor antibodies activate a subset of receptors and reveal an agonist binding site. Neuron 14:755–762
Wagner JJ, Terman GW, Chavkin C (1993) Endogenous dynorphins inhibit excitatory neurotransmission and block LTP induction in the hippocampus. Nature 363:451–454

Watanabe Y, Johnson RS, Butler LS, Binder DK, Spiegelman BM, Papaioannou VE, McNamara JO (1996) Null mutation of c-fos impairs structural and functional plasticities in the kindling model of epilepsy. J Neurosci 16:3827–3836
Weisskopf MG, Zalutsky RA, Nicoll RA (1993) The opioid peptide dynorphin mediates heterosynaptic depression of hippocampal mossy fibre synapses and modulates long-term potentiation. Nature 362:423–427
Westerberg V, Lewis J, Corcoran ME (1984) Depletion of noradrenaline fails to affect kindled seizures. Exp Neurol 84:237–241
Williamson A, Spencer SS, Spencer DD (1995) Depth electrode studies and intracellular dentate granule cell recordings in temporal lobe epilepsy. Ann Neurol 38:778–787
Woldbye DPD, Larsen PJ, Mikkelsen JD, Klemp K, Madsen TM, Bolwig TG (1997) Powerful inhibition of kainic acid seizures by neuropeptide Y via Y5-like receptors. Nature Medicine 3:761–764
Yan Q-S, Jobe PC, Dailey JW (1995) Further evidence of anticonvulsant role for 5-hydroxytryptamine in genetically epilepsy-prone rats. Br J Pharmac 115:1314–1318
Young D, Dragunow M (1994) Status epilepticus may be caused by loss of adenosine anticonvulsant mechanisms. Neuroscience 58:245–261.
Zhang J, Snyder SH (1995) Nitric oxide in the nervous system. Annu Rev Pharmacol Toxicol 35:213–233

CHAPTER 5

Cellular Actions of Antiepileptic Drugs

R.L. MACDONALD

A. Introduction

Antiepileptic drugs have been the mainstays of the treatment of patients with epilepsy. From 1978 to 1993 the primarily used antiepileptic drugs have been phenytoin, carbamazepine, barbiturates and primidone, benzodiazepines, valproic acid and ethosuximide. Recently a number of new antiepileptic drugs have been developed which include gabapentin, lamotrigine, oxcarbazepine, vigabatrin, tiagabine, topiramate and felbamate. Unfortunately, early experience with felbamate was associated with an unacceptably high incidence of aplastic anaemia (PENNELL et al. 1995) and chemical hepatitis, and in August of 1994 the manufacturer and the United States Federal Drug Administration recommended that, if clinically possible, patients be withdrawn from felbamate. Fortunately, the remaining newly developed antiepileptic drugs have been approved in many countries and are currently in use.

Interactions of the established and new antiepileptic drugs with neurotransmitter receptors or ion channels may be responsible for their clinical effects (MACDONALD and KELLY 1994; MACDONALD and MELDRUM 1995; MACDONALD and GREENFIELD 1997). Three primary neurotransmitter receptor or ion channels are targeted by the established antiepileptic drugs and by some of the newly developed antiepileptic drugs: γ-aminobutyric acid type A ($GABA_A$) receptor channels, voltage-dependent Na^+ channels and voltage-dependent low threshold (T-type) Ca^{2+} channels. The actions of the established and recently developed antiepileptic drugs on specific neurotransmitter receptors or ion channels will be reviewed.

B. Established Antiepileptic Drug Mechanisms of Action

I. Phenytoin and Carbamazepine

Phenytoin and carbamazepine have been shown to interact with voltage-dependent Na^+ channels at concentrations found free in plasma in patients being treated for epilepsy (MACDONALD 1989 and Table 1). These drugs were demonstrated to reduce the frequency of sustained repetitive firing of neurons. A property of these drugs was that they did not reduce the amplitude or duration of single action potentials but reduced the ability of neurons to fire trains

Table 1. Actions of established antiepileptic drugs

	↓ Sodium current	↑ $GABA_A$ receptor current	↓ T-Calcium current
Carbamazepine	++	–	–
Phenytoin	++	–	–
Primidone	+	–	?
Valproic acid	++	?/+	?/–
Barbiturates	+	+	–
Benzodiazepines	+	++	–
Ethosuximide	–	–	++

of action potentials at high frequency. The limitation of high frequency repetitive firing was voltage-dependent, with limitation of firing being increased following depolarization and reduced following hyperpolarization. Once developed, the limitation of firing was prolonged, lasting several hundred milliseconds. The action of the antiepileptic drugs appeared to be due to a shift of Na^+ channels to an inactive state from which recovery was delayed.

Both phenytoin and carbamazepine produced a voltage-dependent block of mammalian myelinated nerve fibre Na^+ channels that could be removed by hyperpolarization, a shift of the steady-state Na^+ channel inactivation curve to more negative voltages and a reduction in the rate of recovery of Na^+ channels from inactivation (SCHWARZ and GRIGAT 1989). Sodium channels recovered from complete inactivation in a few milliseconds following a 500-ms depolarization to 25 mV. In the presence of 100 μM phenytoin or carbamazepine, however, recovery was prolonged to 90 or 40 ms, respectively. Phenytoin and carbamazepine (50 μM) each produced a frequency-dependent block. However, the frequency-dependent block produced by carbamazepine was somewhat less pronounced than that produced by phenytoin. Thus, phenytoin and carbamazepine produced voltage-dependent and frequency-dependent block of Na^+ channels. Of interest was the finding that phenytoin had a longer time-dependence for frequency-dependent block and for recovery from block than carbamazepine. This would result in more a pronounced frequency-dependent block for phenytoin than for carbamazepine. Thus, although phenytoin and carbamazepine have qualitatively similar actions on Na^+ channels, the actions are quantitatively somewhat different. This may explain, at least in part, differences in efficacy for these two drugs in different patients.

Phenytoin had similar effects on human Na^+ channels (TOMASELLI et al. 1989). Total mRNA was extracted from human brain and injected into *Xenopus* oocytes. The human brain Na^+ channels expressed in oocytes were also blocked by phenytoin in a voltage-, frequency-, and time-dependent fashion. On rat hippocampal neuron Na^+ currents, phenytoin (200 μM) produced a 20 mV negative shift in the steady-state inactivation curve and a frequency-dependent block of Na^+ channels (WAKAMORI et al. 1989; KUO and BEAN 1994). Frequency-dependent block was shown at frequencies as low as

1 Hz, and the block increased to 50% at 10 Hz (WAKAMORI et al. 1989). KUO and BEAN also confirmed the general conclusion that phenytoin enhances Na^+ channel inactivation and provided a partial explanation for the effect. They concluded that unbinding of phenytoin from the Na^+ channel is driven by channel deactivation and that phenytoin may not stabilize the "normal" inactivation state. The delay in recovery from apparent inactivation may be due to phenytoin blocking the Na^+ channel by binding to a blocking site on the Na^+ channel that is formed during activation and removed during deactivation, and only slowly dissociating from the blocking site following deactivation. The voltage dependency of the phenytoin block is thus due to the voltage dependency of deactivation. While not studied, it is likely that many other antiepileptic drugs also block sustained repetitive firing of Na^+ action potentials by selectively binding to the blocking site on the Na^+ channel and increasing apparent Na^+ channel inactivation.

Thus both phenytoin and carbamazepine appear to stabilize the Na^+ channel in an inactive form in a voltage-dependent fashion, the effect being lessened at large negative membrane potentials and increased at less negative membrane potentials. Both drugs slow the rate of recovery of the Na^+ channel from the inactive state and shift the steady-state Na^+ inactivation curve to more negative voltages. This stabilization of the Na^+ channel in an inactive form results in a frequency-dependent block of Na^+ channels and in the blockade of sustained high frequency repetitive firing of action potentials when neurons are depolarized. Of interest is the finding that phenytoin has a stronger slowing effect than carbamazepine, suggesting that these antiepileptic drugs would have slightly different actions under different conditions of repetitive firing.

II. Benzodiazepines and Barbiturates

Both benzodiazepines and barbiturates enhance GABAergic inhibition at free serum concentrations found in ambulatory patients (MACDONALD 1989 and Table 1). At the high concentrations achieved in patients in the treatment of status epilepticus, both drugs also limit high frequency repetitive firing of action potentials, presumably by interacting with voltage-gated Na^+ channels (MCLEAN and MACDONALD 1988). Both benzodiazepines and barbiturates interact with $GABA_A$ receptors, which are macromolecular proteins containing binding sites at least for GABA, picrotoxin, neurosteroids, barbiturates and benzodiazepines and which form a Cl^- ion-selective channel (DE LOREY and OLSEN 1992; MACDONALD and OLSEN 1994). GABA binds to $GABA_A$ receptors to regulate gating (opening and closing) of the Cl^- ion channel (MACDONALD et al. 1989a; WEISS and MAGLEBY 1989; TWYMAN et al. 1990). The binding of GABA increases the probability of channel opening and the open channel can close and rapidly reopen to create bursts of openings.

$GABA_A$ receptors are hetero-pentameric glycoproteins of about 275 kDa and are composed of combinations of multiple polypeptide subunits. The sub-

Table 2. Structural properties of $GABA_A$ receptor subunits

Subunits	α	β	γ	δ	ρ
Number of subtypes	6	4	4	1	2
Number of splice variants	0	2	1	0	0
Size range (kDa)	48–64	51	48	48	52
Percent amino acid homology intrafamily	70–80	70–80	70–80	NA	70–80
Percent amino acid homology interfamily	30–40	30–49	30–40	30–40	30–40

units form a quasi-symmetric structure around the ion channel, with each subunit contributing to the formation of the channel (OLSEN and TOBIN 1990). The model is based on the nicotinic acetylcholine receptor, another member of the ligand-gated ion channel gene superfamily, and electron microscopic image analysis of the native $GABA_A$ receptors (NAYEEM et al. 1994). However, the number of each subtype and their stoichiometry remain uncertain. Based on sequence similarity, six different $GABA_A$ receptor subunit families have been identified and have been named the α, β, γ, δ, ε, and π subunits. There is a 30%–40% sequence identity among the subunit families. About 20%–30% sequence homology exists among all $GABA_A$ receptor subunit candidates and other gene products of the superfamily (SCHOFIELD et al. 1987; DE LOREY and OLSEN 1992). Several of the subunit families have multiple members (α1–6; β1–4, γ1–4), and all of the sequences within each subunit family are homologous with about 70%–80% amino acid sequence identity (Table 2). Additional diversity arises from RNA splice variants, described so far for $\gamma2$ and $\beta4$ subunits (MACDONALD and OLSEN 1994). Each $GABA_A$ receptor subunit cDNA encodes for a polypeptide of about 50kDa, with putative *N*-glycosylation sites and 4 α-helical hydrophobic membrane-spanning regions. Between the third and fourth membrane-spanning region is a hydrophilic putative cytoplasmic region of highly variable sequence involved in intracellular regulatory mechanisms such as phosphorylation.

The pharmacological properties of $GABA_A$ receptors are dependent upon their subunit subtype composition. Benzodiazepine sensitivity requires a γ subunit in the $GABA_A$ receptor (PRITCHETT et al. 1989b; MOSS et al. 1990). Analysis of binding of various benzodiazepines to $GABA_A$ receptors from brain regions revealed two subclasses of benzodiazepine binding sites, type I and type II benzodiazepine sites (KLEPNER et al. 1978; BRAESTRUP and NIELSEN 1981; EICHINGER and SIEGHART 1986; GARRET and TABAKOFF 1985; LIPA et al. 1981). The identification of the multiple $GABA_A$ receptor subunit families led to clarification of the basis for this heterogeneity. The benzodiazepine sensitivity of $GABA_A$ receptors differs when different α subtypes are combined with β and γ subunits (Table 3 and PRITCHETT et al. 1989a; PRITCHETT and SEEBERG 1990; WISDEN et al. 1991; DOBLE and MARTIN 1992). The $\alpha1\beta\gamma$

Table 3. Subunit specific pharmacological properties of $GABA_A$ receptors

Pharmacological property	Subtypes
Benzodiazepine sensitivity	α and β with $\gamma 2$
High benzodiazepine affinity (nM BZ affinity)	$\alpha 1$, $\alpha 2$, $\alpha 3$ or $\alpha 5$ with $\gamma 2$, β
BZ 1 pharmacology (high zolpidem affinity)	$\alpha 1$ with $\gamma 2$, β
BZ 2a,b pharmacology (low zolpidem affinity)	$\alpha 2$, $\alpha 3$ with $\gamma 2$, β
BZ 2c pharmacology (zolpidem insensitive)	$\alpha 5$ with $\gamma 2$, β
BZ 3 pharmacology (BZR agonist insensitive)	$\alpha 4$ or $\alpha 6$ with $\gamma 2$, β
High zinc sensitivity ($IC_{50} < 10$ mM)	α and β without $\gamma 2$
Low zinc sensitivity ($IC_{50} > 100$ mM)	$\alpha 1$ and β with $\gamma 2$
Moderate zinc sensitivity (IC_{50} 10–100 mM)	δ and $\gamma 2$ with α and β or $\alpha 6$, β, $\gamma 2$
Enhancement by loreclezole	$\beta 2$ or $\beta 3$ present
Reduction by furosemide (frusemide)	$\alpha 4$ or $\alpha 6$ present

subunits produce diazepam and zolpidem sensitive benzodiazepine type1 $GABA_A$ receptors, $\alpha 2\beta\gamma$ and $\alpha 3\beta\gamma$ subunits produce benzodiazepine type 2a, b $GABA_A$ receptors with high diazepam and low zolpidem sensitivity, $\alpha 5\beta\gamma$ subunits produce benzodiazepine type 2c $GABA_A$ receptors with high diazepam that are zolpidem insensitive and $\alpha 4$ or $\alpha 6$ $\beta\gamma$ subunits produce benzodiazepine type 3 $GABA_A$ receptors that are benzodiazepine insensitive. Barbiturates bind to an allosteric regulatory site on the $GABA_A$ receptor, but the subunit location of the barbiturate binding site is unknown.

To enhance the $GABA_A$ receptor current, an antiepileptic drug may increase the channel conductance, increase the channel open frequency, and/or increase the channel open duration. Barbiturates and benzodiazepines each modulate the $GABA_A$ receptor current by regulating a different single-channel property of the receptor. Barbiturates enhance the $GABA_A$ receptor current by binding to a regulatory site on the receptor (Olsen 1987). Single channel recordings of barbiturate-enhanced single $GABA_A$ receptor currents have directly demonstrated that barbiturates increase mean channel open duration but do not alter receptor conductance or opening frequency (Macdonald et al. 1989b; Twyman et al. 1989). $GABA_A$ receptors have a high affinity binding site for benzodiazepines, and benzodiazepine and $GABA_A$ receptor binding sites have been demonstrated to be allosterically coupled (Olsen 1987). Benzodiazepines increase $GABA_A$ receptor current, and single channel recordings have demonstrated that they increase $GABA_A$ receptor opening frequency without altering the mean open time or conductance (Vicini et al. 1987; Rogers et al. 1994).

III. Ethosuximide and Trimethadione

Several antiepileptic drugs modify the properties of voltage-dependent Ca^{2+} channels (Macdonald 1989). Phenytoin, barbiturates and benzodiazepines reduce synaptic terminal Ca^{2+} influx and block the presynaptic release of neurotransmitters. However, these actions occur only at high drug concentrations that are above their therapeutic free serum concentrations in patients treated for epilepsy. Thus, these antiepileptic drugs do not appear to have their primary actions on Ca^{2+} channels. Calcium channels, however, have been shown to be heterogeneous (HUI et al. 1991; MORI et al. 1991; STARR et al. 1991; SNUTCH et al. 1991; WILLIAMS et al. 1992). Multiple types of voltage-dependent Ca^{2+} channels have been characterized physiologically (NOWYCKY et al. 1985; MINTZ et al. 1992) and multiple Ca^{2+} channel subunits have been cloned (ZHANG et al. 1993). The Ca^{2+} channels have been called L-, T-, N-, P-, Q- and R-type channels. Each Ca^{2+} channel has different voltage ranges for activation and inactivation and different rates of activation and inactivation. Each channel type has been cloned and shown to be composed of an ion conducting $\alpha 1$ subunit and several smaller accessory subunits (L-type channels: CATTERALL 1988; CAMPBELL et al. 1988; N-type channels: WILLIAMS et al. 1992; FUJITA et al. 1993; P-type channels: MORI et al. 1991; and T-type channels: SOONG et al. 1993). At least six $\alpha 1$, four β, one $\alpha 2$ and one δ subunits have been cloned (PEREZ-REYES and SCHNEIDER 1994). It is also likely that these are not the only types of Ca^{2+} channels present on neurons.

With the finding that neurons express multiple Ca^{2+} channels, it may be that antiepileptic drugs act upon specific types of channels. Indeed, this has been demonstrated for the antiepileptic drugs ethosuximide, trimethadione and (sodium) valproate, which are effective in the treatment of generalized absence seizures (Table 1). Generalized absence epilepsy is characterized clinically by brief periods of loss of consciousness and electrically by generalized 3 Hz spike and wave discharges recorded on the electroencephalogram. Thalamic relay neurons play a critical role in the generation of the abnormal thalamo-cortical rhythmicity that underlies the 3 Hz spike and wave discharge. Whole cell voltage clamp recordings from acutely dissociated relay neurons from the rat thalamus have demonstrated the presence of low threshold (T-type) and high threshold Ca^{2+} currents (COULTER et al. 1989a). T current activation was necessary and sufficient to cause the generation of low threshold Ca^{2+} spikes in thalamic relay neurons. Ethosuximide and dimethadione, the active metabolite of trimethadione, both reduced the T-type current of thalamic neurons isolated from guinea pigs and rats (COULTER et al. 1989b,c). The reduction of the T-type current was produced at concentrations of ethosuximide and dimethadione that have clinical relevance. Phenytoin and carbamazepine, which are ineffective in the control of generalized absence seizures, had minimal effects on the T-type current. The ethosuximide-induced reduction of the T-type current was voltage-dependent. The reduction was most prominent at negative membrane potentials and less prominent at more positive membrane potentials. Ethosuximide did not alter the voltage dependency of steady-state inactivation or the time course of the recovery from inactivation. Dimethadione reduced the T-type current by a mechanism similar to that of ethosuximide. Another anticonvulsant succinimide, α-methyl-α-phenylsuccinimide, also reduced T-type currents, while a convulsant succinimide, tetramethylsuccinimide, reduced the T-type current only at very high concentrations (COULTER et al. 1990). These results suggest that anticonvulsant succinimides and dimethadione, compounds effective in the treatment of generalized absence epilepsy, may have their primary action by reducing the T-type Ca^{2+} current in thalamic relay neurons.

IV. Valproic Acid

The effect of valproic acid on Na^+ channels has been studied less extensively. It remains uncertain if valproic acid has the same mechanism of action as phenytoin and carbamazepine. While valproic acid blocked sustained high frequency repetitive firing of neurons in culture (MCLEAN and MACDONALD et al. 1986a,b and Table 1), detailed voltage clamp experiments of valproic acid actions on Na^+ currents have not been performed. It cannot be concluded that valproic acid has a mechanism of action similar to that of phenytoin and carbamazepine until these studies have been performed.

Valproic acid is one of the most effective drugs against generalized absence seizures. Interestingly, the initial studies of valproic acid did not demonstrate any effect on the T-type Ca^{2+} current; however subsequently, valproic acid was shown to reduce T-type currents in primary afferent neurons (KELLY et al. 1990 and Table 1). The effect was produced over a concentration range of 100–1000 μM. However, the magnitude of the effect was modest, with a 16% reduction seen at 1 mM valproic acid. Whether this modest reduction in T-type Ca^{2+} current is sufficient to explain the effect of valproic acid on generalized absence seizures is unclear. Furthermore, the basis for the discrepancy between the results obtained in rat thalamic neurons and rat primary afferent neurons remains uncertain. It may be that different neuronal types have different sensitivities to these anti-absence drugs or that the small effect is difficult to characterize. Whether this is a relevant mechanism of action for valproic acid will have to be determined by future investigation.

C. Newly Developed Antiepileptic Drug Mechanisms of Action

I. Gabapentin

Gabapentin, 1-(aminomethyl)cyclohexaneacetic acid, is a cyclic GABA analogue which was designed to mimic a restricted steric conformation of GABA and to have a high lipid solubility for penetration of the blood-brain barrier, and was initially intended to act as a GABA agonist (SCHMIDT 1989). Gabapentin is effective in preventing tonic seizures in response to a number of chemoconvulsants and in the maximal electroshock seizure model in rats (ROGAWSKI and PORTER 1990). It prevents reflex seizures in DBA/2 mice and Mongolian gerbils (BARTOSZYK and HAMER 1987) and genetically epilepsy prone rats (Naritoku et al. 1988), but is ineffective in the kindling model. Gabapentin is clinically active in the treatment of human partial and generalized tonic-clonic seizures, and may have some benefit against generalized absence seizures (Bauer et al. 1989; Rowen et al. 1989).

Although early work suggested an effect of gabapentin on $GABA_A$ receptor systems (Bartoszyk and Reimann 1985), a specific effect on GABAergic neurotransmission has not been demonstrated definitively. Gabapentin inhibited monoamine release in electrically stimulated rabbit caudate nucleus (Reimann 1983) and rat cortex (Schlicker et al. 1985), but this inhibition was not modified by GABA, bicuculline or baclofen, suggesting that gabapentin did not act at $GABA_A$ receptors or $GABA_B$ receptors. Gabapentin did not displace [^{3}H]muscimol or [^{3}H]baclofen binding in rat brain and spinal cord, suggesting that it had no specific affinity for $GABA_A$ receptors or $GABA_B$ receptors, and the drug did not inhibit [^{3}H]diazepam binding at the $GABA_A$ receptor benzodiazepine site (Bartoszyk et al. 1986). In electrophysiological studies of GABAergic mechanisms, gabapentin did not affect currents elicited by GABA in mouse spinal cord neurons in culture (Rock et al. 1993), but decreased inhibition evoked by paired pulse orthodromic stimulation of pyramidal neurons in hippocampal slices in vitro (Dooley et al. 1985; Taylor et al. 1988) by an unknown mechanism. In contrast, prolonged (1 h) exposure to gabapentin enhanced the shunting effect on CA_1 region excitatory postsynaptic potentials induced by the GABA uptake inhibitor, nipecotic acid, which promotes GABA release (Honmou et al. 1995a). The enhancement by gabapentin of the nipecotic acid-stimulated conductance increase was not Ca^{2+} dependent, suggesting that there was a non-vesicular release of GABA from neurons or glia (Honmou et al. 1995b). This model suggests that gabapentin may promote GABA synthesis or release through metabolic mechanisms that may be slow to develop.

The effects of gabapentin at glutamate receptors have also been explored. Gabapentin prolonged the onset latency for seizures and for death in mice following intraperitoneal injection of NMDA, but not kainic acid or quinolinic acid; however, it did not affect seizures when NMDA was injected directly into the cerebral lateral ventricle (Bartoszyk 1983). The anticonvulsant effect was blocked by the administration of serine, an agonist at the strychnine-insenstitive glycine receptor site of the NMDA receptor complex, suggesting possible involvement of the NMDA receptor glycine site in the anticonvulsant activity of gabapentin (Oles et al. 1990). However, gabapentin has shown no effect on whole cell or single channel neuronal responses to the application of glutamate or NMDA, with or without glycine co-application (Rock et al. 1993; Taylor et al. 1988). Moreover, gabapentin did not affect long term potentiation in rat hippocampal slices, and this is blocked by most NMDA receptor antagonists (Taylor et al. 1988). These data suggest that the anticonvulsant effect of gabapentin is unlikely to be mediated by actions at NMDA or other glutamatergic receptors.

Biochemical studies have suggested that gabapentin may alter the metabolism and availability of GABA and/or glutamate. Gabapentin has been shown to increase GABA turnover in several rat brain regions (LOSCHER et al. 1991), and increased the levels of GABA in patients with epilepsy, an effect assessed by magnetic resonance spectroscopy (PETROFF et al. 1996). However, gabapentin showed only weak inhibition (33%) of GABA transaminase, the primary enzyme involved in GABA catabolism, with an IC_{50} of 17–20mM, which is higher than that for GABA and much higher than therapeutic concentrations (GOLDLUST et al. 1995). Gabapentin stimulated activity of glutamate dehydrogenase, involved in a major degradative pathway for glutamate, up to 3.4-fold with an EC_{50} of 1.5mM, and competitively inhibited branched chain amino acid aminotransferase, involved in the synthesis of glutamate from amino acids, with a K_i of 0.8–1.4mM, suggesting that gabapentin at therapeutic levels may reduce the synthesis and hasten the degradation of glutamate. Gabapentin is also a substrate for the large neutral amino acid uptake system (system L) in brain synaptosomes, with a K_m of 160μM, similar to that for the amino acid leucine (THURLOW et al. 1996a). In autoradiographic studies in rat brain, [^{3}H]gabapentin binding was inhibited by leucine and a specific large neutral amino acid uptake ligand, suggesting that gabapentin may specifically bind to the system L transporter (THURLOW et al. 1996b). Gabapentin binding was associated with the projection areas of major excitatory amino acid pathways and areas where epileptiform activity occurs, including the hippocampus, dentate gyrus and outer layers of the cerebral cortex. A decrease in gabapentin binding after excitotoxic lesions in the caudate/putamen suggests that the system L sites may be neuronal, and since this binding was also found in a synaptosome preparation, a presynaptic localization is likely. This binding appears to be different from the high affinity site from homogenized brain at which gabapentin was displaced by the anticonvulsant 3-isobutyl GABA (TAYLOR et al. 1993); this may represent an intracellular site. A [^{3}H]gabapentin binding protein was purified from pig cerebral cortex membranes and partially sequenced, revealing an amino-terminal sequence identical to the $\alpha 2\gamma$ subunit of the L-type voltage-dependent Ca^{2+} channel (GEE et al. 1996). It is unclear whether this Ca^{2+} channel is linked to the large neutral amino acid transporter, or how gabapentin might affect its function. Gabapentin blocked responses to BayK8644, an agonist at the dihydropyridine binding site of L-type Ca^{2+} channels (WAMIL et al. 1991), but did not affect voltage-activated Ca^{2+} channel currents of the T, N or L subtypes in recordings from rat dorsal root ganglion cells (ROCK et al. 1993). If gabapentin were to affect brain L-type Ca^{2+} channels, it would imply the displacement of an endogenous BayK8644-like agonist, which has not been demonstrated.

Gabapentin had no effect on sustained repetitive firing of action potentials in mouse spinal cord neurons (TAYLOR et al. 1988; ROCK et al. 1993). While other studies have shown effects on sustained repetitive firing in the same preparation after prolonged (24–48h) incubation with therapeutically relevant

Table 4. Actions of new antiepileptic drugs

	Sodium current	$GABA_A$ receptor current	Calcium current	Glutamate synaptic function
Gabapentin	+/?	+/?	+/?	+/?
Lamotrigine	++	–/?	+/?	+/?
Oxcarbazepine	++	?	+/?	+/?
Vigabatrin	?	+/?	?	–
Tiagabine	?	+/?	?	–
Topiramate	+/?	+/?	?	–
Felbamate	+/?	+/?	–	+/?

concentrations of gabapentin (WAMIL and MCLEAN 1994), gabapentin had no effect on rat brain type IIA Na^+ channel α subunits expressed in CHO cells with acute intracellular or extracellular delivery or after prolonged (24h) bath exposure to the drug (TAYLOR 1993). While it is conceivable that gabapentin might require additional Na^+ channel regulatory subunits to confer activity, the prolonged incubation time necessary to demonstrate an effect in neuronal preparations suggests that a direct action on voltage-gated Na^+ channels is unlikely. Further characterization of gabapentin's activity at the large neutral amino acid transporter and L-type Ca^{2+} channel may provide new insights into its anticonvulsant mechanism.

In summary, the results of several studies have demonstrated a possible effect of gabapentin to increase GABA release but have not demonstrated a major effect of the drug on ligand- or voltage-gated channels (Table 4). Further work on the high-affinity binding site of gabapentin and the possibility of active transport of gabapentin across neuronal membranes should contribute significantly to the understanding of its mechanism of action.

II. Lamotrigine

Lamotrigine [3,5,-diamino-6-(2,3-dichlorophenyl)-1,2,4-triazine] is a phenyltriazine with weak antifolate activity. Lamotrigine was developed following the observations that the use of phenobarbitone, primidone and phenytoin resulted in reduced folate levels and that folates could induce seizures in experimental animals (REYNOLDS et al. 1966). It was proposed that antifolate activity might be related to anticonvulsant activity; however, this has not been demonstrated by structure-activity studies (ROGAWSKI and PORTER 1990). Lamotrigine has anticonvulsant activity in several animal seizure models including hind limb extension in maximal electroshock and maximal pentylenetetrazol seizures in rodents (MILLER et al. 1986). Lamotrigine has been effective as add-on therapy in the treatment of human partial and generalized tonic-clonic seizures.

The action of lamotrigine on the release of endogenous amino acids from rat cerebral cortex slices in vitro has been studied. Lamotrigine potently inhibited the release of glutamate and aspartate evoked by the Na^+ channel activator veratrine, and was much less effective in the inhibition of the release of acetylcholine or GABA. At high concentrations, lamotrigine had no effect on spontaneous or potassium-evoked amino acid release. These studies suggested that lamotrigine acted at voltage-dependent Na^+ channels resulting in decreased presynaptic release of glutamate (LEACH et al. 1986). In radioligand studies, the binding of [^{3}H]batrachotoxinin A 20-α-benzoate, a neurotoxin that binds to receptor site 2 on voltage-dependent Na^+ channels, was inhibited by lamotrigine in rat brain synaptosomes (CHEUNG et al. 1992). Several electrophysiological studies have tested the effects of lamotrigine on voltage-dependent Na^+ channels. Lamotrigine blocked sustained repetitive firing in cultured mouse spinal cord neurons in a dose-dependent manner at concentrations which are therapeutic in the treatment of human seizures (CHEUNG et al. 1992). In cultured rat cortical neurons, lamotrigine reduced burst firing induced by glutamate or potassium, but not unitary Na^+ action potentials evoked at low frequencies (LEES and LEACH 1993). In cultured hippocampal neurons, lamotrigine reduced Na^+ currents in a voltage-dependent manner, and at depolarized potentials showed a small frequency-dependent inhibition (MUTOH and DICHTER 1993). Lamotrigine increased steady-state inactivation of currents in rat brain type IIA Na^+ channel α subunit which were expressed in Chinese hamster ovary cells (TAYLOR 1993) and produced both tonic and frequency-dependent inhibition of voltage-dependent Na^+ channels in clonal N4TG1 mouse neuroblastoma cells, but it had no effect on cationic currents induced by stimulation of glutamatergic receptors in embryonic rat hippocampal neurons (WANG et al. 1993).

In cultured rat cortical neurons, lamotrigine at high concentrations was able to inhibit peak high threshold Ca^{2+} currents and appeared to shift the threshold for inward currents to more depolarized potentials (LEES and LEACH 1993). In clonal rat pituitary GH3 cells, lamotrigine at the same concentration did not inhibit high threshold Ca^{2+} currents, caused only slight inhibition of low threshold Ca^{2+} currents, reduced rapidly inactivating voltage-dependent K^+ currents, and had no significant effect on Ca^{2+}-activated K^+ currents (LANG and WANG 1991). In cultured rat cortical neurons, lamotrigine did not appear to mimic the effect of diazepam when tested on GABA-evoked Cl^- currents (LEES and LEACH 1993).

Other studies, however, suggest a possible effect of the drug on voltage-gated Ca^{2+} channels. Lamotrigine inhibited high voltage activated Ca^{2+} currents in rat cortical neurons with an IC_{50} of 12 μM (STEFANI et al. 1996b). This action was blocked by the N-type Ca^{2+} channel blocker ω-conotoxin GVIA and the P-type Ca^{2+} channel blocker ω-agatoxin IVA, but was not blocked by nifedipine (an L-type Ca^{2+} channel blocker), suggesting that lamotrigine at therapeutic concentrations may reduce the release of neurotransmitters in part by acting at presynaptic Ca^{2+} channels. Lamotrigine also blocked NMDA receptor-mediated excitatory postsynaptic potentials in rat amygdala neurons in vitro, evoked by stimulation of the endopyriform nucleus (WANG et al. 1996).

Postsynaptic responsiveness to AMPA was not affected by lamotrigine, but paired pulse excitatory postsynaptic potential facilitation was increased, suggesting a presynaptic mechanism of action of the drug. The presumed presynaptic inhibitory effects of lamotrigine were blocked by ω-conotoxin GVIA, suggesting mediation of the effect by N-type Ca^{2+} channels (WANG et al. 1996). A presynaptic reduction in the release of glutamate may explain the possible neuroprotective effect of lamotrigine in a model of axotomy-induced motoneuron cell death (CASANOVAS et al. 1996) and in a global ischaemia model (SHUAIB et al. 1995), both of which may involve excitotoxic mechanisms. It is unclear, however, why lamotrigine should preferentially reduce presynaptic release of glutamate more than GABA or other neurotransmitters, and more recent studies have not observed this selectivity (WALDMEIER et al. 1996). Moreover, the efficacy of lamotrigine against generalized absence epilepsy is greater than that seen with the other agents that affect the Na^+ channel, suggesting that additional mechanisms may be at work, perhaps involving a reduction of low threshold (T-type) Ca^{2+} channel currents or $GABA_B$ receptor antagonism, though these effects have not been demonstrated.

These results suggest that the antiepileptic effect of lamotrigine is due to a specific interaction at the voltage-dependent Na^+ channel that results in voltage- and frequency-dependent inhibition of the channel (Table 4). These results are similar to those found for phenytoin and carbamazepine. It remains to be determined whether this action results in a significant preferentially decreased release of presynaptic glutamate.

III. Oxcarbazepine

Oxcarbazepine (10,11-dihydro-10-oxo-carbamazepine) is a derivative of the dibenzazepine series and is very similar to carbamazepine in molecular structure. Oxcarbazepine differs from carbamazepine by a keto substitution at the 10,11-position of the dibenzazepine nucleus. The keto substitution causes a different biotransformation pattern and greater tolerability in humans compared to carbamazepine. Oxcarbazepine is rapidly and nearly completely metabolized to 10,11-dihydro-10-hydroxy carbamazepine (GP 47779), the active metabolite which is responsible for the antiepileptic activity of oxcarbazepine (JENSEN et al. 1991). Hydroxy-carbamazepine is a racemate with both enantiomers having approximately equal anticonvulsant activity (SCHMUTZ et al. 1993). Metabolism of oxcarbazepine does not result in the formation of 10,11-epoxy carbamazepine.

Oxcarbazepine and hydroxy-carbamazepine are effective in inhibiting hind limb extension in rats and mice elicited by maximal electroshock, but are approximately 2–3 times less effective against pentylenetetrazole-induced seizures in mice (BALTZER and SCHMUTZ 1978). In studies using rats at different developmental ages, oxcarbazepine, hydroxy-carbamazepine, and carbamazepine dose-dependently reduced the tonic phase of generalized seizures induced by pentylenetetrazole and appeared to have identical anticonvulsant profiles in this model (KUBOVA and MARES 1993). Oxcarbazepine and hydroxy-carbamazepine have relatively poor anticonvulsant efficacy against picrotoxin- and strychnine-induced seizures in mice (BALTZER and SCHMUTZ 1978). Oxcarbazepine was able to completely suppress seizures in rhesus monkeys in a chronic aluminium focus model of partial seizures. At comparable doses, hydroxy-carbamazepine was less effective in suppressing seizures in this model (JENSEN et al. 1991). Oxcarbazepine is effective in the treatment of human generalized tonic-clonic seizures and partial seizures with and without secondary generalization (DAM and JENSEN 1989).

In electrophysiological studies of rat hippocampal slices, oxcarbazepine and the hydroxy-carbamazepine enantiomers dose-dependently decreased epileptic-like discharges induced by penicillin. Additionally, the drugs' abilities to suppress discharges was decreased by 4-amino-pyridine, a K^+ channel blocker (SCHMUTZ et al. 1993). Oxcarbazepine and hydroxy-carbamazepine have been shown to reduce sustained high frequency repetitive firing of voltage-dependent Na^+ action potentials in mouse spinal cord neurons (MCLEAN et al. 1994), thus suggesting that oxcarbazepine's mechanism of action is similar to that of carbamazepine and phenytoin (Table 2).

More recently, hydroxy-carbamazepine (3–100 μM) was shown to inhibit glutamatergic excitatory postsynaptic potentials in intracellular recordings of striatal neurons in rat brain corticostriatal slices (CALABRESI et al. 1995). The postsynaptic sensitivity to glutamate was unchanged, implying a presynaptic mechanism for the effect. In isolated cortical pyramidal cells, hydroxy-carbamazepine produced a reversible, concentration-dependent decrease in high voltage-activated Ca^{2+} currents (STEFANI et al. 1995). This effect was not blocked by nifedipine, but other, more specific, Ca^{2+} channel toxins were not tested. Together, these data suggest that oxcarbazepine and its metabolites may reduce the presynaptic release of glutamate by blocking a presynaptic high voltage activated Ca^{2+} channel, an effect that may also contribute to its antiepileptic efficacy. The relative contribution of this action at voltage-dependent Ca^{2+} channels is unclear, and other as yet unknown mechanisms may also be involved

IV. Vigabatrin

Vigabatrin (γ-vinyl GABA; 4-amino-hex-5-enoic acid) is a synthetic derivative and structural analogue of GABA. Vigabatrin was developed to be an enzyme-activated, irreversible inhibitor of GABA-transaminase, the primary presynaptic degradative enzyme for GABA. Vigabatrin's selective inhibition of GABA transaminase was intended to have potential therapeutic value by increasing GABA levels in the brain and thereby enhancing GABAergic transmission. Vigabatrin is a racemic mixture of S(+)- and R(–)-enantiomers. The S(+)-enantiomer potently inhibits GABA transaminase whereas the R(–)-enantiomer has minimal activity (LARSSON et al. 1986). The molecular mechanism of action of vigabatrin's inhibition of GABA transaminase was proposed by Lippert et al. (1977). Vigabatrin is accepted as a substrate of GABA transaminase by forming a Schiff base with pyridoxal phosphate in the active site of the enzyme that then abstracts a proton from the Schiff base. The resulting charge stabilization by the pyridine ring induces the aldimine to ketimine tautomerism that occurs in the normal transamination process. The reactive unsaturated ketimine forms a stable bond with a nucleophilic residue at GABA transaminase's active site, resulting in irreversible inhibition of the enzyme, thus terminating its ability to transaminate new substrate.

Numerous animal studies have described the effects of vigabatrin's inhibition of GABA transaminase. Vigabatrin inhibited mouse whole brain GABA transaminase activity and increased whole brain GABA concentrations (Jung et al. 1977; Schecter et al. 1977). These actions were seen in all brain areas assayed and were quantitatively different corresponding to the relative regional distribution of GABAergic neurons (Chapman et al. 1982). In rat cortex, vigabatrin markedly increased the synaptosomal GABA pool compared with non-synaptosomal GABA (Sarhan and Seiler 1979), suggesting a greater effect of vigabatrin on neuronal GABA transaminase than on glial GABA transaminase. This effect is consistent with the finding that neurons have a high affinity GABA uptake system whereas astrocytes have a low affinity system (Schousboe et al. 1986). In human studies, vigabatrin dose-dependently increased cerebrospinal fluid levels of free and total GABA (Grove et al. 1981; Schechter et al. 1984; Ben-Menachem 1989) but did not significantly affect other neurotransmitter systems (Schechter et al. 1984; Riekkinen et al. 1989). In recent studies with healthy subjects, nuclear magnetic resonance spectroscopy showed that occipital lobe GABA concentrations were elevated after taking vigabatrin (Petroff et al. 1993).

Vigabatrin has been shown to be an effective anticonvulsant in a variety of animal models of epilepsy. In studies with rodents, vigabatrin inhibited strychnine-induced and audiogenic seizures (Schechter et al. 1977). Other studies showed that only the active S(+)-enantiomer of vigabatrin was effective in inhibiting audiogenic seizures in mice (Meldrum and Murugaiah 1983). Vigabatrin inhibited epileptic responses in photosensitive baboons (Meldrum and Horton 1978) and inhibited the development of kindling (Shin et al. 1986; Loscher et al. 1987) as well as of fully developed generalized seizures in the amygdala-kindled rat (Kalichman et al. 1982). Vigabatrin was less effective in inhibiting seizures caused by bicuculline and picrotoxin (Schechter and Tranier 1977). Vigabatrin has been effective in the treatment of human partial seizures with or without secondary generalization.

In summary, vigabatrin is a selective irreversible inhibitor of GABA transaminase, the main degradative enzyme for GABA. Inhibition of GABA transaminase produces greater available pools of presynaptic GABA for release in central nervous system synapses. Increased activity of GABA at postsynaptic GABA receptors can cause increased inhibition of neurons which are important in controlling the abnormal electrical activity of seizures (Table 2). These actions probably account for the clinical antiepileptic effects of vigabatrin.

V. Tiagabine

Tiagabine, R(–)-*N*-[4,4-di(3-methyl-thien-2-yl)-but-3-enyl] nipecotic acid hydrochloride, is a nipecotic acid derivative that selectively and potently inhibits neuronal and glial GABA uptake (Braestrup et al. 1990). Unlike nipecotic acid, tiagabine is not a substrate for the uptake transporter, and therefore does not act as a false transmitter. Tiagabine specifically inhibits the GABA transporter GAT-1, which has been cloned (Borden et al. 1994). It interacts only weakly with the GABA and benzodiazepine sites on $GABA_A$ receptors and does not bind to other neurotransmitter receptors (Suzdak and Jansen 1995). Unlike vigabatrin, its actions are reversible and do not result in a general elevation of CSF GABA levels. However, microdialysis studies reveal regional extracellular GABA overflow in the globus pallidus, ventral pallidum, and substantia nigra in awake rats (Fink-Jensen et al. 1992). Curiously, tiagabine pretreatment resulted in increases in $[^3H]$GABA binding to $GABA_A$ receptors in the prefrontal, motor, sensory, pyriform and cingulate cortex, and reductions in $GABA_B$ receptor binding in regions including a number of cortical areas (prefrontal, motor, striate, entorhinal, retrosplenial and temporal cortex) and in the medial geniculate and anteroventral thalamic nuclei, superior colliculus and molecular layer of the cerebellar cortex (Thomsen and Suzdak 1995). It is unclear whether these changes represent alterations in receptor number, affinity or subunit composition. In CA_1 pyramidal cells recorded from hippocampal slices in vitro, tiagabine increased the half-width of inhibitory postsynaptic currents, suggesting a prolonged effect of GABA at inhibitory synapses (Roepstorff and Lambert 1992). In contrast, nipecotic acid reduced the amplitude of inhibitory postsynaptic currents while only modestly prolonging the declining phase of the current; the reduced amplitude presumably results from nipecotic acid entering the presynaptic terminal and acting as a false transmitter.

Tiagabine blocked pentylenetetrazole as well as audiogenic seizures in DBA/2 mice and amygdala- or hippocampal-kindled seizures in rats (Dalby and Nielsen 1990; Morimoto et al. 1997). It also blocked reflex epileptic seizures in the genetically epilepsy-prone rat and photosensitive baboon (*Papio papio*) animal models (Smith et al. 1995). Tiagabine prevented generalized clonic seizures in the perforant path stimulation model of status epilepticus and reduced the loss of pyramidal cells in hippocampal CA_3 and CA_1 regions, but did not protect somatostatin-immunoreactive neurons in the dentate hilus (Halonen et al. 1996). Tiagabine also slowed neuronal death in the gerbil hippocampus in a model of postischemic excitotoxic cell death (Inglefield et al. 1995).

Decreased uptake of GABA, and the possible increases in $GABA_A$ receptors and reductions in $GABA_B$ receptors, does not always imply increased inhibition; the effect depends on the neuronal circuitry involved. Increased GABA can facilitate spike-wave discharges in animal models of generalized absence seizure (Vergnes et al. 1984; Peeters et al. 1989). In WAG/Rij rats, tiagabine enhanced the number and duration of spike-wave discharges and provoked expression of a second type of epileptiform discharge (COENEN et al. 1995). In a rat model of status epilepticus produced by homocysteine injection after a cobalt lesion, tiagabine was effective in controlling generalized tonic-clonic seizures; but tiagabine induced an abnormal hyporeactive behavioural state associated with rhythmic high amplitude bifrontal 3–5 Hz spike and wave activity which may have represented a form of non-convulsive status epilepticus (WALTON et al. 1994). A similar syndrome may also occur in humans. Although tiagabine is effective against partial and generalized convulsive seizures, it may be contraindicated in patients with generalized absence epilepsy.

VI. Topiramate

Topiramate, 2,3:4,5-bis-*O*-(1-methylethylidine)-β-D-fructopyranose sulfamate, is a sulfamate derivative structurally unique among anticonvulsants, with clinical efficacy as adjunctive therapy against partial seizures (FAUGHT et al. 1996; PRIVATERA et al. 1996; REIFE and PLEDGER 1997) and possible when used as monotherapy (ROSENFELD et al. 1997).

Topiramate blocked audiogenic seizures in a rat model of ischemia-induced epilepsy in which three seizure types reflected the degree of severity, progressing from wild running through clonic seizures to tonic hind limb extension (EDMONDS et al. 1996). Topiramate and phenytoin blocked these seizure types with similar ED_{50}s. Topiramate was also effective in reducing seizure activity in an amygdala kindling model (WAUQUIER and ZHOU 1996) and in maximal electroshock seizures but was ineffective against pentylenetetrazol, bicuculline and picrotoxin seizures (MARYANOFF et al. 1987; WHITE et al. 1997).

In in vitro electrophysiological studies, topiramate reversibly decreased the number of action potentials in spontaneous epileptiform bursts and reduced the burst duration in cultured hippocampal neurons and (at 20 μM) also reduced the number of action potentials elicited by a 1 s depolarization (COULTER et al. 1993). Topiramate suppressed the intrinsic bursting of proximal subiculum neurons in rat hippocampal slices and reduced the tonic repetitive firing of these neurons during depolarizing pulses (KAWASAKI et al. 1996). Topiramate also reduced voltage-gated Na^+ currents in cultured cerebellar granule cells without changing the voltage dependency of activation, though these effects were observed at high (200–500 μM) drug concentrations (ZONA et al. 1996). The steady state inactivation curve was shifted to the left, suggesting an effect on the inactivated form of the channel. These findings suggest that the anticonvulsant mechanism of the drug may be similar to that of phenytoin, and that its effect may be to prevent the propagation of seizure activity.

Additional mechanisms of action may also be important. In a microdialysis study of spontaneously epileptic rats (SER), an epileptic double mutant derived from the Wistar strain, topiramate reduced the basal levels of glutamate and aspartate from two- to threefold above normal to near normal with the same concentration-response relationship and time course as that with which it suppressed tonic seizures (KANDA et al. 1996). There was no effect on glutamate levels in normal Wistar rats. The mechanism underlying the reduction in elevated levels of excitatory amino acids was unclear, but thought to be presynaptic in its site. Topiramate also reversibly enhanced postsynaptic $GABA_A$ receptor currents measured by Cl^- flux or by electrophysiological recordings (WHITE et al. 1997), perhaps explaining its modest activity against pentylenetetrazole seizures (at low topiramate doses) (WHITE et al. 1996), and the reduction in spike-wave discharges in a rodent model of absence seizures (NAKAMURA et al. 1994). It is as yet unclear whether topiramate's postsynaptic effect on $GABA_A$ receptors requires a specific $GABA_A$ receptor subunit subtype or isoform.

VII. Felbamate

Felbamate, 2-phenyl-1,3-propanediol dicarbamate, is a dicarbamate with a structure similar to that of the antianxiety agent meprobamate. It was effective against seizures elicited by maximum electroshock, pentylenetetrazole and picrotoxin (SWINYARD et al. 1986) and blocked bicuculline- but not strychnine-induced seizures (SOFIA et al. 1991). Felbamate also reduced seizures produced by cortical aluminium lesions in rhesus monkeys (LOCKARD et al. 1987) and inhibited seizures induced by NMDA and also inhibited kainate-induced status epilepticus (WHITE et al. 1992; CHRONOPOULOS et al. 1993). More recently, felbamate was shown to block the development of chemical kindling in rats given repeated subconvulsive doses of pentylenetetrazole (GIORGI et al. 1996). These studies suggest that felbamate increases the seizure threshold and prevents the electrical spread of seizure activity. In humans, felbamate has been effective against partial seizures with and without secondary generalization, and was particularly useful in patients with partial and generalized seizures associated with the Lennox-Gastaut syndrome. Unfortunately an unacceptably high incidence of aplastic anaemia (1 in 20,000) and severe hepatotoxicity have precluded the use of felbamate except in special circumstances (PENNELL et al. 1995; STABLES et al. 1995).

Felbamate in subprotective doses enhanced the protective effects of diazepam against seizures induced by maximum electroshock, pentylenetetrazole and isoniazid, but not seizures induced by bicuculline, suggesting a possible action at $GABA_A$ receptors (GORDON et al. 1991). Early studies failed to find an effect of felbamate on ligand binding to the GABA, benzodiazepine or picrotoxin binding sites on $GABA_A$ receptors in rat brain cortical membranes, and felbamate did not affect GABA-induced $[^{36}Cl^-]$ flux in cultured mouse spinal cord neurons (TICKU et al. 1991). However, in cultured hippocampal neurons, felbamate at relatively high concentrations (1–3 mM) potentiated GABA-evoked Cl^- currents, an effect not antagonized by the benzodiazepine antagonist flumazenil (RHO et al. 1994). Felbamate inhibited binding of [^{3}H]t-butylbicycloorthobenzoate, a picrotoxin site ligand, in rat brain slices with an IC_{50} of 250 μM, and produced small enhancements of GABA-induced Cl^- currents which were not affected by flumazenil or pentobarbitone but blocked by picrotoxin or bicuculline (KUME et al. 1996).

Felbamate also prevented NMDA- and quisqualate-induced seizures in mice, suggesting a possible effect at glutamatergic receptors, though it did not inhibit the binding of MK-801, an NMDA receptor antagonist (SOFIA et al. 1991). However, intra-cerebro-ventricular administration of D-serine, an NMDA receptor glycine site agonist, produced a shift to the right of the felbamate anticonvulsant concentration-response curve in audiogenic seizure-susceptible mice (HARMSWORTH et al. 1993). Felbamate also inhibited the binding of [^{3}H]5,7-dichlorokynurenic acid, a competitive antagonist at the strychnine-insensitive glycine site of the NMDA receptor (MCCABE et al. 1993), which further suggests that felbamate may act in part as an NMDA glycine site antagonist. Both felbamate and kynurenic acid derivatives blocked the expression of epileptiform activity induced by kainic acid in hippocampal slices, while antagonists at other NMDA receptor sites (MK-801, ketamine, CGS19755) were ineffective. In hippocampal neurons in culture, felbamate inhibited NMDA receptor mediated responses with an IC_{50} of about 1.8 mM (RHO et al. 1994). This inhibition did not appear to be mediated by antagonism at either the NMDA or glycine binding sites, but was more consistent with open channel block (SUBRAMANIAM et al. 1995). In rat striatal neurons in slices, felbamate inhibited both extracellular field potentials and intracellular excitatory postsynaptic potentials only when Mg^{2+} was absent, consistent with NMDA-mediated responses, and in acutely isolated striatal neurons felbamate blocked currents elicited by bath or focal application of NMDA (PISANI et al. 1995). Felbamate inhibited extracellularly recorded excitatory postsynaptic potentials in hippocampal slices at moderate concentrations (200–700 μM), reducing both AMPA- and NMDA-receptor mediated responses (PUGLIESE and CORRADETTI 1996). It also blocked long term potentiation, but only at concentrations (700–1300 μM) higher than those needed for antiepileptic activity.

Felbamate may also affect voltage gated Na^+ and/or Ca^{2+} channels. In mouse spinal cord neurons, felbamate produced a 50% inhibition of repetitive firing of action potentials at 67 μM (PISANI et al. 1995; WHITE et al. 1992). In striatal neurons, felbamate blocked repetitive current-evoked action potentials and inhibited depolarization-evoked Na^+ currents with an IC_{50} of 28 μM (PISANI et al. 1995). Felbamate (30 μM) also shifted the steady-state inactivation curve to the left by 10.4 mV without affecting the slope, consistent with an effect on the inactivated state of the Na^+ channel. In guinea pig olfactory cortex neurons, felbamate also reduced the slow excitation and blocked sustained repetitive firing elicited by muscarinic receptor or metabotropic glutamate receptor agonists (LIBRI et al. 1996), possibly by blocking Ca^{2+} influx through voltage-gated Ca^{2+} channels, as felbamate also reduced the duration of Ca^{2+} spikes elicited by cesium loading. Felbamate blocked high voltage-activated Ca^{2+} currents in acutely isolated cortical and neostriatal neurons with an IC_{50} of 504 nM (STEFANI et al. 1996a). The felbamate-mediated inhibition was blocked by nifedipine but not by ω-conotoxin GVIA or ω-agatoxin IVA, suggesting that felbamate inhibits L-type, dihydropyridine-sensitive Ca^{2+} channels. Blockade of L-type channels might be effective in controlling spike discharges from epileptic foci, and may be neuroprotective by limiting Ca^{2+} loading.

Several recent studies have demonstrated a neuroprotective effect of felbamate in transient forebrain ischaemia in gerbils (SHUAIB et al. 1996; WASTERLAIN et al. 1996), in fluid percussion trauma (WALLIS and PANIZZON 1995) and after kainate-induced status epilepticus (CHRONOPOULOS et al. 1993). In each case, there was significant protection of hippocampal CA_1 neurons that would have otherwise undergone apoptosis, and the neuroprotective effect was observed when felbamate was administered after the neuronal injury. Felbamate also blocked excitotoxic neuronal injury in cultured cortical neurons (KANTHASAMY et al. 1995), decreasing NMDA- and glutamate-induced Ca^{2+} influx. This effect was not antagonized by glycine, suggesting that the effect might result from an action of felbamate at an NMDA receptor site distinct from the strychnine-insensitive glycine receptor. Blockade of Ca^{2+} entry, whether at voltage- or ligand-gated channels, appears to be crucial to the neuroprotective effect. In the circumstance of an acute cerebral infarct, injury or neurosurgery, a brief exposure to felbamate may be an acceptable risk if it provides significant neuroprotective benefit; this possible therapeutic modality is deserving of further controlled study.

References

Baltzer V, Schmutz M (1978) Experimental anticonvulsive properties of GP 47 680 and of GP 47 779, its main human metabolite; compounds related to carbamazepine. In: Meinardi H, Rowan AJ (eds) Advances in Epileptology. Lisse: Swets and Zeitlinger, Amsterdam, pp. 295–299

Bartoszyk GD (1983) Gabapentin and convulsions provoked by excitatory amino acids. Naunyn-Schmiedeberg's Arch Pharmacol 324:R24

Bartoszyk GD, Hamer M (1987) The genetic animal model of reflex epilepsy in the Mongolian gerbil: differential efficacy of new anticonvulsive drugs and prototype antiepileptics. Pharmacol Res Commun 19:429–440

Bartoszyk GD, Reimann W (1985) Preclinical characterization of the anticonvulsant gabapentin. 16th Epilepsy International Congress, Hamburg

Bartoszyk GD, Meyerson N, Reimann W, Satzinger G, von Hodenberg A (1986) Gabapentin. In: Meldrum BS, Porter RJ (eds) Current problems in epilepsy: new anticonvulsant drugs. John Libbey & Company, London, pp. 147–164

Bauer G, Bechinger D, Castell M (1989) Gabapentin in the treatment of drug-resistant epileptic patients. Adv Epileptol 17:219–221

Ben-Menachem E (1989) Pharmacokinetic effects of vigabatrin on cerebrospinal fluid amino acids in humans. Epilepsia 30 [Suppl 3]:S12–S14

Borden LA, Dhar TGM, Smith KE, Weinshank RL, Branchek TA, Gluchowski C (1994) Tiagabine, SKF89976-A, CI-966 and NNC-711 are selective for the cloned GABA transporter GAT-1. Eur J Pharmacol 269:219–224

Braestrup C, Nielsen MJ (1981) [^{3}H]-propyl-β-carboline-3-carboxylate as a selective radioligand for the BZI benzodiazepine receptor subclass. J Neurochem 37: 333–341

Braestrup C, Nielsen EB, Sonnewald U et al. (1990) R(-)-N-[4,4-di(3-methylthien-2-yl)-but-3-en-1-yl] nipecotic acid binds with high affinity to the brain γ-aminobutyric acid uptake carrier. J Neurochem 54:639–648

Calabresi P, De Murtas M, Stefani A, Pisani A, Sancesario G, Mercuri NB, Bernardi G (1995) Action of GP 47779, the active metabolite of oxcarbazepine, on the corticostriatal system. I. Modulation of corticostriatal synaptic transmission. Epilepsia 36:990–996

Campbell KP, Leung AT, Sharp AH (1988) The biochemistry and molecular biology of the dihydropydrine-sensitive calcium channel. Trends Neurosci 11:425–430

Casanovas A, Ribera J, Hukkanen M, Riveros-Moreno V, Esquerda JE (1996) Prevention by lamotrigine, MK801 and N-omega-nitro-L-arginine methyl ester of motoneuron cell death after neuronal axotomy. Neuroscience 71:313–325

Catterall WA (1988) Structure and function of voltage-sensitive ion channels. Science 242:50–61

Chapman AG, Riley K, Evans MC, Meldrum BS (1982) Acute effects of sodium valproate and γ-vinyl GABA on regional amino acid metabolism in the rat brain: incorporation of 2-$^{[14C]}$glucose into amino acids. Neurochem Research 7:1089–1105

Cheung H, Kamp D, Harris E (1992) An in vitro investigation of the action of lamotrigine on neuronal voltage-activated sodium channels. Epilepsy Res 13:107–112

Chronopoulos A, Stafstrom C, Thurber S, Hyde P, Mikati M, Holmes, GL (1993) Neuroprotective effect of felbamate after kainic acid-induced status epilepticus. Epilepsia 34:359–366

Coenen AML, Blezer EHM, van Luijtelaar ELJM (1995) Effects of the GABA-uptake inhibitor tiagabine on electroencephalogram, spike-wave discharges and behaviour of rats. Epilepsy Res 21:89–94

Coulter DA, Hugenard JR, Prince DA (1989a) Calcium currents in rat thalamocortical relay neurones: kinetic properties of the transient low-threshold current. J Physiol 414:587–604

Coulter DA, Hugenard JR, Prince DA (1989b) Specific petit mal anticonvulsants reduce calcium currents in thalamic neurons. Neurosci Lett 98:74–78

Coulter DA, Hugenard JR, Prince DA (1989c) Characterization of ethosuximide reduction of low-threshold calcium current in thalamic neurons. Ann Neurol 25:582–593

Coulter DA, Hugenard JR, Prince DA (1990) Differential effects of petit mal anticonvulsants and convulsants on thalamic neurones: calcium current reduction. Br J Pharmacol 100:800–806

Dalby NS, Nielsen EB (1990) Tiagabine exerts an anti-epileptogenic effect in amygdala kindling epileptogenesis in the rat. Neurosci Lett 229:135–137

Dam M, Jensen PK (1989) Potential antiepileptic drugs: oxcarbazepine. In: Levy RH, Driefuss FE, Mattson RH, Meldrum BS, Penry JK (eds) Antiepileptic drugs, 3rd edn. Raven Press, New York, pp. 913–924

De Lorey TM, Olsen RW (1992) γ-Aminobutyric acida receptor structure and function. J Biol Chem 267:16747–16750

Doble A, Martin IL (1992) Multiple benzodiazepine receptors – no reason for anxiety. Trends Pharmacol Sci 13:76–81

Dooley DJ, Bartoszyk GD, Rock DM, Satzinger G (1985) Preclinical characterization of the anticonvulsant gabapentin. 16th Epilepsy International Congress, Hamburg

Edmonds HL, Jiang YD, Zhang PY, Shank RP (1996) Anticonvulsant activity of topiramate and phenytoin in a rat model of ischemia-induced epilepsy. Life Sci 59:127–131

Eichinger A, Sieghart W (1986) Postnatal development of proteins associated with different benzodiazepine receptors. J Neurochem 46:173–180

Faught E, Wilder BJ, Ramsey RE, Reife RA, Kramer LD, Pledger GW, Karim RM, and the Topiramate YD Study Group (1996) Topiramate placebo-controlled dose-ranging trial in refractory partial epilepsy using 200-, 400-, and 600-mg daily dosages. Neurology 46:1684–1690

Fink-Jensen A, Suzdak RD, Sweberg MD, Judge ME, Hansen L, Nielsen PG (1992) The GABA uptake inhibitor, tiagabine, increases extracellular brain levels of GABA in awake rats. Eur J Pharmacol 220:197–201

Fujita Y, Mynlieff M, Kirksen RT et al. (1993) Primary structure and functional expression of the ω-conotoxin-sensitive N-type calcium channel from rabbit brain. Neuron 10:585–598

Garret KM, Tabakoff B (1985) The development of type I and type II benzodiazepine receptors in the mouse cortex and cerebellum. Pharmacol Biochem Behav 22:985–992

Gee NS, Brown JP, Dissanayake VUK, Offord J, Thurlow R, Woodruff GN (1996) The novel anticonvulsant drug, gabapentin (Neurontin), binds to the 2 subunit of a calcium channel. J Biol Chem 271:5768–5776

Giorgi O, Carboni G, Frau V, Orlandi M, Valentini V, Feldman A, Corda MG (1996) Anticonvulsant effect of felbamate in the pentylenetetrazol kindling model of epilepsy in the rat. Naunyn Schmiedebergs Arch Pharmacol 354:173–178

Goldlust A, Su T-Z, Welty DF, Taylor CP, Oxender DL (1995) Effects of anticonvulsant drug gabapentin on the enzymes in metabolic pathways of glutamate and GABA. Epilepsy Res 22:1–11

Gordon R, Gels M, Diamantis W, Sofia RD (1991) Interaction of felbamate and diazepam against maximal electroshock seizures and chemoconvulsants in mice. Pharmacol Biochem Behav 40:109–113

Grove J, Schechter PJ, Tell G et al. (1981) Increased gamma-aminobutyric acid (GABA), homocarnosine and β-alanine in cerebrospinal fluid of patients treated with gamma-vinyl GABA (4-amino-hex-5-enoic acid). Life Sci 28: 2431–2439

Halonen T, Nisssinen J, Jansen JA, Pitkänen A (1996) Tiagabine prevents seizures, neuronal damage and memory impairment in experimental status epilepticus. Eur J Pharmacol 299:69–81

Harmsworth WL, Wolf HH, Swinyard EA, White HS (1993) Felbamate modulates glycine receptor function. Epilepsia 34 [Suppl 2]:92–93

Honmou O, Oyelese AA, Kocsis JD (1995a) The anticonvulsant gabapentin enhances promoted release of GABA in the hippocampus: a field potential analysis. Brain Res 692:273–277

Honmou O, Kocsis JD, Richerson GB (1995b) Gabapentin potentiates the conductance increase induced by nipecotic acid in CA1 pyramidal neurons in vitro. Epilepsy Res 20:193–202

Hui A, Ellinor PT, Krizanova O, Wang JJ, Diebold RJ, Schwartz A (1991) Molecular cloning of multiple subtypes of a novel rat brain isoform of the 1 subunit of the voltage-dependent calcium channel. Neuron 7:35–44

Inglefield JR, Perry JM, Schwartz RD (1995) Postischemic inhibition of GABA reuptake by tiagabine slows neuronal death in the gerbil hippocampus. Hippocampus 5:460–468

Jensen PK, Gram L, Schmutz M (1991) Oxcarbazepine. In: Pisani F, Perucca E, Avanzini G, Richens A (eds) New antiepileptic drugs (Epilepsy Res, Suppl 3). Elsevier, Amsterdam, pp. 135–140

Jung MJ, Lippert B, Metcalf B, Bohler P, Schechter PJ (1977) γ-Vinyl GABA (4-amino-hex-5-enoic acid), a new irreversible inhibitor of GABA-T: effects on brain GABA metabolism in mice. J Neurochem 29:797–802

Kalichman MW, Burnham WM, Livingstone KE (1982) Pharmacological investigation of gamma-aminobutyric acid (GABA) and fully developed generalized seizures in the amygdala-kindled rat. Neuropharmacology 21:127–131

Kanda T, Kurokawa M, Tamura S et al. (1996) Topiramate reduces abnormally high extracellular levels of glutamate and aspartate in the hippocampus of spontaneously epileptic rats. Life Sci 59:1607–1616

Kanthasamy AG, Matsumoto RR, Gunasekar PG, Truong DD (1995) Excitoprotective effect of felbamate in cultured cortical neurons. Brain Res 705:97–104

Kawasaki H, Lopantsev V, Zona C, Avoli M (1996) Topiramate depresses intrinsic bursts in the rat subiculum in vitro. Epilepsia (Abstract) 37 [Suppl 5]:26

Kelly KM, Gross RA, Macdonald RL (1990) Valproic acid selectively reduces the low-threshold (T) calcium in rat nodose neurons. Neurosci Lett 116:233–238

Klepner CA, Lippa AS, Benson DI, Sano MC, Beer B (1978) Resolution of two biochemically and pharmacologically distinct benzodiazepine receptors. Pharmacol Biochem Behav 11:457–462

Kubova H, Mares P (1993) Anticonvulsant action of oxcarbazepine, hydroxycarbamazepine, and carbamazepine against metrazol-induced motor seizures in developing rats. Epilepsia 34:188–192

Kume A, Greenfield LJ Jr, Macdonald RL, Albin RL (1996) Felbamate inhibits [^{3}H]t-butylbicycloorthobenzoate binding and enhances Cl^- current at the γ-aminobutyric acidA receptor. J Pharmacol Exp Therap 277:1784–1792

Kuo C-C, Bean BP (1994) Na^+ channels must deactivate to recover from inactivation. Neuron 12:819–829

Lang DG, Wang CM (1991) Lamotrigine and phenytoin interactions on ionic currents present in N4TG1 and GH3 clonal cells. Soc Neurosci Abs 17:1256

Larsson OM, Gram L, Schousboe I, Schousboe A (1986) Differential effect of gamma-vinyl GABA and valproate on GABA-transaminase from cultured neurones and astrocytes. Neuropharmacol 25:617–625

Leach MJ, Marden CM, Miller AA (1986) Pharmacological studies on lamotrigine, a novel potential antiepileptic drug: II. Neurochemical studies on the mechanism of action. Epilepsia 27:490–497

Lees G, Leach MJ (1993) Studies on the mechanism of action of the novel anticonvulsant lamotrigine (Lamictal) using primary neuroglial cultures from rat cortex. Brain Res 612:190–199

Libri V, Constanti A, Zibetti M, Nistico S (1996) Effects of felbamate on muscarinic and metabotropic glutamate agonist-mediated responses and magnesium-free or 4-aminopyridine-induced epileptiform activity in guinea pig olfactory cortex neurons in vitro. J Pharmacol Exp Therap 277:1759–1769

Lipa AS, Beer B, Sano MC, Vogel RA, Myerson LR (1981) Differential ontogeny of type I and type II benzodiazepine receptors. Life Sci 28:2343–2347

Lippert B, Metcalf BW, Jung MJ, Casara P (1977) 4-Amino-hex-5-enoic acid, a selective catalytic inhibitor of 4-aminobutyric-acid aminotransferase in mammalian brain. Eur J Biochem 74:441–445

Lockard JS, Levy RH, Moore DF (1987) Drug alteration of seizure cyclicity. Adv Epileptol 16:725–732

Loscher W, Czuczwar SJ, Jackel R, Schwarz M (1987) Effect of microinjections of gamma-vinyl GABA or isoniazid into substantia nigra on the development of amygdala kindling in rats. Exp Neurol 95:622–638

Loscher W, Honack D, Taylor CP (1991) Gabapentin increases aminooxyacetic acid-induced GABA accumulation in several regions of rat brain. Neurosci Lett 128:150–154

Macdonald RL (1989) Antiepileptic drug actions. Epilepsia 30:S19–S28

Macdonald RL, Greenfield LJ Jr (1997) Mechanisms of action of new antiepileptic drugs. Curr Opinion Neurol 10:121–128

Macdonald RL, Kelly K (1994) New antiepileptic drug mechanisms of action. In: Trimble M (ed) An appraisal of some new anticonvulsants – a clinical perspective. John Wiley & Sons, New York, pp. 35–50

Macdonald RL, Meldrum BS (1995) Principles of antiepileptic drug action. In: Levy RH, Mattson RH, Meldrum B (eds) Antiepileptic drugs, 4th edn., Raven Press, New York, pp. 61–77

Macdonald RL, Olsen RW (1994) GABAA receptor channels. Ann Rev Neurosci 17:569–602

Macdonald RL, Rogers CJ, Twyman RE (1989a) Kinetic properties of the GABAA receptor main-conductance state of mouse spinal cord neurons in culture. J Physiol 410:479–499

Macdonald RL, Rogers CJ, Twyman RE (1989b) Barbiturate regulation of kinetic properties of the GABAA receptor channel of mouse spinal neurones in culture. J Physiol 417:483–500
Maryanoff BE, Nortey SO, Gardocki JF, Shank RP, Dodgson SP (1987) Anticonvulsant O-alkyl sulfamates. 2,3:4,5-bis-O-(1-methylethylidine)-β-D-fructopyranose sulfamate and related compounds. J Med Chem 30:880–887
McCabe RT, Wasterlain CG, Kucharczyk N, Sofia RD, Vogel JR (1993) Evidence of anticonvulsant and neuroprotective action of felbamate mediated by strychnine-insensitive glycine receptors. J Pharmacol Exp Therap 264:248–252
McLean MJ, Macdonald RL (1986a) Sodium valproate, but not ethosuximide, produces use- and voltage-dependent limitation of high frequency repetitive firing of action potentials of mouse central neurons in cell culture. J Pharmacol Exp Ther 237:1001–1011
McLean MJ, Macdonald RL (1986b) Carbamazepine and 10,11-epoxycarbamazepine produce use- and voltage-dependent limitation of rapidly firing action potentials of mouse central neurons in cell culture. J Pharmacol Exp Ther 238:727–732
McLean MJ, Macdonald RL (1988) Benzodiazepines, but not beta carbolines, limit high frequency repetitive firing of action potentials of spinal cord neurons in cell culture. J Pharmacol Exp Ther 244:789–795
McLean MJ, Schmutz M, Wamil AW, Olpe H-R, Portet C, Feldmann KF (1994) Oxcarbazepine: mechanisms of action. Epilepsia 35 [Suppl 3]:S5–S9
Meldrum BS, Horton R (1978) Blockade of epileptic responses in photosensitive baboon Papio papio by two irreversible inhibitors of GABA-transaminase, gamma-acetylenic GABA (4-amino-hex-5-ynoic acid) and gamma-vinyl GABA (4-amino-hex-5-enoic acid). Psychopharmacologia 59:47–50
Meldrum BS, Murugaiah K (1983) Anticonvulsant action in mice with sound-induced seizures of the optical isomers of gamma vinyl GABA. Eur J Pharmacol 89:149–152
Miller AA, Wheatley P, Sawyer DA, Baxter MG, Roth B (1986) Pharmacological studies on lamotrigine, a novel potential antiepileptic drug: I. Anticonvulsant profile in mice and rats. Epilepsia 27:483–489
Mintz IM, Adams ME, Bean BP (1992) P-Type calcium channels in rat central and peripheral neurons. Neuron 9:85–95
Mori Y, Friedrich T, Man-Suk K et al. (1991) Primary structure and functional expression from complementary DNA of a brain calcium channel. Nature 350:398–402
Morimoto K, Sato H, Tamamota Y, Watanabe T, Suwaki H (1997) Antiepileptic effects of tiagabine, a selective GABA uptake inhibitor, in the rat kindling model of temporal lobe epilepsy. Epilepsia 38:966–974
Moss SJ, Smart TA, Porter NM (1990) Cloned GABA receptors are maintained in a stable cell line: allosteric and channel properties. Eur J Pharmacol 189:77–88
Mutoh K, Dichter MA (1993) Lamotrigine blocks voltage-dependent Na currents in a voltage-dependent manner with a small use-dependent component. Epilepsia 34 [Suppl 6]:87
Nakamura J, Tamura S, Kanda T et al. (1994) Inhibition by topiramate of seizures in spontaneously epileptic rates and DBA/2 mice. Eur J Pharmacol 254:83–89
Naritoku DK, Stryker MT, Mecozzi LB, Copley CA, Faingold CL (1988) Gabapentin reduces the severity of audiogenic seizures in the genetic epilepsy-prone rat. Epilepsia 29:693
Nayeem N, Green TP, Martin IL, Barnard EA (1994) Quaternary structure of the native GABAA receptor determined by electron microscopic image analysis. J Neurochem 62:815–818
Nowycky MC, Fox AP, Tsien RW (1985) Three types of neuronal calcium channels with different agonist sensitivity. Nature 316:440–443
Oles RJ, Singh L, Hughes J, Woodruff GN (1990) The anticonvulsant action of gabapentin involves the glycine/NMDA receptor. Soc Neurosci 16:783

Olsen RW (1987) The γ-aminobutyric acid/benzodiazepine/barbiturate receptor-chloride ion channel complex of mammalian brain. In: Edelman, Gall and Cowan (eds) Synaptic function. John Wiley & Sons, New York, pp. 257–271

Olsen RW, Tobin AJ (1990) Molecular biology of GABAA receptors. FASEB J 4:1469–1480

Peeters BWMM, van Rijn CM, Vossen JMH, Coenen AML (1989) Effects of GABAergic agents in spontaneous non-convulsive epilepsy, EEG and behaviour, in the WAG/Rij inbred strain of rats. Life Sci 45:1171–1176

Pennell PB, Mohammed SO, Macdonald RL (1995) Aplastic anemia in a patient receiving felbamate for partial complex seizures. Neurology 45:456–460

Perez-Reyes E, Schneider T (1994) Calcium channels: structure, function and classification. Drug Develop Res 33:295–318

Petroff OAC, Rothman DL, Behar KL, Mattson RH (1993) Effect of vigabatrin on GABA levels in human brain measured in vivo with [^{1}H] NMR spectroscopy. Epilepsia 34 [Suppl 6]:68

Petroff OAC, Rothman DL, Behar KL, Lamoureux D, Mattson RH (1996) The effect of gabapentin on brain gamma-aminobutyric acid in patients with epilepsy. Ann Neurol 39:95–99

Pisani A, Stefani A, Siniscalchi A, Mercuri NB, Bernardi G, Calabresi P (1995) Electrophysiological actions of felbamate on rat striatal neurones. Br J Pharmacol 116:2053–2061

Pritchett DB, Seeburg PH (1990) Gamma-aminobutyric acidA receptor 5-subunit creates novel type II benzodiazepine receptor pharmacology. J Neurochem 54:1802–1804

Pritchett DB, Luddens H, Seeburg PH (1989a) Type I and Type II GABAA-benzodiazepine receptors produced in transfected cells. Science 245:1389–1392

Pritchett DB, Sontheimer H, Shivers BD (1989b) Importance of a novel GABAA receptor subunit for benzodiazepine pharmacology. Nature 338:582–584

Privatera M, Fincham R, Penry J, Reife R, Kramer L, Pledger G, Karim R, and the Topiramate YD Study Group (1996) Topiramate placebo-controlled dose-ranging trial in refractory partial epilepsy using 600-, 800-, and 1000-mg daily dosages. Neurology 46:1678–1683

Pugliese AM, Corradetti R (1996) Effects of the antiepileptic drug felbamate on long term potentiation in the CA1 region of rat hippocampal slices. Neurosci Lett 215:21–24

Reife RA, Pledger GW (1997) Topiramate as adjunctive therapy in refractory partial epilepsy: pooled analysis of data from five double-blind, placebo-controlled trials. Epilpesia 38:S31–S33

Reimann W (1983) Inhibition by GABA, baclofen and gabapentin of dopamine release from rat caudate nucleus: are there common or different sites of action? Eur J Pharmacol 94:341–344

Reynolds EH, Milner G, Matthews DM, Chanarin I (1966) Anticonvulsant therapy, megaloblastic haemopoiesis and folic acid metabolism. Quart J Med 35:521–537

Rho JM, Donevan SD, Rogowski MA (1994) Mechanism of action of the anticonvulsant felbamate: opposing effects on N-methyl-D-aspartate and γ-aminobutyric acidA receptors. Ann Neurol 35:229–234

Riekkinen PJ, Pitkanen A, Ylinen A, Sivenius J, Halonen T (1989) Specificity of vigabatrin for the GABAergic system in human epilepsy. Epilepsia 30 [Suppl 3]:S18–S22

Rock DM, Kelly KM, Macdonald RL (1993) Gabapentin actions on ligand- and voltage-gated responses in cultured rodent neurons. Epilepsy Res 16:89–98

Roepstorff A, Lambert JDC (1992) Comparison of the effect of the GABA uptake blockers, tiagabine and nipecotic acid, on inhibitory synaptic efficacy in hippocampal CA1 neurones. Neurosci Lett 146:131–134

Rogawski MA, Porter RJ (1990) Antiepileptic drugs: pharmacological mechanisms and clinical efficacy with consideration of promising developmental stage compounds. Pharmacol Rev 42:223–286
Rogers CJ, Twyman RE, Macdonald RL (1994) Benzodiazepine and β-carboline regulation of single GABAA receptor channels of mouse spinal neurones in culture. J Physiol 475:69–82
Rosenfeld WE, Sachdeo RC, Faught RE, Privitera M (1997) Long-term experience with topiramate as adjunctive therapy and as monotherapy in patients with partial onset seizures: retrospective survey of open-label treatment. Epilepsia 38:S34–S36
Rowen AJ, Schear MJ, Wiener JA, Luciano D (1989) Intensive monitoring and pharmacokinetic studies of gabapentin in patients with generalized spike-wave discharges. Epilepsia 30:30
Sarhan S, Seiler N (1979) Metabolic inhibitors and subcellular distribution of GABA. J Neuroscience Res 4:399–421
Schechter PJ, Tranier Y (1977) Effects of elevated brain GABA concentrations on the action of bicuculline and picrotoxin in mice. Psychopharmacology 54:145–148
Schechter PJ, Trainier Y, Jung MJ, Bohlen P (1977) Audiogenic seizure protection by elevated brain GABA concentration in mice: effects of γ-acetylenic GABA and γ-vinyl GABA, two irreversible GABA-T inhibitors. Eur J Pharmacol 45:319–328
Schechter PJ, Hanke NFJ, Grove J, Huebert N, Sjoerdsma A (1984) Biochemical and clinical effects of gamma-vinyl GABA in patients with epilepsy. Neurology 34:182–186
Schlicker PJ, Reimann W, Gothert M (1985) Gabapentin decreases monoamine release without affecting acetylcholine release in the brain. Arzneim-Forsch/Drug Res 35:1347–1349
Schmidt D (1989) Potential antiepileptic drugs: gabapentin. In: Levy RH, Driefuss FE, Mattson RH, Meldrum BS, Penry JK (eds) Antiepileptic drugs. Raven Press, New York, pp. 925–935
Schmutz M, Ferret T, Heckendorn R, Jeker A, Portet Ch, Olpe HR (1993) GP 47779, the main human metabolite of oxcarbazepine (Trileptal), and both enantiomers have equal anticonvulsant activity. Epilepsia 34 [Suppl 2]:122
Schofield PR, Darlison MG, Fujita N et al. (1987) Sequence and functional expression of the GABA A receptor shows a ligand-gated receptor super-family. Nature 328:221–227
Schousboe A, Larsson OM, Seiler N (1986) Stereoselective uptake of the GABA-transaminase inhibitors gamma-vinyl GABA and gamma-acetylenic GABA into neurons and astrocytes. Neurochem Res 11:1497–1505
Schwarz J, Grigat G (1989) Phenytoin and carbamazepine: Potential- and frequency-dependent block of Na currents in mammalian myelinated nerve fibers. Epilepsia 30:286–294
Shin C, Rigsbee LC, McNamara JO (1986) Anti-seizure and anti-epileptogenic effect of gamma-vinyl gamma-aminobutyric acid in amygdaloid kindling. Brain Res 398:370–374
Shuaib A, Mahmood RH, Wishart T, Kanthan R, Murabit MA, Ijaz S, Miyashita H, Howlett W (1995) Neuroprotective effects of lamotrigine in global ischemia in gerbils: a histological in vivo microdialysis and behavioral study. Brain Res 702:199–206
Shuaib A, Waqaar T, Ijaz MS, Kanthan R, Wishart T, Howlett W (1996) Neuroprotection with felbamate: a 7 and 28-day study in transient forebrain ischemia in gerbils. Brain Res 727:65–70
Sofia RD, Kramer L, Perhach JL, Rosenberg A (1991) Felbamate. In: Pisani F, Perucca E, Avanzini G, Richens A (eds) New antiepileptic drugs. Elsevier, Amsterdam, pp. 103–108
Soong TW, Stea A, Hodson CD, Dubel SJ, Vincent SR, Snutch TP (1993) Structure and functional expression of a member of the low voltage-activated calcium channel family. Science 260:1133–1136

Smith SE, Parvez NS, Chapman AG, Meldrum BS (1995) The γ-aminobutyric acid uptake inhibitor, tiagabine, is anticonvulsant in two animal models of reflex epilepsy. Eur J Pharmacol 273:259–265

Snutch TP, Tomlinson WJ, Leonard JP, Gilbert MM (1991) Distinct calcium channels are generated by alternative splicing and are differentially expressed in the mammalian CNS. Neuron 7:45–57

Stables JP, Bialer M, Johannessen SI, Kupferberg HJ, Levy RH, Loiseau P, Perucca E (1995) Progress report on new antiepileptic drugs: a summary of the Second Eilat Conference. Epilepsy Res 22:235–246

Starr TVB, Prystay W, Snutch TP (1991) Primary structure of a calcium channel that is highly expressed in the rat cerebellum. Proc Natl Acad Sci USA 88:5621–5625

Stefani A, Pisani A, De Murtas M, Mercuri NB, Marciani MG, Calabresi P (1995) Action of GP 47779, the active metabolite of oxcarbazepine, on the corticostriatal system. II. Modulation of high-voltage-activated calcium currents. Epilepsia 336:997–1002

Stefani A, Calabresi P, Pisani A, Mercuri NB, Siniscalchi A, Bernardi G (1996a) Felbamate inhibits dihydropyridine-sensitive calcium channels in central neurons. J Pharmacol Exp Therap 277:121–127

Stefani A, Spadoni F, Siniscalchi A, Bernardi G (1996b) Lamotrigine inhibits Ca^{2+} currents in cortical neurons: functional implications. Eur J Pharmacol 307:113–116

Subramaniam S, Rho JM, Peniz L, Donevan SD, Feilding RP, Rogawski MA (1995) Felbamate block of the N-methyl-D-aspartate receptor. J Pharmacol Exp Therap 273:878–886

Suzdak PD, Jansen JA (1995) A review of the preclinical pharmacology of tiagabine: a potent and selective anticonvulsant GABA uptake inhibitor. Epilepsia 36:612–626

Swinyard EA, Sofia RD, Kupferberg HJ (1986) Comparative anticonvulsant activity and neurotoxicity of felbamate and four prototype antiepileptic drugs in mice and rats. Epilepsia 27:27–34

Taylor CP (1993) The anticonvulsant lamotrigine blocks sodium currents from cloned alpha-subunits of rat brain Na^+ channels in a voltage-dependent manner but gabapentin does not. Soc Neurosci Abs 19:1631

Taylor CP, Rock DM, Weinkauf RJ, Ganong AH (1988) In vitro and in vivo electrophysiology effects of the anticonvulsant gabapentin. Soc Neurosci Abs 14:866

Taylor CP, Vartanian MG, Yuen PW, Bigge C (1993) Potent and stereospecific anticonvulsant activity of 3-isobutyl GABA relates to in vitro binding at a novel site labeled by tritiated gabapentin. Epilepsy Res 14:11–15

Thomsen C, Suzdak PD (1995) Effects of chronic tiagabine treatment on [^{3}H]GABAA, [^{3}H]GABAB and [^{3}H]tiagabine binding to sections from mice brain. Epilepsy Res 21:79–88

Thurlow RJ, Hill DR, Woodruff GN (1996a) Comparison of the uptake of [^{3}H]-gabapentin with the uptake of L-[^{3}H]-leucine into rat brain synaptosomes. Br J Pharmacol 118:449–456

Thurlow RJ, Hill DR, Woodruff GN (1996b) Comparison of the autoradiographic binding distribution of [^{3}H]-gabapentin with excitatory amino acid receptor and amino acid uptake site distributions in rat brain. Br J Pharmacol 118:457–465

Ticku MK, Kamatchi GL, Sofia RD (1991) Effect of anticonvulsant felbamate on GABAA receptor system. Epilepsia 32:389–91

Tomaselli G, Marban E, Yellen G (1989) Sodium channels from human brain RNA expressed in Xenopus oocytes basic electrophysiologic characteristics and their modifications by diphenylhydantoin. J Clin Invest 83:1724–1732

Twyman RE, Rogers CJ, Macdonald RL (1989) Differential regulation of γ-aminobutyric acid receptor channels by diazepam and phenobarbital. Ann Neurol 25:213–220

Twyman RE, Rogers CJ, Macdonald RL (1990) Intraburst kinetic properties of the GABAA receptor main conductance state of mouse spinal cord neurones in culture. J Physiol 423:193–219
Vergnes M, Marescaux C, Micheletti G, Depaulis A, Rumbach L, Warter J-M (1984) Enhancement of spike and wave discharges by GABA mimetic drugs in rats with spontaneous petit mal-like epilepsy. Neurosci Lett 44:91–94
Vicini S, Mienville JM, Costa E (1987) Actions of benzodizapine and β-carboline derivatives on γ-aminobutyric acid-activated C1- channels recorded from membrane patches of neonatal rat cortical neurons in culture. J Pharm Exper Therap 243:1195–1201
Wakamori M, Kaneda M, Oyama Y, Akaike N (1989) Effects of chlordiazepoxide, chlorpromazine, diazepam, diphenylhydantoin, flunitrazepam and haloperidol on the voltage-dependent sodium current of isolated mammalian brain neurons. Brain Res 494:374–378
Waldmeier PC, Martin P, Stocklin K, Portet C, Schmutz M (1996) Effect of carbamazepine, oxcarbazepine and lamotrigine on the increase in extracellular glutamate elicited by veratridine in rat cortex and striatum. Naunyn Schmiedeberg's Arch Pharmacol 354:164–172
Wallis RA, Panizzon KL (1995) Felbamate neuroprotection against CA1 traumatic neuronal injury. Eur J Pharmacol 294:475–482
Walton NY, Gunawan S, Treiman DM (1994) Treatment of experimental status epilepticus with the GABA uptake inhibitor, tiagabine. Epilepsy Res 19:237–244
Wamil AW, McLean MJ (1991) Limitation by gabapentin of high frequency action potential firing by mouse central neurons in cell culture. Epilepsy Res 17:1–12
Wamil AW, McLean MJ (1994) Limitation by gabapentin of high frequency action potential firing by mouse central neurons in cell culture. Epilepsy Res 17:1–10
Wamil AW, McLean MJ, Taylor CP (1991) Multiple cellular actions of gabapentin. Neurology 41 [Suppl 1]:140
Wang CM, Lang DG, Cooper BR (1993) Lamotrigine effects on ion channels in cultured neuronal cells. Epilepsia 34 [Suppl 6]:117–118
Wang SJ, Huang CC, Hsu KS, Tsai JJ, Gean PW (1996) Presynaptic inhibition of excitatory neurotransmission by lamotrigine in the rat amygdalar neurons. Synapse 24:248–255
Wasterlain CG, Adams LM, Wichmann JK, Sofia RD (1996) Felbamate protects CA1 neurons from apoptosis in a gerbil model of global ischemia. Stroke 27:1236–1240
Wauquier A, Zhou S (1996) Topiramate: a potent anticonvulsant in the amygdala-kindled rat. Epilepsy Res 24:73–77
Weiss DS, Magleby K (1989) Gating scheme for single GABA-activated Cl- channels determined from stability plots, dwell-time distributions, and adjacent-interval durations. J Neurosci 9:1314–1324
White HS, Wolf HH, Swinyard EA, Skeen GA, Sofia RD (1992) A neuropharmacologic evaluation of felbamate as a novel anticonvulsant. Epilepsia 33:564
White HS, Woodhead JS, Wolf HH (1996) Effect of topiramate (TMP) on pentylenetetrazol (PTZ) seizure threshold. Epilepsia (Abstract) 37 [Suppl 5]:26
White HS, Brown D, Woodhead JH, Skeen GA, Wolf HH (1997) Topiramate enhances GABA-mediated chloride flux in murine brain neurons and increases seizure threshold. Epilepsy Res 28:167–179
Williams ME, Feldman DH, McCue AF, Brenner R, Velicelebi G, Ellis SB, Harpold MM (1992) Structure and functional expression of $\alpha 1$ subunits of a novel human neuronal calcium channel subtype. Neuron 8:71–84
Wisden W, Herb A, Wieland H, Keinanen K, Luddens H, Seeburg PH (1991) Cloning, pharmacological characteristics and expression pattern of the rat GABAA receptor $\alpha 4$ subunit. FEBS Lett 289:227–230

Zhang JF, Randall AD, Ellinor PT, Horne WA, Sather WA, Tanabe T, Schwarz TL, Tsien RW (1993) Distinctive pharmacology and kinetics of cloned neruonal Ca^{2+} channels and their possible counterparts in mammalian CNS neurons. Neuropharmacol 32:1075–1088

Zona C, Barbarosie M, Kawasaki H, Avoli M (1996) Effects induced by the anticonvulsant drug topiramate on voltage-gated sodium currents generated by cerebellar granule cells in tissue culture. Epilepsia (Abstract) 37 [Suppl 5]:24

CHAPTER 6

The Search for New Anticonvulsants

D. SCHMIDT

A. Introduction

Any review of the rational search for new anticonvulsants runs the danger of neglecting the informality that may lie at the heart of drug discovery – the flashes of insight, inspiration, fruitful discussion and, last but not least, serendipity. While recognizing the possibility of the accidental discovery of new drugs, the aim of this chapter is to compare critically the pharmacological strategies which are currently used in antiepileptic drug development. In particular, the modern rational approach to the development of new drugs, which is based on knowledge of the basic events involved in epilepsy, will be compared with the more traditional approaches of random screening and devising structural variants of known antiepileptic drugs.

The ultimate goal of the discovery of a drug for the treatment of epilepsy is to find a compound that completely controls all seizures and does not cause any intolerable adverse events. Although a large number of antiepileptic drugs have been marketed, they have shown a surprising lack of efficacy for many of the various seizure types, and none has proven free from adverse effects. Approximately 20%–30% of patients with epilepsy have seizures that are resistant to treatment with standard antiepileptic drugs (SCHMIDT and MORSELLI 1986). Therefore, there is a pressing need for new antiepileptic drugs which should be more effective than existing drugs in patients with intractable epilepsies, such as those with complex partial seizures and the Lennox-Gastaut syndrome. Furthermore, because of growing concern about the acute and chronic toxicity of currently used antiepileptic drugs, newly developed drugs should be less toxic than existing drugs. Any new drug will eventually undergo rigorous clinical comparison against standard drugs such as carbamazepine, phenytoin or valproate, in terms of both efficacy and tolerability. The outcome of this comparison will ultimately determine the success of the preclinical (and clinical) development strategy chosen. In addition, the efficacy observed in controlled clinical trials can be compared to that seen during the testing of the drug in animal models during preclinical development. Thus, the predictive ability of individual experimental models can be reassessed. Finally, promising strategies for future antiepileptic drug discovery will be discussed briefly. Since a prerequisite to all approaches is the choice of adequate experimental seizure models (LÖSCHER and SCHMIDT 1988; WHITE and KUPFERBERG 1996), these will first be discussed, briefly.

For preclinical evaluation and development of new antiepileptic drugs, animal models are needed that are predictive both in terms of antiepileptic efficacy against the different seizure types and in terms of adverse effects occurring at anticonvulsant dosages. The most popular and widely used of these models are the maximal electroshock seizure (MES) test, a model for generalized tonic-clonic seizures of human epilepsy, the pentylenetetrazole (PTZ) seizure test, a model for generalized myoclonic seizures, and amygdaloid kindling, a model for complex partial seizures with or without secondarily generalized tonic-clonic seizures (LÖSCHER and SCHMIDT 1994). Furthermore, kindling renders the brain more susceptible to adverse effects of certain anticonvulsants and thus avoids overestimation of the tolerability of new drugs (LÖSCHER and HÖNACK 1991; HÖNACK and LÖSCHER 1995). It should be noted, however, that no animal models currently exist for several difficult-to-treat epilepsies such as the West syndrome or the Lennox-Gastaut syndrome. A detailed discussion of animal models of epilepsy and epileptic seizures is provided in Chap. 2 of this volume. In any event, in view of the diverse types of epileptic seizures mentioned above, more than one seizure model has to be used in the search for new antiepileptic drugs. Based on experience with major antiepileptic drugs, such as valproate or the novel drug vigabatrin, not only traditional seizure tests with stimuli clearly above the individual seizure threshold for animals within a group should be used; drugs such as valproate or vigabatrin would have been missed if only such tests had been employed. In addition, models with the determination of individual seizure thresholds should be used, especially when models with supramaximal stimulation have failed to show anticonvulsant activity. An example of a battery of seizure models, and of models for the detection of adverse effects, is presented in Table 1.

B. Pharmacological Strategies in the Search for New Anticonvulsants

There are at least three strategies which are currently used for the development of new antiepileptic drugs: (1) random screening of newly synthesized chemical compounds of diverse structural categories for the presence of anticonvulsant activity, (2) molecular structural variation of known antiepileptic drugs, and (3) rational drug design (or rational drug development) based on knowledge of the basic pathophysiological events responsible for epilepsy (Tables 2, 3). All three strategies are generating clinically useful antiepileptic drugs, although many scientists currently believe that the strategy of rational ('modern') drug development has important advantages over the more traditional alternative strategies (PORTER and ROGAWSKI 1992).

Historically, all standard antiepileptic drugs have been found or developed by serendipity, by screening or by structural variation of known drugs. The first

Table 1. Preclinical seizure models used for the development of new anticonvulsants. A test hierarchy proposed for the evaluation of antiepileptic drugs (modified from LÖSCHER and SCHMIDT 1988, 1994)

1. Models of primary generalized seizures in human epilepsy:
   a) Tonic-clonic seizures: maximum electroshock seizure (MES) test with tonic hind limb seizures induced by corneal and/or transauricular stimulation in mice (50 mA) and rats (150 mA)
   b) Clonic seizures: s.c. pentylenetetrazole seizure test with clonic convulsions in mice (80 mg/kg) and rats (90 mg/kg); doses are CD_{97} for seizure induction (doses may vary among strains)
   c) Tonic seizures: threshold for tonic seizures induced by electrical stimulation in mice and rats via corneal and/or transauricular electrodes
   d) Myoclonic, tonic and tonic-clonic seizures: thresholds for myoclonic, clonic and tonic seizures induced by i.v. infusion of pentylenetetrazole (PTZ) in mice
2. Models of complex partial seizures with or without secondary generalization in human epilepsy:
   a) Threshold for induction of afterdischarges (ADT) induced by electrical stimulation of the amygdala in fully amygdala-kindled rats; recording of seizure severity (stage 1, 2: complex partial seizures; stage 4,5: secondarily generalized seizures), seizure duration and afterdischarge duration at threshold current
   b) Suprathreshold stimulation of amygdala-kindled rats; recording of seizure severity (stage 1,2:complex partial seizures; stage 4,5: secondarily generalized seizures), seizure duration and afterdischarge duration at suprathreshold current (500 μA)
3. Models for the detection of motor impairment and other adverse effects:
   a) Rotarod and chimney test in mice and rats, including kindled rats
   b) Open field behaviour in mice and rats, including kindled rats
4. Models for chronic efficacy testing:
   Chronic drug experiments in mice (MES, PTZ) and fully amygdala-kindled rats
5. Models for detection of antiepileptogenic effects:
   Chronic drug administration during kindling development
6. Further (more specialized) models if test drug looks promising: e.g. models for drug resistant seizure types, e.g. complex partial seizures such as phenytoin-resistant amygdala-kindled rats, genetic animal models of absence seizures such as lethargic mice or rat strains with spontaneous spike wave discharges (e.g. GAERS), and models for the detection of antipsychotic and cognition enhancing drug effects

drugs for epilepsy were bromides, introduced by Sir Charles LOCOCK for the treatment of seizures in 1857. Bromides were the only useful therapy for about 60 years until the serendipitous discovery of the antiepileptic efficacy of phenobarbitone by HAUPTMANN in 1912. Whereas both bromides and barbiturates were introduced without experimental evaluation prior to their clinical use, phenytoin was the result of a search by MERRITT and PUTNAM in 1937 for a non-sedating analogue of phenobarbitone capable of suppressing maximal electroshock seizures in animals. For about 50 years following the discovery of phenytoin, the main research effort was devoted to the development of phenytoin-like drugs. This was determined partly by the choice of an animal model (the maximum electroshock seizure test) which is selective for

Table 2. Pharmacological strategies for the development of new anticonvulsants. Drugs developed by rational drug design. Experimental activity refers to the traditional maximum electroshock seizure (MES) and pentylenetetrazole (PTZ) tests and electrical amygdala or hippocampal kindling. Inefficacy in the MES or PTZ test does not exclude the respective drug being active on MES or PTZ thresholds (LÖSCHER and SCHMIDT 1988, 1994). Clinical efficacy relates to placebo-controlled randomized add-on trials in patients with partial seizures inadequately treated with standard drugs, while open-label randomized trials were used for comparison of the new drug with a standard drug, mostly carbamazepine, during monotherapy in previously untreated patients with partial seizures and generalized tonic-clonic seizures. As discussed above, gabapentin may not be a selective GABA-mimetic drug (see text). Data are from LÖSCHER and SCHMIDT (1988, 1994), ROGAWSKI and PORTER (1990), PISANI et al. (1991), HANDFORTH et al. (1995) and BIALER et al. (1996)

New drug	Animal models (MES/PTZ/kindling)	Add-on therapy vs. placebo	Monotherapy vs. AEDs
GABA-mimetic drugs			
Gabapentin (see legend)	±/±/±	Yes	Yes
Progabide	–/–/–	No	WD
THIP	–/–/–	No	WD
Tiagabine	±/+/+	Yes	N/A
Vigabatrin	–/±/+	Yes	Yes
NMDA-antagonists			
MK-801 (dizocilpine)	+/±/–	WD, confusion, poor efficacy	WD
D-CPP-ene	+/±/–	WD, confusion, poor efficacy	N/A
Dextromethorphan	+/±/–	Unimpressive efficacy	N/A
Selective ion channel drugs			
Flunarizine	+/–/+	WD, modest efficacy	N/A
Ralitoline, designed as phenytoin-like	+/–/+	WD, unremarkable efficacy	N/A

+, active; –, inactive; ±, weakly active; yes, more effective than placebo as add-on or broadly similar in efficacy or better tolerated during monotherapy; no, not more effective than placebo as add-on or less effective or less well tolerated during monotherapy; WD, development was discontinued, mostly because of adverse effects; N/A, no data available

phenytoin-like drugs and partly by an emphasis on molecular structures related to that of phenytoin (MELDRUM and PORTER 1986). Interestingly, the latter emphasis led to the development of two classes of compounds, i.e. the oxazolidinediones (e.g. trimethadione) and the succinimides (e.g. ethosuximide) whose mechanisms of action and antiepileptic activities are totally different from that of phenytoin. From that point on, the development of new drugs concentrated on different molecular structures, resulting in the marketing of carbamazepine, valproate, and the benzodiazepines. The iminostilbene carbamazepine was the product of a structure-activity study carried out in the

Table 3. Pharmacological strategies for the development of new anticonvulsants. Drugs developed by random screening (RS) and structural variation (SV). For legend and abbreviations see Table 2. Data are from ROGAWSKI and PORTER (1990); PISANI et al. (1991); OWEN (1993), CRAWFORD et al. (1992), RUNGE et al. (1993); SCHMUTZ et al. (1993); LÖSCHER and SCHMIDT (1994); WALKER and PATSALOS (1995); BIALER et al. (1996); HARIA and BALFOUR (1997). As discussed above, gabapentin may actually belong to the group of drugs developed by molecular structure variation (see text)

New drug	Animal models (MES/PTZ/kindling	Polytherapy vs. placebo	Monotherapy vs. AEDs	Comments
Clobazam	+/+/+	Yes	Yes	SV of diazepam
Eterobarb	+/+/N/A	N/A	N/A	SV of phenobarbitone
Felbamate	+/+/N/A	Yes	N/A	SV of meprobamate
Fosphenytoin	N/A	N/A	Yes	Pro-drug of phenytoin
Levetiracetam	±/±/+	Yes	N/A	SV of piracetam
Lamotrigine	+/–/+	Yes	Yes	RS, based on erroneous "folate hypothesis"
MHD	+/±/N/A	N/A	N/A	Active metabolite of oxcarbazepine
Losigamone	+/+/N/A	Yes	N/A	RS
Oxcarbazepine	+/+/N/A	Yes	Yes	SV of carbamazepine
Remacemide	+/–/N/A	Yes	N/A	SV of phenytoin
Rufinamide	+/±/N/A	Yes	N/A	RS
Stiripentol	+/+/N/A	WD, drug interaction	WD	RS
Topiramate	+/–/N/A	Yes	N/A	RS
Zonisamide	+/–/+	Yes	N/A	SV

late 1950s in the Geigy laboratories to maximize the anticonvulsant activity of a series of iminodibenzyl derivatives (ROGAWSKI and PORTER 1990). The anticonvulsant properties of valproate against pentylenetetrazole-induced seizures were serendipitously discovered in France by PEYMARD in 1962 (LÖSCHER and SCHMIDT 1988, 1994). Subsequent clinical trials substantiated the anticonvulsant activity of valproate in epileptic patients, and it is now one of the major drugs for the treatment of different types of epileptic seizures. The benzodiazepines were initially developed in the late 1950s as tranquillizers and sedatives, but their anticonvulsant properties were readily noted during early animal and clinical studies (LÖSCHER and SCHMIDT 1988, 1994).

All of these important categories of antiepileptic drugs were developed before 1965. The unquestionable improvement in seizure control that accrued in many epileptic patients from the availability of these effective antiepileptic drugs convinced the drug industry and many clinicians that the marketed drugs were adequate for the successful therapy of the epilepsies (KRALL et al. 1978a).

As a consequence, only few new drugs were then in preclinical development for the treatment of epilepsy (KRALL et al. 1978b). The single most frequent reason cited for this situation was financial; the cost of development was prohibitive when compared with the expected return from marketing. In an attempt to increase the involvement of both industry and academia in the discovery and development of new anticonvulsant drugs, the Epilepsy Branch of the National Institute for Neurological and Communication Disorders and Stroke (NINCDS) established an Anticonvulsant Screening Project in 1975 and began screening new chemical compounds for anticonvulsant activity and potential development as antiepileptic agents (KUPFERBERG 1989). Since then, many thousands of compounds have been screened by the Antiepileptic Drug Development Program of the NINCDS (about 15,000 till 1993) and in industrial laboratories (KUPFERBERG 1989). In an explosion of activity, a large number of active compounds with novel structures have been identified and are at various stages of preclinical and clinical development (see below). The screening program of the NINCDS has, at least initially, relied heavily on the capacity of the drugs to modify the convulsive effects of maximal electric shock and pentylenetetrazole (WHITE and KUPFERBERG 1996). However, as mentioned above, there are a number of important exceptions to the predictive value of these models of epilepsy. Continued development of model systems for the detection and evaluation of potential therapeutic agents is needed, and the use of genetically based or kindling models is currently being emphasized. Furthermore, it should be noted that in addition to the screening efforts initiated by the NINCDS program, many pharmaceutical firms and academic groups have developed new anticonvulsant drugs by other strategies, including molecular variation and rational drug design.

The past decades have witnessed an increase in our knowledge of the pathophysiology of brain diseases and the basic mechanisms of drug activity that is without precedent. It might be imagined that this knowledge would generate rational strategies for drug development. The most important resultant strategies for the rational design of antiepileptic drugs have been enhancement of GABA-mediated neuronal inhibition, diminution of glutamate-mediated neuronal excitation, and modulation of Na^+, K^+, and particularly Ca^{2+} channels (DICHTER 1989; MUTANI et al. 1991; PORTER and ROGAWSKI 1992). Various drugs which increase GABAergic inhibition, decrease glutamatergic excitation, or block Ca^{2+} ion channels were developed rationally on the basis of such basic knowledge. The most important drugs thus developed in the last decades will be reviewed in the following sections, followed by reviews of novel antiepileptic drugs developed by random screening or by molecular structural variation. For detailed preclinical and clinical descriptions of the individual drugs and their mechanism of action, the interested reader is referred to the relevant chapters of this volume. Furthermore, in this chapter, it is not possible to describe in full all the novel compounds that have been developed in recent decades and which are already marketed or will be marketed in the near future. For interested readers, the recent reviews by LÖSCHER and SCHMIDT (1988, 1994), ROGAWSKI and PORTER (1990), PISANI et al. (1991) and BIALER et al. (1996) are recommended. With some exceptions, new antiepileptic drugs with proven clinical efficacy as seen during placebo-controlled add-on trials will therefore be described briefly in the following sections. In view of the numerous novel anticonvulsant drugs in early development, it will not be possible to cover all of these, and only the most important compounds that have progressed from their initial development stages through to clinical trials in patients with epilepsy will be reviewed. Some relevant data concerning the novel drugs which are reviewed in the following sections are summarized in Tables 2 and 3. With regards to the allocation of drugs to the respective sections, it is important to note that only the initial stages of drug recognition were used as the basis of this allocation. In other words, a drug which was found serendipitously by random screening, but was subsequently discovered to block glutamatergic transmission, will be allocated to the random screening section rather than to the glutamate antagonist subsection of the section on rational drug design.

I. Rational Drug Design

As mentioned above, the preferred strategies for rational drug discovery primarily involve the selective enhancement of inhibitory GABAergic neurotransmission, the selective attenuation of excitatory amino acid neurotransmission and the selective modulation of ion channels.

1. Selective Enhancement of GABAergic Neurotransmission

The realization that impairment of GABAergic inhibitory processes in the brain might be involved in the generation of seizures led to the first rational strategy for antiepileptic drug design, i.e. the development of drugs which selectively increase GABAergic functions (MELDRUM 1995). Drugs developed by this rational strategy have now been evaluated experimentally and clinically for more than 30 years (LÖSCHER and SCHMIDT 1988, 1994). In recent decades, the increase of brain GABA concentrations by inhibition of the GABA degrading enzyme GABA transaminase (GABA-T) has been investigated both experimentally and clinically. The search for selective inhibitors of GABA degradation resulted in the development and marketing of vigabatrin. In traditional animal models of seizures, vigabatrin is ineffective against maximum electroshock seizures and shows equivocal efficacy against pentylenetetrazole after acute systemic administration; in contrast, vigabatrin is a potent anticonvulsant in the kindling model (Table 2). Thus, vigabatrin is one example of a drug which would not have been discovered by the use of traditional seizure models, such as the maximum electroshock seizure and the pentylenetetrazole models (LÖSCHER and SCHMIDT 1988).

Other earlier pharmacological strategies for GABA potentiation involved postsynaptic potentiation of GABA responses by the use of $GABA_A$ receptor agonists such as progabide or gabaxadol (THIP), which failed due to lack of clinical efficacy and, in the case of progabide, because of hepatic toxicity (Schmidt and Utech 1986; Dam et al. 1991). Interestingly, both progabide and THIP were almost inactive in standard models of seizures, such as the maximum electroshock seizure and subcutaneous pentylenetetrazole tests, and amygdala-kindling (Table 2).

The most thoroughly evaluated and clinically useful GABAmimetic drugs to date are the GABA-transaminase inhibitor vigabatrin (see above), the GABA uptake blocker tiagabine and gabapentin, although the exact mechanism of action of the latter is still elusive. Tiagabine is a potent anticonvulsant in several rodent models, including amygdala-kindling. An exception is the maximum electroshock seizure test, in which tiagabine exerts only weak efficacy (Table 2). Gabapentin was developed at Goedecke in the late 1970s as a GABA-related amino acid which passes the blood-brain barrier and appears to increase human brain GABA levels (Petroff et al. 1996a). In addition it inhibits voltage-dependent Na^+ currents (Wamil and McLean 1994). Thus gabapentin may not be a selective GABA-mimetic drug after all and may be better categorized as a drug developed by structural variation. Gabapentin is a potent anticonvulsant in several chemical and electrical seizure models in rodents and against audiogenic seizures in DBA/2J mice. However, it was only weakly effective against pentylenetetrazole-induced clonic seizures in rodents and partial seizures in the kindling model in rats (Dalby and Nielsen 1997). A detailed discussion of vigabatrin, tiagabine and gabapentin is beyond the scope of the present review, and the interested reader is referred to the relevant chapters of this volume.

Alternative strategies for selectively enhancing GABAergic neurotransmission include pharmacological enhancement of GABA synthesis in GABAergic nerve terminals (Löscher and Schmidt 1988, 1994), development of partial agonists at benzodiazepine receptors (Haefely et al. 1990), such as the 1,4-benzodiazepine bretazenil and the non-benzodiazepine DN-2327, or benzodiazepine subreceptor selective agonists, such as the β-carboline abecarnil. The evidence was fully reviewed recently (Löscher and Schmidt 1988, 1994). In addition to the benzodiazepine "receptor", the $GABA_A$ receptor complex comprises various other drug-binding sites through which the effect of GABA on Cl^- conductance can be modulated pharmacologically. Several steroids, such as the anaesthetic alphaxolon, or the sedative-hypnotic and anxiolytic 3*O*-hydroxylated, 5*O*-reduced metabolites of progesterone and desoxycortisone, were found to exert barbiturate-like effects, i.e. to enhance GABA-stimulated Cl^- conductance by prolonging the open time of the ion channel, via a distinct steroid recognition site within the $GABA_A$ receptor complex (Sieghardt 1992).

The most recent development in the field of GABA research is the development of selective $GABA_B$ receptor blockers (Bowery and Pratt 1992), such as CGP-35348 (P-(3-aminopropyl)-P-di-ethoxymethyl-phosphinic acid). The $GABA_B$ antagonist CGP-35348 is ineffective in several models of convulsive seizures, including maximum electroshock seizures and pentylenetetrazole-induced clonic seizures (LÖSCHER and SCHMIDT 1988, 1994), but has been shown to exert anticonvulsant activity in a model of generalized nonconvulsive (absence) epilepsy (MARESCAUX et al. 1992). Speculatively, the mechanism of action of CGP-35348 might involve T-type Ca^{2+} channels, which are probably primed for activation by $GABA_B$ receptor-mediated synaptic potentials (PORTER and ROGAWSKI 1992). In this regard, it is interesting to note that the anti-absence effect of ethosuximide is also thought to relate to its ability to block T-type Ca^{2+} channels, which have been shown to mediate the burst firing of thalamic neurons involved in the genesis of absence seizures (COULTER et al. 1989).

2. Selective Attenuation or Blockade of Excitatory Aminoacidergic Neurotransmission

There is increasing evidence that an abnormality of glutamate-mediated neurotransmission may contribute to epileptic phenomena in various animal and human syndromes. This is more fully discussed in Chap. 4 of this volume and by DINGLEDINE et al. (1990) and MELDRUM (1995). Drugs, such as phencyclidine (PCP) and ketamine, which non-competitively block the NMDA subtype of glutamate receptor and which were originally developed as anaesthetic agents in the 1950s and 1960s, induce psychotomimetic effects in humans and therefore cannot be used for chronic treatment of epilepsy or other forms of chronic brain dysfunction (ROGAWSKI and PORTER 1990). The present discussion will be limited to a review of compounds for which enough evidence exists to allow evaluation of their clinical usefulness. These drugs include the noncompetitive NMDA receptor antagonists MK 801 and dextromethorphan, and the competitive NMDA antagonists such as D-CPP-ene which have been thought preferable to traditional non-competitive antagonists (ROGAWSKI and PORTER 1990). Unfortunately, clinical development of both MK 801 and D-CPP-ene had to be stopped because of psychomimetic adverse effects and unimpressive efficacy (WATKINS et al. 1990; SVEINBJORNSDOTTIR et al. 1993; Table 2). Furthermore, treatment with dextromethorphan yielded equivocal results (FISHER et al. 1990). In view of these disappointing clinical data, the whole strategy of developing glutamate antagonists as potential novel antiepileptic therapies has to be reconsidered. In addition, these data demonstrate that the current preclinical strategies of evaluating an anticonvulsant only in non-epileptic animals may exaggerate its potential clinical usefulness. Instead, testing in kindled animals may be better suited to uncover motor impairment and psychomimetic adverse effects of certain drugs, such as NMDA-antagonists (HÖNACK and LÖSCHER 1995).

3. Selective Modulation of Ion Channels

The ionic environment is vital to the excitability of neurons, and all anticonvulsant drugs may ultimately exert their action on synapses and membranes at the ionic level, either by indirect or direct actions on neuronal ion conductances. The evidence is more fully discussed in Chap. 5 of this volume. With regard to the role of voltage-gated ion channels in the cellular mechanisms of epilepsy and antiepileptic drug actions, voltage-gated cationic channels, particularly for Na^+, K^+ and Ca^{2+}, are of special interest (CATTERALL 1987; FAINGOLD 1992). Two investigational drugs have been evaluated clinically, but the clinical development of both was discontinued, mainly due to their unimpressive efficacy in the treatment of refractory partial seizures (Table 2). More recently, the dihydropyridine calcium antagonist nimodipine proved ineffective in an add-on trial for intractable epilepsy (MEYER et al. 1995). In view of these disappointing results, the strategy of developing new anticonvulsants for selective modulation of ion channels needs to be re-examined.

4. Other Strategies for Rational Drug Design

In addition to finding drugs which act on GABAergic or glutamatergic neurotransmission, several other pharmacological attempts to manipulate neurotransmitters and neuromodulators involved in brain excitability have been evaluated. Only two drugs, milacemide (a prodrug for glycine) and taltrimide (a derivative of taurine), have been evaluated to a significant extent and were then deemed not effective enough to warrant further development (ROGAWSKI and PORTER 1990; LÖSCHER and SCHMIDT 1994).

II. Random Screening or Molecular Structural Variation of Known Compounds

As described earlier in this review, serendipity and screening processes, as well as structural variation of already known drugs, led to the discovery of all the clinically established antiepileptic drugs, i.e. the barbiturates, primidone, the hydantoins, the oxazolidinediones, the succinimides, carbamazepine, valproate and the benzodiazepines. Despite the development of mechanism-related strategies of rational drug design, "irrational drug design" by random screening of newly synthesized chemical structures is still a very successful strategy in modern pharmacology so that it is not surprising that various novel antiepileptic drugs were developed in this way during recent decades. Furthermore, variants of clinically established drugs may also provide very useful new compounds. The list of drugs developed by structure variation or random screening includes clinically useful drugs such as clobazam, felbamate, lamotrigine, oxcarbazepine, topiramate and zonisamide (Table 3). For a detailed discussion of the individual drugs, the reader is referred to other chapters of this volume. In addition, a number of drugs such as losigamone, remacemide and levetiracetam are rapidly progressing towards marketing (Table 3). Finally, several compounds either have been discontinued from further development or their future development is currently being reconsidered. These investigational compounds include flupirtine, nafimidone, stiripentol, *trans*-2-en valproate, and eterobarbitone (Table 3). A detailed discussion of these compounds is also beyond the scope of the present chapter. Interested readers are referred to recent reviews (LÖSCHER and SCHMIDT 1988, 1994; ROGAWSKI and PORTER 1990; PISANI et al. 1991; BIALER et al. 1996). In addition to the drugs described above, various other anticonvulsant drugs have been developed by screening strategies and are currently in the preclinical pipeline, but it is not possible to review all of them here. Some examples are mentioned below.

1. Retigabine

A derivative of flupirtine, retigabine (5-(*p*-fluoro-benzylamino)-2-etoxy-carbonylamino)-aniline), has recently been reported to exert a broad spectrum of anticonvulsant activity in different seizure models, including the amygdala-kindling one (ROSTOCK et al. 1996). Clinical testing is under way.

2. TV 1901

TV 1901 (*n*-valproyl glycinamide) was developed from structure-pharmacokinetic-pharmacodynamic relationship studies of a series of *n*-valproyl derivatives of GABA and glycine (BIALER et al. 1996). The drug is active in the maximum electroshock seizure, subcutaneous pentylenetetrazole and corneal kindling tests. Studies in volunteers showed no significant adverse effects.

3. Dezinamide

Dezinamide is a member of a unique chemical class of antiepileptic drugs, the 3-(aryloxy)-azetidine-1-carboxamides), and has undergone successful preclinical and preliminary clinical evaluation for the treatment of complex partial seizures (BIALER et al. 1996).

4. MDL 27,192

The compound 5-(4-chlorophenyl)-2,4-dihydro-4-ethyl-3h-1,2,4-triazol-3-one possesses a broad spectrum preclinical anticonvulsant profile and, interestingly, also has potential neuroprotective activity (KEHNE et al. 1997).

Since the ultimate goal of any drug development is to provide clinically useful agents, it is appropriate to compare the efficacy and the tolerability of drugs generated by rational drug design with those developed through random screening or molecular structural variation.

C. Clinical Evaluation of Preclinical Development Strategies

There is general agreement that, in the absence of confounding drug interactions, a randomized controlled trial comparing add-on treatment of the new anticonvulsant with use of a placebo in patients with refractory disease is the gold-standard for the initial clinical evaluation of the drug (GRAM and SCHMIDT 1993). Recently, the efficacy of 6 new antiepileptic drugs was assessed through careful meta-analysis of 28 placebo-controlled add-on trials. The drugs studied were gabapentin, tiagabine, and vigabatrin, all developed through rational design, and lamotrigine, topiramate, and zonisamide, which were developed by random screening and structural variation (MARSON et al. 1996). Each drug was significantly better than placebo, but none was significantly different from the others in terms of efficacy or tolerability. It should also be noted that several new drugs failed to be more effective than a placebo (Tables 2, 3).

In recent add-on trials, the highest percentages of patients with refractory partial epilepsy who demonstrated a 100% reduction of seizure frequency compared with baseline values were, respectively, 4% for topiramate (FAUGHT et al. 1966), 6% for zonisamide (SCHMIDT et al. 1993), 8% for vigabatrin (FRENCH et al. 1996) and 2%–8% for levetiracetam (SHORVON 1997). For other new drugs, such as lamotrigine, tiagabine or gabapentin, published data on the proportion of patients becoming seizure free in add-on trials are not available. The drug doses tested in some of these trials, however, may not have been optimal. Although a direct comparison with standard drugs is not available, it is nevertheless of interest that a similar percentage (8%) of patients with refractory epilepsy became seizure free when a standard drug, divalproex (a valproate/valproic acid compound), was tested in a similar trial design (WILLMORE et al. 1996). Understandably, the relatively small effect of new drugs in add-on trials in patients with refractory partial epilepsy is a concern.

Add-on trials have been criticized for testing new drugs in the most difficult-to-treat patients in whom standard drugs have already failed. This may be seen as unfair to new drugs, and comparison with standard drugs during monotherapy in patients with previously untreated epilepsy may be more appropriate for their evaluation, since most patients can be treated adequately with monotherapy. When used alone as first line treatment in previously untreated patients with partial seizures and generalized tonic-clonic seizures, vigabatrin achieved complete seizure control in fewer patients than carbamazepine, although it was better tolerated, mainly because it produced no rashes (KÄLVIÄINEN et al. 1995). It should be pointed out that vigabatrin proved to be more effective and better tolerated than hydrocortisone in patients with infantile spasms due to tuberous sclerosis (CHIRON et al. 1997). This clinically relevant effect of vigabatrin was not foreseen from preclinical data because currently no experimental models are available for studying a number of malignant epilepsy syndromes of childhood, including infantile spasms and the Lennox-Gastaut syndrome. When tiagabine is given alone, preliminary data suggest that fewer patients remain on the drug as compared with carbamazepine. The major reasons for tiagabine withdrawal were poor efficacy and poor tolerability (RICHENS et al. 1997). Preliminary pilot data suggest that gabapentin may also be less effective than carbamazepine when given alone to previously untreated patients with partial seizures (CHADWICK et al. 1997). When lamotrigine was compared with carbamazepine there was no significant difference between the two drugs in the time to the first seizure occurrence (a pure efficacy parameter) after 6 weeks' treatment. In this study, time to withdrawal from the study for any reason – a measure of global effectiveness – showed a preference for lamotrigine over carbamazepine which was statistically significant (BRODIE et al. 1995). The main reason for this was less sedation on lamotrigine. When oxcarbazepine was compared with phenytoin or valproate in adults with previously untreated partial seizures and generalized tonic-clonic seizures (BILL et al. 1997; CHRISTE et al. 1997), no statistically significant differences were found for either efficacy or tolerability.

Based on the published clinical evidence reviewed here, rational drug design has generated clinically useful GABAmimetic drugs such as vigabatrin, tiagabine and gabapentin, while drug design based on the modification of glutamatergic neurotransmission and selective alteration of ion channel function has failed, up to now, to provide clinically useful new drugs. Random variation and screening has been successful in providing clinically useful new drugs such as clobazam, felbamate, lamotrigine, oxcarbazepine and zonisamide. A fair clinical assessment of all new drugs, regardless of their mode of preclinical development, has to acknowledge that, compared with the standard drugs such as carbamazepine, phenytoin or valproate, in terms of efficacy none of them has provided a quantum leap towards finding the ideal anticonvulsant. In fact, based on the present evidence, some of the new drugs such as vigabatrin, tiagabine and gabapentin may be even less effective than the standard drugs when given alone. In terms of tolerability, some of the new drugs such as lamotrigine, gabapentin, vigabatrin or levatiracetam may have advantages such as being less sedative or, in the case of gabapentin, causing fewer hypersensitivity reactions than standard drugs. When discussing potential benefits of the new drugs in terms of better tolerability, it should be kept in mind, however, that rare but serious adverse events have occurred with several of the new drugs, e.g. aplastic anaemia and hepatic failure (felbamate) and the hypersensitivity reactions seen with lamotrigine, especially when given with a high titration rate or in combination with valproate (SCHMIDT and KRÄMER 1994). Direct comparison between the new drugs at their optimal clinical doses is required, however, to demonstrate any differences in efficacy and tolerability between them and the standard drugs, if any such differences should exist. Even an optimistic observer would agree that there is a clear need for additional and better new antiepileptic drugs. It is therefore appropriate to review promising future strategies for the development of new anticonvulsants.

D. Strategies for Future Drug Development

Progress in elucidating the basis of epilepsy will vastly increase the number of potential drug targets. A number of potentially useful strategies for the development of better new antiepileptic drugs in the future will be briefly reviewed.

I. Chemical Systems for Delivery of Antiepileptic Drugs to Regions of the Brain

An alternative strategy to that of the traditional structural variation of known drugs is the development of transportable forms of known neuroactive compounds to facilitate drug distribution into the brain. Chemical delivery systems are biologically inert molecules which enhance drug delivery to a particular organ or site and require several steps (chemical or enzymatic reactions) in order to release the active substances (POP and BODOR 1992). By preferential delivery of the drug to the site of action, the overall toxicity of the drug may be significantly reduced while maintaining its therapeutic benefits. Several chemical delivery systems have been designed, synthesized and tested for some traditional (phenytoin, valproate) and novel (stiripentol) antiepileptic drugs, as well as for some neurotransmitters or neuromodulators (GABA, adenosine) with potential roles in epileptogenesis (POP and BODOR 1992). Such chemical delivery systems could be developed to yield antiepileptic drugs with practical uses, thus providing a new strategy for improved epilepsy treatment. Other, more conventional attempts to facilitate the distribution of anticonvulsant drugs into the brain include the implantation of minipumps, or drug entrapment in liposomes. For instance, liposome-entrapped GABA was shown to penetrate the blood-brain barrier and exert anticonvulsant effects in seizure models (LOEB et al. 1989). Finally, intracerebral grafting of inhibitory neurons (or possibly other cells producing inhibitory neurotransmitters) is a new strategy for seizure suppression in the central nervous system (LINDVALL and BJÖRKLUND 1992).

II. Rational Polytherapy

The theoretical and/or experimental basis for choosing specific antiepileptic drug combinations is compromised mainly by the current lack of a full understanding of the chain of events leading from molecular mechanisms to specific seizure types and the progression of seizures into human epilepsy syndromes (SCHMIDT 1996a). Animal models may be useful both in studying basic mechanisms of seizure propagation and in defining targets for rational drug design and rational polytherapy (LÖSCHER and EBERT 1996). Furthermore, in view of the fact that possible combinations of standard and newly developed antiepileptic drugs have not been studied in controlled clinical trials, animal models might be used to preselect potentially interesting drug combinations. The maximum electroshock seizure and kindling models may be especially interesting in this regard. The disappointing clinical effectiveness of add-on therapy in refractory epilepsy (SCHMIDT and GRAM 1995) may be due to inappropriate drug combinations, which are also ineffective experimentally. In experimental seizure models, compounds that block excitatory neurotransmission or voltage-dependent Ca^{2+} channels enhance the effectiveness of certain antiepileptic drugs (CZUCZWAR et al. 1996). The goal of rational polytherapy would be to devise drug combinations which are better than either drug used alone and, even more important, are more effective and less toxic than standard drugs.

III. Predictive Identification of Responders

The physician needs to know those patients in whom a specific drug is likely to be ineffective and to be able to identify those patients who are most likely to benefit from its use. Unfortunately, this information is difficult to retrieve from clinical trial data. Future efforts to search for new anticonvulsants should also attempt to establish diagnostic measures which will allow the prediction of responders. For GABA-mimetic drugs, measuring the GABA concentration in regions of the brain by ^{1}H spectroscopy using a 2.1-T magnetic resonance imager-spectrometer (PETROFF et al. 1996b), or monitoring the plasma GABA concentration, may be useful (LÖSCHER et al. 1993a). Identifying responders may allow new drugs to prove unequivocally more effective and better tolerated for such pre-selected individual patients.

IV. Strategies for the Development of Drugs for Unresponsive Epilepsies

At present, most strategies for the discovery of new drugs centre on animal models which respond to standard drugs. Animal models for drug-resistant epilepsies such as the catastrophic epilepsies of early childhood or partial epilepsies which become drug-resistant over the years, may support the development of new drugs which are better suited to the treatment of unresponsive epilepsies than the current generation of new drugs (LÖSCHER et al. 1993b; HEINEMANN et al. 1994).

V. Identification of Genetic Defects in Epilepsy

Advances in molecular genetics and molecular medicine may become a source of promise for the therapy of diseases previously unresponsive to all treatments. In the case of the epilepsies, identification of mutant genes underlying familial epilepsies may lead to a new pharmacology, through the development of in vitro expression systems permitting the rapid search for novel drugs, the creation of specific animal models based on expression of the precise mutation involved and the correction of disease phenotypes by introducing novel and highly specific genetic information into the person with epilepsy (MCNAMARA 1994).

E. Conclusions

As is apparent from this chapter, numerous novel, effective anticonvulsants have been developed during recent years. Many of these are in clinical trial or have already been introduced into clinical practice. It can also be seen that, in spite of some 30 years of "modern" neuroscientific research in epilepsy, most novel antiepileptic drugs have been developed by screening or as molecular structural variants of known drugs and not by rational strategies based on knowledge of epilepsy mechanisms. The fact that several of the novel drugs that emerged from screening projects were subsequently found to act by one or several of the mechanisms proposed to constitute novel strategies for drug development only demonstrates that serendipity is still an important factor in drug discovery.

Although various drugs which increase GABAergic inhibition, decrease glutamatergic excitation, or block Ca^{2+} channels were developed rationally on the basis of modern neuroscientific research in epilepsy, most of these drugs do not seem to have achieved the expected optimal results, either in epileptic patients resistant to conventional anticonvulsants, or in previously untreated patients. This failure could be due to the following reasons (MUTANI et al. 1991; LÖSCHER and SCHMIDT 1994):

1. Though empirically developed, conventional antiepileptic drugs act by several of the mechanisms on which rational developmental strategies are based (ROGAWSKI and PORTER 1990). Thus, phenobarbitone, valproate and benzodiazepines enhance GABA-mediated inhibition, and excitatory aminoacidergic transmission is decreased by phenobarbitone, phenytoin, carbamazepine, valproate and benzodiazepines. Phenytoin, carbamazepine, and valproate decrease Na^{+} conductance, thus inhibiting repetitive neuronal firing. Furthermore, phenobarbitone, phenytoin and carbamazepine block voltage-dependent Ca^{2+} entry into neurons, and ethosuximide blocks T-type Ca^{2+} currents in thalamic neurons. Thus, there would appear to be no real qualitative difference between these conventional drugs and new drugs developed by the rational strategies described above. One important difference, however, is that most conventional antiepileptic drugs possess more than one mechanism of action, while several of the novel agents are often selective for one particular mechanism. Since epileptic seizures must be viewed as multifactorial in their pathogenesis, antiepileptic drugs with several mechanisms of actions, such as valproate, clearly would have advantages in terms of antiepileptic efficacy when compared with drugs with a more selective effect, e.g. on a single ion channel. Successful treatment of specific seizure types such as generalized myoclonic seizures may require drugs with several cellular mechanisms of action (SCHMIDT et al. 1996). In addition, the optimal use of a compound with a single selective mechanism of action would ideally require the development of predictive markers, suggesting that this particular mechanism is operative in producing the epilepsy of the individual patient. Indeed, almost all the novel antiepileptic drugs with proven clinical efficacy reviewed above were not developed by rational strategies but rather by screening or by molecular variation of

known drugs. For many of these novel effective drugs, even the exact mechanism of action is not known.
2. Newly developed antiepileptic drugs are mostly tested in patients with severe refractory epilepsy with a long history of partial and/or generalized seizures, which might explain the lower than expected degree of efficacy of the drugs that have been found (PLEDGER and SCHMIDT 1994). New guidelines for the clinical testing of antiepileptic drugs have been presented recently and provide a framework of suggestions for the flexible and adaptive evaluation of novel compounds. Innovative trial designs allow early evaluation of efficacy during monotherapy with novel antiepileptic drugs (COMMISSION 1989; GRAM and SCHMIDT 1993). Although one alternative to evaluating new drugs in patients with chronic refractory epilepsy would be to carry out studies in patients not yet treated or at an early phase in the history of their epilepsy, it should be kept in mind that the most important goal of antiepileptic drug development is the eventual availability of more effective medications for patients whose disorders are refractory to current antiepileptic drugs. In that regard, testing of investigational drugs in animal models of refractory partial epilepsy is encouraged. Furthermore, very effective drugs may be successful at low doses which are less prone to cause adverse effects.

In addition to those with refractory epilepsy, newly diagnosed patients expect help from new anticonvulsants. Approximately 40% of those with newly diagnosed partial seizures will not become seizure-free on monotherapy with established anticonvulsants (SCHMIDT and GRAM 1995). Although not requiring withdrawal of their medication, many patients may have inconvenient adverse effects such as mild sedation or subtle cognitive impairment. It is a challenge for new anticonvulsants to help such patients. The current preliminary evidence, discussed above, suggests that none of the new drugs is more effective than the standard anticonvulsants, although patients may benefit from fewer adverse effects such as sedation if the new drugs are used.

Apart from these important points, which may be responsible for the apparent failure of most rational strategies to produce new, effective antiepileptic drugs, an additional reason might be that the way in which modern approaches are applied to drug discovery are still too simplistic, ignoring the complex alterations of brain functions, particularly the disturbances of behaviour and cognition, induced by chronic epilepsy (LÖSCHER 1993). Most of the events that contribute to epileptogenesis appear to be exaggerated aspects of normal physiology, so that many possible pharmacotherapeutic interventions may interfere with normal neural excitability or synaptic transmission (DICHTER 1989). Furthermore, in view of the fact that the most clinically useful antiepileptic drugs are those that possess two or more mechanisms of action, the current strategy of developing drugs with a selective effect on a single neurotransmitter system or even neurotransmitter receptor subtypes may yield drugs with narrow spectra of anticonvulsant activity and an unfavourable risk-benefit ratio in general use. Drug developers traditionally aim towards more and more selective targets, but it has been pointed out recently that an absolute selectivity in a drug may in fact not be desirable in a clinical situation that involves complex adaptive changes (Fredholm and Abbott 1990). Thus, there are various recent examples from different fields of pharmacotherapy where the development of drugs with a more selective biochemical action has proved disappointing in providing a more selective therapy with fewer side-effects and improved clinical efficacy. On the other hand, highly selective drugs are indispensable as research tools to increase our knowledge of physiological and pathophysiological mechanisms. Greater understanding of basic brain pharmacology and mechanisms of epilepsy may allow the development of new treatment strategies. In view of the fact that patients with the same types of clinical seizure respond differentially to antiepileptic drugs, the pathophysiological events underlying epileptic seizures apparently not only differ between different seizure types but are multifactorial for the same type of seizure. In order to achieve improved therapy of epilepsy, the real challenge for the future will be to create novel, broadly acting, antiepileptic drugs with multiple mechanisms of actions and with better efficacy and decreased adverse effect potentials compared to the currently used medical therapies.

Acknowledgement. I would like to thank Professor Dr. Wolfgang Löscher (Hannover, Germany) for critical revision of the manuscript.

References

Bialer M, Johannessen SI, Kupferberg HJ, Levy RH, Loiseau P, Perucca E (1996) Progress report on new antiepileptic drugs: a summary of the third Eilat conference. Epilepsy Res 25:299–307

Bill PA, Vigonius U, Pohlmann H, Guerreiro CAM, Kochen S, Saffer D, Moore A (1997) A double-blind controlled trial of oxcarbazepine versus phenytoin in adults with previously untreated epilepsy. Epilepsy Res 27:205–214

Bowery NG, Pratt GD (1992) GABAB receptors as targets for drug action. Arzneim Forsch 42:215–223

Brodie MJ, Richens A, Yuen AWC (1995) Double blind comparison of lamotrigine and carbamazepine in newly diagnosed epilepsy. Lancet 345:476–479

Catterall WA (1987) Common modes of drug action on Na^+ channels: local anesthetics, antiarrhythmics and anticonvulsants. Trends Pharmacol Ther 8:57–65

Chadwick D, Anhut H, Murray G, Greiner M, Alexander INT J (1997) Gabapentin Monotherapy Study Group (945–077). Gabapentin (GBP); (Neurontin) monotherapy in patients with newly-diagnosed epilepsy. Results of a double-blind fixed dose study comparing three dosages of gabapentin and open-label carbamazepine. Epilepsia 38 [Suppl 3]:34

Chiron C, Dumas C, Jambaque I, Mumford J, Dulac O (1997) Randomised trial comparing vigabatrin and hydrocortisone in infantile spasms due to tuberous sclerosis. Epilepsy Res 26:389–395

Christe W, Krämer G, Vigonius U, Pohlmann H, Steinhoff BJ, Brodie MJ, Moore A (1997) A double-blind controlled clinical trial: oxcarbazepine versus valproate in adults with newly diagnosed epilepsy. Epilepsy Res 26:451–460

Commission on Antiepileptic Drugs of the International League Against Epilepsy (1989) Guidelines for the clinical evaluation of antiepileptic drugs. Epilepsia 30:400–406

Coulter DA, Huguenard JR, Prince DA (1989) Characterization of ethosuximide reduction of low-threshold calcium current in thalamic neurones. Ann Neurol 25:582–593

Crawford P, Richens A, Mawer G, Cooper P, Hutchison JB (1992) A double-blind placebo controlled cross-over study of remacemide hydrochloride as adjunctive therapy in patients with refractory epilepsy. Seizure 1 [Suppl A]:7–13

Croucher MJ, Collins JF, Meldrum BS (1982) Anticonvulsant action of excitatory amino acid antagonists. Science 216:899–901

Czuczwar SJ, Kleinrok Z, Turski WA (1996) Interaction of calcium channel blockers and excitatory amino acid antagonists with conventional antiepileptic drugs. CNS Drug Reviews (2/4):452–467

Dalby NO, Nielsen EB (1997) Comparison of the preclinical anticonvulsant profiles of tiagabine, lamotrigine, gabapentin and vigabatrin. Epilepsy Res 28:63–72

Dam M, Reeh Petersen R, Jensen I et al. (1982) GABA-agonists in the treatment of epilepsy. Acta Neurol Scand 65 [Suppl 90]:191–192

Dichter MA (1989) Cellular mechanisms of epilepsy and potential new treatment strategies. Epilepsia 30 [Suppl 1]:S3–S12

Dichter MA, Brodie MJ (1996) New antiepileptic drugs. N Engl J Med (334):1583–1590

Dingledine R, McBain CJ, McNamara JO (1990) Excitatory amino acid receptors in epilepsy. Trends Pharmacol Sci 11:334–338

Faingold CL (1992) Overview of ion channels, antiepileptic drugs, and seizures. In: Faingold CL, Fromm GH (eds) Drugs for control of epilepsy: actions on neuronal networks involved in seizure disorders. CRC Press, Boca Raton, pp. 57–68

Faught E, Wilder BJ, Ramsay RE et al. (1996) Topiramate placebo controlled dose ranging trial in refractory partial epilepsy using 200-, 400-, and 600-mg daily dosages. Topiramate YD Study Group. Neurology 46:1684–1690

Fisher RS, Cysyk BJ, Lesser RP et al. (1990) Dextromethorphan for treatment of complex partial seizures. Neurology 40:547–549

Fredholm B, Abbott A (1990) New targets for drug action: is high selectivity always beneficial? Trends Pharmacol Ther 11:175–178

French JA, Mosier M, Walker S, Sommerville K, Sussman N and the Vigabatrin Protocol 024 Investigative Cohort (1996) A double-blind, placebo-controlled study of vigabatrin three g/day in patients with uncontrolled complex partial seizures. Neurology 46:54–61

Gram L, Schmidt D (1993) Innovative designs of controlled clinical trials in epilepsy. Epilepsia 34 [Suppl 79]:S1–S6

Haefely W, Martin JR, Schoch P (1990) Novel anxiolytics that act as partial agonists at benzodiazepine receptors. Trends Pharmacol Sci 11:452–456

Handforth A, Mai T, Treiman DM (1995) Rising dose study of safety and tolerance of flunarizine. Eur J Clin Pharmacol 49:91–94

Haria M, Balfour JA (1997) Levetiracetam. CNS Drugs 7:159–164

Heinemann U, Draguhn A, Ficker E, Strabel J, LiZhang C (1994) Strategies for the development of drugs for pharmacoresistant epilepsies. Epilepsia 35 [Suppl 5]:S10–S21

Holland KD, McKeon AC, Canney DJ, Covey DF, Ferrendelli JA (1992) Relative anticonvulsant effects of GABAmimetic and GABA modulatory agents. Epilepsia 33:981–986

Hönack D, Löscher W (1995) Kindling increases the sensitivity of rats to adverse effects of certain antiepileptic drugs. Epilepsia 36:763–771

Kälviäinen R, Äikiä M, Saukkonen AM, Mervaala E, Riekkinen PJ (1995) Vigabatrin vs. carbamazepine monotherapy in patients with newly diagnosed epilepsy. Arch Neurol 52:889–996

Kehne JH, Kane JM, Chaney SF, Hurst G, McCloskey TC, Petty MA, Senyah Y, Wolf HH, Zobrist R, White HS (1997) Preclinical characterisation of MDL 27,192 as a

potential broad spectrum anticonvulsant agent with neuroprotective properties. Epilepsy Res 27:41–45
Krall RL, Penry JK, Kupferberg HJ, Swinyard EA (1978a) Antiepileptic drug development: I. History and a program for progress. Epilepsia 19:393–408
Krall RL, Penry JK, White BG, Kupferberg HJ, Swinyard EA (1978b) Antiepileptic drug development: II. Anticonvulsant drug screening. Epilepsia 19:409–428
Kupferberg HJ (1989) Antiepileptic drug development program: a cooperative effort of government and industry. Epilepsia 30 [Suppl 1]:S51–S56
Lindvall O, Björklund A (1992) Intracerebral grafting of inhibitory neurons. A new strategy for seizure suppression in the central nervous system. Adv Neurol 57:561–569
Loeb C, Marinari UM, Benassi E et al. (1989) Phosphatidylserine increases in vivo the synaptosomal uptake of exogenous GABA in rats. Exp Neurol 99:440–446
Löscher W (1984) Genetic animal models of epilepsy as a unique resource for the evaluation of anticonvulsant drugs. A review. Meth Find Experiment Clin Pharmacol 6:531–547
Löscher W (1993) Basic aspects of epilepsy. Current Opinion Neurol Neurosurg 6:223–232
Löscher W, Ebert U (1996) Basic mechanisms of seizure propagation: targets for rational drug design and rational polypharmacy. In: Homan RW, Leppik IE, Lothman EW, Penry JK, Theodore WH (eds) Rational polypharmacy. Epilepsy Res [Suppl 11]:17–44
Löscher W, Hönack D (1991) Responses to NMDA receptor antagonists altered by epileptogenesis. Trends Pharmacol Sci 12:52
Löscher W, Schmidt D (1988) Which animal models should be used in the search for new antiepileptic drugs? A proposal based on experimental and clinical considerations. Epilepsy Res 2:145–181
Löscher W, Schmidt D (1994) Strategies in antiepileptic drug development: is rational drug design superior to random screening and structural variation? Epilepsy Res 17:95–134
Löscher W, Fassbender CP, Gram L, Gramer M, Hörstermann D, Zahner B, Stefan H (1993a) Determination of GABA and vigabatrin in human plasma by a rapid and simple HPLC method: correlation between clinical response to vigabatrin and increase in plasma GABA. Epilepsy Res 14:245–255
Löscher W, Rundfeldt C, Hönack D (1993b) Pharmacological characterization of phenytoin-resistant amygdala-kindled rats, a new model of drug-resistant partial epilepsy. Epilepsy Res 15:207–220
Macdonald RL (1989) Antiepileptic drug actions. Epilepsia 30 [Suppl 1]:S19–S28
Marescaux C, Vergnes M, Bernasconi R (1992) GABAB receptor antagonists: potential new anti-absence drugs. J Neural Transm Suppl 35:179–188
Marson AG, Kadir ZA, Chadwick DW (1996) New antiepileptic drugs: a systematic review of their efficacy and tolerability. Brit Med J 313:1169–1176
McNamara JO (1994) Identification of genetic defect of an epilepsy: strategies for therapeutic advances. Epilepsia 35 [Suppl1]:S51–S57
Meldrum BS (1995) Neurotransmission in epilepsy. Epilepsia 36 [Suppl 1]:S30–S35
Meldrum BS, Porter RJ (1986) New anticonvulsant drugs. Libbey, London, pp. 147–164
Meyer FB, Cascino GD, Whisnant JP, Sharbrough FW, Ivnik RJ, Gorman DA, Windschitl WL, So EL, O'Fallon WM (1995) Nimodipine as an add-on therapy for intractable epilepsy. Mayo Clinic Proc 70:623–627
Mutani R, Cantello, R, Gianelli M, Bettucci D (1991) Rational basis for the development of new antiepileptic drugs. In: Pisani F, Perucca E, Avanzini G, Richens A (eds) New antiepileptic drugs. Epilepsy Res Suppl 3:23–28
Owen RT (1993) Development of lamotrigine. Drugs News Perspec 6:304–307
Petroff OA, Rothman DL, Behar KL, Lamoureux D, Mattson RH (1996a) The effect of gabapentin on brain gamma-aminobutyric acid in patients with epilepsy. Ann Neurol 39:95–99

Petroff OAC, Rothman Dl, Behar KL, Mattson RH (1996b) Low brain GABA level is associated with poor seizure control. Ann Neurol 40:908–911
Pisani F, Perucca E, Avanzini G, Richens A (1991) New antiepileptic drugs. Epilepsy Res Suppl 3:141–146
Pledger G, Schmidt D (1994) Problems in the evaluation of antiepileptic drug efficacy. Drugs 48:498–509
Pop E, Bodor N (1992) Chemical systems for delivery of antiepileptic drugs to the central nervous system. Epilepsy Res 13:1–16
Porter RJ, Rogawski MA (1992) New antiepileptic drugs: from serendipity to rational discovery. Epilepsia 33 [Suppl 1]:S1–S6
Richens A, Chadwick D, Duncan I, Dam M, Morrow I, Gram L, Mengel H, Shu V, Pierce M (1992) Tiagabine: safety and efficacy as adjunctive treatment for complex partial seizures. Seizure 1 [Suppl A]:S37–S44
Richens A, Sommerville KW, Lyby K, Deaton R (1997) Efficacy of tiagabine in all partial seizure types. Abstract of a company sponsored symposium at the 22nd International Epilepsy Congress, 1997 Dublin, pp. 1–6
Rogawski MA (1993) Therapeutic potential of excitatory amino acid antagonists: channel blockers and 2,3-benzodiazepines. Trends Pharmacol Sci 14:325–331
Rogawski MA, Porter RJ (1990) Antiepileptic drugs: pharmacological mechanisms and clinical efficacy with consideration of promising developmental stage compounds. Pharmacol Rev 42:223–285
Rostock A, Tober C, Rundtfeldt C et al. (1996) D-23129. A new anticonvulsant with a broad spectrum activity in animal models of epileptic seizures. Epilepsy Res 23:211–223
Runge U, Rabending G, Röder H, Dienel A (1993) Losigamone: first results in patients with drug-resistant focal epilepsy. Epilepsia 34 [Suppl 2]:6
Schmidt D (1966) Rational polytherapy. In: Brodie MJ, Treiman DM (eds) Bailliere's clinical neurology: modern management of epilepsy 5:757–764
Schmidt D, Gram L (1995) Monotherapy versus polytherapy in epilepsy: a reappraisal. CNS Drugs 3:194–208
Schmidt D, Krämer G (1994) The new antiepileptic drugs. Implications for avoidance of adverse effects. Drug Safety 11:422–431
Schmidt D, Morselli PL (eds) (1986) Intractable epilepsy: experimental and clinical aspects. Raven Press, New York
Schmidt D, Utech K (1986) Progabide for refractory partial epilepsy: a controlled add-on trial. Neurology 36:217–221
Schmidt D, Jacob R, Loiseau P et al. (1993) Zonisamide for add-on treatment of refractory partial epilepsy: a European double-blind trial. Epilepsy Res 15:67–73
Schmidt D, Straub HB, Meenke HJ (1996) Putative dual (or multiple) cellular mechanism of anti-myoclonic epilepsy medication. Epilepsia 38 [Suppl 3]:44
Schmutz M, Allgeier H, Jeker A et al. (1993) Anticonvulsant profile of CGP 33101 in animals. Epilepsia 34 [Suppl 2]:122
Shorvon S (1997) Analysis of the European and US clinical studies. Findings and perspectives (abstract). Satellite symposium at the 22nd International Epilepsy Congress, pp. 8–9
Sieghart W (1992) GABAA receptors: ligand-gated Cl^- ion channels modulated by multiple drug binding sites. Trends Pharmacol Ther 13:446–450
Sveinbjornsdottir S, Sander JWAS, Upton D et al. (1993) The excitatory amino acid antagonist D-CPP-ene (SDZ EAA-494) in patients with epilepsy. Epilepsy Res 16:165–174
Walker MC, Patsalos PN (1995) Clinical pharmacokinetics of new antiepileptic drugs. Pharmacol Ther 67:351–384
Wamil AW, McLean MJ (1994) Limitation by gabapentin of high frequency action potential firing by mouse cerebral neurones in cell cultures. Epilepsy Res 17:1–11

Watkins JC, Krogsgaard-Larsen P, Honoré T (1990) Structure-activity relationships in the development of excitatory amino acid receptor agonists and competitive antagonists. Trends Pharmacol Sci 11:25–33

White HS, Kupferberg HJ (1996) Preclinical identification of novel anticonvulsant substances. Epilepsy. Advances in understanding and latest drug developments. February 1996, Orlando, Fl. Abstract

Willmore LJ, Shu V, Wallin B and the M88-194 Study Group (1996) Efficacy and safety of add-on divalproex sodium in the treatment of complex partial seizures. Neurology 46:49–53

CHAPTER 7

Measurement of Anticonvulsants and Their Metabolites in Biological Fluids

W.D. HOOPER and L.P. JOHNSON

A. Introduction

There seems to be a greater volume of literature dealing with the assay of antiepileptic drugs and their metabolites than with the assay of almost any other class of drugs. Many factors have contributed to this situation, including (1) the older antiepileptic drugs have been studied over a long period, (2) several antiepileptic drugs have unusual and interesting disposition characteristics, which have warranted extensive study, (3) antiepileptic drugs are probably the drug class to which therapeutic drug monitoring (TDM) is most commonly applied, and (4) there are a large number of antiepileptic drugs in clinical use or under development. There is a great diversity of analytical methods, and to a large extent the choice of method is governed by the application to which the method will be put. It is often the case that a method which is suitable for therapeutic drug monitoring will not meet the requirements of clinical pharmacokinetic or metabolic studies, while methods which meet these latter requirements may be inappropriate in terms of cost, speed or convenience in the therapeutic drug monitoring laboratory. While it is not possible in the space available to give a comprehensive survey of all methods for all drugs, we have attempted to provide a contemporary outline of the most commonly used methods, to indicate their attributes, limitations and areas of applicability, and to provide references in which further information may be located. Analytical methodologies for antiepileptic drug analyses have been reviewed previously (KUMPS 1982; MEIJER et al. 1983; ALBANI et al. 1992).

Unless specified, the analysis of antiepileptic drugs throughout this chapter refers to the substances in plasma or serum. Although not routinely used, analysis of antiepileptic drugs in hair has been reported (KINTZ et al. 1995; MEI and WILLIAMS 1997), as has their measurement in other non-conventional biological fluids (PICHINI et al. 1996). Saliva is now used routinely by some laboratories and is discussed later in this chapter.

B. Chromatographic Methods

The various chromatographic techniques are without doubt the most broadly applicable to the assay of antiepileptic drugs or indeed drugs generally. The combination of the separation power of chromatography with the versatile array of either relatively specific or almost universally encompassing detectors, makes chromatography often the method of first (or only) choice for the demanding requirements of metabolic or pharmacokinetic studies. While chromatographic methods have been extensively applied in therapeutic drug monitoring laboratories, there are now preferred alternatives (see below) for many of the most commonly monitored drugs.

There are a large number of techniques under the broad heading of "chromatographic". All are separation techniques involving the differential distribution of solutes (analytes) between a stationary phase (solid or viscous liquid) and a mobile phase (liquid, gas or supercritical fluid). The mechanisms involved include partitioning, adsorption, size exclusion and ion pairing. While some techniques like thin-layer chromatography have been more widely applied in the past, the two major methods of gas chromatography (GC) and high performance liquid chromatography (HPLC) have maintained or increased their ranges of application over the past couple of decades. More recently, efforts have been made to establish supercritical fluid chromatography (Smith 1988) as a practical method, but this method will not be discussed here since there have been few specific applications in which supercritical fluid chromatography has demonstrated superiority to either gas chromatography or high performance liquid chromatography (Wong 1993; Scott 1994).

I. Gas Chromatography and High Performance Liquid Chromatography

While there are significant differences between these two techniques, some of which are mentioned below, there is sufficient in common that it is appropriate to discuss them together. We have not described the elements of the techniques, since these will be familiar to most readers. There are, in any case, numerous monographs and reviews devoted to both gas chromatography (Freeman 1981; Grant 1995; Jennings et al. 1997) and high performance liquid chromatography (Johnson and Stevenson 1978; Snyder et al. 1988; McMaster 1994; Scott 1994).

Since, as noted above, chromatographic techniques are fundamentally separation methods, their major advantages result from their capacity to separate and concurrently assay a drug and its metabolites, or multiple antiepileptic drugs, in the same sample. This also underlines the immense flexibility and adaptability of chromatographic methods: there are few organic compounds which cannot, at least in principle, be assayed by gas chromatography and/or high performance liquid chromatography. This contrasts sharply with the immune-based procedures, which are, or are intended to be, highly specific. The strength and versatility of gas chromatography for assay of a drug and multiple metabolites is well illustrated in the case of valproic acid. The drug and 14 of its metabolites have been co-assayed by gas chromatography/mass spectrometry (gas chromatography MS), using either electron impact ionization with monitoring of positively charged ions (Rettenmeier et al. 1989) or chemical ionization and monitoring of negatively charged ions (KASSAHUN et al. 1989). The application of high performance liquid chromatography to concurrent assay of carbamazepine plus five metabolites (in urine) was carried out by BERNUS et al. (1995). These latter authors also illustrated the capacity of high performance liquid chromatography to co-assay multiple drugs, since the same method incorporated the assay of phenytoin, methylphenobarbitone and two of their metabolites. Numerous methods have been described for the simultaneous assay of multiple antiepileptic drugs (in some cases up to eight drugs) in plasma by high performance liquid chromatography (e.g. REIDMANN et al. 1981; ROMANYSHYN et al. 1994). An excellent summary covering 16 methods has been published (KAPETANOVIC 1990). There are many published gas chromatography and/or high performance liquid chromatography methods for the older, established antiepileptic drugs and, in most cases, for their metabolites. However, in the therapeutic drug monitoring context, as shown below, it is preferable to adopt immune-based techniques for which suitable methods are commercially available for most of the established antiepileptic drugs. On the other hand, immune-based methods are generally unavailable for the many new antiepileptic drugs which have either recently reached the market or are in the latter stages of clinical development. In these cases a chromatographic technique will be the best option for pharmacokinetic and other studies conducted during drug development, and for therapeutic drug monitoring following marketing, at least initially, should that be shown to offer clinical advantages.

Although gas chromatography and high performance liquid chromatography techniques have been applied to the assay of antiepileptic drugs (and other drugs) over many years, there are a number of recent developments in these areas which impact positively on their utility. These include the shorter assay times and high resolution made possible by capillary gas chromatography columns (GRANT 1995), microbore and restricted access media columns and automated extraction procedures which are now commercially available for high performance liquid chromatography (ALBANI et al. 1992) and the increasing availability and affordability of the extremely specific and sensitive techniques of gas chromatography MS (KITSON et al. 1996), liquid chromatography mass spectrometry and especially liquid chromatography mass spectrometry/mass spectrometry (NIESSEN and VANDERGREEF 1992).

C. Capillary Electrophoresis and Micellar Electrokinetic Capillary Electrophoresis

Capillary electrophoresis and micellar electrokinetic capillary electrophoresis are relatively new analytical techniques which have promising potentials for the analysis of antiepileptic drugs. Comprehensive presentations of the theory and application of these techniques, including their use in therapeutic drug monitoring, can be found in a number of texts (LUNTE and RADZIK 1996;

Shintani and Polanski 1996). General clinical applications of capillary electrophoresis including therapeutic drug monitoring have been discussed (Shihabi 1992) and an educational article on the application of capillary electrophoresis to therapeutic drug monitoring and drug toxicology has been published (Rosenzweig 1996).

Capillary electrophoresis is a technique which separates analytes in a buffer-filled open-tubular fused silica capillary tube, with separation being achieved on the basis of analyte electrophoretic mobility, hydrophobicity and stereospecificity. Ionic and neutral species migrate toward the cathode due to the process of electroendosmosis, the process whereby a solvent moves toward an electrode under the influence of hydrated ions in a buffer. Buffers are an integral part of capillary electrophoresis and micellar electrokinetic capillary electrophoresis in that they solubilize the solute, carry the applied current and adjust the pH, and can be modified to enhance the specificity including the separation of enantiomers (e.g. by the addition of cyclodextrins).

Micellar electrokinetic capillary electrophoresis separates compounds on the basis of their physicochemical properties using partitioning between aqueous and organic phases of a buffer which is usually a surfactant (e.g. sodium dodecylsulphate) added at a concentration greater than the critical micelle concentration.

The advantages of capillary electrophoresis for therapeutic drug monitoring are its high resolution enabling analysis of complex drug/drug metabolite mixtures, small sample volumes (5–15 nl injected), relatively simple instrumentation, low solvent usage and reduced sample preparation. Methods involving both pretreatment and direct injection have been reviewed by Lloyd (1996). Capillary electrophoresis can also be fully automated and coupled to detectors such as variable ultraviolet, photodiode array, laser induced fluorescence and mass spectrometric ones. These have recently been reviewed by Naylor et al. (1996).

I. Antiepileptic Drug Analysis by Capillary Electrophoresis and Micellar Electrokinetic Capillary Electrophoresis

General applications of capillary electrophoresis to therapeutic drug monitoring have been reported by Evenson and Wiktorowicz (1992). Concerns that suitable internal and external quantitation methods have not been reliably validated for these techniques in general, and that the small injection volumes used in capillary electrophoresis/micellar electrokinetic capillary electrophoresis may result in poor precision and accuracy seem unfounded, at least on the basis of the reported applications of capillary electrophoresis and micellar electrokinetic capillary electrophoresis for the analysis of antiepileptic drugs. The assay of felbamate has been reported by Shihabi and Oles (1994), using micellar electrokinetic capillary electrophoresis direct injection, and the results correlated well with the sensitivity and precision of high performance liquid chromatography. Schmutz and Thorman (1993) compared micellar electrokinetic capillary electrophoresis with high performance liquid chromatography and immunoassay techniques for phenobarbitone, ethosuximide and primidone. They found a good correlation between all methods with the results being validated against international quality assurance program specimens. Similar results have been obtained by LEE et al. (1992), who demonstrated the separation of six commonly prescribed antiepileptic drugs, and by GARCIA et al. (1995), who described a rapid and precise capillary electrophoresis method for the serum analysis of the newer antiepileptic drug gabapentin.

D. Stereoselective Drug Analysis

Many drugs exist in stereoisomeric forms. The most commonly encountered situation is a molecule with one centre of asymmetry, giving rise to two stereoisomers which differ only in the spatial orientation of the groups bound to the stereogenic centre. These stereoisomers are mirror images of each other, and are termed enantiomers. Many such drugs are marketed as a mixture of enantiomers in equal parts, called a racemic mixture. Anticonvulsants in this category include ethosuximide and its analogues, ethotoin, methylphenobarbitone, vigabatrin, remacemide and stiripentol. Other new antiepileptic drugs, for example, tiagabine and topiramate, are being developed as single stereoisomers.

It is generally accepted that the study of the pharmacokinetics, metabolism and other dispositional aspects including drug-drug interactions of drugs administered as racemates requires enantioselective analytical methods.

There are essentially two approaches to the chromatographic separation of enantiomers. The first approach involves direct separation, which uses analytical columns coated with an optically active (chiral) stationary phase. A variety of chiral columns is commercially available for both high performance liquid chromatography and gas chromatography applications. One limitation of these columns for gas chromatography work is their thermal instability at higher operating temperatures (offset to some degree by functional chemical derivatization of analytes prior to analysis) and their susceptibility to contamination, requiring specimen cleanup prior to analysis.

The second approach involves indirect separation where the enantiomers are first converted to diastereoisomers by derivatization with optically active reagents which themselves must be of high optical and chemical purity, thereby placing some limitations on certain derivatization processes. Diastereoisomers are stereoisomers which have the same chemical composition but distinctly different physicochemical properties, allowing them to be separated on standard non-chiral chromatographic systems. Derivatization affords other advantages including improved chromatographic properties and enhanced sensitivity via derivatives responsive to specific detectors such as ultraviolet, fluorescence, electron capture and electrochemical. Comprehensive reviews of enantiomeric derivatization for biomedical chromatography have been presented (GOROG and GAZDAG 1994; SRINIVAS et al. 1995) as have various texts on chiral separations using high performance liquid chromatography (SUBRAMANIAN 1994) and capillary electrophoresis (CHANKVETADZEE 1997).

There is ongoing debate as to whether such methods are required for therapeutic drug monitoring applications. Vigabatrin enantiomers have been studied extensively (SHEANN et al. 1992; SCHRAMM et al. 1993), including the kinetics of both enantiomers (HAEGLE et al. 1986), the interaction with felbamate (REIDENBERG et al. 1995) and in children where results indicated altered enantiomer ratios compared with adults (REY et al. 1990; NAGARAJAN et al. 1993). It is well known that the S-enantiomer of vigabatrin contributes all of the pharmacological activity of the drug and it might seem in principle that this isomer should be assayed specifically. However, there is little difference in the disposition of the enantiomers, and also no indication that therapeutic drug monitoring would improve the clinical use of this drug since its antiepileptic drug effects do not correlate well with its plasma concentrations at a given time. We are not aware that a compelling case for the stereoselective assay of any chiral antiepileptic drug in the therapeutic drug monitoring context has yet been established.

E. Immunoassay Methods

Immunoassays are now ubiquitous in clinical laboratories which routinely perform antiepileptic drug monitoring. The reasons are quite simply that today's assays are easy to perform, being fully automated on both dedicated and general clinical chemistry analysers, and in most cases have adequate sensitivity and specificity for the commonly prescribed antiepileptic drugs. Although generally not reagent cost effective compared with chromatographic procedures, they are easily performed in both batch and statim analysis, with a rapid turnaround. Over the last few decades the range of analytes covered by commercial immunoassays has changed little, in stark contrast to the variety of immunoassay methodologies and instrumentation currently used. Commercial assays still are limited to phenytoin, carbamazepine, valproic acid and their corresponding free fractions, as well as primidone, phenobarbitone and ethosuximide.

For the purposes of this article immunoassays can generally be classified as heterogeneous or homogeneous, and competitive or non-competitive. Heterogeneous immunoassays are capable of measuring both small and large analytes. They include a specific step for the separation of the antibody-bound labelled fraction and unlabelled fraction, generally have greater specificity and sensitivity than homogeneous immunoassays and include all radioimmunoassays. Radioimmunoassays are generally not used in the routine measurement of antiepileptic drugs for reasons which include safety in handling radioisotopes, long turn-around times, and the need for frequent calibration and specialized equipment, to name but a few.

The homogeneous immunoassays widely used in clinical chemistry do not require physical separation of the antibody-bound labelled fraction from the unlabelled fraction. There is an extensive variety of commercial homogeneous assay systems available. A feature of these assays is their calibration stability, which may range from a few weeks to a few months. Reagent systems are relatively simple, the turn-around is fast and the universal acceptance of such assays means that there is generally considerable participation in external quality assurance programs for the majority of antiepileptic drugs monitored in routine therapeutic drug monitoring.

Enzymatic and fluorescence immunoassay techniques which have been applied to the measurement of antiepileptic drugs include for example, enzyme multiplied immunoassay technique (EMIT; Syva Corporation), radial partition enzyme immunoassay, cloned enzyme donor immunoassay (CEDIA), fluorescence polarization immunoassay (FPIA) and substrate labelled fluorescence immunoassay. Other methods include particle enhanced turbidimetric inhibition nephelometric immunoassay (PETINIA) and latex particle agglutination inhibition procedures. A method based on immunolysis of liposomes has also been reported (Kubotsu et al. 1992).

A non-homogeneous competitive immuno-rate assay for phenytoin is offered by Johnson and Johnson which uses dry-slide technology. In a fully automated process, anti-drug antibody is immobilized between specific layers of reagents on a multilayered polyester support slide. The reagents include a drug specific peroxidase conjugate. The patient drug and the conjugate compete for antibody binding in a separate layer of the slide, with the reaction being stopped after a pre-determined time by washing the slide to remove unbound drug-peroxidase conjugate whilst also providing a substrate for the enzyme-mediated oxidation of a leuco dye. The rate of dye formation, measured by reflectance spectrophotometry, is inversely proportional to the drug concentration in the specimen.

A novel non-isotopic carbonyl metallo-immunoassay has recently been developed for carbamazepine (Varenne et al. 1995), phenobarbitone (Salmain et al. 1992) and phenytoin (Varenne et al. 1994). This technique uses a metal carbonyl complex as a tracer and Fourier transform infra-red spectroscopy as the detection method. The method requires only a few microlitres of serum and has the exciting potential of developing an immunoassay method for the simultaneous analysis of multiple antiepileptic drugs.

It is beyond the scope of this chapter to provide a comprehensive description of immunoassay procedures for the analysis of antiepileptic drugs and the various analytical problems associated with each methodology. For more in depth information various texts (Wild 1993; Price and Newman 1996) may be consulted.

I. Immunoassay Instrumentation

Immunoassay instrumentation has recently been reviewed (Chan 1995) and described effectively as an open or closed system. Open systems consist of general purpose clinical chemistry analysers which can be adapted to different immunoassay systems, providing that the assay is homogeneous and that the analyser has reagent handling and detection systems compatible with the assay protocols. Closed systems are inherently restricted to specific manufacturer protocols and often to specific instrumentation. Instrumentation can be batch, random-access or continuous access. The variety of both open and closed instrumental systems in combination with different immunoassay procedures is quite substantial and information concerning the different systems for therapeutic drug monitoring and toxicology has been summarized (SASSE 1997).

II. Analytical Performance

Despite the variety of assay procedures and instrumentation currently available, antibody specificity is perhaps the single most significant factor which affects immunoassay analytical performance. The introduction of monoclonal antibodies has improved some assays but these may still suffer from varying degrees of non-specific cross-reactivity with endogenous substances, metabolites and/or other drugs. Analytical performance may also be affected, for example, by specimen preservatives, haemolysis, bilirubin and lipids. A well researched problem which has recently been re-evaluated is that related to the major metabolites of phenytoin, namely 5-(*p*-hydroxyphenyl)-5-phenylhydantoin and its glucuronic acid conjugate (SCHWENZER et al. 1995; RAINEY et al. 1996). Both these compounds significantly cross-reacted with the Abbott fluorescence polarization immunoassay system and originally with the EMIT system. This has significant clinical relevance in uraemic patients where free drug levels may need to be measured. Modification of these assays by the manufacturers via the introduction of more specific antibodies resulted in metabolite cross-reactivity which was clinically insignificant. However, the improved Abbott fluorescence polarization immunoassay system has recently been withdrawn due to another cross-reactivity problem with a non-steroidal anti-inflammatory drug, oxaprozin.

Lack of antibody specificity can in certain instances be taken advantage of to provide measurement of active metabolites via modification of assays targeted to a particular drug. For example, desmethylmethsuximide has been measured using both fluorescence polarization immunoassay and EMIT assays designed to measure ethosuximide (MILES et al. 1989). The procedure was carefully validated against high performance liquid chromatography and shown to provide reliable measurement of desmethylmethsuximide.

The vast array of instruments and methodologies for the measurement of antiepileptic drugs by immunoassay has inevitably led to a plethora of method comparisons and evaluations. In nearly all comparisons, good correlation, precision, accuracy and specificity have been shown, although not all immunoassay methods have been compared with a specific reference method. For example, fluorescence polarization immunoassay and cloned enzyme donor immunoassay phenytoin assays compared on Hitachi and TDx instruments showed good agreement (KURZE et al. 1995), as did phenobarbitone analysis on a Dimension instrument using PETINIA compared with TDx (FLEMING et al. 1995). Similarly, cloned enzyme donor immunoassay for phenytoin and phenobarbitone was comparable with high performance liquid chromatography (VAN DER WEIDE et al. 1993) and a multi-centre investigation involving high performance liquid chromatography, fluorescence immunoassays and EMIT on various Hitachi models (KLEIN et al. 1995) also showed good correlations. A dry film multilayer fluorescence immunoassay has been compared with a fluorescence polarization immunoassay on different instruments (O'CONNELL et al. 1995) and the results correlated well.

III. Non-laboratory Immunoassay Antiepileptic Drug Monitoring

A number of non-laboratory immunoassay systems have been developed which offer the convenience of small specimen size (finger-prick) and on-site drug level determination. The Acculevel enzyme immunochromatography system (Syntex Medical Diagnostics, USA) uses whole blood and chromatographic paper coated with monoclonal antibodies to the drug of interest. It is a single analyte system with the measurement based on a colour bar retention factor which is converted to a plasma concentration using special conversion tables. The assay is available for carbamazepine, phenytoin and phenobarbitone. Another system, Biotrack (Ciba Corning Diagnostics, USA), is based on a turbidimetric latex agglutination inhibition reaction and uses an electronic monitor to measure whole blood drug levels which are converted to plasma concentrations based on a measured haemoglobin concentration and known relationships between blood and plasma. These methods have been evaluated and shown to perform to acceptable standards although requiring strict adherence to procedural detail and manufacturer's instructions. The Acculevel (OLES et al. 1989; NIELSEN et al. 1992) and the Biotrack (RAMBECK et al. 1994) systems have been evaluated against EMIT, fluorescence polarization immunoassay and high performance liquid chromatography and both showed acceptable agreement in all comparisons. Another system, the Seralyser (Ames, Miles Laboratories, USA), is a portable system which uses an apoenzyme reactivation immunoassay with reflectance photometry. Serum phenytoin and phenobarbitone concentrations have been evaluated against fluorescence polarization immunoassay using this system and showed good correlations (BRETTFELD et al. 1989).

F. Free Drug Monitoring

Many methods exist for the characterization of protein bound and unbound drugs in physiological fluids including equilibrium dialysis, microdialysis, gel filtration, ultracentrifugation and ultrafiltration. These methods have been reviewed extensively (WRIGHT et al. 1996). The most commonly used method for the separation of free drugs in clinical evaluation of drug therapy is ultrafiltration, which uses a membrane filter to separate free and protein bound drugs under the forces of centrifugation. The advantages of this technique are that it is quick, requires standard laboratory centrifuges, albeit ideally with temperature control and fixed angle rotors, and gives a direct free drug fraction which can be used subsequently with the total levels to determine the extent of protein binding. The concentration of free drug remains unaltered during the filtration process and is independent of the serum volume. The limitations of ultrafiltration include possible non-specific adsorption of drugs to the separation membrane. However, in any analytical procedure, these potential effects should always be investigated. Commercial ultrafiltration devices are available (e.g. Centrifree system; Amicon Danvers, MA, USA). Despite the perception that ultrafiltration requires highly sensitive analytical methods to measure the free levels, modern analytical systems have more than adequate sensitivity for free antiepileptic drug monitoring in typical clinical situations. High performance liquid chromatography has been used for the measurement of free drug levels (TAYLOR and ACKERMAN 1987), including fully automated sample preparation and analysis of free and total drug concentrations using in-line equilibrium dialysis (JOHANSEN et al. 1995), direct serum analysis using restricted access media high performance liquid chromatography (GURLEY et al. 1995) and high performance liquid chromatography for free valproic acid, with a critical evaluation of the ultrafiltration systems and comparisons with enzyme immunoassays (LIU et al. 1992).

I. Saliva

Saliva is a natural ultrafiltrate of blood plasma and as such can be used for the evaluation of certain antiepileptic drug free drug levels including carbamazepine, phenytoin and phenobarbitone. The clinical utility of routine salivary therapeutic drug monitoring (STDM) has been demonstrated (KNOTT and REYNOLDS 1984, 1989), whilst a detailed critique of salivary therapeutic drug monitoring in general has been presented (DROBITCH and SVENSSON 1992). From an analytical viewpoint, several important factors need to be considered. Sample collection can be achieved with or without the stimulation of salivary secretions. Although citric acid stimulation is commonly used there is minimal need for it due to the fact that most analytical procedures today have sufficient sensitivity to analyse the drugs in small volumes of saliva. A method for collecting pre-purified saliva ultrafiltrate using an oral osmotic device has been shown to be simple and reliable in the determination of free antiepileptic drug levels (SCHRAMM et al. 1991). A similar device is commercially available (Saliva Sac, BioQuant Inc., Ann Arbor, USA). A simple collection device which uses a gauze-wrapped cotton ball with attached string has been shown to be effective in children (CHEE et al. 1993). The presence of residual drug from previously administered tablets or syrup may give spurious results unless a sufficient lag-time between administration and sampling is allowed (Dickinson et al. 1985). After collection, it is common to measure the salivary pH and to centrifuge the sample, using the supernatant for analysis. Freezing saliva can also improve dispensing accuracy by reducing sample viscosity. Correction for the effects of pH is important for some ionic drugs (e.g. phenobarbitone).

Analytical methodologies for salivary therapeutic drug monitoring are mainly chromatographic. Although immunoassay methods designed for plasma have been used with modification, they require careful validation. The effect of citric acid on interference in the EMIT immunoassay has been debated (Paton and Logan 1986; Knott and Reynolds 1987). A dry phase apoenzyme reactivation method modified for saliva has been compared with fluorescence polarization immunoassay (Miles et al. 1990): both methods were proven suitable for salivary therapeutic drug monitoring of antiepileptic drugs, as were gas chromatography and EMIT after comparison (Goldsmith and Ouvrier 1981).

G. Quality Assurance

Comparison of analytical methods for measuring antiepileptic drugs has been aided by the greater availability of external quality assurance programs throughout the world, and an increasing and almost mandatory participation by clinical laboratories in these programs. Consequently, more objective assessment of comparisons of analytical precision, accuracy, sensitivity and specificity has been possible (Wilson et al. 1989). However, care is required in interpreting results from different quality control programs, especially with respect to matrix effects. The preferred material is human serum or plasma to which weighed-in amounts of drug have been added (Tsanaclis et al. 1990; Witte 1993). Pre-analytical variation caused by various sampling procedures is also important. Criteria for therapeutic drug monitoring of antiepileptic drugs including sampling, storage and collection have been reviewed (Li and Nichols 1997). Studies of widely used serum or plasma separator tubes have shown varying analyte losses of antiepileptic drugs due to absorption to the gel in one manufacturer's tubes under certain conditions (Mauro and Mauro 1991; Dasgupta et al. 1996) but clinically insignificant losses in different manufacturer's tubes (Koch and Platoff 1990). This highlights the obvious requirement that laboratories must evaluate new clinical products thoroughly, and have input into sampling procedures.

References

Albani F, Riva R, Baruzzi A (1992) Therapeutic drug monitoring of antiepileptic drugs II. Analytical Techniques. Il Farmaco 47 [Suppl 5]:671–680

Bernus I, Hooper WD, Dickinson RG, Eadie MJ (1995) Metabolism of carbamazepine and co-administered anticonvulsants during pregnancy. Epilepsy Res 21:65–75

Brettfeld C, Gobrogge R, Massoud N, Munzenberger P, Nigro M, Sarnaik A (1989) Evaluation of the Ames Seralyser for the therapeutic drug monitoring of phenobarbital and phenytoin. Ther Drug Monit 11:612–615

Chan DW (1995) Clinical Instrumentation (Immunoassay Analysers). Anal Chem 67:519R–524R

Chankvetadzee B (1997) Capillary electrophoresis in chiral analysis. Wiley, London

Chee KY, Lee D, Byron D, Naidoo D, Bye A (1993) A simple collection method for saliva in children: potential for home monitoring of carbamazepine therapy. Br J Clin Pharmacol 35:311–313

Dasgupta A, Blackwell W, Bard D (1996) Stability of therapeutic drug measurement in specimens collected in VACUTAINER plastic blood – collection tubes. Ther Drug Monit 18:306–309

Dickinson RG, Hooper WD, King AR, Eadie MJ (1985) Fallacious results from measuring salivary carbamazepine concentrations. Ther Drug Monit 7:41–45

Drobitch RK, Svensson CK (1992) Therapeutic drug monitoring in saliva – an update. Clin Pharmacokinet 23:365–379

Evenson MA, Wiktorowicz JE (1992) Automated capillary electrophoresis applied to therapeutic drug monitoring. Clin Chem 38:1847–1852

Fleming CS, Waller SJ, Craig AR, Chu VP, Reiner JA (1995) A phenobarbital method on the Dimension clinical chemistry system. Ther Drug Monit 17:391

Freeman RR (ed) (1981) High resolution gas chromatography, 2nd edn. Hewlett-Packard Company, California

Garcia LL, Shihabi ZK, Oles K (1995) Determination of gabapentin in serum by capillary electrophoresis. J Chromatogr B Biomed Appl 669:157–162

Goldsmith RF, Ouvrier RA (1981) Salivary anticonvulsant levels in children: a comparison of methods. Ther Drug Monit 3:151–157

Gorog S, Gazdag M (1994) Enantiomeric derivatisation for biomedical chromatography. J Chromatogr B Biomed Appl 659:51–84

Grant DW (1995) Capillary gas chromatography. Wiley, New York

Gurley BJ, Marx M, Olsen K (1995) Phenytoin free fraction determination: comparison of an improved direct serum injection HPLC method to ultrafiltration coupled with FPIA. J Chromatogr B Biomed Appl 670:358–364

Haegele KD, Schecter P (1986) Kinetics of the enantiomers of vigabatrin after an oral dose of the racemate or the active S enantiomer. Clin Pharmacol Ther 40:581–586

Jennings W, Mittlefehldt E, Stremple P (1997) Analytical gas chromatography, 2nd edn. Academic Press, New York

Johansen K, Krogh M, Andersen AT, Christophersen AS, Lehne G, Rasmussen KE (1995) Automated analysis of free and total concentrations of three antiepileptic drugs in plasma with on-line dialysis and hplc. J Chromatogr B Biomed Appl 669:281–288

Johnson EL, Stevenson R (1978) Basic liquid chromatography. Varian Associates, Palo Alto, California

Kapetanovic IM (1990) Analysis of antiepileptic drugs. J Chromatogr 531:421–457

Kassahun K, Burton R, Abbott FS (1989) Negative ion chemical ionization gas chromatography/mass spectrometry of valproic acid metabolites. Biomed Environ Mass Spectrom 18:918–926

Kintz P, Marescaux C, Mangin P (1995) Testing human hair for carbamazepine in epileptic patients: is hair investigation suitable for drug monitoring? Hum Exp Toxicol 14:812–815

Kitson FG, Larsen BS, McEwen CN (1996) Gas chromatography and mass spectrometry: a practical guide. Academic Press, New York

Klein G, Lehman P, Coty W (1995) Multicentre evaluation of the CEDIA immunoassay for carbamazepine, phenytoin, phenobarbital and valproic acid on Hitachi 704, 717 and 911 analysers. Ther Drug Monit 17:409

Knott C, Reynolds F (1984) The place of saliva in antiepileptic drug monitoring. Ther Drug Monitor 6:35–41

Knott C, Reynolds F (1987) Citrate and salivary drug measurement. Lancet 97
Knott C, Reynolds F (1989) Saliva monitoring of anticonvulsants Report on the workshop conference "Application of saliva in laboratory medicine". J Clin Chem Clin Biochem 27:226–228
Koch TR, Platoff G (1990) Suitability of collection tubes with separator gels for therapeutic drug monitoring. Ther Drug Monitor 12:277–280
Kubotsu K, Goto S, Fujita M, Tuchiya H, Kid M, Takano S, Matsuura S, Sakurabayashi I (1992) Automated homogeneous liposome immunoasssay systems for anticonvulsant drugs. Clin Chem 38:808–812
Kumps A (1982) Therapeutic drug monitoring: A comprehensive and critical review of analytical methods for anticonvulsant drugs. J Neurol 228:1–16
Kurze S, Hamwi A, Soregi G, Schweiger CR, Vukovich TH (1995) Comparison of FPIA and CEDIA method for determination of digitoxin, theophylline and phenytoin. Ther Drug Monit 17:391
Lee Kong-Joo, Heo GS, Kim NJ, Moon DC (1992) Analysis of antiepileptic drugs in human plasma using micellar electrokinetic capillary chromatography. J Chromatogr A 608:243–250
Li D, Nichols J (1997) Specimen collection and stability for therapeutic drug monitoring. AACC Therapeutic Drug Monitoring and Toxicology In-Service training and continuing education program. 8:3–9
Liu H, Montoya JL, Forman LJ, Eggers CM, Barham CF, Delgado M (1992) Determination of free valproic acid and evaluation of the Centrifree system and comparison between HPLC and EIA. Ther Drug Monit 14:513–521
Lloyd DK (1996) Capillary electrophoretic analysis of drugs in body fluids: sample pretreatment and methods for direct injection of biofluids. J Chromatogr A 735:29–42
Lunte SM, Radzik DM (eds) (1996) Pharmaceutical and biomedical applications of capillary electrophoresis. Progress in pharmaceutical and biomedical analysis. Vol 2, Elsevier Science, Oxford
Mauro LS, Mauro VF (1991) Effect of serum separator tubes on free and total phenytoin and carbamazepine serum concentrations. Ther Drug Monit 13:240–243
McMaster MC (1994) HPLC: a practical users' guide. Wiley, New York
Mei Z, Williams J (1997) Simultaneous determination of phenytoin and carbamazepine in human hair by high performance liquid chromatography. Ther Drug Monit 19:92–94
Meijer JWA, Rambeck B, Reidmann M (1983) Antiepileptic drug monitoring by chromatographic methods and immunometric techniques – Comparison of analytical performance, practicability and economy. Ther Drug Monit 5:39–53
Miles MV, Howlett CM, Tennison MB, Greenwood RS, Cross RE (1989) Determination of n-desmethylmethsuximide serum concentrations using enzyme multiplied and fluorescence polarisation immunoassays. Ther Drug Monit 11:337–342
Miles MV, Tennison MB, Greenwood RS, Benoit SE, Thorn MD, Messenheimer JA, Ehle AL (1990) Evaluation of the Ames Seralyser for the determination of carbamazepine, phenobarbital and phenytoin concentrations in saliva. Ther Drug Monit 12:501–510
Nagarajan L, Schramm T, Appleton DB, Burke CJ, Eadie MJ (1993) Plasma vigabatrin enantiomer ratios in adults and children. Clin Exper Neurol 30:127–136
Naylor S, Benson LM, Tomlinson AJ (1996) Application of capillary electrophoresis and related techniques to drug metabolism studies. J Chromatogr A 735:415–438
Nielsen IM, Gram L, Dam M (1992) Comparison of the Acculevel and TDx: evaluation of on-site monitoring of antiepileptic drugs. Epilepsia 33:558–563
Niessen W, Vandergreef J (1992). Liquid chromatography-mass spectrometry. Marcel Dekker, New York
O'Connell MT, Ratnaraj N, Elyas AA, Doheny MH, Darsot S, Patsalos PN (1995) A comparison of the OPUS and TDx analysers for antiepileptic drug monitoring. Ther Drug Monit 17:549–555

Oles KS, Penry JK, Dyer RD (1989) Evaluation of an enzyme immunochromatography method for carbamazepine: a comparison with enzyme-multiplied immunoassay technique, fluorescence polarisation immunoassay and high performance liquid chromatography. Ther Drug Monit 11:471–476

Paton RD, Logan RW (1986) Salivary drug measurement: A cautionary tale. Lancet 1340

Pichini S, Altieri I, Zuccaro P, Pacifici R (1996) Drug monitoring in non-conventional biological fluids and matrices. Clin Pharmacokinet 30:211–228

Price CP, Newman DJ (1996) Principles and practice of immunoassay. 2nd edn, Stockton Press, New York

Rainey PM, Rogers KE, Roberts WL (1996) Metabolite and matrix interference in phenytoin immunoassays. Clin Chem 42:1645–1653

Rambeck B, May TW, Jurgens U, Blankenhorn V, Jurges U, Korn-Merker E, Salke-Kellermann A (1994) Comparison of phenytoin and carbamazepine serum concentrations measured by high performance liquid chromatography, the standard TDx assay, the Enzyme Multiplied Immunoassay Technique and a new patient-side immunoassay cartridge system. Ther Drug Monit 16:608–612

Reidenberg P, Glue P, Banfield C et al. (1993) Pharmacokinetic interaction studies between felbamate and vigabatrin. Br J Clin Pharmacol 40:157–160

Reidmann M, Rambeck B, Meijer JWA (1981) Quantitative simultaneous determination of eight common antiepileptic drugs and metabolites by liquid chromatography. Ther Drug Monit 3:397–413

Rettenmeier AW, Howald WN, Levy RH, Witek DJ, Gordon WP, Porubek DJ, Baillie TA (1989) Quantitative metabolic profiling of valproic acid in humans using automated gas chromatographic/mass spectrometric techniques. Biomed Environ Mass Spectrom 18:192–199

Rey E, Pons G, Richard MO et al. (1990) Pharmacokinetics of the individual enantiomers of vigabatrin (gamma-vinyl GABA) in epileptic children. Br J Clin Pharmacol 30:253–257

Romanyshyn LA, Wichmann JK, Kucharczyk N, Shumaker RC, Ward D, Sofia RD (1994) Simultaneous determination of felbamate, primidone, phenobarbital, carbamazepine, two carbamazepine metabolites, phenytoin and one phenytoin metabolite in human plasma by high-performance liquid chromatography. Ther Drug Monit 16:90–99

Rosenzweig B (1996) Capillary electrophoresis: A new methodology for therapeutic drug monitoring and drugs of abuse. AACC Continuing Education Therapeutic Drug Monitoring and Toxicology 17:143–160

Salmain M, Vessieres A, Brossier P, Butler IS, Jaouen G (1992) Carbonyl metalloimmunoassay (CMIA) a new type of non-radioisotope immunoassay. Principles and application to phenobarbital assay. J Immunol Methods 148:65–75

Sasse EA (1997) Immunoassays and immunoassay analysers for analytical toxicology. In: Wong SHY, Sunshine I (eds) Handbook of analytical therapeutic drug monitoring and toxicology. CRC Press, Boca Raton, pp. 223–235

Schmutz A, Thormann W (1993) Determination of phenobarbital, ethosuximide and primidone in human serum by micellar electrokinetic capillary chromatography with direct sample injection. Ther Drug Monit 15:310–316

Schramm TM, McKinnon GE, Eadie MJ (1993) Gas chromatographic assay of vigabatrin enantiomers in plasma. J Chromatogr B Biomed Appl 616:39–44

Schramm W, Annesley TM, Seigel GJ, Sackellares JC, Smith RH (1991) Measurement of phenytoin and carbamazepine in ultrafiltrate of saliva. Ther Drug Monit 13:452–460

Schwenzer K, Liu-Allison L, Motter K (1995) Application of the new monoclonal COBAS FP phenytoin and valproic acid reagents for the analysis of free phenytoin and free valproic acid on the Cobas Integra and Cobas Farah. Ther Drug Monit 17:409

Scott RPW (1994) Liquid chromatography for the analyst. Marcel Dekker, New York

Sheean G, Schramm T, Anderson DS, Eadie MJ (1992) Vigabatrin plasma enantiomer concentrations and clinical effects. Clin Exp Neurol 29:107–116
Shihabi ZK (1992) Clinical applictions of capillary electrophoresis. Ann Clin Lab Sci 22:398–405
Shihabi ZK, Oles KS (1994) Felbamate measured in serum by two methods: HPLC and capillary electrophoresis. Clin Chem 40:1904–1908
Shintani H, Polanski J (eds) (1996) Analytical applications of capillary electrophoresis. Blackie Academic, London
Smith RM (ed) (1988) Supercritical fluid chromatography. Royal Society of Chemistry, London
Snyder LR, Glajch JL, Kirkland JJ (1988) Practical HPLC method development. Wiley, New York
Srinivas NR, Shyu WC, Barbhaiya RH (1995) Gas chromatographic determination of enantiomers as diastereoisomers following pre-column derivatisation and applications to pharmacokinetic studies: a review. Biomed Chromatogr 9:1–9
Subramanian G (ed) (1994) A practical approach to chiral separations by liquid chromatography. VCH, Weinheim
Taylor EH, Ackerman BH (1987) Free drug monitoring by liquid chromatography and implications for therapeutic drug monitoring. J Liq Chromatogr 10:323–343
Tsanaclis LM, Wilson JF, Williams J, Perrett JE, Richens A (1990) Comparison of human, bovine and new-born calf serum in the preparation of external quality assurance samples for therapeutic drugs. Ther Drug Monit 12:373–377
Van der Weide J, Luiting HK, Veerfkind AH (1993) Evaluation of the cloned enzyme donor immunoassay for measurement of phenytoin and phenobarbital in serum. Ther Drug Monit 15:344–348
Varenne A, Vessieres A, Brossier P, Jaouen G (1994) Application of the non-radioisotopic carbonyl metallo-immunoassay (CMIA) to diphenylhydantoin. Res Commun Chem Pathol Pharmacol 84:81–92
Varenne A, Vessieres A, Salmain M, Brossier P, Jaouen G (1995) Production of specific antibodies and development of a non-isotopic immunoassay for carbamazepine by the carbonyl metallo-immunoassay (CMIA) method. J Immunol Methods 186:195–204
Wild D (ed) (1993) The immunoassay handbook. MacMillan, London
Wilson JF, Tsanaclis TM, Williams J, Tedstone JE, Richens A (1989) Evaluation of assay techniques for the measurement of antiepileptic drugs in serum: A study based on external quality assurance measurements. Ther Drug Monit 11:185–195
Witte DL (1993) Matrix effects in therapeutic drug monitoring surveys. Proposed protocol to identify error components and quality improvement opportunities. Arch Pathol Lab Med 117:373–380
Wong SHY (1993) Advances in chromatography for clinical drug analysis: supercritical fluid chromatography, capillary electrophoresis, and selected high-performance liquid chromatography techniques. Ther Drug Monit 15:576–580
Wright JD, Boudinot FD, Ujhelyi MR (1996) Measurement and analysis of unbound drug concentrations. Clin Pharmacokinet 30:445–462

CHAPTER 8

Older Anticonvulsants Continuing in Use but with Limited Advance in Knowledge

M.J. EADIE and F.J.E. VAJDA

A. Introduction

Several relatively long-established anticonvulsants continue in clinical use though there has been comparatively little advance in knowledge of their pharmacologies. Whilst more effective and less toxic alternatives are now available, significant numbers of patients continue to be satisfactorily managed with these older drugs and they are sometimes extremely helpful after their more modern counterparts prove inadequate. Such agents include phenobarbitone and its congeners, the succinimides, sulthiame and acetazolamide, and the bromides. The various oxazolidinediones (principally troxidone – trimethadione), formerly important for treating absence epilepsy, now seem to have almost completely disappeared from clinical use, though they are still employed in experimental laboratory studies.

B. Phenobarbitone and Congeners

Phenobarbitone has been used as an anticonvulsant since 1912 (HAUPTMANN 1912). Subsequently, two congeners, *N*-methylphenobarbitone and primidone (desoxy-phenobarbitone), came into moderately widespread use for treating epilepsy. These latter substances are both biotransformed to phenobarbitone and act largely, though not exclusively, though this substance. All three congeners are here discussed together.

In Western medicine the barbiturate anticonvulsants are now often regarded as largely superseded. However, phenobarbitone remains widely used in developing countries (ISMAEL 1990). Another barbiturate anticonvulsant, eterobarbitone, has been studied but has not come into general use. It is not discussed further.

I. Chemistry and Use

1. Chemistry

Phenobarbitone (5-ethyl-5-phenyl-barbituric acid: phenobarbital) is a white crystalline material, molecular weight 232.23, pK_a 7.3, sometimes prescribed as its sodium salt. *N*-Methylphenobarbitone (5-ethyl-1-methyl-5-phenyl-barbituric acid: mephobarbital) is chiral around the C atom at the 5-position of the barbiturate ring, because of the methyl substituent on the 1-position of the ring. It is supplied commercially as the racemate (molecular weight 246.26, pK_a 7.8). It is more lipophilic than phenobarbitone. Primidone (2-desoxyphenobarbitone; molecular weight 218.25, pK_a 13) is another white crystalline material. Chemically, strictly speaking, it is not a barbiturate, but 5-ethyldihydro-5-phenyl-4,6-(1*H*, 5*H*)-pyrimidine-dione.

2. Use

Phenobarbitone and methylphenobarbitone are now employed almost exclusively as anticonvulsants, and sometimes to treat neonatal hyperbilirubinaemia. Primidone too is employed mainly as an anticonvulsant, but is sometimes used for essential (hereditary, senile) tremor (FINDLEY et al. 1985; SASSO et al. 1988, 1991; KOLLER et al. 1994; METZER 1994) and primary writing tremor (BAIN et al. 1995), lithium tremor (GELENBERG and JEFFERSON 1995), orthostatic tremor (WILLEIT 1991) and theophylline-resistant apnoea of prematurity (MILLER et al. 1994). Several lines of evidence suggest that primidone itself, and not phenobarbitone derived from it (SASSO et al. 1988, 1991; SEYFERT et al. 1988), benefits essential tremor.

The three barbiturates are effective for all partial epilepsies, for generalized epilepsies with bilateral tonic-clonic seizures, including juvenile myoclonic epilepsy (but not for myoclonic epilepsies which begin earlier in life) and for benign febrile convulsions of infancy (FAERO et al. 1972; THIOTAMMAL et al. 1993).

II. Pharmacodynamics

Methylphenobarbitone and primidone are both biotransformed to phenobarbitone. Most of their anticonvulsant actions appear to depend on this metabolite. There is some indirect evidence that (R,S)-methylphenobarbitone (CRAIG and SHIDEMANN 1971), probably its (S)-enantiomer (BUCH et al. 1968), primidone (LÖSCHER and HÖNACK 1989), and its metabolite phenylethylmalonamide (BAUMEL et al. 1973) have antiepileptic effects in their own rights, though the mechanisms of these effects have been relatively little investigated. Only the mechanisms of action of phenobarbitone are discussed below.

1. Animal Models of Epilepsy

GALLAGHER and FREER (1985) considered this topic. Phenobarbitone protects against maximum and minimum electroshock seizures in several animal species (GOODMAN et al. 1953), and against chemically induced bilateral myoclonic seizures (SWINYARD and CASTELLION 1966), light-induced seizures in *Papio papio* (MELDRUM et al. 1975) and amygdaloid electrically kindled seizures (WADA 1977).

2. Electrophysiological Actions

The electrophysiological actions of phenobarbitone were reviewed by PRICHARD and RANSON (1995). Phenobarbitone limits the spread of seizure activity from experimental epileptic foci, probably by interfering with synaptic neurotransmission (ESPLIN 1975). It increases the cortical stimulation threshold for inducing local and generalized seizure activity (HOOGERKAMP et al. 1994). It and (S)(+)-methylphenobarbitone facilitate inhibition in rat hippocampal slices (DUNWIDDIE et al. 1986).

3. Biochemical Actions

Certain biochemical effects of phenobarbitone, e.g. inhibition of mitochondrial electron transport (COWGER and LABBE 1967), occur only at drug concentrations higher than those needed for an antiepileptic effect in humans. Phenobarbitone (and certain other barbiturates) produce prolonged opening of postsynaptic Cl^- channels which are components of $GABA_A$ receptors (BARKER and MCBURNEY 1979), thus facilitating Cl^- entry through neuronal cell membranes (ALLAN and HARRIS 1986). This entry hyperpolarizes the cell membrane, thus inhibiting neurotransmission. SCHWARTZ et al. (1985) showed that (R,S)-methylphenobarbitone, but not phenobarbitone, enhanced Cl^- efflux from rat synaptoneurosomes.

At supratherapeutic concentrations phenobarbitone inhibits neuronal NMDA-induced responses (DANIELL 1994), reduces intraneuronal Na^+ concentrations (PINCUS et al. 1970) and increases Na^+ channel opening in frog skin (FONESCA et al. 1994).

The biochemical mechanisms of action of primidone itself are not known (FREY 1995).

III. Pharmacokinetics

The following pharmacokinetic data refer to humans, except where specified. Pharmacokinetic information is available for phenobarbitone in dogs (RAVIS et al. 1989; THURMAN et al. 1990), cats (COCHRAN et al. 1990) and horses (RAVIS et al. 1987; KNOX et al. 1992).

1. Absorption

a) Phenobarbitone

Oral phenobarbitone is reasonably fully bioavailable (NELSON et al. 1982), with a mean absorption half-time of 1.37 h (EADIE et al. 1976) but a relatively late T_{max} value of 6–18 h (LOUS 1954), which has sometimes led to claims that the drug is slowly absorbed. However, the late T_{max} is due to the drug's slow elimination. The T_{max} after intramuscular administration is 1–3 h (VISWANATHAN et al. 1978; GRAHAM 1978). Rectal phenobarbitone is about 90% bioavailable (GRAVES et al. 1989).

b) Methylphenobarbitone

Empirically, twice as much methylphenobarbitone as phenobarbitone is needed to achieve the same steady-state plasma phenobarbitone concentrations in patients. This has sometimes led to an assumption that oral methylphenobarbitone is only 50% bioavailable. HOOPER et al. (1981a,b) showed that oral (R,S)-methylphenobarbitone was 75% bioavailable and later showed that (R)-methylphenobarbitone was so rapidly cleared that it probably underwent significant presystemic elimination (LIM and HOOPER 1989), thus explaining the incomplete oral bioavailability of the racemate. In two subjects, the absorption half-times for oral (R,S)-methylphenobarbitone were 0.48 and 0.38 h (HOOPER et al. 1981a). The mean T_{max} for (R)-methylphenobarbitone was 2.29 ± SD 1.03 h, and for (S)-methylphenobarbitone 3.50 ± SD 1.52 h (LIM and HOOPER 1989).

c) Primidone

As judged from urinary output data, oral primidone is at least 92% bioavailable (KAUFMANN et al. 1977). The drug's T_{max} after oral intake is 0.5–7 h (GALLAGHER et al. 1972), 3.2 ± 1.0 h (BOOKER et al. 1970) or 4–6 h (KAUFMANN et al. 1977).

2. Distribution

a) Phenobarbitone

In adults, the apparent volume of distribution of phenobarbitone is 0.5–0.6 l/kg (MARTIN et al. 1979; NELSON et al. 1982; WILENSKY et al. 1982). It is higher in neonates (0.97 ± 0.15 l/kg – PAINTER et al. 1977; 0.81 l/kg – FISCHER et al. 1981), and intermediate in infants (0.667 l/kg – MINAGAWA et al. 1981). In adults 50%–60% of the phenobarbitone in plasma is protein bound (BAUMEL et al. 1972; MC AULIFFE et al. 1977; LÖSCHER 1979). In neonates 36%–43% is bound (BOSSI 1982). The plasma protein binding of the drug decreases in late pregnancy (YERBY et al. 1990).

Phenobarbitone concentrations in CSF are 43%–47% of those in whole plasma (VAJDA et al. 1974; HOUGHTON et al. 1975; SCHMIDT and KUPFERBERG 1975), and salivary concentrations 30%–38% (SCHMIDT and KUPFERBERG 1975; KNOTT and REYNOLDS 1984). With correction for the effects of salivary pH on drug distribution, the salivary phenobarbitone concentration is 43.1 ± 5.2% of that in whole plasma (MC AULIFFE et al. 1977). Concentrations of the drug in milk are 35%–45% of those in plasma (KANEKO et al. 1979). Reported brain to plasma concentration ratios for phenobarbitone range from 0.59:1 (VAJDA et al. 1974) to 1.13:1 (HOUGHTON et al. 1975).

b) Methylphenobarbitone

(R,S)-Methylphenobarbitone has a higher apparent volume of distribution than phenobarbitone (mean 1321 in adults – EADIE et al. 1978). The mean apparent volumes of distribution of the (R)- and the (S)-enantiomers were 5.32 ± SD 3.33 l/kg and 1.73 ± SD 0.31 l/kg respectively (LIM and HOOPER 1989), but the value for the (R)-enantiomer probably represents that of V/F. In plasma, (R)-methylphenobarbitone is approximately 67%, and (S)-methylphenobarbitone approximately 59% bound to plasma proteins (LIM and HOOPER 1989). In rats, the brain concentration of (R,S)-methylphenobarbitone is some 8 times its blood concentration (CRAIG and SHIDEMAN 1971).

c) Primidone

Primidone has an apparent volume of distribution of 0.6 l/kg (VAN DER KLEIJN et al. 1975) and its metabolite phenylethylmalonamide one of 0.69 ± 0.20 l/kg (PISANI and RICHENS 1983). Little (6%–7% – LÖSCHER 1979) or no primidone is bound to plasma proteins, and its CSF, salivary and plasma concentrations are similar. CSF primidone concentrations average 80% (SCHMIDT and KUPFERBERG 1975) or 81% (HOUGHTON et al. 1975) and salivary concentrations average 75% (MC AULIFFE et al. 1977) to 108% (TROUPIN and FRIEL 1975) of its plasma ones. The drug's concentration in milk is 70%–80% of that in plasma (KANEKO et al. 1984), while its concentrations in human temporal lobectomy specimens averaged 87% of its concentrations in plasma (HOUGHTON et al. 1975).

3. Elimination

The barbiturate anticonvulsants are eliminated mainly by metabolism.

a) Metabolism

α) Phenobarbitone

At steady state, a mean of 25% or 27% of a phenobarbitone dose is excreted in human urine unmetabolized (WHYTE and DEKABAN 1977; BERNUS et al. 1994b). In humans, phenobarbitone undergoes (Fig. 1):

1. Oxidation at the *p*-position on its benzene ring, forming a phenolic derivative (*p*-hydroxy-phenobarbitone), most of which then undergoes glucuronide conjugation before being excreted into urine. Such glucuronidation is poorly developed in neonates (BOREUS et al. 1978). The phenolic metabolite has relatively little biological activity (CRAIG et al. 1960). This metabolic pathway accounted for 25% (WHYTE and DEKABAN 1977), 21% (VISWANATHAN et al. 1978) or 16 ± SD 10% (BERNUS et al. 1994a) of a phenobarbitone dose.
2. *N*-Glucoside formation (TANG et al. 1979), resulting in (R)- and (S)-enantiomers of the glucoside. At steady state 14 ± SD 11% of a phenobarbitone dose was excreted as (S)-phenobarbitone-*N*-glucoside, with the (R)-enantiomer accounting for less than 4% of the dose and being unmeasurable in

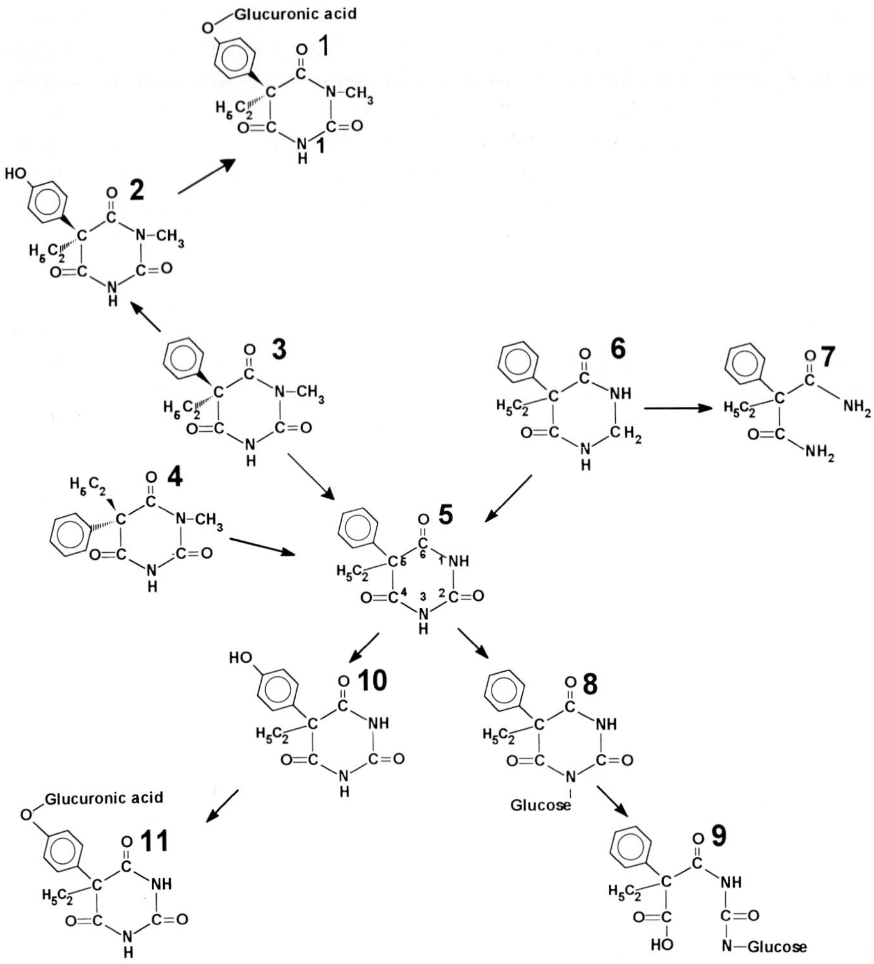

Fig. 1. Interrelationships and major metabolic pathways for phenobarbitone, methylphenobarbitone and primidone. *1*, *p*-hydroxy-(R)-methylphenobarbitone glucuronide; *2*, *p*-hydroxy-(R)-methylphenobarbitone; *3*, (R)-methylphenobarbitone; *4*, (S)-methylphenobarbitone; *5*, phenobarbitone; *6*, primidone; *7*, phenylethylmalonamide; *8*, (R,S)-phenobarbitone-*N*-glucoside; *9*, first stage barbiturate ring-opened derivative of (R,S)-phenobarbitone-*N*-glucoside; *10*, *p*-hydroxyphenobarbitone; *11*, *p*-hydroxyphenobarbitone glucuronide

nearly one-third of subjects (Bernus et al. 1994a). The *N*-glucosides of phenobarbitone are pH labile, and begin to decompose at pH values above 5, yielding barbiturate ring-opened derivatives whose subsequent fates are unknown (Vest et al. 1989). In vitro, at 37°C and pH 7.4, the half-life of (S)-phenobarbitone-*N*-glucoside is about 15h (Bernus et al. 1994a). Therefore phenobarbitone-*N*-glucosides may decompose to as yet untraced derivatives while still present in tissue fluids and in urine in the bladder.

This decomposition may contribute to the discrepancy between the phenobarbitone dose and the amounts of drug and metabolites traceable in urine. The N-glucosidation pathway is inactive in the first 2 weeks of postnatal life (BHARGAVA and GARRETTSON 1985).

3. At least in mice, *N*-glucuronides of phenobarbitone form (NEIGHBORS and SOINE 1995) and, in rats and mice, a 1-hydroxyethyl metabolite (HARVEY et al. 1972).

β) Methylphenobarbitone

Less than 3% of a methylphenobarbitone dose is excreted in urine unmetabolized (EADIE et al. 1978). (R,S)-Methylphenobarbitone undergoes relatively stereoselective biotransformation (LIM and HOOPER 1989). The (R)-enantiomer is metabolized by CYP2C19, the same P_{450} isoenzyme which catalyses (S)-mephenytoin oxidation (KUPFER and BRANCH 1985; HALL et al. 1987; WRIGHT et al. 1995). 4-Hydroxymethylphenobarbitone (*p*-hydroxymethylphenobarbitone) forms and is excreted in urine mainly as its glucuronide conjugate. This, predominantly as the (R)-enantiomer, accounts for some 35% of an oral dose of (R,S)-methylphenobarbitone (HOOPER et al. 1981b). Some 4-hydroxymethylphenobarbitone is probably further metabolized to dihydrodiol (HARVEY et al. 1972) and *O*-methyl catechol derivatives (TRESTON et al. 1987). As well, a small amount of (R)-methylphenobarbitone is oxidatively dealkylated to phenobarbitone. In contrast, (S)-methylphenobarbitone does not undergo aromatic hydroxylation, but is oxidatively dealkylated to phenobarbitone, some of which is further metabolized along the biotransformation pathways for that substance, described above. Between 8% and 25% of a dose of (R,S)-methylphenobarbitone ultimately appears in urine as phenobarbitone (EADIE et al. 1978). It is not known whether *N*-glucosides of either methylphenobarbitone enantiomer are formed.

γ) Primidone

From 15% to 66% of a primidone dose appears in urine unmetabolized (KAUFMANN et al. 1977). In those not previously exposed to antiepileptic drugs, 64% of a primidone dose appeared in urine unmetabolized; in those with prior antiepileptic drug exposure only 39.6% was excreted intact (ZAVADIL and GALLAGHER 1976). Primidone is oxidized at the 2-position on its heterocyclic ring, forming phenobarbitone, whose possible patterns of further metabolism are described above. Between 1% and 8% of a primidone dose is excreted in urine as phenobarbitone (KAUFMANN et al. 1977). The primidone molecule also undergoes heterocyclic ring opening, forming phenylethylmalonamide which, excreted as such in urine, accounts for 16%–65% of a primidone dose (KAUFMANN et al. 1977). Unlike phenobarbitone, primidone undergoes very little aromatic hydroxylation (HOOPER et al. 1983). Neonates and infants cannot oxidize primidone to phenobarbitone until they have been exposed to the drug for 3 or 4 months (POWELL et al. 1984).

b) Elimination Parameters

α) Phenobarbitone

The half-life of phenobarbitone varies with age. BATTINO et al. (1995) and DODSON and RUST (1995) have tabulated the available data relating the drug's elimination to the ages of the individuals studied. In infants the half-life averaged 114.2 ± 40.3 h in the first 10 postnatal days, 73.19 ± 24.17 h on days 11–30, and 41.23 ± 13.95 h from days 31 to 70 (ALONSO-GONZALEZ et al. 1993). In childhood, the half-life is shorter than in adult life, e.g. 37 h compared to 73 h (GARRETTSON and DAYTON 1970). Other half-life values in adults include 4 days (BUCHTHAL and LENNOX-BUCHTHAL 1972), 5 days (VAN DER KLEIJN et al. 1975), 5.8 days (NELSON et al. 1982) and 75–126 h (WILENSKY et al. 1982). The half-life may decrease with repeated administration of phenobarbitone, consistent with some autoinduction of metabolism, though WILENSKY et al. (1982) found no evidence of this.

Phenobarbitone has a relatively low clearance (0.0053 ± 0.0038 l/kg/h – GUELEN et al. 1975). The clearance decreases from 0.0012 l/kg/h in young children to 0.0040 l/kg/h by the age of 12–14 years, but after that does not alter much with age. Other published figures for the clearance in adults are 0.003 l/kg/h (NELSON et al. 1982) and 0.0038 ± 0.00077 l/kg/h (WILENSKY et al. 1982). Most investigators have found that the apparent clearance of the drug increases during pregnancy (LANDER et al. 1977; BARDY et al. 1982; HOSOKOWA et al. 1984; KAN et al. 1984; LANDER and EADIE 1991), but there have been findings to the contrary (LEVY and YERBY 1985).

β) Methylphenobarbitone

In adults, the half-life of (S)-methylphenobarbitone averaged 69.8 ± SD 14.8 h and that of (R)-methylphenobarbitone 7.5 ± SD 1.7 h (LIM and HOOPER 1989). The apparent clearances were, respectively, 0.017 ± SD 0.001 l/kg/h and 0.47 ± SD 0.18 l/kg/h. Details of the effects of age and gender on the disposition of the individual enantiomers of methylphenobarbitone are available (HOOPER and QING 1990). The half-life of (R,S)-methylphenobarbitone in adults was 49.0 ± 18.8 h (EADIE et al. 1978). Its clearance is increased in pregnancy (LANDER et al. 1977).

γ) Primidone

Tabulated data for the elimination parameters of primidone in various animal species are available (FREY 1985). In humans primidone has a half-life of 6–12 h (BOOKER et al. 1970; GALLAGHER et al. 1972; KAUFMANN et al. 1977). In the neonate, the half-life is 23 ± 10 h (NAU et al. 1980). Phenylethylmalonamide, the metabolite of primidone, has a half-life of 15.7 ± 3.4 h (PISANI and RICHENS 1983). The clearance of primidone is 0.0355 l/kg/h after the first dose of the drug (CLOYD et al. 1981), and may increase during long-term intake of the drug. The clearance of phenylethylmalonamide averaged 0.0313 ± 0.0066 l/kg/h (PISANI and RICHENS 1983).

4. Applied Pharmacokinetics

a) Phenobarbitone

Because of phenobarbitone's relatively long half-life, steady-state conditions may not apply for 3 weeks after a dosage change in adults, and after 1.5 weeks in children (SVENSMARK and BUCHTHAL 1963).

The generally accepted therapeutic range of plasma phenobarbitone concentrations for treating epilepsy is 15–25 (LOISEAU et al. 1977) or 15–40 mg/l (FELDMAN et al. 1975). Some have set the lower limit of the range at 10 mg/l (BUCHTHAL and LENNOX-BUCHTHAL 1972; AIRD and WOODBURY 1974; FEELEY et al. 1980). Levels above 15 mg/l appear necessary to prevent benign febrile convulsions of infancy (FAERO et al. 1972; HOJO et al. 1979; HERRANZ et al. 1984). During withdrawal of phenobarbitone (or primidone) over a 5-week period, seizures tended to recur when plasma phenobarbitone concentrations had declined to between 20 and 15 mg/l (THEODORE et al. 1987). SCHMIDT et al. (1986) noted that plasma phenobarbitone concentrations of 18 mg/l would control bilateral tonic-clonic seizures, whereas concentrations of 37 mg/l were needed for full control of simple or complex partial seizures, whether or not they became secondarily generalized. Patients often become drowsy with plasma phenobarbitone concentrations in the range 30–50 mg/l (LIVINGSTONE et al. 1975), but some tolerate higher concentrations without apparent ill effect.

EADIE et al. (1977a) showed that, in the individual, steady-state plasma phenobarbitone concentrations tended to increase more than proportionately to dosage increase.

Relative to body weight, children need higher phenobarbitone doses than adults to achieve the same steady-state plasma drug concentrations. Excluding neonates, EADIE et al. (1976, 1977a) found that phenobarbitone doses of 3.1, 2.3, 1.75 and 0.9 mg/kg/day yielded an average plasma phenobarbitone concentration of 15 mg/l in persons up to 4 years, from 4 to 14 years, from 15 to 40 years, and over 40 years of age, respectively. Females required lower phenobarbitone doses than males in the under 4 years age group only.

Phenobarbitone clearance tends to rise during pregnancy, and increasing drug doses are needed to maintain plasma phenobarbitone concentrations at their pre-pregnancy value (LANDER and EADIE 1991).

b) Methylphenobarbitone

Steady-state conditions should occur sooner for (S)-methylphenobarbitone than for its (R)-counterpart when (R,S)-methylphenobarbitone is prescribed. However, the simultaneous plasma phenobarbitone concentrations are more relevant clinically.

At steady state, plasma (R,S)-methylphenobarbitone concentrations are 1/7th to 1/10th of the simultaneous phenobarbitone concentrations (EADIE et al. 1978). No therapeutic range of plasma methylphenobarbitone concentrations has been suggested, plasma phenobarbitone concentrations providing a satisfactory alternative. In the individual, steady-state plasma phenobarbitone concentrations increase in direct proportion to methylphenobarbitone dose (EADIE et al. 1977a). To achieve an average plasma phenobarbitone concentration of 15 mg/l, a methylphenobarbitone dose of around 5 mg/kg/day is required in persons under 14 years of age, a dose of 4 mg/kg/day in persons 15–40 years, and a dose of around 2 mg/kg/day in older persons. Methylphenobarbitone doses need to be increased to maintain previous steady-state plasma phenobarbitone concentrations during pregnancy (LANDER et al. 1977).

c) Primidone

The phenobarbitone derived from primidone has a much longer half-life than the parent drug, and under steady-state conditions achieves plasma concentrations 2 or 3 times those of primidone. The phenobarbitone levels show much less interdosage fluctuation than steady-state primidone levels (BOOKER et al. 1970; GALLAGHER et al. 1972). Therefore plasma phenobarbitone concentrations are often preferred to plasma primidone ones in managing human epilepsy, though therapeutic ranges of primidone concentrations are quoted, e.g. 8–12 mg/l (VAN DER KLEIJN et al. 1975). Because of primidone's relatively short half-life, its steady-state plasma concentrations can vary from measurement to measurement simply because of inconsistent timing of blood collections in relation to drug intake.

In treated populations, plasma phenobarbitone concentrations tend to increase in proportion to increasing primidone doses (EADIE et al. 1977a). Steady-state plasma phenobarbitone to primidone concentration ratios are lower in children than adults, and plasma concentrations of both substances, relative to primidone dose, increase with age (BATTINO et al. 1983). Primidone apparent clearance may increase in pregnancy (NAU et al. 1982; RATING et al. 1982; OTANI et al. 1984), necessitating higher primidone dosages to maintain previous plasma phenobarbitone concentrations (LANDER et al. 1977). Plasma primidone to phenobarbitone concentration ratios tend to increase in pregnancy (BATTINO et al. 1984).

IV. Interactions

Derived phenobarbitone mediates much of the effect of methylphenobarbitone and primidone, so that interactions involving phenobarbitone are likely when its congeners are prescribed.

1. Pharmacodynamic Interactions

Combining phenobarbitone with other sedative drugs, including other antiepileptic drugs and alcohol, may cause increased sedation. Prescribing phenobarbitone with anticonvulsants which act through mechanisms other than blocking postsynaptic Cl^- channels might be expected to yield additional antiepileptic effects. Combining carbamazepine (a voltage-dependent Na^+

channel blocker) with phenobarbitone has yielded improved seizure control (CEREGHINO et al. 1973).

2. Pharmacokinetic Interactions

Interactions involving phenobarbitone are referenced below only when not listed in EADIE and TYRER (1989) or PATSALOS and DUNCAN (1993).

a) Phenobarbitone Affecting Other Substances

Phenobarbitone is a classical inducer of various cytochrome P450 isoenzymes (CONNEY 1967), e.g. CYP3A4 (BOLT 1994). This induction increases the body's capacity to eliminate certain endogenous substances and numerous drugs. It increases the clearances of bile salts, biotin (KRAUSE et al. 1985), cholesterol, lipids, bilirubin, cortisol, folate, renin, unconjugated oestriol and vitamin E. It also increases the clearances (or reduces the plasma concentrations) of various co-administered drugs, e.g. aminopyrine, amitriptyline (PERUCCA et al. 1984), antipyrine (phenazone), bishydroxycoumarin, carbamazepine, chloramphenicol, chlorpromazine, cimetidine, clobazam, clonazepam (KHOO et al. 1980), cyclosporin, cyproheptadine, cyclophosphamide (JAO et al. 1972), diazepam, dicophane, dicoumarol, digitoxin, dipyrone, doxycycline, ethinylestradiol, felodipine, flunarazine, glyceryl trinitrate (BOGAERT et al. 1971), griseofulvin, haloperidol, isoniazid (LEVI et al. 1968), itraconazole (BONAY et al. 1993), lignocaine, mesoridazine, methadone, methsuximide, metoprolol (HAGLAND et al. 1979), nimodipine, nortriptyline, oral contraceptives, paracetamol (acetaminophen), pethidine (meperidine), phenylbutazole, phenytoin (however, its plasma levels are sometimes raised), prednisolone (BROOKS et al. 1976), propranolol (ROWLAND 1970), quinidine (DATA et al. 1976), theophylline, thioridazine, valproate and warfarin. Whether phenobarbitone administration lowers plasma folate levels is uncertain. Impaired absorption from the alimentary tract possibly contributes to the interactions involving cyclosporin, cimetidine and griseofulvin (PATSALOS and DUNCAN 1993).

b) Other Substances Affecting Phenobarbitone

Plasma phenobarbitone concentrations may be raised by intake of acetazolamide, chloramphenicol, dicoumarol (HANSEN et al. 1966), felbamate (GIDAL and ZUPANC 1994; REIDENBERG et al. 1995), frusemide, methylphenidate, methsuximide, phenylacetylurea, phenytoin (LAMBIE and JOHNSON 1981), though this interaction is not consistent (EADIE and TYRER 1989), phenothiazines (HAIDUKEWYCH and RODIN 1985), propoxyphene, quinine (AMABEOKU et al. 1993), stiripentol (FAREWELL et al. 1990), and valproate (BRUNI et al. 1980; PATEL et al. 1980), the latter due to impaired formation of phenobarbitone-*N*-glucoside (BERNUS et al. 1994b). Co-administration of folate, pyridoxine, chloramphenicol, dicoumarol and phenylbutazole lowers plasma phenobarbitone concentrations.

Alkalinizing the urine, e.g. by giving ammonium chloride, increases phenobarbitone excretion, thus lowering its plasma concentrations (PATSALOS and DUNCAN 1993). Activated charcoal ingestion impairs phenobarbitone absorption from the alimentary tract (NEUVONEN et al. 1980; MODI et al. 1994).

α) Methylphenobarbitone

Reports of interactions affecting plasma methylphenobarbitone concentrations have not been found. The drug competitively inhibits the metabolism of mephenytoin (methoin), as explained above.

β) Primidone

FINCHAM and SCHOTTELIUS (1995) tabulated many reported primidone interactions. As well as interactions involving phenobarbitone formed from it, primidone enhances the clearance of dexamethasone (YOUNG and HUGHES 1991) and raises plasma concentrations of urate (FICHSEL et al. 1993) and total and HDL cholesterol (REDDY 1985). Phenytoin (SATO et al. 1992) and carbamazepine (BATTINO et al. 1983; PIPPENGER 1987) increase the conversion of primidone to phenobarbitone. Acetazolamide sometimes decreases primidone absorption (SYVERSEN et al. 1977). Clonazepam raises plasma primidone concentrations (WINDORFER and SAUER 1977) and isoniazid inhibits primidone oxidation to phenobarbitone (SUTTON and KUPFERBERG 1975).

V. Adverse Effects

Phenobarbitone appears within a few hours of initial intake of methylphenobarbitone or primidone. Therefore whether or not the latter substances have adverse effects in their own rights, they exhibit similar unwanted effects to phenobarbitone.

1. Idiosyncratic Effects

Phenobarbitone may cause various uncommon, presumably idiosyncratic, unwanted effects involving (1) the skin, with rashes ranging from fine punctate erythema through large erythematous macules, erythroderma (SAKAI et al. 1993) and localized subepidermal bullae (HAROUN et al. 1987) to major dermatoses such as erythema multiforme (SALOMON and SAURAT 1990), exfoliative dermatitis (MCGEACHY and BLOOMER 1953) and epidermal necrolysis (BOURGALT et al. 1991); (2) the connective tissues, resulting in fibromyalgia (GOLDMAN and KRINGS 1995), the shoulder-hand syndrome (TAYLOR and POSNER 1989) and certain other disorders (MATTSON et al. 1989) including lupus erythematosus; (3) nervous system, resulting in bucco-lingual dyskinesia (SECHI et al. 1988), Tourette's syndrome (SANDUK 1986), tics (BURD et al. 1987) and reflex sympathetic dystrophy (FASCALA et al. 1994); (4) bone marrow, causing agranulocytosis and aplastic anaemia; (5) the liver, causing hepatitis and jaundice (JEAVONS 1983; GRAM and BENTSEN 1985; ROBERTS et al.

1990; SAWAISHI et al. 1992); and (6) kidneys, producing nephritis (SAWAISHI et al. 1992). In those predisposed, phenobarbitone may precipitate attacks of porphyria.

2. Dose-Determined Effects

Phenobarbitone and its congeners cause sedation, though some tolerance to the sedation appears to develop, especially when the drug's dose is increased gradually. It is not certain that true pharmacological tolerance occurs. Before sedation becomes overt, phenobarbitone may impair concentration and slow intellectual processes. At higher dosages drowsiness becomes obvious, dysequilibrium, ataxia of gait and nystagmus develop, and consciousness is increasingly impaired. Paradoxically, low plasma phenobarbitone concentrations in children may be associated with hyperactivity and disordered behaviour, and higher concentrations with depression (HERRANZ et al. 1988). This does not recur when the same individuals are re-exposed to the drug in adult life.

The various sedative type adverse effects of phenobarbitone may develop insidiously, and go unnoticed. At therapeutic dosage, there may be impaired learning performance in children, and reversible deterioration in the results of intelligence testing (VINING et al. 1987; CALANDRE et al. 1990; FARWELL et al. 1990; DE SILVA et al. 1996). Prenatal exposure to phenobarbitone has been associated with lowered verbal IQ scores in adult males (REINISCH et al. 1995). In studies of comparative drug efficacy, these various sedative effects make phenobarbitone and primidone more likely to be ceased than other major anticonvulsants (SMITH et al. 1987; HELLER et al. 1995). Rarely, the initial dose of primidone may cause severe and prolonged drowsiness.

A cross-over study failed to support anecdotal evidence that methylphenobarbitone is less sedating than phenobarbitone in equally effective anticonvulsant doses (YOUNG et al. 1986). MATTSON et al. (1985) considered primidone to be more likely than phenobarbitone to cause intolerable adverse effects in potentially equi-effective anticonvulsant doses. Primidone is more likely than other anticonvulsants to cause impotence, though phenobarbitone may cause it (CRAMER and MATTSON 1995).

Phenobarbitone may cause subclinical peripheral neuropathy, detectable electrophysiologically (BALDINI et al. 1991), folate depletion and a subacute combined degeneration-like syndrome (RAVAKHAH and WEST 1995) and macrocytic anaemia (CHANARIN et al. 1958; DAVIS and WOODLIFF 1971).

Long continued intake of phenobarbitone (and presumably its congeners) can cause radiological and clinical osteomalacia. Bone mineral density may be measurably decreased in children after 3 years' intake of the drug (CHUNG and AHN 1994). Heel-pad thickening (SCHMIDT 1983), Dupuytren's contracture (CRITCHLEY et al. 1976), and a peculiar thickening of facial features may develop insidiously.

Plasma primidone concentrations over 80 mg/l may be associated with crystalluria (LEHMANN 1987).

3. Effects on the Foetus and Neonate

Over 20 years ago, an association was reported between maternal phenobarbitone intake during pregnancy and various malformations in the offspring (MEADOW 1970; SPEIDEL and MEADOW 1972). Unfortunately, data on the malformation rate from a control population of pregnant women with untreated epilepsy of equal severity are not yet available. SHAPIRO et al. (1976) reported no increase in the foetal malformation rate in non-epileptic Finnish women who took phenobarbitone as a sedative during pregnancy; however, the incidence of foetal malformations was increased when pregnant American women used the drug mainly as an anticonvulsant. The risk of malformation in the offspring appears greater if phenobarbitone is taken together with phenytoin during pregnancy (LINDHOUT et al. 1982; MAJEWSKI et al. 1980), but the drug combinations may have been used because of more severe maternal epilepsy. Certain Japanese data suggest that phenobarbitone is the least teratogenic of the commonly used anticonvulsants (KANEKO and KONDO 1995). Curiously, KANEKO et al. (1992) found that the risk of teratogenesis was related to the dose of methylphenobarbitone, but not to the dose of other anticonvulsants. In addition to the malformations, exposure to phenobarbitone during pregnancy may be associated with smaller head circumferences in the offspring, and decreased cognitive development (VAN DER POL et al. 1991).

Maternal phenobarbitone intake during pregnancy can also be associated with coagulation factor deficiency in the newborn, which may be manifested as subependymal, intraventricular or intracerebral haemorrhages (KUBAN et al. 1986). Intra-partum administration of vitamin K can prevent these phenomena (MOUNTAIN et al. 1970). Infants born to mothers who were treated with phenobarbitone during pregnancy may be hypotonic and irritable during their first 3 postnatal days, possibly as the result of drug withdrawal (ERITH 1975). If low birth weight infants receive phenobarbitone there is an increased risk that they will develop pneumothorax or interstitial pulmonary oedema (KUBAN et al. 1987).

C. Succinimides

Since 1951, three succinimide anticonvulsants have become available. Of these phensuximide and methsuximide are now virtually superseded drugs. Ethosuximide provides satisfactory treatment for absence (petit mal) seizures in humans, and remains in clinical use. There has been relatively little advance in knowledge of its pharmacology in recent years.

I. Chemistry and Use

1. Chemistry

Ethosuximide (2-ethyl-2-methylsuccinimide), a weak acid (pK_a 9.3), is a water-soluble white crystalline material (MW 141.2). Phensuximide

(*N*-methyl-2-phenylsuccinimide; MW 189.21) and methsuximide (*N*,2-dimethyl-2-phenylsuccinimide; MW 203.23) are poorly water-soluble crystalline materials.

All three succinimides contain a chiral C atom at the 2-position of the succinimide ring.

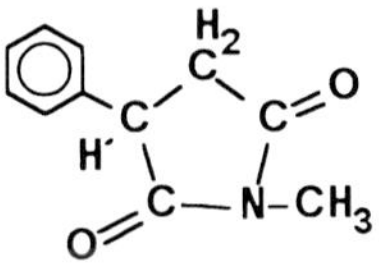

Phensuximide

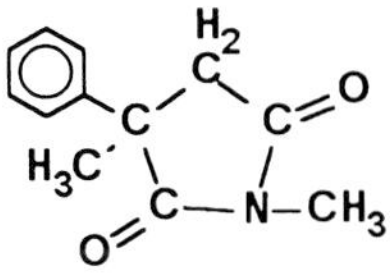

Methsuximide

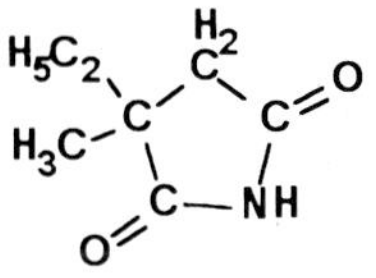

Ethosuximide

2. Use

Ethosuximide is as effective as valproate for pure absence seizures (Chadwick 1988) but has no other use in human medicine. It is efficacious in 85% of patients who have absence seizures only (Covanis et al. 1992), but is less successful if bilateral tonic-clonic seizures also occur, when a drug effective against this type of seizure must be co-prescribed, or valproate substituted. Ethosuximide appeared potentially useful in an animal model of Parkinsonian tremor, but failed in the human disease (Gomez-Mancilla et al. 1992; Pourcher et al. 1992). Phensuximide is less effective than ethosuximide in suppressing absence seizures, but methsuximide has been reported useful for both absence seizures and, added to other anticonvulsants, for refractory partial seizures (Brown et al. 1983; Tennison et al. 1991). Pharmacokinetic interactions may have contributed to the latter outcome.

II. Pharmacodynamics

1. Animal Models of Epilepsy

Earlier studies on the animal pharmacology of ethosuximide were reviewed by Teschendorf and Kretzschmar (1985). The drug protects against generalized convulsive seizures induced by systemically administered convulsants, e.g. pentylenetetrazole (Chen et al. 1963; Becker et al. 1995) and penicillin (Guberman et al. 1975) but not against photomyoclonic seizures in the baboon *Papio papio* (Meldrum et al. 1975). It inhibits absence-like seizures in the double-mutant spontaneously epileptic rat (Sasa et al. 1988), in the homozygous tremor rat (Hayana et al. 1995), the Wistar rats of Micheletti et al. (1985) and the tottering mutant mouse (Heller et al. 1983). It offers relatively little protection against maximum electroshock seizures in mice (Anonymous 1976) but reduces their severity and does not raise the threshold for their electrical or chemical provocation (Piredda et al. 1985).

2. Electrophysiological Studies

The thalamo-cortical circuits involved in the genesis of generalized spike-wave activity have now been defined (SNEAD 1995). Ethosuximide inhibits burst firing in populations of reciprocally interconnected relay and thalamic reticular nuclear neurons. It thus desynchronizes the circuits which generate the 3 Hz spike-wave phenomenon (HUGUENARD and PRINCE 1994). In the pentylenetetrazole rat model, ethosuximide is ineffective after intercollicular brain stem transection, so that the drug's action is at least influenced by more caudal levels of the brain stem (MARES et al. 1994). Other evidence (PELLEGRINI et al. 1989) is consistent with the drug's having an anti-inhibitory action in the cortex and thalamus and activating the mid-brain reticular formation or, alternatively, depressing reticular inhibitory pathways (FROMM 1985). The drug's overall effect alters the activity of the spontaneous thalamic synchronizing mechanisms, thus ablating spike-wave activity.

3. Biochemical Effects

A number of biochemical effects of ethosuximide were described prior to 1989, though they did not explain the drug's anti-absence effects adequately (EADIE and TYRER 1989). Since 1989 it has been increasingly accepted that ethosuximide, at the concentrations at which it has an anti-absence effect in humans, reduces low threshold Ca^{2+} currents in thalamic neurons (COULTER et al. 1989a,b). These neurons include the generators of normal thalamo-cortical rhythms. At relevant concentrations the drug appears to function as an antagonist at "T" but not at "L" type Ca^{2+} channels (MACDONALD 1989; MACDONALD and KELLY 1993; 1994) in thalamic ventro-basal complex (COULTER et al. 1989a) and dorsal root ganglia neurons (KOSTYUK et al. 1992). It does not block Ca^{2+} currents in isolated neocortical neurons (SAYER et al. 1993). This action on thalamic "T" type Ca^{2+} channels appears to explain the anti-absence action of the drug.

Little information is available concerning the mechanisms of action of the other succinimides.

III. Pharmacokinetics

Pharmacokinetic data for ethosuximide in various animal species are summarized by BAILER et al. (1995).

1. Absorption

Ethosuximide has an oral T_{max} of between 1 and 4 h (WECHSELBERG and HUBEL 1967; GLAZKO 1975; EADIE et al. 1977b). No data for its absolute bioavailability in humans are available. Peak plasma phensuximide levels occur 0.5–1.5 h after oral intake (KINKEL 1971).

2. Distribution

The apparent volume of distribution of ethosuximide in adults is approximately 50 l (BUCHANAN et al. 1973), or from 0.67 to 0.72 l/kg (EADIE et al. 1977; BAUER et al. 1982). In humans, ethosuximide is not bound to plasma proteins (LÖSCHER 1979; LEVY and SCHMIDT 1985). Cerebrospinal fluid and serum levels of the drug are similar (WECHSELBERG and HUBEL 1967; PIREDDA and MONACO 1981), as are salivary and whole plasma levels (HORNING et al. 1977; MC AULIFFE et al. 1977). CORADELLO (1973) found no ethosuximide in the milk of mothers taking the drug but KANEKO et al. (1984) reported a milk/plasma ratio of 0.7832 ± 0.1038:1.0, and KUHNZ et al. (1984) a ratio of 0.86 ± 0.08:1.0. KOUP et al. (1978) stated that milk and plasma ethosuximide concentrations were equal. In rats, brain and plasma ethosuximide concentrations were reasonably similar (DILL et al. 1965; PATEL et al. 1977).

3. Elimination

The elimination of the succinimide anticonvulsants occurs mainly through metabolism.

a) Metabolism

Some 17%–38% (GLAZKO 1975) or 20% (GOULET et al. 1976) of an ethosuximide dose is excreted in urine unmetabolized. MILLERSHIP et al. (1993) reviewed earlier studies of the metabolism of ethosuximide in animals and humans. The known biotransformation pathways for ethosuximide in humans are shown in Fig. 2. Ethosuximide contains a chiral C atom at the 2-position of the succinimide ring. The main metabolites in urine are the enantiomers of 2-(1-hydroxyethyl)-2-methylsuccinimide, present chiefly as glucuronide conjugates. Oxidation of the ethyl group adds a further centre of chirality, at the 1-position on the 2-ethyl side chain. In a subsequent study in rats, MILLERSHIP et al. (1995) found in urine (1) both enantiomers of ethosuximide, (2) all four stereoisomers of 2-(1-hydroxyethyl)-2-methylsuccinimide and (3) one stereoisomer of 2-ethyl-3-hydroxy-2-methylsuccinimide (derived from (R)-ethosuximide). At least in rats, (R)-ethosuximide yields the two diasteromers of 2-(1-hydroxyethyl)-2-methylsuccinimide in equal proportions, but the corresponding oxidation products of (S)-ethosuximide appear in unequal proportions. The various 2-(1-hydroxy ethyl) oxidation products, the 3-hydroxy derivatives, 2-hydroxyethyl-2-methylsuccinimide and 2-carboxymethyl-2-methylsuccinimide have been found in human urine, but two previously identified metabolites probably are not genuine (2-ethyl-2-hydroxy methylsuccinimide and 2-acetyl-2-methylsuccinimide). In rats, the oxidations of ethosuximide are catalysed by CYP 3 A and CYP 2 E (BACHMANN et al. 1992).

Phensuximide is N-desmethylated in humans, while methsuximide undergoes oxidative N–desmethylation in both animals and man (MUNI et al. 1973), a reaction catalysed by CYP 2C19 (BACHMANN et al. 1992).

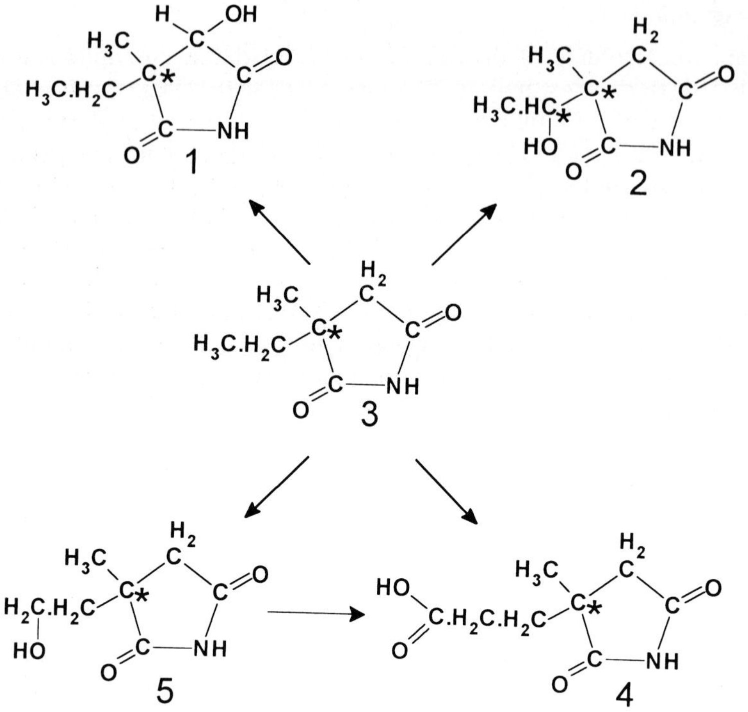

Fig. 2. Major metabolic pathways for ethosuximide. *1,* 2-ethyl-3-hydroxy-2-methylsuccinimide; *2,* 2-(1-hydroxyethyl)-2-methylsuccinimide; *3,* ethosuximide (2-ethyl-2-methylsuccinimide); *4,* 2-carboxymethyl-2-methylsuccinimide; *5,* 2-hydroxymethyl-2-methylsuccinimide

b) Elimination Parameters

Mean half-life values for ethosuximide in adults range from 30 or 36h (BUCHANAN et al. 1969) to 56h (GLAZKO 1975). BROWNE et al. (1975) found the half-life was shorter in patients taking lower drug doses and did not change during 8 weeks of ethosuximide intake. The half-life is shorter in children (mean values 33.4h for capsules and 29.7h for a solution – BUCHANAN et al. 1969). KOUP et al. (1978) found a mean ethosuximide half-life of 41.3h in neonates.

Plasma ethosuximide clearance values were: 0.016 and 0.013 l/kg/h in two children (BUCHANAN et al. 1969), and in adults 0.010 ± 0.004 l/kg/h (EADIE et al. 1977), 0.0131 ± .0043 l/kg/h (BAUER et al. 1982) and 0.0091 ± 0.0023 l/kg/h (BACHMANN et al. 1986).

In man, phensuximide forms an *N*-desmethyl metabolite whose half-life is similar to that of the parent drug (average 7.8h; range 4.5–12.0h – PORTER et al. 1977), raising the possibility that the metabolite has a shorter half-life, and its formation half-life has been interpreted as its elimination one. Methsuximide has a half-life of 1.0–2.6h (PORTER et al. 1979; STRONG et al. 1974), but its *N*-desmethyl metabolite is more slowly eliminated (half-life 34–80h).

4. Applied Pharmacokinetics

Steady-state conditions take more than 7 or 10–12 days to develop after commencement of ethosuximide therapy (BUCHANAN and SMITH 1972). Similar mean daily ethosuximide doses (20.7, 20.6 and 21.7mg/kg) yield, respectively, mean steady-state plasma concentrations of 40 ± 14.9, 63.2 and 63.5mg/l (HAERER et al. 1970; SOLOW and GREEN 1971; PENRY et al. 1972). Steady-state plasma ethosuximide concentrations vary widely in individual patients relative to the ethosuximide dose (BATTINO et al. 1982).

BROWNE et al. (1975) and BATTINO et al. (1982) noted that plasma ethosuximide concentrations increased more rapidly relative to dose in adults than in children. Also relative to dose, steady-state plasma ethosuximide levels in females increase more rapidly than in males (EADIE and TYRER 1989).

In individual patients given increasing doses of ethosuximide, EADIE (1976), SMITH et al. (1979) and BAUER et al. (1982) all noted that steady-state plasma concentrations of the drug increase more than proportionately relative to an increased dose of ethosuximide. This non-linearity is unexplained.

PENRY et al. (1972) stated that ethosuximide plasma levels of 40–60mg/l were associated with complete control of absence seizures. SHERWIN and ROBB (1972) quoted a therapeutic range of 40–120mg/l, BROWNE et al. (1975) one of 40–100mg/l, WINEK (1976) one of 25–75mg/l, and CALLAGHAN et al. (1982) one of 15–88mg/l. STEAD et al. (1983) found that 50% of the specimens referred to their laboratory from patients with controlled absence seizures had plasma ethosuximide levels below 44mg/l, with 90% having levels below 71mg/l.

Phensuximide is less effective than ethosuximide against human absence seizures. At a dose of 3000mg/day, its steady-state plasma level averages 5.7mg/l, and levels of its *N*-desmethyl metabolite 1.7mg/l.

Steady-state plasma levels of *N*-desmethyl methsuximide are 73–2800 times those of methsuximide itself (STRONG et al. 1974). Suggested provisional therapeutic ranges for the metabolite are 10–40mg/l (STRONG et al. 1974) or 10–30mg/l (BROWN et al. 1983).

IV. Interactions

1. Pharmacodynamic Interactions

Ethosuximide and valproate share a common molecular mechanism of action against absence seizures, viz. blocking low threshold thalamic "T" type Ca^{2+} channels, and the two agents used together can control absence seizures refractory to either agent used alone (PERUCCA 1995).

Adding ethosuximide to phenobarbitone therapy may exacerbate absence seizures (TODOROV et al. 1978).

2. Pharmacokinetic Interactions

Ethosuximide does not alter the plasma protein binding of phenytoin (PATSALOS and LASCELLES 1977), carbamazepine (HOOPER et al. 1975) or phenobarbitone (PATSALOS and LASCELLES 1982).

Ethosuximide does not induce the liver mono-oxygenase enzyme system in humans. FRANTZEN et al. (1967), but not RICHENS and HOUGHTON (1975), found that the drug caused raised plasma phenytoin levels in humans. Ethosuximide did not alter the conversion of primidone to phenobarbitone (SCHMIDT 1975). Serum pyridoxal phosphate levels fell in persons taking ethosuximide long-term (REINKEN 1973).

Carbamazepine (PIPPENGER 1987; DUNCAN et al. 1991), phenobarbitone (BACHMANN and JAUREGUI 1993), primidone (BATTINO et al. 1982) and rifampicin (BACHMANN and JAUREGUI 1993) increase the clearance of ethosuximide while methylphenobarbitone (SMITH et al. 1979) and isoniazid (VAN WIERINGEN and VRITLAND 1983) reduce it. Valproate intake may increase (BATTINO et al. 1982; MATTSON and CRAMER 1980) or not alter ethosuximide plasma levels (BAUER et al. 1982).

Methsuximide interacts with phenytoin, phenobarbitone and primidone, raising plasma phenytoin and phenobarbitone concentrations (RAMBECK 1979). It lowers plasma carbamazepine levels (BROWNE et al. 1983). Felbamate alters the pharmacokinetics of methsuximide (WAGNER 1994).

V. Adverse Effects

Ethosuximide, particularly large individual doses (DOOLEY et al. 1990), may irritate the stomach, causing gastric discomfort, anorexia, nausea and vomiting. Other dose-related unwanted effects include tiredness, headache and feelings of dysequilibrium. Ethosuximide use may precipitate episodes of acute intermittent porphyria (REYNOLDS and MISKA 1981). Occasionally it appears to precipitate bilateral tonic-clonic seizures when used alone for absence seizures, though this may only be coincidence (DREIFUSS 1995).

The idiosyncratic unwanted effects of ethosuximide mainly involve the skin (PELEKANOS et al. 1991). It may cause systemic lupus erythematosus and related syndromes (ANSELL 1993; DRORY and KORCZYN 1993) and rarely leucopenia, pancytopenia and aplastic anaemia (KIORBOE et al. 1964; COHN 1968; SEIP 1983; MASSEY et al. 1994). There is little evidence of teratogenicity in humans.

BROWNE (1995) has tabulated the reported adverse effects of methsuximide and their incidences in humans. Phensuximide may cause haemorrhagic cystitis and mild nephrotoxicity (RANKIN et al. 1992).

D. Sulthiame

I. Chemistry and Use

Sulthiame (tetrahydro-2-(*p*-sulphamoylphenyl)-1,2–thiazine 1,1-dioxide), a sulphonamide derivative, is a non-competitive inhibitor of carbonic anhydrase

(MATSUMOTO et al. 1989) lacking antibacterial activity. It is an acidic white crystalline substance (molecular weight 290.37). Sulthiame came into use as an anticonvulsant, principally for partial epilepsies, over 30 years ago (SUTHERLAND and BOWMAN 1963) but began to fall from favour after GREEN et al. (1974) showed that it was less satisfactory than phenytoin in a head to head comparison. In most centres the drug is now largely ignored, but it has recently been suggested to be the agent of choice for all types of benign partial epilepsy in childhood (GROSS-SELBECK 1995). It may also have some efficacy in otherwise refractory juvenile myoclonic epilepsy (LERMAN and NUSSBAUM 1975). FEELY et al. (1982) showed that sulthiame monotherapy fully controlled generalized and partial seizures in 8 of 14 newly diagnosed epileptics.

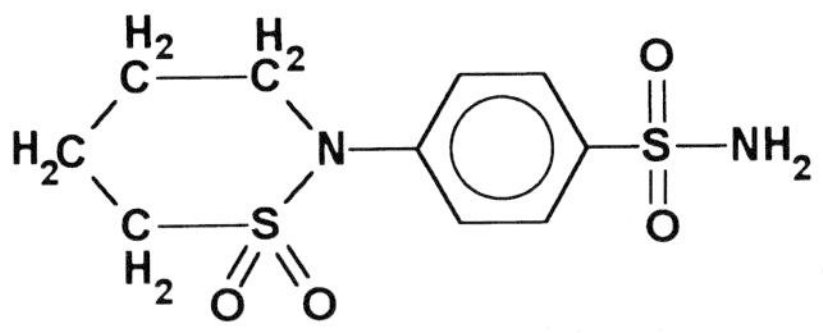

II. Pharmacodynamics

Sulthiame protects rats and mice against pentylenetetrazole-induced seizures and maximum electroshock seizures, but not against strychnine-provoked seizures (WIRTH et al. 1960). Despite its anticonvulsant efficacy, sulthiame is only about 1/16th as potent as acetazolamide as a carbonic anhydrase inhibitor (WIRTH et al. 1961). Its mechanism of anticonvulsant action is inadequately understood. GEETS and PINON (1971) correlated successful treatment with sulthiame correlated with a lowering of plasma pH while GRAY and RAUH (1967) showed that the presence of noradrenaline was required for carbonic anhydrase inhibitors to have anticonvulsant effects.

III. Pharmacokinetics

Relatively little pharmacokinetic information is available for sulthiame in humans and animals. Over 90% of the dose is absorbed in humans (DIAMOND and LEVY 1963). In rats, sulthiame concentrations were reasonably similar in brain and serum, but higher in tissues and red blood cells than in serum (DUHM et al. 1963). Sulthiame displaced phenytoin from serum albumin, raising the possibility that it may bind to plasma proteins (HOOPER et al. 1973). The mean half-life of sulthiame in humans is 8.65 ± 3.1 h (MAY et al. 1994). It is eliminated more quickly in children (half-life 7 ± 2 h) than in adults (half-life 12 ± 2 h). DIAMOND and LEVY (1963) found that 60%–70% of a sulthiame dose is excreted in human urine unmetabolized, some 25%–50% being present as metabolites, including a 2-hydroxylated derivative lacking in anticonvulsant activity (DUHM et al. 1963). OLESEN (1968) found 32% of a sulthiame dose was excreted unchanged in human urine over the 24 h following intake.

Adequate data are not available to define a "therapeutic" or "toxic" range of plasma sulthiame concentrations (FEELY et al. 1982). STEAD et al. (1983) reported that, of those whose seizures were controlled by the drug, plasma sulthiame levels below 2.8 mg/l were associated with control in only 10%, while levels below 9.2 mg/l were associated with control in 90%.

IV. Interactions

No reports of pharmacodynamic interactions involving sulthiame have been traced. Sulthiame intake increases plasma phenytoin concentrations (NATION et al. 1990; PISANI et al. 1990). In rats sulthiame inhibits the *p*-hydroxylation of phenytoin (PATSALOS and LASCELLES 1984). It also raises plasma phenobarbitone and primidone levels (PERUCCA 1982).

V. Adverse Effects

Sulthiame taken by mouth may cause upper abdominal distress and nausea. In many patients, once a sufficient dose is taken, hyperpnoea with dyspnoea, and paraesthesiae of the extremities develop (SUTHERLAND and BOWMAN 1963). These symptoms may limit the sulthiame dosage that can be tolerated. Sulthiame may sometimes produce headache, drowsiness, ataxia, anorexia and occasionally mental changes (e.g. hallucinations). Transient catatonia has been reported (MYKYTA 1968) and increased salivation has occurred occasionally. Other probably idiosyncratic unwanted effects are known, e.g. acute renal tubular necrosis (AVIRAM et al. 1965).

There do not appear to be reports of dysmorphogenesis associated with sulthiame.

E. Acetazolamide

Although more commonly used for other disorders, acetazolamide is occasionally prescribed as an anticonvulsant.

I. Chemistry and Use

Acetazolamide (5-acetamido-1,3,4-thiadiazole-2-sulphonamide; MW 222; pK_a 7.4) is a potent non-competitive inhibitor of carbonic anhydrase II. Details of the X-ray crystallographic structure of the drug-enzyme complex have been published (VIDGREN et al. 1990). Acetazolamide is used to treat various disorders, e.g. glaucoma, macular oedema, periodic paralysis syndromes and periodic cerebellar ataxia, and is a diuretic. It has been employed for various types of epilepsy, though it tends to lose its efficacy in the patient as its duration of use increases. It probably is most effective for absence epilepsy, though it is sometimes helpful in preventing convulsive seizures in juvenile myoclonic

(RESOR and RESOR 1990) and other epilepsies and in treating refractory partial epilepsy (OLES et al. 1989). It has often been used as add-on therapy, in which case possible pharmacokinetic interactions may have complicated the interpretation of its efficacy. RESOR et al. (1995) have reviewed data for its efficacy in human epilepsy.

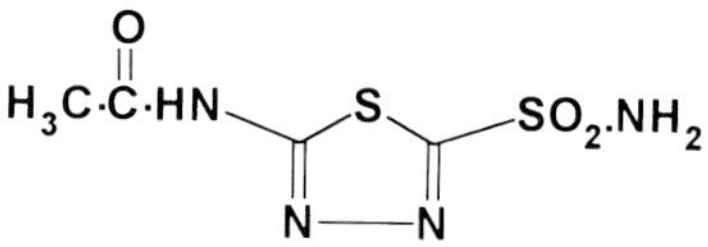

II. Pharmacodynamics

Carbonic anhydrase-deficient mutant mice are less susceptible to induced seizures than their normal littermates (VELISEK et al. 1993). Acetazolamide elevates the electroshock seizure threshold in mice (ANDERSON et al. 1986), the elevation correlating with inhibition of carbonic anhydrase activity in myelin. The drug also inhibits carbonic anhydrase in glia and, at higher concentrations, in red blood cells. The inhibition causes CO_2 accumulation in neurons, and decreased pH and HCO_3 concentrations in glia. The inhibition seems to mediate the antiepileptic effect of the drug. The exact molecular mechanisms involved are unclear.

III. Pharmacokinetics

At usual doses, acetazolamide is reasonably fully absorbed from the alimentary tract, but at higher doses its absorption may be incomplete (MAREN and ROBINSON 1960). Its disposition parameters in humans and various animal species have been tabulated by RESOR et al. (1995). The apparent volume of distribution in humans is 0.2 l/kg. Much of the drug in the body is bound to tissue (mainly red blood cell) carbonic anhydrase. In plasma 90%–95% of the drug is protein bound; the amount bound falls as the plasma acetazolamide concentration rises. The binding is less in the elderly (CHAPRON et al. 1985). Acetazolamide has a mean phase α half-life of 1.6 h, and a β phase one of 10–12 h. It is eliminated by renal excretion, unmetabolized.

Over 1–2 months from the commencement of intake, plasma acetazolamide concentrations fall relative to drug dose (INUI et al. 1982), due to increased synthesis of carbonic anhydrase which results in transfer of the drug from extracellular fluid to binding sites in the tissues. This contributes to the tolerance which develops to the drug.

Very preliminary data suggest that the therapeutic range of plasma acetazolamide concentrations may be around 8–14 mg/l in plasma, and 49–53 mg/l in red blood cells (INUI et al. 1982).

IV. Interactions

Probenicid co-administration raises plasma acetazolamide concentrations. Salicylate causes increased plasma unbound concentrations of acetazolamide (SWEENEY et al. 1989) and inhibits its renal tubular secretion (SWEENEY et al. 1986). Acetazolamide impairs primidone absorption (SYVERSEN et al. 1977), and increases the renal excretion of phenobarbitone by alkalizing the urine (KELLEY et al. 1966). It may raise plasma concentrations of phenytoin (NORELL et al. 1975) and carbamazepine (FORSYTHE et al. 1980).

V. Adverse Effects

Very occasionally hypersensitivity reactions to acetazolamide occur, and there have been rare instances of renal failure, agranulocytosis, thrombocytopenia and aplastic anaemia (KEISU et al. 1990). Dysgeusia is very common and facial and peripheral paraesthesiae are frequent (GRABER and KELLEHER 1988), while some patients experience intermittent dyspnoea. There is an increased risk of renal calculus formation in those taking the drug (KASS et al. 1981; RESOR and RESOR 1990). Some patients complain of tiredness, malaise and anorexia (EPSTEIN and GRANT 1977). High dosages may cause metabolic acidosis, particularly in the elderly (CHAPRON et al. 1989).

F. Bromides

Bromide salts (mainly potassium bromide) were the first effective antiepileptic agents found. LOCOCK (1857) originally described their efficacy but it seems clear that WILKS (1878) recognized their effectiveness independently, and probably played a more influential part in popularizing their use. With the advent of newer anticonvulsants, and recognition of their toxicity, bromides had largely faded from use in humans by the middle of the present century. In recent years there has been some interest in resurrecting them for patients whose epilepsies prove resistant to all other appropriate therapies (SCHNEBLE 1993).

I. Chemistry and Use

Given alone or, more often, as "add-on" therapy, bromides appear most successful for bilateral tonic-clonic seizures, irrespective of the underlying epileptic syndrome. They have been used mainly in therapeutically-refractory childhood epilepsies with bilateral tonic-clonic seizures as well as other epileptic manifestations (ERNST et al. 1988; WOODY 1990; STEINHOFF and KRUSE 1992; OGUNI et al. 1994). Adverse effects have occurred, but have not proved prohibitive.

II. Pharmacodynamics

Suzuki et al. (1994) showed that therapeutic concentrations of Br^- (10–20 mM), substituted for Cl^-, potentiate GABA-activated currents at $GABA_A$ receptors, thus increasing postsynaptic membrane hyperpolarization. This finding correlates with the old observation that chloride loading reversed the adverse effects of bromides, but also their anticonvulsant effects (Shaw et al. 1996). Bromides thus resemble barbiturates in their probable mechanism of anticonvulsant action. However, bromides at anticonvulsant concentrations are also carbonic anhydrase inhibitors (Maren 1967).

III. Pharmacokinetics

Bromides (potassium, sodium) have an oral bioavailability of 0.75–1.18 (Vaiseman et al. 1986); Br^- is distributed throughout body water (similarly to Cl^-). The anion is not bound to plasma proteins and is eliminated from the body by renal excretion unmetabolized, with a half-life of around 12 days (SOREMARK et al. 1960).

Woody (1990) reported a mean therapeutic serum Br^- concentration of 14.1 mmol/l (range 4–30.5 mmol/l). Toxicity is unusual at levels below 2 g/l (27 mmol/l).

IV. Interactions

Chloride competitively displaces Br^- from body fluids, thus enhancing its excretion and reducing its effects.

V. Adverse Effects

Bromides are sedatives and may cause hallucinations and pseudo-dementia but also restlessness, headache and insomnia. They produce skin rashes, commonly resembling acne, but also other dermatoses such as bromoderma tuberosum (Pfeifle et al. 1992) and necrotizing panniculitis (Diener et al. 1993). There is little contemporary information concerning their teratogenic potential.

References

Aird RB, Woodbury DM (1974) The management of epilepsy. Thomas, Springfield

Allan AM, Harris RA (1986) Anesthetic and convulsant barbiturates alter gamma-aminobutyric acid-stimulated chloride flux across brain membranes. J Pharmacol Exp Therap 238:763–768

Alonso-Gonzalez AC, Ortega-Valin L, Santos-Buelga D, Garcia-Sanchez MJ, Santos-Borbujo J, Monzon-Corral L (1993) Dosage programming of phenobarbital in neonatal seizures. J Clin Pharm Ther 18:267–270

Amabeoku GJ, Chikuni O, Akino C, Mutetwa S (1993) Pharmacokinetic interaction of single doses of quinine and carbamazepine, phenobarbitone and phenytoin in healthy volunteers. East Afr Med J 70:90–93
Anderson RE, Howard RA, Woodbury DM (1986) Correlation between effects of acute acetazolamide administration to mice on electroshock seizure threshold and maximal electroshock seizure pattern, and on carbonic anhydrase activity in subcellular fraction of brain. Epilepsia 27:504–509
Anonymous (1976) Anticonvulsant screening project. Department of Health Education and Welfare Publication No (NIH) 76–1093
Ansell BM (1993) Drug-induced systemic lupus erythematosus in a nine-year old-boy. Lupus 2:193–194
Aviram A, Czaczkes JW, Rosenmann E (1965) Acute renal failure associated with sulthiame. Lancet 1:818
Bachmann KA, Jauregui L (1993) Use of single sample clearance estimates of cytochrome P450 substrates to characterize human hepatic CYP status in vivo. Xenobiotica 23:307–315
Bachmann K, Schwartz J, Sullivan T, Jauregui L (1986) Single sample estimate of ethosuximide clearance. Int J Clin Pharmacol Ther Toxicol 24:546–550
Bachmann K, Chu CA, Greear V (1992) In vivo evidence that ethosuximide is a substrate for cytochrome P450IIIA. Pharmacology 45:121–128
Bailer M, Xiaodong S, Perucca E (1995) Ethosuximide. Absorption, distribution and excretion. In: Levy RH, Mattson RH, Meldrum BS (eds) Antiepileptic drugs, 4th edn. Raven Press, New York, pp. 659–665
Bain PG, Findley LJ, Britton TC, Rothwell JC, Gresty MA, Thompson PD, Marsden CD (1995) Primary writing tremor. Brain 118:1461–1472
Baldini S, Carenini L, Leone M, D'Alessandro G, Bottacchi E (1992) Peripheral neuropathy caused by antiepileptic drugs. Neurophysiological study of the A delta and C fibres. Ital J Neurol Sci 13:233–238
Bardy AH, Teramo K, Hiilesmaa VK (1982) Apparent clearances of phenytoin, phenobarbitone, primidone and carbamazepine during pregnancy: results of the prospective Helsinski study. In: Janz D, Bossi L, Helge H, Richens A, Schmidt D (eds) Epilepsy, pregnancy, and the child. Raven Press, New York, pp. 141–145
Barker JL, McBurney RN (1979) Phenobarbitone modulation of postsynaptic GABA receptor function on cultured mammalian neurons. Proc Roy Soc, Ser B Biol Sci 206:319–327
Battino D, Cusi C, Franceschetti S, Moise A, Spina S, Avanzini G (1982) Ethosuximide plasma concentrations: Influence of age and associated concomitant therapy. Clin Pharmacokinet 7:176–180
Battino D, Avanzini G, Bossi L, Croci D, Cusi C, Gomeni C, Moise A (1983) Plasma levels of primidone and its metabolite phenobarbital: effects of age and associated therapy. Ther Drug Monit 5:73–79
Battino D, Binelli S, Bossi L, Como ML, Croci D, Cusi C, Avanzini G (1984) Changes in primidone/phenobarbitone ratio during pregnancy and the puerperium. Clin Pharmacokinet 9:252–260
Battino D, Estienne M, Avanzini G (1995) Clinical pharmacology of antiepileptic drugs in paediatric patients. Part I: Phenobarbital, primidone, valproic acid, ethosuximide and methsuximide. Clin Pharmacokinet 29:257–286
Bauer LA, Harris C, Wilensky AJ, Raisys VA, Levy RH (1982) Ethosuximide kinetics: possible interaction with valproic acid. Clin Pharmacol Ther 31:741–745
Baumel IP, Gallagher BB, Mattson RH (1972) Phenylethylmalonamide (PEMA). An important metabolite of primidone. Arch Neurol 27:34–41
Baumel IP, Gallagher BB, DiMicco J, Goico H (1973) Metabolism and anticonvulsant properties of primidone in the rat. J Pharmacol Exp Therap 186:305–314
Becker A, Greeksch G, Brosz M (1995) Antiepileptic drugs – their effects on kindled seizures and kindling-induced learning impairments. Pharmacol Biochem Behav 52:453–459

Bernus I, Dickinson RG, Hooper WD, Eadie MJ (1994a) Urinary excretion of phenobarbitone and its metabolites in chronically treated patients. Europ J Clin Pharmacol 46:473–475
Bernus I, Dickinson RG, Hooper WD, Eadie MJ (1994b) Inhibition of phenobarbitone-N-glucosidation by valproate. Br J Clin Pharmac 38:411–416
Bhargava VO, Garrettson LK (1988) Development of phenobarbital glucosidation in the human neonate. Dev Pharmacol Ther 11:8–13
Bogaert MG, Rosseel MT, Belpaine FM (1971) Metabolism of nitroglycerine in man: influence of phenobarbital. Arch Internat Pharmacodyn Therap 24:1303–1311
Bolt HM (1994) Interactions between clinically used drugs and oral contraceptives. Environ Health Perspect 102 [Suppl 9]:35–38
Bonay M, Jonville-Bera AP, Diot P, Lemaire E, Lavandier M, Autret E (1993) Possible interaction between phenobarbital, carbamazepine and itraconazole. Drug Safety 9:309–311
Booker HE, Hosokowa K, Burdette RD, Darcey B (1970) Clinical study of serum primidone levels. Epilepsia 11:395–402
Boreus LO, Jalling B, Kallberg N (1975) Clinical pharmacology of phenobarbital in the neonatal period. In: Morselli PL, Garrattini S, Sereni F (eds) Basic and therapeutic aspects of perinatal pharmacology. Raven Press, New York, pp. 331–340
Bossi L (1982) Neonatal period including drug disposition in newborns: review of the literature. In: Janz D, Bossi L, Dam M, Helge H, Richens A, Schmidt D (eds) Epilepsy, pregnancy, and the child. Raven Press, New York, pp. 327–341
Bourgault I, Prost C, Andre C, Villada G, Wechsler J, Chosidow O, Revuz J (1991) Transient intraepidermal bullous reaction after skin graft for toxic epidermal necrolysis. Ultrastructural and immunohistochemical features similar to those of inherited epidermolysis bullosa simplex. Arch Dermatol 127:1369–1374
Brooks PM, Buchanan WW, Grove M, Downie HW (1976) Effects of enzyme-induction on metabolism of prednisolone. Ann Rheum Dis 35:339–343
Browne TR (1995) Other succinimides. Methsuximide. In: Levy RH, Mattson RH, Meldrum BS (eds) Antiepileptic drugs, 4th edn. Raven Press, New York, pp. 681–687
Browne TR, Dreifuss FE, Dyken PR et al. (1975) Ethosuximide in the treatment of absence (petit mal) seizures. Neurology 25:515–524
Browne TR, Feldman RG, Buchanan RA et al. (1983) Methsuximide for complex partial seizures: Efficacy, toxicity, clinical pharmacology, and drug interactions. Neurology 33:414–418
Bruni J, Wilder BJ, Perschalski RJ, Hammond EJ, Villareal HJ (1980) Valproic acid and plasma levels of phenobarbital. Neurology 30:94–97
Buch H, Buzello W, Neurohr O, Rummel W (1968) Vergleich von Verteilung, narkotischer Wirksamkeit und metabolischer Elimination der optischen Antipoden von Methylphenobarbital. Biochem Pharmacol 17:2391–2398
Buchanan RA, Fernandez L, Kinkel AW (1969) Absorption and elimination of ethosuximide in children. J Clin Pharmacol 9:393–398
Buchanan RA, Smith TC, cited by Chang T DWA, Glazko AJ (1972) Ethosuximide. Absorption, distribution and excretion. In: Woodbury DM, Penry JK, Schmidt RP (eds) Antiepileptic drugs, 1st edn. Raven Press, New York, pp. 417–423
Buchanan RA, Kinkel AW, Smith TC (1973) The absorption and excretion of ethosuximide. J Clin Pharmac Ther Toxicol 7:213–218
Buchthal F, Lennox-Buchthal M (1972) Phenobarbital. Relation of serum concentration to control of seizures. In: Woodbury DM, Penry JK, Schmidt RP (eds) Antiepileptic drugs, 1st edn. Raven Press, New York, pp. 335–343
Burd L, Kerbeshian J, Fisher W (1987) Does the use of phenobarbital as an anticonvulsant permanently exacerbate hyperactivity? Can J Psychiatry 32:10–13
Calandre EP, Dominguez-Granados R, Gomez-Rubio M, Molina-Font JA (1990) Cognitive effects of long-term treatment with phenobarbital and valproic acid in school children. Acta Neurol Scand 81:504–506

Callaghan N, O'Hare J, O'Driscoll D, O'Neill B, Daly M (1982) Comparative study of ethosuximide and sodium valproate in the treatment of typical absence seizures (petit mal). Develop Med Child Neurol 24:830–836

Cereghino JJ, Van Meter JC, Brock JT, Penry JK, Smith LD, White BG (1973) Preliminary observations of serum carbamazepine concentrations in epileptic patients. Neurology 23:357–366

Chadwick D (1988) Comparison of monotherapy with valproate and other antiepileptic drugs in the treatment of seizure disorders. Amer J Med 84:3–6

Chanarin I, Mollin DL, Anderson BB (1958) Folic acid and the megaloblastic anaemia. Proc Roy Soc Med 51:757

Chapron DJ, Sweeney KR, Feig PU, Kramer PA (1985) Influence of age on the disposition of acetazolamide. Br J Clin Pharmacol 19:363–371

Chapron DJ, Gomolin IH, Sweeney KR (1989) Acetazolamide blood concentrations are excessive in the elderly: propensity for acidosis and relationship to renal failure. J Clin Pharmacol 29:348–353

Chen G, Weston JK, Bratton AC Jr (1963) Anticonvulsant activity and toxicity of phensuximide, methsuximide and ethosuximide. Epilepsia 4:66–76

Chung S, Ahn C (1994) Effect of anti-epileptic drug therapy on bone mineral density in ambulatory epileptic children. Brain Develop 16:382–385

Cloyd JC, Miller KW, Leppik IE (1981) Primidone kinetics: effect of concurrent drugs and duration of therapy. Clin Pharmacol Ther 29:402–407

Cochrane SM, Black WD, Parent JM, Allen DG, Lumsden JH (1990) Pharmacokinetics of phenobarbital in the cat following intravenous and oral administration. Can J Vet Res 54:132–138

Cohn R (1968) Neuropathological study of a case of petit mal epilepsy. Electroencephalog Clin Neurophysiol 24:282

Conney AH (1967) Pharmacological implications of microsomal enzyme induction. Pharmacol Rev 19:317–366

Coradello H (1973) Ueber die Ausscheidung von Antiepileptika in die Muttermilch. Weiner Klin Wochenschr 85:695–697

Coulter DA, Huguenard JR, Prince DA (1989a) Characterization of ethosuximide reduction of low-threshold calcium currents in thalamic neurons. Ann Neurol 25:582–593

Coulter DA, Huguenard JR, Prince DA (1989b) Specific petit mal anticonvulsants reduce calcium currents in thalamic neurons. Neurosci Lett 98:74–78

Covanis A, Skiadas K, Loli N, Lada C, Theodorou V (1992) Absence epilepsy: early prognostic signs. Seizure 1:281–289

Cowger ML, Labbe RF (1967) The inhibition of terminal oxidation by porphyrinogenic drugs. Biochem Pharmacol 16:2189–2199

Craig C, Hirano K, Shideman F (1960) Anticonvulsant activity of a metabolite of phenobarbital. Federation Proc 19:280

Craig CR, Shideman FE (1971) Metabolism and anticonvulsant properties of mephobarbital and phenobarbital in rats. J Pharmacol Exp Therap 176:35–41

Cramer JA, Mattson RH (1995) Phenobarbital. Toxicity. In: Levy RH, Mattson RH, Meldrum BS (eds) Antiepileptic drugs, 4th edn. Raven Press, New York, pp. 409–420

Critchley EMR, Vakil SD, Hayward HW, Owen VMH (1976) Dupuytren's contracture in epilepsy: result of prolonged administration of anticonvulsants. J Neurol Neurosurg Psychiat 39:498–503

Daniell-LC (1994) Effect of anesthetic and convulsant barbiturates on N-methyl-D-aspartate receptor-mediated calcium flux in brain membrane vesicles. Pharmacology 49:296–307

Data JL, Wilkinson GR, Nies AS (1976) Interaction of quinidine with anticonvulsant drugs. New Eng J Med 294:699–702

Davis RE, Woodliff HJ (1971) Folic acid deficiency in patients receiving anticonvulsant drugs. M J Australia 2:1070–1072

Deiner W, Kruse R, Berg P (1993) Halogenpannikulitis auf Kaliumbromid. Monatsschr Kinderheilkd 141:705–707

de Silva M, Mac Ardle B, McGowan M et al. (1996) Randomized comparative monotherapy trial of phenobarbitone, phenytoin, carbamazepine, or sodium valproate for newly diagnosed childhood epilepsy. Lancet 347:709–713

Diamond S, Levy L (1963) Metabolic studies on a new antiepileptic drug Riker 594. Current Ther Res 5:325–330

Dodson WE, Rust RSJ (1995) Phenobarbital. Absorption, distribution and excretion. In: Levy RH, Mattson RH, Meldrum BS (eds) Antiepileptic drugs, 4th edn. Raven Press, New York, pp. 379–387

Dooley JM, Camfield PR, Camfield PS, Fraser AD (1990) Once-daily ethosuximide in the treatment of absence epilepsy. Pediatr Neurol 6:38–39

Dreifuss FE (1995) Ethosuximide. Toxicity. In: Levy RH, Mattson RH, Meldrum BS (eds) Antiepileptic drugs, 4th edn. Raven Press, New York, pp. 675–679

Drory VE, Korczyn AD (1993) Hypersensitivity vasculitis and systemic lupus erythematosus induced by anticonvulsants. Clin Neuropharmac 16:19–29

Duhm B, Maul W, Medenwald H, Patzchke K, Wegner LA (1963) Tierexperimentelle Untersuchungen mit 35S-markiertem N-(4'-sulfamylphenyl)-(1,4). Zeitschr fur Naturforsch 18:475–492

Duncan JS, Patsalos PN, Shorvon SD (1991) Effects of discontinuation of phenytoin, carbamazepine, and valproate on concomitant antiepileptic medication. Epilepsia 32:101–115

Dunwiddie TV, Worth TS, Olsen RW (1986) Facilitation of recurrent inhibition in rat hippocampus by barbiturate and related nonbarbiturate depressant drugs. J Pharmacol Exp Therap 238:564–575

Eadie MJ (1976) Plasma level monitoring of anticonvulsants. Clin Pharmacokinet 1:52–66

Eadie MJ, Tyrer JH (1989) Anticonvulsant therapy: pharmacological basis and practice, 3rd edn. Churchill-Livingstone, Edinburgh

Eadie MJ, Bochner F, Hooper WD, Tyrer JH (1978) Preliminary observations on the pharmacokinetics of methylphenobarbitone. Clin Exptl Neurol 15:131–144

Eadie MJ, Lander CM, Hooper WD, Tyrer JH (1976) The effect of phenobarbitone dose on plasma phenobarbitone levels in epileptic patients. Proc Austn Assoc Neurol 13:89–96

Eadie MJ, Lander CM, Hooper WD, Tyrer JH (1977a) Factors influencing plasma phenobarbitone levels in epileptic patients. Br J Clin Pharmac 4:541–547

Eadie MJ, Tyrer JH, Smith GA, McKauge L (1977b) Pharmacokinetics of drugs used for petit mal absence. Clin Exptl Neurol 14:172–183

Epstein DL, Grant WM (1977) Carbonic anhydrase inhibitor side effects: serum chemical analysis. Arch Ophthalmol 95:1378–1382

Erith MJ (1975) Withdrawal symptoms in newborn infants of epileptic mothers. Brit Med J 3:40

Ernst JP, Doose H, Baier WK (1988) Bromides were effective in intractable epilepsy with generalized tonic-clonic seizures and onset in early childhood. Brain Develop 10:385–388

Esplin DW (1975) Criteria for assessing effects of depressant drugs on spinal cord synaptic transmission, with examples of drug selectivity. Arch Internat Pharmacodyn Therap 143:479–497

Faero O, Kastrup KW, Lykkegaard Nielsen E, Melchior JC, Thorn I (1972) Successful prophylaxis of febrile convulsions with phenobarbital. Epilepsia 13:279–285

Falasca GF, Toly TM, Reginato AJ, Schraeder PL, O'Connor CR (1994) Reflex sympathetic dystrophy associated with antiepileptic drugs. Epilepsia 35:394–399

Farwell JR, Lee YJ, Hirtz DG, Sulzbacher SI, Ellenberg JH, Nelson KB (1990) Phenobarbital for febrile seizures – effects on intelligence and on seizure recurrence. New Eng J Med 322:364–369

Feely MP, O'Callaghan M, Duggan B, Callaghan N (1980) Phenobarbitone in previously untreated epilepsy. J Neurol Neurosurg Psychiat 43:365–368
Feely MP, O'Callaghan M, O'Driscoll D, Callaghan N (1982) Sulthiame in previously untreated epilepsy. Irish J Med Sci 151:175–179
Feldman RG, Pippenger CE, Florence ML (1975) The relation of anticonvulsant drug levels to complete seizure control. Epilepsia 16:203–204
Fichsel G, Fichsel H, Liappis N (1993) Harnsaureserumkonzentration und antiepileptische Therapie im Kindesalter [serum uric acid concentration and anticonvulsant therapy in childhood]. Klin Pediatr 205:429–431
Fincham RW, Schottelius DD (1995) Primidone. Interactions with other drugs. In: Levy RH, Mattson RH, Meldrum BS (eds) Antiepileptic drugs, 4th edn. Raven Press, New York, pp. 467–475
Findley LJ, Cleeves L, Calzetti S (1985) Primidone in essential tremor of the hands and head: a double blind controlled study. J Neurol Neurosurg Psychiat 48:911–915
Fischer JH, Lockman LA, Zaske D, Kriel R (1981) Phenobarbital maintenance dose requirements in treating neonatal seizures. Neurology 31:1042–1044
Fonseca PD, Moura TF, Ferreira KT (1994) Opening of frog skin sodium channels by phenobarbital. Arch Internat Pharmacodyn Therap 328:106–124
Forsythe WI, Owens JR, Toothill C (1981) Effectiveness of acetazolamide in the treatment of carbamazepine-resistant epilepsy in children. Develop Med Child Neurol 23:761–769
Frantzen E, Hansen JM, Hansen OE, Kristensen M (1967) Phenytoin (Dilantin[R]) intoxication. Acta Neurol Scand 43:440–446
Frey H-H (1985) Primidone. In: Frey H-H, Janz D (eds) Antiepileptic drugs, 1st edn. Springer-Verlag, Berlin, pp. 449–477
Frey HH (1995) Primidone. Mechanisms of action. In: Levy RH, Mattson RH, Meldrum BS (eds) Antiepileptic drugs, 4th edn. Raven Press, New York, pp. 439–447
Fromm GH (1985) Effects of different classes of antiepileptic drugs on brain-stem pathways. Federation Proc 44:2432–2435
Gallagher BB, Freer LS (1985) Barbituric acid derivatives. In: Frey H-H, Janz D (eds) Antiepileptic drugs, 1st edn. Springer-Verlag, Berlin, pp. 421–447
Gallagher BB, Baumel IP, Mattson RH (1972) Metabolic disposition of primidone and its metabolites in epileptic subjects after single and repeated administration. Neurology 22:1186–1192
Garrettson LK, Dayton PG (1970) Disappearance of phenobarbital and diphenylhydantoin from serum of children. Clin Pharmacol Ther 11:674–679
Geets W, Pinon A (1971) L'action metabolique et antiepileptique de l'Ospolot. Acta Neurol Belg 71:164–172
Gelenberg AJ, Jefferson JW (1995) Lithium tremor. J Clin Psychiatry 56:283–287
Gidal BE, Zupanc ML (1994) Potential pharmacokinetic interaction between felbamate and phenobarbital. Ann Pharmacother 28:455–458
Glazko AJ (1975) Antiepileptic drugs: biotransformation, metabolism and serum half-life. Epilepsia 16:367–391
Goldman SI, Krings MS (1995) Phenobarbital-induced fibromyalgia as the cause of bilateral shoulder pain. J Am Osteopath Assoc 95:487–490
Gomez-Mancilla B, Latulippe JF, Boucher R, Bedard PJ (1992) Effect of ethosuximide on rest tremor in the MPTP monkey model. Mov Disord 7:137–141
Goodman LS, Swinyard EA, Brown WC, Schiffman DO, Grewal MS, Bliss EL (1953) Anticonvulsant properties of 5-phenyl-5-ethyl-hexahydropyrimidine-4,6-dione (Mysoline), a new anticonvulsant. J Pharmacol Exp Therap 108:428–436
Goulet JR, Kinkel AW, Smith TC (1976) Metabolism of ethosuximide. Clin Pharmacol Ther 20:213–218
Graber M, Kelleher S (1988) Side effects of acetazolamide. The champagne blues. Amer J Med 84:979–980
Graham J (1978) A comparison of the absorption of phenobarbitone given via the oral and the intramuscular route. Clin Exptl Neurol 15:154–158

Gram L, Bentsen KD (1985) Hepatic toxicity of antiepileptic drugs: a review. Acta Neurol Scand 68 [Suppl 97]:81–90
Graves NM, Holmes GB, Kriel RL, Jones-Saete C, Ong B, Ehresman DJ (1989) Relative bioavailability of rectally administered phenobarbital sodium parenteral solution. DICP 23:565–568
Gray WD, Rauh CE (1967) The anticonvulsant action of inhibitors of carbonic anhydrase: relation to endogenous amines in brain. J Pharmacol Exp Therap 155:127–134
Green JR, Troupin AS, Halpern LM, Friel P, Kanarek P (1974) Sulthiame: evaluation as an anticonvulsant. Epilepsia 15:329–349
Gross-Selbeck G (1995) Treatment of "benign" partial epilepsies of childhood, including atypical forms. Neuropediat 26:45–50
Guberman A, Gloor P, Sherwin AL (1975) Response of generalised penicillin epilepsy in the cat to ethosuximide and diphenylhydantoin. Neurology 25:758–764
Guelen PJM, van der Kleijn E, Woudstra U (1975) Statistical analysis of pharmacokinetic parameters in epileptic patients chronically treated with antiepileptic drugs. In: Schneider H, Janz D, Gardner-Thorpe C, Meinardi H, Sherwin AL (eds) Clinical pharmacology of antiepileptic drugs. Springer, Berlin, pp. 2–10
Haerer AF, Buchanan RA, Wiygul FM (1970) Ethosuximide blood levels in epileptics. J Clin Pharmacol 10:370–374
Hagland K, Seidman P, Collote P, Von Bahr C (1979) Influence of phenobarbital on metoprolol plasma levels. Clin Pharmacol Ther 26:326–329
Haidukewych I, Rodin EA (1985) Effect of phenothiazines on serum antiepileptic drug concentrations in psychiatric patients with seizure disorder. Ther Drug Monit 7:401–404
Hall SD, Guengerich FP, Branch RA, Wilkinson GR (1987) Characterization and inhibition of mephenytoin 4-hydroxylase activity in human liver microsomes. J Pharmacol Exp Therap 240:216–222
Hansen JM, Kristensen M, Skovsted L, Christensen LK (1966) Dicoumarol induced diphenylhydantoin intoxication. Lancet ii:265–266
Haroun M, Jakubovic HR, Nethercott JR (1987) Localized subepidermal bullae after intravenous phenobarbital. Cutis 39:233–234
Harvey DJ, Glazener L, Stratton C, Nowlin J, Hill RM, Horning MG (1972) Detection of a 5-(3,4-dihydroxy-1,5-cyclohexadien-1-yl)-metabolite of phenobarbital and mephobarbital in rat, guinea pig and human. Res Commun Chem Pathol Pharmacol 3:557–565
Hauptmann A (1912) Luminal bei Epilepsie. Munch Med Wochenschr 59:1907–1909
Hayana R, Sasa M, Ujihara H et al. (1995) Effect of antiepileptic drugs on absence-like seizures in the tremor rat. Epilepsia 36:938–942
Heller AH, Dichter MA, Sidman RL (1983) Anticonvulsant sensitivity of absence seizures in the tottering mutant mouse. Epilepsia 25:25–34
Heller AJ, Chesterman P, Elwes RD, Crawford P, Chadwick D, Johnson AL, Reynolds EH (1995) Phenobarbitone, phenytoin, carbamazepine, or sodium valproate for newly diagnosed adult epilepsy: a randomised comparative monotherapy trial. J Neurol Neurosurg Psychiat 58:44–50
Herranz JL, Armijo JA, Arteaga R (1984) Effectiveness and toxicity of phenobarbital, primidone, and sodium valproate in the prevention of febrile convulsions, controlled by plasma levels. Epilepsia 25:89–95
Hojo H, Nakano S, Kataoka K (1979) Serum levels of phenobarbital and carbamazepine in children with convulsive disorders, with reference to therapeutic levels of phenobarbital to prevent recurrence of febrile and afebrile convulsions. Brain Develop 11:10–17
Holmes EL, Lane AZ, cited by Chang T DWA, Glazko AJ (1972) Ethosuximide. Absorption, distribution and excretion. In: Woodbury DM, Penry JK, Schmidt RP (eds) Antiepileptic drugs, 1st edn. Raven Press, New York, pp. 417–423

Hoogerkamp A, Vis PW, Danhof M, Voskuyl RA (1994) Characterization of the pharmacodynamics of several antiepileptic drugs in a direct cortical stimulation model of anticonvulsant effect in the rat. J Pharmacol Exp Therap 269:521–528
Hooper WD, Du Betz DK, Bochner F, Cotter LM, Smith GA, Eadie MJ, Tyrer JH (1975) Plasma protein binding of carbamazepine. Clin Pharmacol Ther 17:433–440
Hooper WD, Qing MS (1990) The influence of age and gender on the stereoselective metabolism and pharmacokinetics of methylphenobarbital in humans. Clin Pharmacol Ther 48:633–640
Hooper WD, Sutherland JM, Bochner F, Tyrer JH, Eadie MJ (1973) The effect of certain drugs on the plasma protein binding of diphenylhydantoin. Aust N Z J Med 3:377–381
Hooper WD, Kunze HE, Eadie MJ (1981a) Pharmacokinetics and bioavailability of methylphenobarbitone in man. Ther Drug Monit 3:39–44
Hooper WD, Kunze HE, Eadie MJ (1981b) Qualitative and quantitative studies of methylphenobarbital metabolism in man. Drug Metabol Disposit 9:381–385
Hooper WD, Treston AM, Jacobsen NW, Dickinson RG, Eadie MJ (1983) Identification of p-hydroxyprimidone as a minor metabolite of primidone in rat and man. Drug Metabol Disposit 11:607–610
Horning MG, Brown L, Nowlin J, Letratangangkoon K, Kellaway P, Zion E (1977) Use of saliva in therapeutic drug monitoring. Clinical Chemistry 23:157–164
Hosokowa K, Takahashi S, Yamomoto M (1984) Plasma concentrations of antiepileptic drugs during pregnancy. In: Sato T, Shinagawa S (eds) Antiepileptic drugs and pregnancy. Excerpta Medica, Amsterdam, pp. 3–11
Houghton GW, Richens A, Toseland PA, Davidson S, Falconer MA (1975) Brain concentrations of phenytoin, phenobarbitone and primidone in epileptic patients. Europ J Clin Pharmacol 9:73–78
Huguenard JR, Prince DA (1994) Intrathalamic rhythmicity studied in vitro: nominal T-current modulation causes robust antioscillatory effects. J Neurosci 14: 5485–5502
Inui M, Azuma H, Nishimura T, Hatada N (1982) The concentration of acetazolamide in blood and saliva. In: Akimoto H, Kazamatsuri H, Seino M, Ward AAJ (eds) The XIIIth epilepsy international symposium. Raven Press, New York, pp. 307–309 (Advances in Neurology 13:307–309)
Ismael S (1990) The efficacy of phenobarbital in controlling epilepsy in children. Paediatr Indones 30:97–110
Jao JY, Jusko WJ, Cohen JL (1972) Phenobarbital effects on cyclophosphamide pharmacokinetics. Cancer Res 32:2761–2764
Jeavons PM (1983) Hepatotoxicity of antiepileptic drugs. In: Oxley J, Janz D, Meinardi H (eds). Chronic toxicity of antiepileptic drugs. New York, Raven, pp. 1–45
Kan R, Masubuchi Y, Nikaido T, Yoshijima T, Ono T, Takahashi Y, Kumashiro H (1984) Antiepileptic drug trends during pregnancy. In: Sato T, Shinagawa S (eds) Antiepileptic drugs during pregnancy. Excerpta Medica, Amsterdam, pp. 12–19
Kaneko S, Kondo Y (1995) Antiepileptic agents and birth defects: incidence, mechanism and prevention. CNS Drugs 3:41–55
Kaneko S, Sato T, Suzuki K (1979) The levels of anticonvulsants in breast milk. Br J Clin Pharmac 7:624–627
Kaneko S, Fukushima Y, Sato T, Ogawa Y, Nomura Y, Shinagawa S (1984) Breast feeding in epileptic mothers. In: Sato T, Shinagawa S (eds) Antiepileptic drugs and pregnancy. Excerpta Medica, Amsterdam, pp. 38–45
Kaneko S, Otani K, Kondo T et al. (1992) Malformations in infants of mothers with epilepsy receiving antiepileptic drugs. Neurology 42 [Suppl 5]:68–74
Kass MA, Kolker AE, Gordon M et al. (1981) Acetazolamide and urolithiasis. Ophthalmology 88:261–265
Kaufmann RE, Habersang R, Lansky L (1977) Kinetics of primidone metabolism and excretion in children. Clin Pharmacol Ther 22:200–206

Keisu M, Wiholm BE, Ost A, Mortimer O (1990) Acetazolamide-associated aplastic anaemia. J Intern Med 228:627–632
Kelley WN, Richardson AP, Mason MR, Rector FC (1966) Acetazolamide in phenobarbital intoxication. Arch Intern Med 117:64–69
Khoo KC, Mendels J, Rothart M et al. (1980) Influence of phenytoin and phenobarbital on the disposition of a single dose of clonazepam. Clin Pharmacol Ther 28:368–375
Kinkel A, cited by Glazko AJ (1972) In: Woodbury DM, Penry JK, Schmidt RP (eds) Antiepileptic drugs, 1st edn. Raven Press, New York, pp. 455–464
Kiorboe E, Paludan J, Trolle E, Overvad E (1964) Zarontin (ethosuximide) in the treatment of petit mal and related disorders. Epilepsia 5:83–89
Knott C, Reynolds F (1984) The place of saliva in antiepileptic drug monitoring. Ther Drug Monit 6:35–41
Knox DA, Ravis WR, Pedersoli WM, Spano JS, Nostrandt AC, Krista LM, Schumacher J (1992) Pharmacokinetics of phenobarbital in horses after single and repeated oral administration of the drug. Am J Vet Res 53:706–710
Koller WC, Busenbark K, Miner K (1994) The relationship of essential tremor to other movement disorders: report on 678 patients. Ann Neurol 35:717–723
Kostyuk PG, Molokanova EA, Pronchuk NF, Savchenko AN, Verkhratsky AN (1992) Different action of ethosuximide on low- and high-threshold calcium currents in rat sensory neurons. Neuroscience 51:755–758
Koup JR, Rose JQ, Cohen ME (1978) Ethosuximide pharmacokinetics in a pregnant patient and her newborn. Epilepsia 19:535–539
Krause KH, Bonjour JP, Berlit P, Kochen W (1985) Biotin status of epileptics. Ann N Y Acad Sci 447:297–313
Kuban KC, Leviton A, Krisnamoorthy KS et al. (1986) Neonatal intracranial hemorrhage and phenobarbital. Pediatrics 77:443–450
Kuban KC, Leviton A, Brown ER, Krishnamoorthy K, Baglivo J, Sullivan KF, Allred E (1987) Respiratory complications in low-birth-weight infants who received phenobarbital. Amer J Dis Child 141:996–999
Kuhnz W, Koch S, Jakob S, Hartmann A, Helge H, Nau H (1984) Ethosuximide in epileptic women during pregnancy and lactation period. Placental transfer, serum concentrations in nursed infants and clinical status. Br J Clin Pharmac 18:671–677
Kupfer A, Branch RA (1985) Stereoselective mephobarbital hydroxylation cosegregates with mephenytoin hydroxylation. Clin Pharmacol Ther 38:414–418
Lambie DG, Johnson RH (1981) The effect of phenytoin on phenobarbitone and primidone metabolism. J Neurol Neurosurg Psychiat 44:148–151
Lander CM, Eadie MJ (1991) Plasma antiepileptic drug concentrations during pregnancy. Epilepsia 32:257–266
Lander CM, Edwards VE, Eadie MJ, Tyrer JH (1977) Plasma anticonvulsant concentrations during pregnancy. Neurology 27:128–131
Lehmann DF (1987) Primidone crystalluria following overdose. Med Toxicol Adverse Drug Exp 2:383–387
Lerman P, Nussbaum E (1975) The use of sulthiame in myoclonic epilepsy of childhood and adolescence. Acta Neurol Scand [Suppl] 60:7–12
Levi AJ, Sherlock S, Walker D (1968) Phenylbutazone and isoniazid metabolism in patients with liver disease in relation to previous drug therapy. Lancet ii:1275–1279
Levy RH, Schmidt D (1985a) Utility of free level monitoring of antiepileptic drugs. Epilepsia 26:199–205
Levy RH, Yerby MS (1985b) Effects of pregnancy on antiepileptic drug utilization. Epilepsia 26 [Suppl 1]:S52–S57
Lim W, Hooper WD (1989) Stereoselective metabolism and pharmacokinetics of methylphenobarbitone in humans. Drug Metabol Disposit 17:212–217
Lindhout D, Meinardi H, Barth P (1982) Hazard of fetal exposure to drug combinations. In: Janz D, Bossi L, Helge H, Richens A, Schmidt D (eds) Epilepsy, pregnancy, and the child. New York, Raven, pp. 275–281

Livingstone S, Berman W, Pauli LL (1975) Anticonvulsant blood drug levels. Practical applications based on 12 years experience. J Amer Med Assoc 232:60–62
Locock C (1857) Discussion of paper by E.H. Sieveking. Analysis of fifty-two cases of epilepsy observed by the author. Lancet 1:527–528
Loiseau P, Brachet Liermain A, Legroux M, Jogeix M (1977) Interet du dosage des anticonsulsivants dans le traitment des epilepsies. Nouvelle Presse Medicale 16:813–817
Löscher W (1979) Comparative study of the protein binding of anticonvulsant drugs in serum of dog and man. J Pharmacol Exp Therap 208:429–435
Löscher W, Hönack D (1989) Comparison of the anticonvulsant efficacy of primidone and phenobarbital during chronic treatment of amygdaloid-kindled rats. Eur J Pharmacol 162:309–322
Lous P (1954) Plasma levels and urinary excretion of three barbituric acids after oral administration to man. Acta Pharmacol Toxicol 10:147–165
Macdonald RL (1989) Antiepileptic drug actions. Epilepsia 30 [Suppl 1]:S19–S28
Macdonald RL, Kelly KM (1993) Antiepileptic drug mechanisms of action. Epilepsia 34 [Suppl 5]:S1–S8
Macdonald RL, Kelly KM (1994) Mechanism of action of currently prescribed and newly developed antiepileptic drugs. Epilepsia 36 [Suppl 4]:S41–S50
Majewski F, Raff W, Fischer P, Huenges R, Petruch F (1980) Zur Teratogenitat von Antikonvulsiva. Deutsch Med Wochenschr 105:719–723
Maren TH (1967) Carbonic anhydrase: chemistry, physiology. and inhibition. Physiol Rev 47:595–781
Maren TH, Robinson B (1960) The pharmacology of acetazolamide as related to cerebrospinal fluid and the treatment of hydrocephalus. Bull Johns Hopkins Hosp 106:1–24
Mares P, Pohl M, Kubova H, Zelizko M (1994) Is the site of action of ethosuximide in the hindbrain? Physiol Res 43:51–56
Martin PR, Kapur BM, Whiteside EA, Sellers EM (1979) Intravenous phenobarbital therapy in barbiturate and other hypnosedative withdrawal reactions: a kinetic approach. Clin Pharmacol Ther 26:256–264
Massey GV, Dunn NL, Heckel JL, Myer EC, Russell EC (1994) Aplastic anaemia following therapy for absence seizures with ethosuximide. Pediatr Neurol 11:59–61
Matsumoto K, Miyazaki H, Fujii T, Hashimoto M (1989) Binding of sulfonamides to erythrocytes and their components. Chem Pharm Bull Tokyo 37:1913–1915
Mattson RH, Cramer JA (1980) Valproic acid and ethosuximide interaction. Ann Neurol 7:583–584
Mattson RH, Cramer J, McCutchen CB (1989) Barbiturate-related connective tissue disorders. Arch Intern Med 149:911–914
May TW, Korn-Merker E, Rambeck B, Boenigt HE (1994) Pharmacokinetics of sulthiame in epileptic patients. Ther Drug Monit 16:251–257
Mc Auliffe JJ, Sherwin AL, Leppik IE, Fayle SA, Pippenger CE (1977) Salivary levels of anticonvulsants: a practical approach to drug monitoring. Neurology 27:409–413
McGeachy TE, Bloomer WE (1953) The phenobarbital sensitivity syndrome. Amer J Med 14:600–604
Meadow SR (1970) Congenital abnormalities and anticonvulsant drugs. Proc Roy Soc Med 63:48–49
Meldrum BS, Horton RW, Toseland PA (1975) Primate model for testing anticonvulsant drugs. Arch Neurol 32:289–294
Metzer WS (1994) Essential tremor: an overview. J Ark Med, Soc 90:587–590
Micheletti G, Vergnes M, Marescaux C, Reis J, Depaulis A, Rumbach L, Warter JM (1985) Antiepileptic drug evaluation in a new animal model: spontaneous petit mal epilepsy in the rat. Arzneim Forsch 35:483–485
Miller CA, Gaylord M, Lorch V, Zimmerman AW (1994) The use of primidone in neonates with theophylline-resistant apnea. Amer J Dis Child 147:183–186

Millership JS, Mifsud J, Collier PS (1993) The metabolism of ethosuximide. Eur J Drug Metab Pharmacokinet 18:349–353
Millership JS, Collier PS, Hamilton JT, McRoberts WC, Mifsud J (1995) Chiral aspects of the metabolism of ethosuximide. Chirality 7:173–180
Minagawa K, Miura H, Chiba K, Ishizaki T (1981) Pharmacokinetics and relative bioavailability of intramuscular phenobarbital sodium or acid in infants. Pediatric Pharmacology 1:279–289
Modi NB, Veng-Pedersen P, Wurster DE, Berg MJ, Schottelius DD (1994) Phenobarbital removal characteristics of three brands of activated charcoal: a system analysis approach. Pharm Res 11:318–323
Mountain KR, Hirsch J, Gallus AS (1970) Neonatal coagulation defect due to anticonvulsant drug treatment in pregnancy. Lancet 1:265–268
Muni IA, Altschuler CH, Neicheril JC (1973) Identification of blood metabolite of methsuximide by GLC-mass spectrometry. J Pharm Sci 62:1820–1823
Mykyta GJ (1968) A case of sulthiame overdosage. M J Australia 2:118–119
Nation RL, Evans AM, Milne RW (1990) Pharmacokinetic drug interactions with phenytoin. Clin Pharmacokinet 18:37–60 and 131–150
Nau H, Rating D, Haeuser I, Jager E, Koch S, Helge H (1980) Placental transfer and pharmacokinetics of primidone and its metabolites phenobarbital, PEMA and hydroxyphenobarbital in neonates and infants of epileptic mothers. Europ J Clin Pharmacol 18:31–42
Nau H, Schmidt D, Beck-Mannagetta G, Rating D, Koch S, Helge H (1982) Pharmacokinetics of primidone and metabolites during human pregnancy. In: Janz D, Bossi L, Helge H, Richens A, Schmidt D (eds) Epilepsy, pregnancy, and the child. Raven Press, New York, pp. 121–129
Neighbors SM, Soine WH (1995) Identification of phenobarbital N-glucuronides as urinary metabolites of phenobarbital in mice. Drug Metabol Disposit 23:548–552
Nelson E, Powell JR, Conrad K, Likes K, Byers J, Baker S, Perrier D (1982) Phenobarbital pharmacokinetics and bioavailability in adults. J Clin Pharmacol 22:141–148
Neuvonen PJ, Elonen E (1980) Effect of activated charcoal on absorption and elimination of phenobarbitone, carbamazepine and phenylbutazone in man. Europ J Clin Pharmacol 17:51–57
Norell E, Lilienberg G, Gamstorp I (1975) Systematic determination of the serum phenytoin level as an aid in the management of children with epilepsy. Eur Neurol 13:232–244
Nowack WJ, Johnson RN, Englander RW, Hanna GR (1979) Effects of valproate and ethosuximide on thalamocortical excitability. Neurology 29:96–99
Oguni H, Hayashi K, Oguni M et al. (1994) Treatment of severe myoclonic epilepsy in infants with bromide and its borderline variant. Epilepsia 335:1140–1145
Oles KS, Penry JK, Cole DL, Howard G (1989) Use of acetazolamide as an adjunct to carbamazepine in refractory partial seizures. Epilepsia 30:74–78
Olesen OV (1968) Determination of sulthiame (Ospolot) in serum and urine by thin-layer chromatography: serum levels and urinary output in patients under long term treatment. Acta Pharmacol Toxicol 26:22–28
Otani K, Kaneko S, Shimada S, Fukushima Y, Sato T, Ogwana Y, Nomura Y (1984) The pharmacokinetics of primidone during pregnancy. In: Sato T, Shinagawa S (eds) Antiepileptic drugs and pregnancy. Excerpta Medica, Amsterdam, pp. 33–37
Painter MJ, Pippenger C, Carter G, Pitlick W (1977) Metabolism of phenobarbital and phenytoin by neonates with seizures. Neurology 27:370
Patel IH, Levy RH, Rapport RL (1977) Distribution characteristics of ethosuximide in discrete areas of rat brain. Epilepsia 18:533–541
Patel IH, Levy RH, Cutler RE (1980) Phenobarbital-valproic acid interaction. Clin Pharmacol Ther 27:515–521
Patsalos PN, Duncan JS (1993) Antiepileptic drugs. A review of clinically significant drug interactions. Drug Safety 9:156–184

Patsalos PN, Lascelles PT (1977) Effect of sodium valproate on plasma protein binding of diphenylhydantoin. J Neurol Neurosurg Psychiat 40:570–574
Pelekanos L, Camfield P, Camfield C, Gordon K (1991) Allergic rash due to antiepileptic drugs: clinical features and management. Epilepsia 32:554–559
Pellegrini A, Dossi RC, Dal-Pos F, Ermani M, Zanotto L, Testa G (1989) Ethosuximide alters intrathalamic and thalamocortical synchronizing mechanisms: a possible explanation of its antiabsence effect. Brain Res 497:344–360
Penry JK, Porter RJ, Dreifuss FE (1972) Ethosuximide. Relation of plasma levels to clinical control. In: Woodbury DM, Penry JK, Schmidt RP (eds) Antiepileptic drugs, 1st edn. Raven Press, New York, pp. 431–441
Perucca E (1982) Pharmacokinetic interactions with antiepileptic drugs. Clin Pharmacokinet 7:57–84
Perucca E (1995) Pharmacological principles as a basis for polytherapy. Acta Neurol Scand [Suppl] 162:31–34
Perucca E, Hedges A, Makki KA, Ruprah M, Wilson JF, Richens A (1984) A comparative study of the relative enzyme inducing properties of anticonvulsant drugs in epileptic patients. Br J Clin Pharmac 18:401–410
Pfeifle J, Greiben U, Bork K (1992) Bromoderma tuberosum durch antikonvulsive Behandlung mit Kaliumbromid. Hautarzt 43:792–794
Pincus JH, Grove I, Marino BB, Glaser GE (1970) Studies on the mechanism of action of diphenylhydantoin. Arch Neurol 22:566–571
Pippenger CE (1987) Clinically significant carbamazepine drug interactions. Epilepsia 28 [Suppl 3]:S71–S76
Piredda S, Monaco F (1981) Ethosuximide in tears, saliva and cerebrospinal fluid. Ther Drug Monit 3:321–323
Piredda SG, Woodhead JH, Swinyard EA (1985) Effect of stimulus intensity on the profile of anticonvulsant activity of phenytoin, ethosuximide and valproate. J Pharmacol Exp Therap 232:741–745
Pisani F, Richens A (1983) Pharmacokinetics of phenylethylmalonamide (PEMA) after oral and intravenous administration. Clin Pharmacokinet 8:272–276
Pisani F, Perucca E, Di Perri R (1990) Clinically relevant anti-epileptic drug interactions. J Int Med Res 18:1–15
Porter RJ, Penry JK, Lacy JR, Newmark ME, Kupferberg HJ (1977) The clinical efficacy and pharmacokinetics of phensuximide and methsuximide. Neurology 27:375
Porter RJ, Penry JK, Lacey JR, Newmark ME, Kupferberg HJ (1979) Plasma concentrations of phensuximide, methsuximide, and their metabolites in relation to clinical efficacy. Neurology 29:1509–1513
Pourcher E, Gomez-Mancilla B, Bedard PJ (1992) Ethosuximide and tremor in Parkinson's disease: a pilot study. Mov Disord 7:132–136
Powell C, Painter MJ, Pippenger CE (1984) Primidone therapy in refractory neonatal seizures. J Pediat 105:651–654
Pranzatelli MR (1988) Effect of antiepileptic and antimyoclonic drugs on serotonin receptors in vivo. Epilepsia 29:412–419
Prichard JW, Ransom BR (1995) Phenobarbital. Mechanisms of action. In: Levy RH, Mattson RH, Meldrum BS (eds) Antiepileptic drugs, 4th edn. Raven Press, New York, pp. 359–369
Rambeck B (1979) Pharmacological interaction of methsuximide with phenobarbital and phenytoin in hospitalised epileptic patients. Epilepsia 20:147–156
Rankin GO, Beers KW, Nicoll DW, Anestis OK, Shih HC, Brown PI, Hubbard JL (1992) Role of para-hydroxylation in phensuximide-induced urotoxicity in the Fischer 334 rat. Toxicology 74:77–88
Rating D, Nau H, Jager-Roman E et al. 1982 Teratogenic and pharmacokinetic studies of primidone during pregnancy and in the offspring of (epileptic) women. Acta Paediatrica Scandinavica 71:301–311
Ravakhah K, West BC (1995) Case report: subacute combined degeneration of the spinal cord from folate deficiency. Am J Med Sci 310:214–216

Ravis WR, Duran SH, Pedersoli WM, Schumacher J (1987) A pharmacokinetic study of phenobarbital in mature horses after oral dosing. J Vet Pharmacol Ther 10:283–289
Ravis WR, Pedersoli WM, Wike JS (1989) Pharmacokinetics of phenobarbital in dogs given multiple doses. Am J Vet Res 50:1343–1347
Reddy MN (1985) Effect of anticonvulsant drugs on plasma total cholesterol, high-density lipoprotein cholesterol, and apolipoproteins A and B in children with epilepsy. Proc Soc Exp Biol Med 180:359–363
Reidenberg P, Glue P, Banfield CR et al. (1995) Effects of felbamate on the pharmacokinetics of phenobarbital. Clin Pharmacol Ther 58:279–287
Reinisch JM, Sanders SA, Mortensen EL, Rubin DB (1995) In utero exposure to phenobarbital and intelligence deficits in adult men. J Amer Med Assoc 274:1518–1525
Reinken L (1973) Die Wirkung von Hydantoin und Succinimid auf den Vitamin B6 Stoffwechsel. Clin Chim Acta 48:435–436
Resor SRJ, Resor LD (1990) Chronic acetazolamide monotherapy in the treatment of juvenile myoclonic epilepsy. Neurology 40:1677–1681
Resor SRJ, Resor LD, Woodbury DM, Kemp JW (1995) Other antiepileptic drugs. Acetazolamide. In: Levy RH, Mattson RH, Meldrum BS (eds) Antiepileptic drugs, 4th edn. Raven Press, New York, pp. 969–985
Reynolds NC Jr, Miska RM (1981) Safety of anticonvulsants in hepatic porphyrias. Neurology 31:480–484
Richens A, Houghton GW (1975) Effect of drug therapy on the metabolism of phenytoin. In: Schneider H, Janz D, Gardner-Thorpe C, Meinardi H, Sherwin AL (eds) Clinical pharmacology of antiepileptic drugs. Springer, Berlin, pp. 87–95
Roberts EA, Spielberg SP, Goldbach M, Phillips MJ (1990) Phenobarbital hepatotoxicity in an 8-month-old infant. J Hepatol 10:235–239
Rowland M (1972) Influence of route of administration on drug availability. J Pharm Sci 61:70–74
Sakai C, Takagi T, Oguro M, Tanabe N, Wakatsuki S (1993) Erythroderma and marked atypical lymphocytosis mimicking cutaneous T-cell lymphoma probably caused by phenobarbital. Intern Med 32:182–184
Salomon D, Saurat JH (1990) Erythema multiforme major in a 2-month-old child with human immunodeficiency (HIV) infection. Br J Dermat 123:797–800
Sanduk R (1986) Phenobarbital-induced Tourette-like symptoms. Pediatr Neurol 2:54–55
Sasa M, Ohno Y, Ujihara H et al. (1988) Effects of antiepileptic drugs on absence-like and tonic seizures in the spontaneously epileptic rat, a double mutant rat. Epilepsia 29:505–513
Sasso E, Perucca E, Calzetti S (1988) Double-blind comparison of primidone and phenobarbital in essential tremor. Neurology 38:808–810
Sasso E, Perucca E, Fava R, Calzetti S (1991) Quantitative comparison of barbiturates in essential hand and head tremor. Mov Disord 6:65–68
Sato J, Sekizawa Y, Yoshida A et al. (1992) Single-dose kinetics of primidone in human subjects: effect of phenytoin on formation and elimination of active metabolites of primidone. J Pharmacobiodyn 15:467–472
Sawaishi Y, Komatsu K, Takeda O, Tazawa Y, Takahashi I, Hayasaka K, Takada G (1992) A case of tubulo-interstitial nephritis with exfoliative dermatitis and hepatitis due to phenobarbital hypersensitivity. Eur J Pediatr 151:69–72
Sayer RJ, Brown AM, Schwindt PC, Crill WE (1993) Calcium currents in acutely isolated neocortical neurons. J Neurophysiol 69:1596–1606
Schmidt D (1975) The effect of phenytoin and ethosuximide on primidone metabolism in patients with epilepsy. J Neurol 209:115–123
Schmidt D (1983) Connective tissue disorders induced by antiepileptic drugs. In: Oxley J, Janz D, Meinardi H (eds). Chronic toxicity of antiepileptic drugs. New York, Raven, pp. 115–124

Schmidt D, Kupferberg HJ (1975) Diphenylhydantoin, phenobarbital and primidone in saliva, plasma and cerebrospinal fluid. Epilepsia 16:735–741

Schmidt D, Einicke I, Haenel F (1986) The influence of seizure type on the efficacy of plasma concentrations of phenytoin, phenobarbital, and carbamazepine. Arch Neurol 43:263–265

Schneble H (1993) Antiepileptische Bromtherapie einst und jetzt. Nervenartz 64:730–735

Schwartz RD, Jackson JA, Weigert D, Skolnick P, Paul SM (1985) Characterization of barbiturate-stimulated chloride efflux from rat brain synaptoneurosomes. J Neurosci 5:2963–2970

Sechi GP, Piras MR, Rosati G, Zuddas M, Ortu R, Tanca S, Agnetti V (1988) Phenobarbital-induced buccolingual dyskinesia in oral apraxia. Eur Neurol 28:139–141

Seip M (1983) Aplastic anaemia during ethosuximide medication. Treatment with bolus-methylprednisolone. Acta Paediatr Scandinav 72:927–929

Seyfert S, Hone A, Holl G (1988) Primidone and essential tremor. J Neurol 235:168–170

Shapiro S, Hartz SC, Siskind V et al. (1976) Anticonvulsants and parental epilepsy in the development of birth defects. Lancet 1:272–275

Shaw AN, Trepanier LA, Center SA, Garland S (1996) High dietary chloride content associated with loss of therapeutic serum bromide concentrations in an epileptic dog. J Am Vet Med Assoc 208:234–236

Sherwin AL, Robb JP (1972) Ethosuximide. Relation of plasma level to clinical control. In: Woodbury DM, Penry JK, Schmidt RP (eds) Antiepileptic drugs, 1st edn. Raven Press, New York, pp. 443–448

Smith DB, Mattson RH, Cramer JA, Collins IF, Novelly RA, Craft B (1987) Results of a nationwide Veterans Administration Cooperative Study comparing the efficacy and toxicity of carbamazepine, phenobarbital, phenytoin, and primidone. Epilepsia 28 [Suppl 3]:S50–S58

Smith GA, McKauge L, Du Betz DK, Tyrer JH, Eadie MJ (1979) Factors influencing plasma concentrations of ethosuximide. Clin Pharmacokinet 4:38–52

Snead OC III (1988) Gammahydroxybutyrate model of generalized absence seizures: further observations and comparison with other absence models. Epilepsia 29:361–368

Snead OC III (1995) Basic mechanisms of generalized absence seizures. Ann Neurol 37:146–157

Solow EB, Green JB (1972) The simultaneous determination of multiple anticonvulsant drug levels by gas-liquid chromatography. Method and clinical application. Neurology 22:540–550

Soremark R (1960) Excretion of bromide ions by human urine. Acta Physiol Scand 50:119–123

Speidel BD, Meadow SR (1972) Maternal epilepsy and abnormalities of the fetus and newborn. Lancet 2:839–843

Stead AH, Hook W, Moffat AC, Berry D (1983) Therapeutic, toxic and fatal blood concentration ranges of antiepileptic drugs as an aid to the interpretation of analytical data. Human Toxicol 2:135–147

Steinhoff BJ, Kruse R (1992) Bromide treatment of pharmaco-resistant epilepsies with generalised tonic-clonic seizures: a clinical study. Brain Develop 14:144–149

Strong JM, Abe T, Gibbs EL, Atkinson AJ Jr (1974) Plasma levels of methsuximide and N-desmethylmethsuximide during methsuximide therapy. Neurology 24:250–255

Sutherland JM, Bowman DA (1963) Sulthiame (Ospolot) in the treatment of temporal lobe epilepsy. M J Australia 2:532–533

Sutton G, Kupferberg HJ (1975) Isoniazid as an inhibitor of primidone metabolism. Neurology 25:1179–1181

Suzuki S, Kawakami K, Nakamura F, Nishimura S, Yagi K, Seino M (1994) Bromide, in therapeutic concentration, enhances GABA-mediated currents in cultured neurons of rat cerebral cortex. Epilepsy Res 19:89–97

Svensmark O, Buchthal F (1963) Accumulation of phenobarbital in man. Epilepsia 4:199–206
Sweeney KR, Chapron DJ, Brandt JL, Gromolin IH, Feig PU, Kramer PA (1986) Toxic interaction between acetazolamide and salicylate: case report and a pharmacokinetic explanation. Clin Pharmacol Ther 40:518–524
Sweeney KR, Chapron DJ, Antal EJ, Kramer PA (1989) Differential effects of flurbiprofen and aspirin on acetazolamide disposition in humans. Br J Clin Pharmac 27:866–869
Swinyard EA, Castellion AW (1966) Anticonvulsant properties of some benzdiazepines. J Pharmacol Exp Therap 151:369–375
Syversen GB, Morgan JP, Weintraub M, Myers GJ (1977) Acetazolamide-induced interference with primidone absorption: case reports and metabolic studies. Arch Neurol 34:80–84
Tang BK, Kalow W, Grey AA (1979) Metabolic fate of phenobarbital in man. N-glucoside formation. Drug Metabol Disposit 7:315–318
Taylor LP, Posner JB (1989) Phenobarbital rheumatism in patients with brain tumor. Ann Neurol 25:92–94
Tennison MB, Greenwood RS, Moles MV (1991) Methsuximide for intractable childhood seizures. Pediatrics 87:186–189
Teschendorf HJ, Kretzschmar R (1985) Succinimides. In: Frey H-H, Janz D (eds) Antiepileptic drugs, 1st edn. Springer-Verlag, Berlin, pp. 557–574
Theodore WH, Porter RJ, Raubertas RF (1987) Seizures during barbiturate withdrawal: relation to blood level. Ann Neurol 22:644–647
Thilothammal N, Kannan, Krishamurthy PV, Kamala KG, Ahamed S, Banu K (1993) Role of phenobarbitone in preventing recurrence of febrile convulsions. Indian Pediatr 30:637–642
Thurman GD, McFadyen ML, Miller R (1990) The pharmacokinetics of phenobarbitone in fasting and non-fasting dogs. J S Afr Vet Assoc 61:86–89
Todorov AB, Lenn NJ, Gabor AJ (1978) Exacerbation of generalised convulsive seizures with ethosuximide therapy. Arch Neurol 35:389–391
Treston AM, Phillipides A, Jacobsen NW, Eadie MJ, Hooper WD (1987) Identification and synthesis of O-methylcatechol metabolites of phenobarbital and some N-alkyl derivatives. J Pharm Sci 76:496–501
Troupin A, Friel P (1975) Anticonvulsant levels in saliva, serum, and cerebrospinal fluid. Epilepsia 16:223–227
Vaiseman N, Koren G, Pencharp P (1986) Pharmacokinetics of oral and intravenous bromide in normal volunteers. Clin Toxicol 23:403–413
Vajda F, Williams FM, Davidson S, Falconer MA, Breckenridge A (1974) Human brain, cerebrospinal fluid and plasma concentrations of diphenylhydantoin and phenobarbital. Clin Pharmacol Ther 15:597–603
van der Kleijn E, Guelen PJM, van Wijk C, Baars J (1975) Clinical pharmacokinetics in monitoring chronic medication with anti-epileptic drugs. In: Schneider H, Janz D, Gardner-Thorpe C, Meinardi H, Sherwin AL (eds) Clinical pharmacology of antiepileptic drugs. Springer, Berlin, pp. 11–33
van der Pol MC, Hadders-Algra M, Huisjes HJ, Touowen BC (1991) Antiepileptic medication in pregnancy: late effects in the children's central nervous system development. Am J Obstet Gynecol 164:121–128
Van Wieringen A, Vritland CM (1983) Ethosuximide intoxication caused by interaction with isoniazid. Neurology 33:1227–1228
Velisek L, Moshe SL, Xu SG, Cammer W (1993) Reduced susceptibility to seizures in carbonic anhydrase II deficient mutant mice. Epilepsy Res 14:115–121
Vest FB, Soine WH, Westkaemper RB, Soine PJ (1989) Stability of phenobarbital N-glucosides: Identification of hydrolysis products and kinetics of decomposition. Pharmacol Res 6:458–465
Vidgren J, Liljas A, Walker NP (1990) Refined structure of the acetazolamide complex of human carbonic anhydrase II at 1.9 A. Int J Biol Macromol 12:342–344

Vining EP, Mellitis ED, Dorsen MM, Cataldo MF, Quaskey SA, Spielberg SP, Freeman JM (1987) Psychologic and behavioural effects of antiepileptic drugs in children: a double-blind comparison between phenobarbital and valproic acid. Pediatrics 80:165–174
Viswanathan CT, Booker HE, Welling PG (1978) Bioavailability of oral and intramuscular phenobarbital. J Clin Pharmacol 18:100–105
Wada JA (1977) Pharmacological prophylaxis in the kindling model of epilepsy. Arch Neurol 34:389–395
Wagner ML (1994) Felbamate: a new antiepileptic drug. Am J Hosp Pharm 51:1657–1666
Wechselberg K, Hubel G (1967) Zur Resorption und Verteilung von methyl-aethyl-succinimid (MAS) im Serum und Liquor bei Kindern. Z Kinderheilkunde 100:10–19
Whyte MP, Dekaban AS (1977) Metabolic fate of phenobarbital. A qualitative study of p-hydroxyphenobarbital elimination in man. Drug Metabol Disposit 5:63–70
Wilensky AJ, Friel PN, Levy RH, Comfort CF, Kaluzny SP (1982) Kinetics of phenobarbital in normal subjects and epileptic patients. Europ J Clin Pharmacol 23:87–92
Wilks S (1878) Lectures on diseases of the nervous system. Churchill, London
Willeit J, Deisenhammer F, Ransmayr G, Gerstenbrand F (1991) Orthostatischer Tremor. Deutsch Med Wochenschr 116:1509–1512
Windorfer AJ, Sauer W (1971) Drug interactions during anticonvulsant therapy in childhood: diphenylhydantoin, primidone, phenobarbital, clonazepam, nitrazepam, carbamazepine and dipropylacetate. Neuropediatrie 8:29–41
Winek CL (1976) Tabulation of therapeutic, toxic, and lethal concentrations of drugs and chemicals in blood. Clin Chemistry 22:832–836
Wirth N, Hoffmeister F, Sommer S (1961) The pharmacology of Ospolot. German Medical Monthly 6:309–312
Woody RC (1990) Bromide therapy for pediatric seizure disorder intractable to other antiepileptic drugs. J Child Neurol 5:65–67
Wright JD, Helsby NA, Ward SA (1995) The role of S-mephenytoin hydroxylase (CYP2C19) in the metabolism of the antimalarial biguanides. Br J Clin Pharmacol 39:441–444
Yerby MS, Friel PN, McCormick K, Koerner M, Van Allen M, Leavitt AM, Sells CJ, Yerby JA (1990) Pharmacokinetics of anticonvulsants in pregnancy: alterations in plasma protein binding. Epilepsy Res 5:223–228
Young MC, Hughes IA (1991) Loss of therapeutic control in congenital adrenal hyperplasia due to interaction between dexamethasone and primidone. Acta Paediatr Scandinav 80:120–124
Young RS, Alger PM, Bauer L, Lauderbaugh D (1986) A randomized, double-blind, crossover study of phenobarbital and mephobarbital. J Child Neurol 1:361–363
Zavadil P, Gallagher BB (1976) Metabolism and excretion of ^{14}C-primidone in epileptic patients. In: Janz D (ed) Epileptology. Thieme, Stuttgart, pp. 129–139

CHAPTER 9

Phenytoin and Congeners

H. KUTT and C.L. HARDEN

A. Phenytoin

I. Introduction

The synthesis of 5,5-diphenylhydantoin was reported by BILTZ in 1908. In 1937 PUTNAM and MERRITT reported that it elevated the threshold to electrically induced seizures in cats. In 1938 MERRITT and PUTNAM reported that it provided effective treatment for chronic seizures, without sedation, in patients with convulsive disorders. Since then phenytoin has been one of the mainstays of seizure therapy. In 1968 WALLIS et al. reported success in the treatment of status epilepticus with high doses of phenytoin given intravenously. A water-soluble prodrug was developed in the 1980s to simplify the parenteral administration of phenytoin (see Sect. B on fosphenytoin, below).

In the early 1950s, WOODBURY recognized the importance of Na^+ gradients in the mechanism of action of phenytoin (WOODBURY 1955, 1980). Stereoselective arene oxidation was reported by BUTLER et al. in 1976 to be the initial step in phenytoin metabolism and this was elaborated on by MCLANAHAN and MAGUIRE (1986). Of the cytochrome P450 isoenzymes, CYP2C9 has been identified as the major (VERONESE et al. 1991) and CYP2C19 as the minor (LEVY and BAJPAI 1995) one involved in phenytoin metabolism. SPIELBERG et al. (1981) and KIM and WELLS (1995) have shown that toxic effects with tissue damage may be produced by the arene oxide and free radical intermediates that occur during phenytoin metabolism.

II. Chemistry and Use

1. Chemistry

Phenytoin, 5,5-diphenylhydantoin, is a white crystalline material with a molecular weight of 252.3. A poorly water-soluble weak acid, it has a pK_a value of 8.3. Its sodium salt has a molecular weight of 274.3, so that 100 mg of it is equivalent to 91.8 mg acid phenytoin on a molar basis. For parenteral use, the salt is dissolved in a mixture of propylene glycol, ethanol and water, and the pH is adjusted to 12.0 with sodium hydroxide. The conversion factor from mg/l to μmol/l is 3.96.

2. Indications and Use

Phenytoin is available for oral administration in the form of capsules (usually 100 or 30 mg of the sodium salt), tablets (usually 50 mg acid phenytoin) and suspension (6 or 25 mg/ml acid phenytoin). There are various absorption characteristics of the products from different manufacturers. The strength of the parenteral preparation is usually 50 mg of the sodium salt (46 mg acid phenytoin) per millilitre. Phenytoin is used to prevent generalized tonic-clonic seizures and partial seizures with or without generalization and is also beneficial in the treatment of tic douloureux. The recommended starting dose is 300 mg daily for adults and 5 mg/kg daily for children. The usually effective daily dosages are 300–500 mg in adults and 5–7 mg/kg in children. Increases of dose in the higher dosage range should be made in small instalments because of a non-linear response of plasma phenytoin levels to dose increases. Monitoring of plasma phenytoin levels is helpful in dosage regulation. In the treatment of status epilepticus 1000 mg (18 mg/kg) or more is given intravenously at a rate up to 50 mg/min, while monitoring the blood pressure, ECG, pulse and respiration. The administration rate may be reduced, if indicated. If a rapid effect is desired from oral phenytoin administration, 300 mg may be given every 4 h to a total of 1000–1200 mg.

III. Pharmacodynamics

Phenytoin has been classified as a type I anticonvulsant which modifies maximal electroshock seizures, blocks sustained repetitive firing and prevents tonic-clonic and some partial seizures but is ineffective against pentylenetetrazole-induced convulsions and does not modify GABAergic synaptic transmission or the T-type calcium currents in thalamic relay (pacemaker) nuclei (MACDONALD 1989).

Of the numerous clinical effects of phenytoin, the most useful is its ability to attenuate or control chronic seizures at non-sedative drug concentrations, and to stop ongoing seizures at the high drug concentrations achieved by giving large doses of the drug rapidly. It has this effect mainly by preventing or reducing the propagation of seizure activity from its area of origin rather than by abolishing it in situ. Thus in a patient having partial clonic seizures, phenytoin given intravenously in 250 mg instalments up to a total of 1250 mg gradually decreased and then stopped the clonic movements of the arm while spike activity in the EEG continued unchanged (WALLIS et al. 1968). In the laboratory, in cats rendered epileptic with intracortical penicillin deposits, repeated instalments of phenytoin reduced and finally abolished clonic limb movements, but even very large amounts of phenytoin had little effect on cortical spike activity (LOUIS et al 1964).

The best understood mechanism in the prevention of seizure spread by phenytoin is the drug's ability to reduce post-tetanic potentiation (ESPLIN 1955; RAINES and STANDAERT 1966). Post-tetanic potentiation is a physiological synaptic mechanism that enhances the channeling of nerve impulses of normal activity. It is in a heightened state of activity at the synapses surrounding a seizure focus and at the corresponding active synapses along pathways traversed by impulses from the focus. Reducing the post-tetanic potentiation at each synaptic site in a highly active polysynaptic pathway results in compound attenuation of the impulses. Thus phenytoin can prevent the spread of seizure activity yet has little or no effect on normal functions, which elicit little post-tetanic potentiation activity compared with that which develops near a seizure focus and in its efferent pathways. Exactly how this effect comes about is not yet clear but it is thought to be related to phenytoin's ability to modify ion transport across the cell membrane, particularly that of Na^+ and Ca^{2+}, and to modify transmitter release (WOODBURY 1980). A direct effect of phenytoin on the membranes of neurons and axons is also demonstrable in cultures of cortical and spinal cord neurons (MACDONALD 1989). In these experiments sustained high-frequency repetitive firing elicited by depolarizing pulses applied against a negative membrane potential was markedly reduced by phenytoin at concentrations in the range seen in the drug's clinical usage.

The role of Na^+ in the mechanism of action of phenytoin was first pointed out by WOODBURY in 1955. Subsequent research revealed that phenytoin stimulates Na-K-ATPases in synaptosomes if the Na^+/K^+ ratio is high (near 10), as occurs at sites of heightened activity. Conversely and more importantly, phenytoin also reduces Na^+ entry into neurons (MACDONALD 1989; TUNNICLIFF 1996). In voltage clamp experiments, phenytoin reduced Na^+ currents, suggesting that there was blockage of Na^+ channels. The blockage was shown to be time-, use-, and voltage-dependent. According to the modified receptor hypothesis (COURTNEY and ETTER 1983), the sequence of events would be that use or stimulation would change the resting state (R) of the Na^+ channel, in which it can be activated, to the open state (O), in which the channel conducts Na^+ and allows phenytoin to enter. This, however, turns the channel into an inactive state (I), in which it cannot be activated. The phenytoin within the channel now binds to the inactivatable (I state) channel receptor and prolongs the channel's recovery time. While the channel ordinarily recovers in few milliseconds, in the presence of phenytoin, which dissociates slowly from it, the recovery is extended to 60 or more milliseconds. Thus phenytoin causes time-dependent channel blockage. Repeated depolarization increases the number of channels with phenytoin bound to them and which are therefore incapable of conducting Na^+. Thus the block is also use-dependent. Phenytoin is most effective at sites of high neuronal activity such as at a seizure focus and its emerging pathways, but it has little effect on normal activity. Recovery is enhanced by hyperpolarization, making the ion channel blockage voltage-dependent.

Phenytoin at high concentrations also blocks depolarization-dependent Ca^{2+} uptake in preparations of presynaptic nerve terminals or in intact neuromuscular junctions (MACDONALD 1989; DELORENZO 1995). Similarly, phenytoin blocks sequestration of Ca^{2+} by presynaptic organelles and mitochondria in synaptosome preparations. While the blocking of Ca^{2+} entry has a stabilizing effect on the cell membrane, blocking Ca^{2+} entry into the organelles and altering the intracellular redistribution of Ca^{2+} may increase excitability temporarily. This may account for the increase in seizures which is seen in some patients with high phenytoin plasma levels (Woodbury 1980). It is of interest that phenytoin has little or no effect on T-type Ca^{2+} channels which are present in the thalamic relay nuclei which serve as the pacemaker for the 3 Hz rhythm of absence seizures (Macdonald 1989). Phenytoin inhibits Ca^{2+}-calmodulin-dependent protein phosphorylation and regulates some neurotransmitter release at relatively high concentrations: this may be a factor in the genesis of some unwanted effects of the drug (DeLorenzo 1995). The mechanism of cell damage caused by phenytoin metabolites produced by the cytochrome P450 and tissue peroxidase systems is discussed in the Adverse Effects section below.

IV. Pharmacokinetics

1. Absorption

The absorption rate of phenytoin varies somewhat with different formulations, the peak plasma level usually appearing 4–8 h from oral intake. Generally, the bioavailability of oral phenytoin is about 90%. Calcium sulphate in the formulation and the administration of antacids together with phenytoin retard the drug's absorption. Phenytoin absorption is diminished in enteral feeding, particularly feeding through a nasogastric tube. Little if any phenytoin is absorbed from the rectum, and the drug's absorption from intramuscular injection sites is delayed and erratic.

2. Distribution

The distribution of phenytoin to various tissues is fairly rapid after the drug's intravenous administration and maximum concentrations in the brain are reached in 15 min. Phenytoin passes the placenta, and the umbilical cord plasma concentration of the drug equals that of the mother's plasma (Eadie 1984). Phenytoin concentrations in the CSF usually equal the unbound concentration of the drug in plasma (10% of the concentration in whole plasma), while those in saliva can be somewhat higher (Woodbury 1988; Browne and Le Duc 1995).

The apparent volume of distribution ranges from 0.5 to 0.8 l/kg in adults and from 0.8 to 1.2 l/kg in children. About 90% of the phenytoin in plasma is protein bound. The percentage bound is lower in patients with poor renal function (due mainly to displacement of the drug at its protein binding sites by uraemic products), in patients with chronic liver disease and other conditions which cause reduced serum albumin levels, and in pregnancy. Other drugs such as salicylates and valproate reduce phenytoin binding to plasma proteins by competing for binding sites (Eadie 1984; Yerby et al. 1992).

3. Elimination

Phenytoin is eliminated almost exclusively by metabolism.

a) Metabolism

The metabolism of the symmetrical (prochiral) molecule of phenytoin involves extensive hydroxylation, mostly at one of its phenyl substitutes via an arene oxidation which renders the reaction product asymmetrical, resulting in (S)- and (R)-metabolites. There is evidence that the para-(4)-hydroxylation of the drug is mediated largely by cytochrome P450C2 subfamily isoenzymes, CYP2C9 handling the major portion (90%) of the dose (VERONESE et al. 1991, 1993) and CYP2C19 a minor portion (10% – LEVY and BAJPAI 1995; IEIRI et al. 1997). Epoxide hydrolases and glutathione transferases are involved in the drug's later metabolic steps. The putative sequence of events is that the initial step of arene oxidation produces a transient intermediary arene oxide of phenytoin which converts spontaneously (NIH shift) into the major metabolite, 5-phenyl-5′-*p*-hydroxy-phenylhydantion (*p*HPPH), which accounts for about 60%–80% of the dose. A smaller portion of the arene-oxide becomes phenytoin-epoxide (about 10% of the dose) and this is usually quickly converted to a dihydrodiol (DHD) of phenytoin by epoxide hydrolase activity (MCLANAHAN and MAGUIRE 1986; MAGUIRE et al 1987). Several minor metabolites appear in urine: meta-hydroxy, dihydroxy- and catechol-compounds (mostly as glucuronides), and there is some unmetabolized phenytoin, together usually accounting for less than 1% of the dose (BROWNE and LE DUC 1995; Fig. 1).

In the majority of patients, 75%–95% of the *p*HPPH appears in the (S)-enantiomeric form and 5%–25% in the (R)-form, resulting in an S/R ratio ranging from 20 to 4. The dihydrodiol appears as 75% in the S- and 25% in the R-form with an S/R ratio of about 3 (MAGUIRE et al. 1987). This suggests product selectivity of the isoenzymes involved in the drug's metabolism. The CYP2C9 isoform, which in vitro has proved the most efficient of the CYP2 C subfamily isoenzymes in phenytoin metabolism (VERONESE et al. 1993), is the likely producer of (S)-*p*HPPH. The role of CYP2C19 in the production of (R)-*p*HPPH is indicated by the findings of FRITZ et al. (1987) and IEIRI et al. (1997), which showed that subjects possessing mutant ineffective CYP2C19 (poor mephenytoin metabolizers) produced virtually no (R)-*p*HPPH while their output of (S)-*p*HPPH equaled that of members of the general population. This distinction is relevant in explaining genetic differences in phenytoin metabolism.

The capacity to metabolize phenytoin varies widely among individuals, in part because of their genetic backgrounds, and in part because of environmental factors. The CYP2C isoenzymes are inducible but the extent of induction varies considerably among individuals. Autoinduction takes place in some patients to a modest degree (EDEKI and BRASE 1995) and is relatively greater for CYP2C19 than for CYP2C9, since (R)-*p*HPPH as a percentage of the total *p*HPPH increased during chronic phenytoin administration (FRITZ et al. 1987).

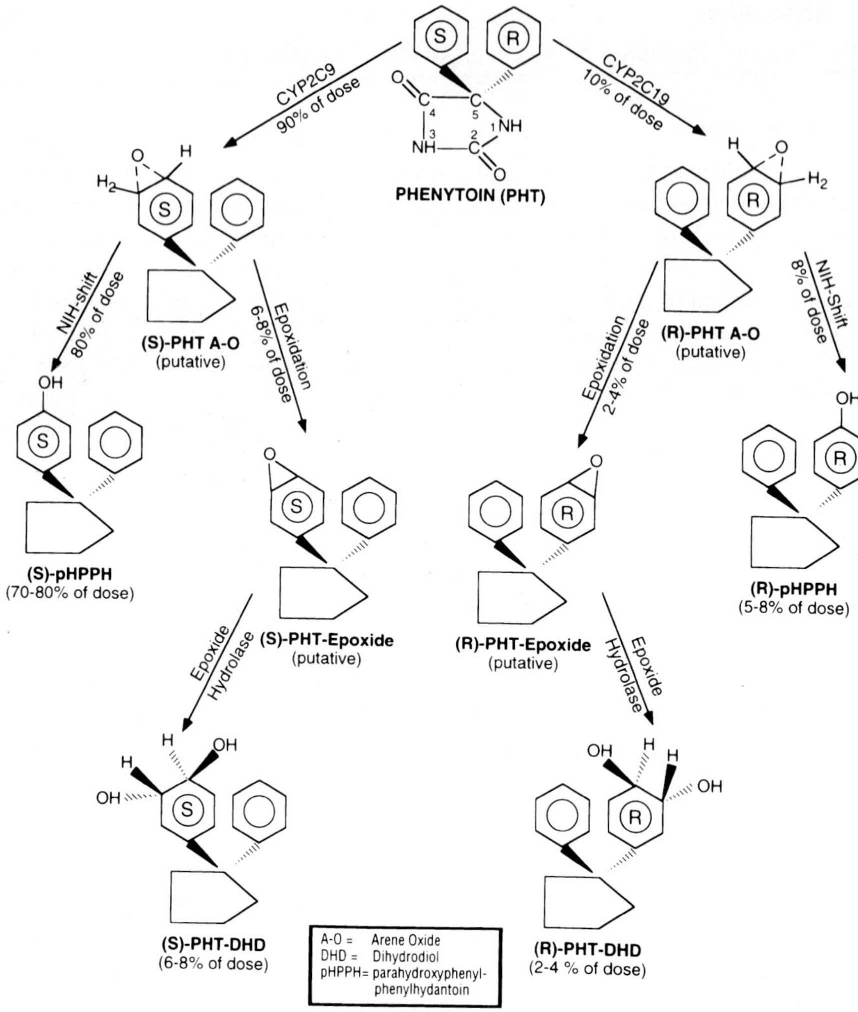

Fig. 1. The major pathways and major enantiomeric [(S)- and (R)-*p*HPPH] and diastereomeric [(S)- and (R)-dihydrodiol] products of phenytoin metabolism in average normal subjects. Based on FRITH et al. (1987), MAGUIRE et al. (1987), VERONESE et al. (1993), LEVY and BAJPAI (1995), BROWN and LE DUC (1995) and IEIRI et al. (1997)

Induction by some other drugs, alcohol and some foods occurs. On the other hand, some other drugs inhibit the enzymes (see Sect. A.V, "Interactions"). In general, the efficiency of phenytoin metabolism (the V_{max}) is low in neonates, increases considerably in children, in adolescents and in pregnancy, and decreases again with advancing age.

The first step of phenytoin parahydroxylation, i.e. arene oxidation, exhibits non-linear enzyme kinetics and follows a Michaelis-Menten model. This becomes significant because clinically effective concentrations of phenytoin are often higher than its K_m in the individual. This results in a non-linear (faster/higher) rise of plasma phenytoin level on increasing the dose. It also has an effect on the phenytoin plasma half-life and clearance: the higher the initial phenytoin level the longer it takes to decline after a decrease in the dose, or to decline by 50% after discontinuation of the drug. The clearance value has an inverse relation to the plasma concentration (BROWNE and LE DUC 1995).

The extrahepatic bioactivation of the phenytoin molecule has been studied extensively in search for causes of phenytoin toxicity. Tissue peroxidases such as prostaglandin H synthetase and the lipoxygenases, using phenytoin as a source of reducing equivalents, convert it to a free radical intermediate, which if not neutralized by glutathionations, may bind covalently to tissue proteins or initiate formation of reactive oxygen species including the hydroxyl (.OH) radical (MIRANDA et al. 1995). In neutrophils activated with hydroperoxidases and incubated with phenytoin, there is production of reactive phenytoin intermediates as well as para-, meta- and ortho-HPPH, implying that arene oxidation had taken place (MAYS et al. 1995).

α) Pharmacogenetics

The wide variations in the dose:plasma level relationships of phenytoin are in part caused by genetic factors. With intake of an average dose of the drug, intoxication due to insufficient parahydroxylation of phenytoin occurred in a patient and several members of his family (KUTT et al. 1964). Since then, several similar patient and family studies have been reported and it appears that deficient phenytoin metabolism occurs as an autosomal recessive trait. INABA (1990) reviewed the reported cases and calculated that the incidence of homozygous slow metabolizers could be about 1 in 500, according to the Hardy-Weinberg law. The pHPPH:phenytoin ratio in urine and the phenytoin:pHPPH ratio in plasma have been used as criteria of the efficiency of phenytoin metabolism; the urinary S/R enantiomeric ratio of *p*HPPH also would be useful. Laboratory evidence for polymorphism in phenytoin metabolism is beginning to emerge: in patients with the Ile/Leu359 mutation in CYP2C9, the V_{max} for phenytoin was 40% lower than average (HASHIMOTO et al. 1996). Other small changes in the amino acid sequence in CYP2C9 have also been found to affect *p*HPPH production significantly (VERONESE et al. 1993; LE DUC et al. 1997). Mutations in CYP2C19, however, which is a minor enzyme in phenytoin metabolism but the major one in mephenytoin hydroxylation, have been identified in poor mephenytoin metabolizers by DE MORAISE et al. (1994). These mutations involve changes from guanine to adenine at positions 681 and 636 in exons 5 and 4 of CYP2C19, producing a truncated non-functional protein. Importantly, the heterozygotes, although considered efficient metabolizers, also have a reduced capacity to parahydroxylate, compared with homozygotes who have two intact genes

(BERTILSSON 1995). Analogous mutation(s) in CYP2C9 might explain the major genetic defect in phenytoin metabolism. Along these lines, it may be postulated that the initial patient of KUTT et al. (1964) probably had inefficient (mutant) CYP2C9 genes, as he was incapable of handling 300 mg of phenytoin daily but had efficient CYP2C19 so that he could handle 100 mg/day of phenytoin to produce 69 mg *p*HPPH (probably all as the R-enantiomer). This is likely in view of the fact that he tolerated easily a daily dose of 300 mg methylphenobarbitone (mephobarbitone), a drug metabolized by CYP2C19 (KUPFER and BRANCH 1985).

b) Elimination Parameters

Clearance values for phenytoin show wide variations, ranging from 0.015 to 0.065 l/kg/h, the higher values being observed in children. Ethnic differences in clearance may exist (EDEKI and BRASE 1995). Published values for the K_m have ranged from 3 to 30 mg/l (average 6.2 mg/l); and those for the V_{max} from 6 to 16 mg/kg/day. The V_{max} values increase in pregnancy and are usually higher in children than in adults (EADIE 1984; WOODBURY 1989). The plasma half-life of phenytoin depends upon the drug dose and the drug's preexisting plasma concentration. A 100 mg test-dose yielded half-life values of 8–15 h and a 250 mg dose values of about 20 h. In patients following large overdoses, phenytoin half-lives of several days have been observed. The often quoted half-life value of 20 h is usually found in adults receiving average phenytoin doses.

4. Clinical Pharmacokinetics

a) Dose-Plasma Level Relationships

The maximum plasma phenytoin level produced by doses of 300–400 mg/day is usually achieved in 5–14 days. The delay is longer with higher drug doses, and the level may reach steady-state values of 10–15 mg/l in compliant adult patients. Wide variations in the dose/plasma level relationship usually indicate unusual rates of phenytoin metabolism or absorption or unreliable drug intake (see also the sections on "Metabolism" and "Interactions"). A phenytoin dose of 500 mg/day usually produces a steady-state plasma level above 20 mg/l (KUTT and MCDOWELL 1968). In general, plasma phenytoin level increases become disproportional to dosage in the higher dosage range because of the saturation elimination kinetics of the drug.

b) Plasma Level-Effects Relationships

α) Beneficial Effects

In the majority of patients, improved seizure control is usually seen when the plasma phenytoin level approaches 10 mg/l. In a prospective study of 32 patients, the average seizure frequency declined from 6 to 1.5 when the phenytoin level was increased from less than 10 to near 15 mg/l (LUND 1974). Of course, there are as many "therapeutic levels" as there are individual patients and a universally applicable therapeutic level is not to be expected. The individual's effective level depends mainly on the severity and nature of his seizure process, and this may change from time to time (KUTT and PENRY 1974). Seizure control has been observed with plasma phenytoin levels as low as 3 mg/l in some patients, but there has also been little improvement in others with levels over 25 mg/l.

β) Acute Toxic Effects

When plasma phenytoin levels approach 20 mg/l, side-effects may start to appear in the form of blurred vision and nystagmus. These become accentuated and associated with disturbances of equilibrium and coordination when the levels approach 30 mg/l; somnolence may be seen with levels near 40 mg/ml (KUTT and MCDOWELL 1968). Coma occurred with a dose of 4 g daily (ROTHENBERG and PUTNAM 1937). The above sequence of events usually takes place when the level increases rapidly. In many patients tolerance develops to these side effects and relatively high plasma phenytoin levels cause little if any discomfort. In disease states with low plasma protein levels and therefore a reduced phenytoin binding capacity, overdosage effects may occur with average total phenytoin plasma levels; in these cases monitoring of the unbound drug level is helpful.

γ) Initial Target Range Concentration (10–20 mg/l)

The use of the term "initial target range" in preference to "therapeutic range" was suggested by Dr. Dixon M. Woodbury in discussions with the first author as a way of avoiding illogical statements such as: "the patient" (with a plasma phenytoin level of 19 mg/l) continued to have seizures despite having a "therapeutic plasma level". Logically, a patient will continue to have seizures until his or her therapeutic level is reached. Aiming to achieve a plasma phenytoin level of 10 mg/l in a patient, whose individual therapeutic level is not yet known, is safe since such a level is usually free of side-effects and is often therapeutically effective. "Limiting" the upper extent of the initial target at the usually trouble-free concentration of 20 mg/l is a policy that can be revised, if indicated clinically.

V. Interactions

Numerous interactions between phenytoin and other drugs have been reported and reviewed periodically (EADIE and TYRER 1980; NATION et al. 1990; KUTT 1995; LEVY and BAJPAI 1995) and are also discussed in Chap. 22 of this book. The most frequently reported interactions involve phenytoin accumulation caused by the intake of another drug; reports of the reduction of the plasma levels of other drugs by phenytoin are somewhat less frequent, while lowering of phenytoin levels or increased levels of other drugs are reported relatively infrequently. In general, there can be wide variations in the extent and incidence, and even in the direction, of an interaction among individual patients receiving the same drugs in combination. This may be somewhat confusing and has led some authors to conclude that the evidence for a given interaction is conflicting. The reasons for the individual variation in the interactions include differences in genetic make-up with regards to the capacity for phenytoin metabolism (mutations in CYP2C9 or CYP2C19 rendering homozygotes impaired and heterozygotes somewhat impaired) or in the genetics of the metabolic handling of the other drug involved, for instance slow isoniazid acetylation. The patient's genetically determined ability to induce microsomal oxidative enzymes also varies (VESELL 1971). The determining factors for clinically evident and significant interactions include the pre-existing state of induction of the enzymes involved as well as the dosages and the pre-existing concentrations of phenytoin and the interacting drug. Not all interactions are detrimental: a modest rise of phenytoin level may improve seizure control; a reduced phenytoin dosage lowers its cost during the use of a drug which inhibits its metabolism. Nearly all reported interacting drugs can still be used with phenytoin, guided by clinical judgement and therapeutic drug monitoring.

LEVY (1995) has suggested that knowing the role of CYP2C9 and CYP2C19 in phenytoin metabolism helps to anticipate the extent and intensity of its interactions. Inhibitors/co-substrates of CYP2C9 (see Table 1A), which catalyze the biotransformation of the larger part of a phenytoin dose, may cause extensive rises in plasma phenytoin levels. Inhibitors/co-substrates of CYP2C19 (Table 1B), which handle a relatively small portion of the phenytoin dose, might be expected to cause smaller and less frequent changes. This hypothesis will apply if the concentration of the inhibitor/co-substrate is high enough when it is used clinically. It is also important to realize that an inhibitor of phenytoin metabolism, which is not itself a substrate for the enzyme it inhibits, is likely to cause a continuing rise in plasma phenytoin level. However, co-substrates which act as competitive inhibitors raise the phenytoin level to a new plateau. Since a co-substrate also often induces the enzymes involved, it may even lower the phenytoin level in subjects who are genetically efficient inducers. Table 1C lists the drugs whose mechanism of inhibiting phenytoin metabolism is not yet established.

Induction of phenytoin metabolism, interference with its absorption or displacement of the drug from its plasma protein binding sites will lower plasma phenytoin levels (see Table 1D). Phenytoin affects other drugs mostly by lowering their plasma levels, primarily by altering their metabolism, and rarely by altering their absorptions (Table 1E). Whatever the mechanism of the interaction, dosage adjustments, if needed, usually solve any clinical problem that develops.

VI. Adverse Effects

1. Acute Toxicity

The acute systemic toxicity of phenytoin is characterized by central nervous system effects and results from a direct action of phenytoin at its receptor site.

Table 1. Drug-drug interactions involving phenytoin (data compiled from the literature)

Drugs reported to elevate phenytoin levels

A. Inhibitors/cosubstrates of CYP2C9: amiodarone, azapropazone, cotrimoxazole, disulphiram, fluconazole, metronidazole, miconazole, phenylbutazone, propoxyphene, stiripentol, sulphaphenazole, tolbutamide, *S*-warfarin

B. Inhibitors/co-substrates of CYP2C19: diazepam, nordiazepam, felbamate, fluoxetine, imipramine, mephenytoin, methylphenobarbitone (mephobarbital), phenobarbitone, proguanyl, propranolol

C. Mechanism not yet established but likely to be inhibition of CYP2 C isoenzymes: chloramphenicol, dicoumarol, diltiazem, ethanol (acute intake), isoniazid, methsuximide, nafimidone, phenylbutazone, progabide, propoxyphene, sulthiame, trazodone, viloxazine

Drugs reported to lower phenytoin levels

D. Interference with phenytoin absorption (abs), protein binding (pb), induction of metabolism (met) or combination mechanisms: antacids in high doses, antineoplastics, calcium sulphate (abs); dexamethazone, ethanol – chronic intake – (met), folic acid, phenobarbitone, rifampicin, salicylates (pb)

Drugs reported to be affected by phenytoin

E. Phenytoin reduces the level of the following drugs, probably by inducing P450 isoenzymes involved in their metabolism: carbamazepine, clobazam, clonazepam, cyclosporin, dexamethasone, dicoumarol, digitalis, disopyramide, doxycycline, folic acid, haloperidol, lamotrigine, methadone, nortriptyline, oral contraceptives, pethidine (meperidine), praziquantel, prednisolone, primidone, quinidine, theophylline, thyroxine, valproate, vitamins D and K, zonisamide

F. Phenytoin may increase the level of the following drugs: chloramphenicol, normethsuximide, phenobarbitone, warfarin

The reversible acute toxicity of the drug is predictable in terms of the drug dose and the drug's plasma concentration. Cerebello-vestibular effects, such as nausea, ataxia, coordination difficulties and dysarthria, occur with mild toxicity. A single oral loading phenytoin dose of 18 mg/kg in a medically supervised setting produced only mild cerebello-vestibular toxicity and some nausea and vomiting; mean serum phenytoin levels of 12.3 mg/l were reached in 6–10 h, and of 15.1 mg/l in 16–24 h (Osborne et al. 1987). As the drug levels rise, toxicity worsens, the mental status is affected and extrapyramidal abnormalities, such as dystonic posturing and choreoathetoid movements, can appear. Seizures may be exacerbated at high plasma phenytoin levels. Extremely high doses cause coma.

Acute prolonged phenytoin intoxication has been reported to produce permanent cerebellar atrophy and ataxia in some patients; this has been clearly documented by pre- and postphenytoin intoxication imaging studies in a report by Kuruvilla and Bharucha (1997). Although cerebellar degeneration has occurred in epileptics who never took phenytoin, it has also been seen in non-epileptic patients taking phenytoin; hence cerebellar atrophy cannot be confidently attributed to an effect of repeated seizures alone (Rapport and

SHAW 1977). Generally the risk of developing permanent cerebellar ataxia and cerebellar atrophy from phenytoin intoxication is not high: the abnormality apparently occurs in subjects who have an individual-specific vulnerability.

The acute local unwanted effects which occur with either intravenous or intramuscular injection of phenytoin include severe irritation, inflammatory and haemorrhagic changes and phlebitis.

2. Idiosyncratic Adverse Effects

Allergic skin rashes are the most frequent idiosyncratic effects of phenytoin, and occur in 5%–10% of patients. Phenytoin infrequently produces a usually reversible, benign lymphadenopathy associated with fever, rash, and hepatosplenomegaly. The mechanism of this form of acute hypersensitivity possibly involves immunogenic metabolites of phenytoin. The evidence for this is the presence of IgG antibodies directed toward a 53-kDa microsomal protein found in the sera of patients taking phenytoin or other aromatic anticonvulsants who develop a hypersensitivity such as a serum sickness-like syndrome (LEEDER et al. 1992). This antigen was also overexpressed in the microsomes of a patient with a fatal hepatotoxic reaction to phenytoin, suggesting that it may be important in the pathogenesis of severe idiosyncratic hypersensitivity to the drug. Hepatic necrosis rarely occurs, nearly always as part of widespread hypersensitivity syndrome, and can be fatal in one-quarter of affected patients. Exfoliative dermatitis, erythema multiforme, toxic epidermal necrolysis, and systemic lupus occur, but are extremely rare.

Decreased immunological function may be the cause of a rare reversible pseudolymphoma syndrome which may occur during phenytoin treatment and which may express depressed cellular and humoral immunity. This idiosyncratic reaction may be confused with Hodgkin's lymphoma. As well, malignant Hodgkin's and non-Hodgkin's lymphomas which do not resolve with discontinuation of phenytoin intake and require chemotherapeutic treatment have been reported in phenytoin-treated patients. A case of Epstein-Barr virus-positive non-Hodgkin's lymphoma was recently reported in a patient who had taken phenytoin for 20 years (GARCIA-SUARES et al. 1996). This report provides clinical evidence for linking a neoplasm with a viral infection possibly facilitated by phenytoin-associated immunodeficiency.

Toxic effects of phenytoin on the haematopoietic systems are not frequent. A modest decline in the white blood cell count has been observed, but agranulocytosis and aplastic anaemia are extremely rare.

3. Teratogenicity

The overall incidence of cleft lip and palate is 2% in the general population, 4% in the offspring of untreated epileptic women and 6% in the offspring of epileptic women treated with average dosages of antiseizure medications. Polypharmacy increases the risk of these major malformations to over 10%.

Cardiac abnormalities such as septal defects can also occur at an increased frequency compared with that in the general population. The foetal hydantoin syndrome differs little from the foetal carbamazepine and phenobarbitone syndromes, and is not clearly distinguished from the foetal alcohol, nicotine and other syndromes. There are several known factors, perhaps genetically regulated, which are involved in teratogenesis. These include a low availability of epoxide hydrolase, glutathione-*S* transferase and other antioxidants, and of folate (YERBY et al. 1992; FINNELL et al. 1995). In susceptible individuals, these factors may act either singly or in various combinations. They are discussed further below under "Mechanisms of Idiosyncratic Toxicity and Teratogenicity".

a) Folate, Anaemia, Teratogenesis

Phenytoin intake usually causes a modest decline of folate levels in serum and red cells, possibly due to interference with folate absorption and biotransformation. Megaloblastic anaemia is quite infrequent during phenytoin therapy and responds to folate administration. Low folate diets and the use of antifolates have caused foetal abnormalities in experimental animals. In clinical evaluations, folate supplementations have not prevented birth defects consistently. However, it may be concluded that folate supplementation helps achieve an optimum outcome to pregnancy (DANSKY et al 1992).

b) Mechanisms of Idiosyncratic Toxicity and Teratogenicity

An untoward idiosyncratic or teratogenic reaction to phenytoin probably indicates the presence of an individual vulnerability caused by a genetically determined low capacity of the drug's detoxification pathways. A low metabolic capacity may not be apparent unless the relevant pathways are saturated, as is more likely to occur in the setting of polypharmacy. These pathways involve substrate specific epoxide hydrolases, glutathione systems and folate systems. Attempts to develop predictive tests to identify high risk subjects are underway. The most advanced of these tests is the identification of subjects with low epoxide hydrolase activities, a test based on finding very low values of epoxide hydrolase activity in fibroblasts and amniocytes from babies exhibiting dysmorphic features, values comparable to those at the lower end of the general population distribution (BUEHLER et al. 1990, FINNELL et al. 1992). A genetic pattern of epoxide hydrolase deficiency was suggested in these studies, but the sample was too small to establish it clearly (LINDHOUT 1992). Another potentially predictive test could be the demonstration of the biotransformation of aspirin to 2,3-dihydroxybenzoic acid by phenytoin-induced hydroxyl radicals; the formation would be increased in the presence of insufficient glutathione activity (KIM and WELLS 1995).

The best studied mechanisms leading to cell and tissue injury are the formations of (1) electrophilic intermediates from CYP2C cytochrome P450 isoenzyme-mediated arene oxidation and (2) the free radical intermediates from tissue perioxidase bioactivation of phenytoin. The arene epoxide intermediate will accumulate in the setting of epoxide hydrolase deficiency and is then available to bind covalently with macromolecules including embryonic nucleic acids, thereby interfering with normal embryogenesis. Support for this theory has been provided experimentally by showing that damage occurs in P450 and phenytoin-containing systems in vivo and in vitro. Cell injury and teratogenesis were increased by epoxide hydrolase inhibitors, and reduced by inhibition of the P450 system (Spielberg et al. 1987; Finnell et al. 1992). Furthermore, in the A/J mouse strain, which is prone to phenytoin teratogenicity, epoxide hydrolase activity is low compared with that in the C57BL/J6 strain, which is relatively resistant to phenytoin teratogenicity. The resistant strain was also capable of greater enzyme induction than the teratogenicity-prone A/J strain (Hartsfield et al. 1995).

The free radical intermediates resulting from the bioactivation of phenytoin by prostaglandin H synthetase or lipoxygenesis will bind covalently to form hydroxyl radicals, which if not neutralized by glutathione and other antioxidants will initiate the oxidation of macromolecules (Miranda et al. 1994; Mays et al. 1995). The evidence for the role of free radicals in toxicity is experimental, there being reduced damage from the use of prostaglandin H synthetase inhibitors as well as free radical trapping agents, whilst inhibitors of glutathione transferase increase the damage (Kim and Wells 1996). The final step to cell injury by the free radical derivatives, which was demonstrated in the hepatic maternal and embryonic nuclei of phenytoin-exposed mice, is oxidation of DNA to form 8-hydroxy-2-deoxyguanosine, thus influencing DNA regeneration (Liu and Wells 1995). Recently, alterations of gene expression by phenytoin were documented by in situ transcription and antisense RNA amplification techniques using phenytoin-exposed mouse embryonic neural tubes (Bennett et al. 1997).

4. Chronic Toxicity

The chronic effects of phenytoin on connective tissue proliferation are troublesome, mainly because of their negative cosmetic impact. Gingival hyperplasia occurs in up to 40% of patients taking the drug and, if present, is evident in the first few months of therapy. It occurs more often in children and adolescents. It may be averted or improved by careful oral hygiene and may be related to a deficiency in salivary IgA (Aarli 1976). Thickening of subcutaneous facial tissue, resulting in a coarsening of facial features, occurs less often and may have a mechanism in common with that of gingival hyperplasia. The changes in facial features are generally more marked in subjects who receive higher phenytoin doses for longer times.

Experimentally, in gingival fibroblast preparations phenytoin promotes tumor necrosis factor-induced production of interleukin-1β and prostaglandin E_2. This effect was further enhanced by prostaglandin H synthetase inhibitors, suggesting that phenytoin rather than its metabolites is the stimulus (Brunius et al. 1996). HAUCK et al. (1972) found that phenytoin caused a decrease in collagen turnover in fibroblast cultures.

Many of the other frequent chronic effects of phenytoin are of minor or minimal clinical significance, e.g. altered thyroid function tests and endogenous steroid levels, and slowing of nerve conduction velocities.

a) Enzyme Induction

Induction of vitamin D metabolism by phenytoin contributes to anticonvulsant osteomalacia in susceptible individuals, such as those with a deficient diet and suboptimal exposure to sunlight (EADIE and TYRER 1980).

B. Fosphenytoin

I. Introduction

Intravenous phenytoin is an effective treatment for status epilepticus, but the existing parenteral preparation is cumbersome, mainly due to phenytoin's low aqueous solubility. In order to make a parenteral formulation, phenytoin is dissolved in 40% propylene glycol and 10% alcohol, with sodium hydroxide added so that the final solution has a pH of 12. These additives and adjustments make phenytoin soluble, but also make the solution severely caustic to tissues should it be extravasated, and this limits the intramuscular use of the drug. Precipitated phenytoin crystals (WILENSKY and LOWDEN 1973) and tissue necrosis (SMITH et al. 1989) have been found at sites of intramuscular injection of the drug. The propylene glycol vehicle is partly responsible for the hypotension and bradyarrhythmias which may occur during intravenous infusion of the drug (LOUIS et al. 1967). Additionally, the solubility of phenytoin in this formulation remains fragile; the drug precipitates readily when mixed into a crystalline solution such as glucose, and precipitates after 1–2h in a saline solution.

Because of these limitations, there had long been a search for a phenytoin "prodrug" which would be rapidly metabolized to phenytoin but would have more favorable solubility properties. Fosphenytoin, first synthesized by STELLA and HIGUCHI (1973), is rapidly and completely converted to phenytoin after parenteral delivery, and has less toxicity than phenytoin due to its better solubility. The compound was synthesized by adding a "synthetic handle" in the form of disodium phosphate attached to a 3-(hydroxymethyl) phenytoin derivative. These improvements over the original parenteral phenytoin formulation led to the eventual marketing of fosphenytoin.

II. Chemistry and Use

1. Chemistry

Fosphenytoin is the disodium phosphate ester of 3-(hydroxymethyl)-phenytoin and has the chemical name 5,5′-diphenyl-3-[(phosphonooxy)methyl]-2,4-imidazolidinedione disodium salt. Its molecular weight of 406.24 is greater than that of phenytoin, but the dose of commercially available fosphenytoin is expressed in terms of the number of milligrams of phenytoin contained in it, i.e. phenytoin equivalents, and will be expressed in this manner in the text that follows. Its solubility is 75,000 mg/l, which is several orders of magnitude greater than that of phenytoin (BROWNE et al. 1993). Fosphenytoin is an off-white agglomerated powder supplied in a premixed solution at a concentration of 50 mg/ml. The solvents are water for injection (USP), and tromethamine (USP) (TRIS) buffer. The pH is adjusted to 8.6–9.0 with either hydrochloric acid or sodium hydroxide (CEREBYX 1996: package insert).

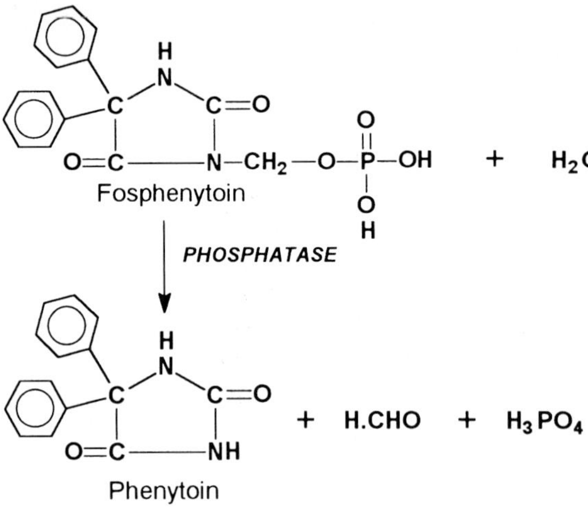

2. Indications and Use

Intravenous fosphenytoin is indicated for the treatment of status epilepticus. Fosphenytoin may be given intramuscularly if other routes of phenytoin delivery are not available. For clinical use, the dose in milligrams of fosphenytoin is the same as that for phenytoin. It can be substituted for oral phenytoin when deemed necessary, but its continuous use for more than 5 days has not been studied systematically (CEREBYX 1996: package insert). In order to obtain total and free plasma phenytoin levels as quickly as those resulting from phenytoin infusion at 50 mg/min, fosphenytoin must be given at 150 mg/min (ELDON et al. 1993). At the maximal delivery rates used in treating status epilepticus, the time to infuse 1000 mg fosphenytoin is 7 min, whereas 20 min is required to infuse 1000 mg phenytoin. An additional factor in achieving desired plasma levels of phenytoin rapidly during fosphenytoin infusion is the near-complete protein binding of fosphenytoin (95%). The drug appears to be more avidly protein-bound than phenytoin. Therefore, at the high concentrations produced by rapid infusion, fosphenytoin will displace phenytoin from its binding sites and transiently raise the level of free phenytoin in plasma (ELDON et al. 1993).

Due to potential adverse cardiovascular effects, fosphenytoin should be given intravenously no faster than at 150 mg/min. When given at this maximal rate, electrocardiographic, blood pressure and respiratory monitoring is needed (data on file: Parke-Davis, Morris Plains, NJ). When given at slower intravenous rates (below 100 mg/min) or intramuscularly using the 50 mg/ml solution, a therapeutic phenytoin level is reached in 30 min (KUGLER et al. 1996). High volumes (9–30 ml) of intramuscular fosphenytoin given at a single injection site were reportedly tolerated well (RAMSAY et al. 1995).

III. Pharmacodynamics

Equimolar doses of fosphenytoin and phenytoin have equivalent anticonvulsant activities against maximal electroshock-induced seizures in mice after intravenous, oral or intraperitoneal administration. The antiarrhythmic properties, effects on blood pressure, acute toxicity and median lethal doses were similar using several animal models given equimolar fosphenytoin and phenytoin doses by the intravenous, intramuscular or intraperitoneal routes. Fosphenytoin produced only inflammation at the intramuscular injection site in five of eight study dogs, in contrast to the haemorrhages and necrosis caused by intramuscular phenytoin (SMITH et al. 1989).

IV. Pharmacokinetics

1. Absorption and Disposition

In intravenous and intramuscular studies in drug-free volunteers and in intravenous studies in patients with therapeutic phenytoin levels, the bioavailability of single doses of fosphenytoin was complete, with AUC ratios of 1.0 (BROWNE et al. 1989, 1993). Since oral phenytoin is ~90% bioavailable, substituting intravenous or intramuscular fosphenytoin at the same dose as that for phenytoin may produce a slight increase in plasma phenytoin levels (CEREBYX 1996: package insert). The apparent volume of distribution is ~0.13 l/kg following a dose of 1200 mg fosphenytoin given at the maximum advised rate of 150 mg/min. Fosphenytoin is a highly plasma-soluble molecule and the majority of the drug achieves rapid equilibria between plasma and associated tissues. The clearance of fosphenytoin is ~250 ml/min at low doses and infusion rates, and increases to ~525 ml/min at higher doses and infusion rates; this increase is probably related to an increased free fraction of the drug at higher plasma concentrations (BROWNE et al. 1996).

2. Metabolism

A major consideration in using fosphenytoin in place of phenytoin in the treatment of status epilepticus is the time to cleave the molecule and convert fosphenytoin to phenytoin. The half-life of fosphenytoin conversion to phenytoin is 8–15 min. It shows little variation among the subjects studied and is not affected by the fosphenytoin or the phenytoin concentration (BROWNE et al.

1996). This complete and rapid conversion is due to the ubiquitous and abundant availability of phosphatases which are present in the liver, red blood cells and other tissues (QUON and STAMPFLI 1987). Besides phenytoin and phosphate, formaldehyde is also formed, but this substance is rapidly metabolized by folate systems. The conversion half-life of fosphenytoin is shorter in patients with hepatic and renal disease, probably due to decreased protein binding in these disease states (AWEEKA et al. 1989). The phenytoin resulting from fosphenytoin infusion is metabolized and eliminated through the same routes as phenytoin normally is (BROWNE et al. 1996). The renal excretion of fosphenytoin is minimal and not significant clinically (BROWNE et al. 1993).

3. Clinical Pharmacokinetics

Whole plasma phenytoin levels of 10–20 mg/l and free drug levels of 1–2 mg/l are the usual goals of therapy. However, plasma phenytoin levels may be overestimated if plasma samples are obtained within 2 h of fosphenytoin infusion and immunoanalytical techniques are used for the measurements, including TDx TDxFLx (fluorescence polarization) and Emit 2000 (enzyme multiplied) methods. Consistent with the vigorous plasma protein-binding of fosphenytoin, the drug also binds to the antibody used in the assays and thus adds to the measured phenytoin level. Therefore, phenytoin levels should be obtained at least 2 h after fosphenytoin infusions, by which time the prodrug conversion has been completed. This problem does not occur with chromatographic analytical methods.

V. Adverse Effects

In clinical trials of fosphenytoin, the most frequent side effects have been ataxia, dizziness, somnolence, nystagmus, headache, pruritus and paraesthesia. Except for pruritus and paraesthesia, these adverse events are probably due to phenytoin and are not specific for fosphenytoin. Pruritus and paraesthesia are seen with other phosphate prodrugs and are transient effects occurring with intravenous administration, and rarely with intramuscular administration. Notably, the paraesthesia have a predilection for the groin, back, head and neck. Compared with phenytoin, fosphenytoin infusion less often needs to be slowed or interrupted because of pain or discomfort at the infusion site, so that the average infusion time may be shorter. Hypotension is known to occur with phenytoin given intravenously, and also occurs with fosphenytoin infusion.

C. Mephenytoin

I. Introduction

In 1933, French and Swiss patents were issued to Sandoz Pharmaceuticals for mephenytoin (MERCK INDEX 1974), in some countries officially named methoin. TAINTER et al. (1943) demonstrated that mephenytoin suppressed electrically induced seizures in rabbits. Success in the use of this new agent to treat epilepsy was first reported by CLEIN (1945), and also by LOSCALZO (1945), who used a preparation consisting of mephenytoin and phenobarbitone. Beneficial effects in treating major motor seizures in particular were found, but frequent toxic reactions to the drug were subsequently reported by KOZOL (1950), LOSCALZO (1952) and ABBOTT and SCHWAB (1954), among others. BUTLER (1952) first described 5-ethyl-5-phenylhydantoin (*N*-desmethylmephenytoin or nor-mephenytoin) as the major metabolite of mephenytoin. This metabolite was later shown to be formed only from the R(–)-mephenytoin, whilst the S(+)-enantiomer is parahydroxylated (KUPFER et al. 1984). Nor-mephenytoin is the major active principle in the antiepileptic effect of mephenytoin and is identical to "Nirvanol". This latter drug had been used to produce nirvanol sickness as an intended cure for chorea in the 1920–1930 decade (JONES et al. 1932) but was eventually abandoned because of its high toxicity. The genetic polymorphism of mephenytoin metabolism was discovered in early 1980s, and poor and extensive metabolizers of the drug have been found (KUPFER et al. 1984). This polymorphism was caused by mutations in the cytochrome P450 isoenzyme CYP2C19 (DE MORAISE et al. 1994).

The current interest in mephenytoin lies mainly in its use as a convenient marker to identify individuals with defective CYP2C19.

II. Chemistry and Use

1. Chemistry

Mephenytoin (methoin: 3-methyl-5-ethyl-5-phenylhydantoin) is a white crystalline material with a molecular weight of 218.25 and a melting point of 137–138°C. It dissolves poorly in water, and the dissociation constant (pK_a) has not been calculated. The drug is moderately soluble in polar organic solvents. The commercially available preparation of the drug is a racemic mixture of its R(–) and S(+) enantiomers in approximate 50:50 proportions. The optical rotations of S(+)-mephenytoin are $[\alpha]125D = +105°$ and $[\alpha]125/365 = +416°$ and those of R(–)-mephenytoin are $[\alpha]125/D = -104°$ and $[\alpha]125/365 = -410°$.

Nirvanol, 5-ethyl-5-phenylhydantoin (identical with nor-mephenytoin, the active metabolite of mephenytoin), has a molecular weight of 204.2 and a melting point of 237°C. It is moderately soluble in organic solvents and reasonably soluble in water, with a pK_a value of 8.4. The optical rotation of each

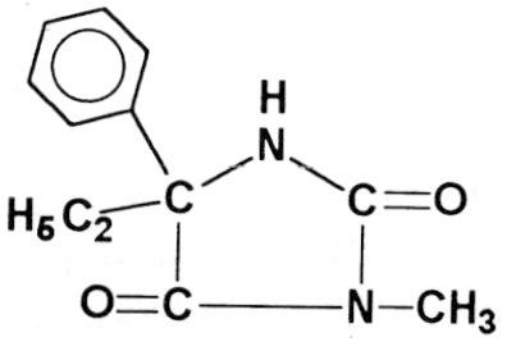

isomer is 115°. The multiplication factors to convert mephenytoin and nor-mephenytoin concentrations from mg/l to μmol/l are 4.58 and 4.90, respectively (MERCK INDEX 1974; KUPFERBERG 1982).

2. Indications and Use

Mephenytoin is most effective in the treatment of generalized convulsive seizures and partial seizures with or without generalization. It is of some benefit for myoclonic seizures (TROUPIN 1992), whereas absence seizures do not respond to it, or may worsen (LOSCALZO 1952). Mephenytoin is available as 100 mg tablets, whilst a tablet containing 100 mg mephenytoin and 20 mg phenobarbitone has been available in some countries. There are no parenteral preparations of the drug available at the present time.

The recommended starting daily dosages of the drug range from 150 mg in children to 300 mg in adults, followed by upward dosage adjustment as needed (LIVINGSTON 1972). Once the dosage has been stabilized, the daily effective amount may be given as a single intake because of the long half-life of the main active principle, nor-mephenytoin. The dose is best taken at bedtime, when any sedation from it would be less of a problem (TROUPIN 1992)

III. Pharmacodynamics

Mephenytoin is effective against maximal electroshock seizures in mice with an ED_{50} of 67 mg/kg. It is also effective against pentylenetetrazole seizures at a lower dose (ED_{50} 40 mg), and protects against bicuculline and picrotoxin-induced seizures with ED_{50} values of 124 and 100 mg/kg, respectively. The antiepileptic profile of the active metabolite, nor-mephenytoin, tested in the form of "Nirvanol", is similar to that of mephenytoin though the metabolite is slightly more potent, with an ED_{50} of 40 mg/kg for maximal electroshock seizures in mice (KUPFERBERG 1982).

IV. Pharmacokinetics

1. Absorption and Disposition

Mephenytoin is absorbed rapidly and fairly completely. The time to peak plasma concentration following ingestion of a 400 mg test dose was 45–120 min. Only about 40% of the mephenytoin and 30% of the nor-mephenytoin in plasma is protein bound (TROUPIN et al. 1972). The plasma half-life of racemic mephenytoin is 11–22 h, while that of nor-mephenytoin is 3–6 days (THEODORE et al. 1982). In the study of BURGEOIS et al. (1986), a very long elimination half-life (175 h) was found in a patient with poor renal function whose creatinine clearance was prolonged at 60.4 ml/min; for the entire group studied the elimination rate constant (k_{el}) for nor-mephenytoin correlated closely with the creatinine clearance. In the same study the renal clearance of nor-mephentoin ranged from 54 to 174 ml/kg/day, the total body clearance from 83 to 198 ml/kg/day, and the apparent volume of distribution from 0.77 to

1.1 l/kg. The nor-mephenytoin clearance is reduced in patients with impaired renal function due either to kidney disease or to old age: lower than average doses of mephenytoin are needed in these circumstances.

2. Metabolism

The oxidative biotransformation of 50:50 racemic commercial mephenytoin is mediated by cytochrome P450 isoenzymes of the CYP2C family. Due to stereospecificity, S(+)-mephenytoin is hydroxylated at the 4-, i.e. para, position of the phenyl ring to produce S(+)-4-hydroxy-mephenytoin, and the R(–)-mephenytoin is *N*-demethylated to produce R(–)-nor-mephenytoin (KUPFER et al. 1982, 1984a). It has now been confirmed that the major catalyst for the metabolism of mephenytoin is the isoenzyme CYP2C19 (WRIGHTON et al. 1993), while the CYP2C8, CYP2C9 and CYP2C18 isoforms may contribute at a 100 times lesser rate (GOLDSTEIN et al. 1994). In the formation of S(+)-4-hydroxy-mephenytoin the arene oxidation pathway is thought to yield an initial arene oxide intermediate, of which the majority (over 80%) quickly rearranges spontaneously (NIH-shift) to (S+)-4-hydroxy-mephenytoin. A minor portion becomes an epoxide which is then converted to a dihydrodiol by epoxide hydrolase activity (KUPFER et al 1984b). This latter enzyme is relevant in the genesis of some mephenytoin side effects. In cases of epoxide hydrolase deficiency, prolonged exposure of tissues to the epoxide occurs, and teratogenicity from the hydantoins has been documented (BUEHLER et al. 1990). Experimentally SPIELBERG et al. (1987) have shown in an in vitro system that inhibitors of epoxide hydrolase increased lymphocyte damage caused by mephenytoin metabolite(s). In the majority of subjects receiving racemic mephenytoin, however, the formation of (S+)-4-hydroxy-mephenytoin and the dihydrodiol is rapid and most of the ingested S(+)-mephenytoin portion of the dose appears in urine as glucuronide conjugates.

R(–)-mephenytoin is demethylated soon after ingestion, but the resulting R(–)-nor-mephenytoin is eliminated slowly, largely (80%–90%) in metabolically unchanged form (KUPFER et al. 1984a). This finding is in accordance with the fact that when R(–)-Nirvanol was given to subjects, 86% of the dose was recovered metabolically unchanged (BURGEOIS et al. 1986). In the average patient receiving racemic mephenytoin, both the S(+)-4-hydroxy and the R(–)-*N*-desmethyl metabolites were recovered in urine in amounts that accounted for about 45% of the dose of the racemate, together with very small amounts of unmetabolized enantiomers (KUPFER et al. 1982, 1984a). The ratio of (S+)- to (R-)-metabolites in the urine can vary, according to the amount of intact isoenzyme CYP2C19 that is present in the individual, and this is genetically regulated (KUPFER and PREISIG 1984; WARD et al. 1987).

a) Pharmacogenetics

Two defects in the CYP2C19 gene have been demonstrated using polymerase chain reaction techniques (DE MORAISE et al. 1994). The mutant m1 results from a guanine to adenine mutation at position 681 (G681 to A) in exon 5 and is seen in Caucasians, blacks and orientals. The mutant m2 (G636 to A) in exon 4 is seen in orientals only. These mutations produce aberrant splice site and truncated non-functional protein which lacks a heme-binding site. Individuals with mutation(s) in CYP2C19, often called poor metabolizers, have a limited capacity to 4-hydroxylate (S+)-mephenytoin, which causes a backup of unmetabolized S(+)-mephenytoin resulting in its eventual shunting into the demethylation pathway, causing an increase in the slowly excreted normephenytoin (KUPFER et al. 1984a). This accumulation of non-mephenytoin leads to intoxication from the high total concentration of active substances. The enzyme deficiency is inherited via a Mendelian autosomal recessive trait controlled by two alleles at a single autosomal gene location (WARD et al. 1987; BERTILSSON 1995). Individuals with very low hydroxylation capacities, the poor metabolizers, represent the homozygous recessive genotype, whereas the efficient metabolizers traditionally include the heterozygous average efficient and the highly efficient homozygous dominant genotypes (WARD et al. 1987; BERTILSSON 1995). The phenotype of an individual subject can be determined by two techniques. In one, the hydroxylation index is calculated by dividing the S(+)-mephenytoin dose (one-half of the amount of the racemate) by the amount of S(+)-OH-mephenytoin recovered in the urine. This gives values of 1–10 in efficient hydroxylators and 50–200 in poor hydroxylators (WEDLUND et al. 1984). The other method is to calculate the S/R ratio from the values of unmetabolized S(+)- and R(–)-mephenytoin recovered from urine 8h after a test dose of the racemic drug. This yields values of 0.1–0.8 in efficient and 0.9–1.2 in poor hydroxylators (TYBRING and BERTILSSON 1992).

The apparent polymorphism of mephenytoin metabolism shows marked variations among ethnic groups, poor (S+)-hydroxylators ranging from 1% to 5% in Caucasians and from 10% to 22% in orientals. The lowest rate (1.3%) was seen in a group of over 300 Spanish Caucasians (REVIRIEGO et al. 1993). Incidences of 3%–6% were reported from Swiss (KUPFER and PREISIG 1984), Estonian (KIIVET et al. 1993), Swedish (BERTILSSON et al. 1992), French (JACQZ et al. 1988) and United States (POLLOCK et al. 1991) Caucasian populations. In a Korean population the incidence was 12.6% (SOHN et al. 1992), in a Chinese one 14.3% and in a Japanese one 23% (BERTILSSON 1992). The incidence of mephenytoin poor hydroxylators in African Americans was 18.5% (POLLOCK et al 1991), but it was only 4% in Zimbabweans (MASIMIREMBWA et al. 1995) and 4%–5% in Nigerians and Tanzanians (SKJELBE at al. 1996). The incidence in Jordanians was 4.6% (HAIDI et al. 1995). BERTILSSON (1995) has suggested that the two mutants occurring in orientals might account for their overall high incidence of poor and intermediate (heterozygous) hydroxylators.

3. Clinical Pharmacokinetics

a) Dose-Plasma Level Relationships

At stable dosage a steady state plasma concentration of mephenytoin is reached in 48–72h, and that of nor-mephenytoin after nearly 2 weeks. The plasma concentration of nor-mephenytoin at steady state can be 5–8 times that of mephenytoin (TROUPIN et al. 1972; THEODORE et al. 1984), and varies with the phenotype. The dose-plasma level relationships are less predictable than for phenytoin. In average (S+)-mephenytoin hydroxylators receiving 400 mg of the drug daily, plasma mephenytoin levels ranged from 1 to 2 mg/l and those of nor-mephenytoin from 17 to 28 mg/l (THEODORE et al. 1984). This relationship becomes complex in poor S(+)-hydroxylators, in whom S(+)-mephenytoin accumulates and is shunted into a demethylation pathway. In such patients the mephenytoin dose has to be titrated individually.

b) Plasma Level-Effect Relationships

α) Beneficial Effects

To evaluate the plasma level/clinical effects relationship, TROUPIN (1992) has suggested adding the values of the plasma concentrations of the parent compound and the metabolite to obtain a "total mephenytoin" level. A reduction in seizures has occurred with such levels below 5 mg/l (THEODORE et al. 1984), but generally 10–35 mg/l is the useful plasma concentration range, and is obtained with a mephenytoin dose of 5–7 mg/kg daily (TROUPIN 1992).

β) Acute Toxic Effects

Overdosage effects begin to appear with plasma mephenytoin levels over 40 mg/l and are first manifested by drowsiness. Patients may accommodate to this effect and it may lessen with time (TROUPIN 1992).

V. Interactions

The concomitant use of carbamazepine and various barbiturates lowered the plasma levels of mephenytoin metabolic products, while elevations in level were produced by succinimides, phenacemide and nordiazepam (TROUPIN 1992). It is important to point out that the CYP2C19 isoenzyme involved in mephenytoin biotransformation is also utilized in, or contributes to, the biotransformation of chloroguanyl (SKJELBO et al. 1996), cimetidine (LEVY 1995), diazepam (ANDERSSON et al. 1994), fluoxetine, imipramine (MADSEN et al. 1995), methylphenobarbitone (mephobarbitone) (KUPFER and BRANCH 1985), omeprazole (CHANG et al. 1995), proguanyl and propranolol (BERTILSSON 1995) among other drugs. These drugs, when used together with mephenytoin, would be expected to compete for the available CYP2C19 and to cause accumulation of mephenytoin products in subjects with a marginal supply of efficient enzyme.

VI. Adverse Effects

The early signs and symptoms related to high mephenytoin and non-mephenytoin concentrations are sedation and confusion; with further increase in their plasma levels, disturbances of equilibrium and coordination occur. Double vision and nystagmus are less of a problem than with phenytoin (TROUPIN et al. 1972, 1973). One advantage of mephenytoin over phenytoin is that it rarely causes hirsutism and gum hypertrophy. Nausea may be present at the onset of therapy with the drug (LIVINGSTON 1972).

It has been pointed out that many of the serious and/or fatal effects of mephenytoin therapy have occurred in the setting of polypharmacy and that the real culprit may not have always been identified. The most alarming event is depression of the haematopoietic system. It may start with leucopenia and thrombocytopenia and may progress to pancytopenia and aplastic anaemia (ENGLAND and MCEACHERN 1962; ROBINS 1962). Haematological toxicity may appear within 6–8 months of the onset of therapy but may occur at any time subsequently. The precise incidence of aplastic anaemia from mephenytoin is not known but LIVINGSTON (1972) traced from the world literature 32 cases of aplastic anaemia in patients whose medication included mephenytoin; 20 had a fatal outcome. We have observed two patients who had received mephenytoin for over 10 years uneventfully but then developed thrombocytopenia after reaching their early seventies. The complication subsided upon changing the medication.

Dermatological complications of mephenytoin occur relatively frequently. Simple morbilliform rashes may occur in about 8%–12% of patients, usually appearing 10–14 days after the initiation of therapy. They may become associated with a serum sickness-like syndrome including lymphadenopathy, fever, leucopenia and eosinophilia. In most cases this "Nirvanol-sickness" like picture subsides after discontinuation of the drug (SHICK et al. 1933; KOZOL 1950; ABBOTT and SCHWAB 1954). The rash, particularly if of a purpuric variety, may proceed to exfoliative dermatitis or a Stevens-Johnson syndrome (LIVINGSTON 1972). These disorders were potentially fatal before the advent of steroid therapy. Renal toxicity from the drug is not common and liver damage occurs during severe allergic involvement. Insufficient data are on hand to evaluate the teratogenicity of mephenytoin, but LOSCALZO (1952) observed no complications in the baby or the mother in 15 pregnancies.

D. Ethotoin

I. Introduction

The synthesis of ethotoin was first reported by PINNER (1888); a commercial patent to manufacture ethotoin in the United States was issued to Abbott Laboratories in 1957 (MERCK INDEX 1974). SCHWADE et al. (1956) and LIVINGSTON (1956) first reported the effectiveness and low toxicity of ethotoin in the treatment of various types of seizures, including absences. Maintenance of seizure control, however, was difficult because of the low potency and the short half-life of the drug. More recent knowledge of ethotoin kinetics has enhanced its effectiveness clinically (CARTER et al. 1984; RITTER 1992).

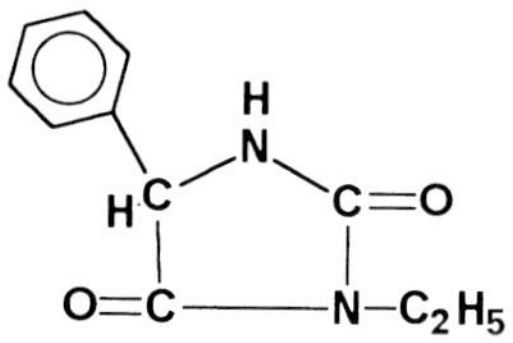

II. Chemistry and Use

1. Chemistry

Ethotoin (3-ethyl-5-phenylhydantoin) is a white crystalline material. Its molecular weight is 204.22 and its melting point is 94°C. Ethotoin is insoluble in cold water but dissolves in polar organic solvents. The optical rotation of R(–)-ethotoin is 88° (MERCK INDEX 1974). The conversion factor from mg/l to μmol/l for the drug is 4.9.

2. Indications and Use

Like phenytoin, ethotoin is effective against generalized tonic-clonic and partial seizures, but unlike phenytoin, it also has had some effectiveness in the treatment of absence and myoclonic seizures (SCHWADE et al. 1956). It is available only in tablets of 250 and 500 mg. The commonly recommended daily doses for adults range from 2000 to 4000 mg (LIVINGSTON 1972). Recently RITTER (1992) has pointed out that for some refractory seizures, up to 6000 mg a day are needed. In children, daily doses of 20–50 mg/kg have been effective (CARTER et al. 1984; RITTER 1992). Ethotoin therapy should be started at the low dose of 10–20 mg/kg, and the dose should be increased slowly every 5–7 days. High initial loading doses cause unacceptable side effects. The administration of the daily dose in three to four instalments is generally recommended and in some patients the bedtime dose needs to be higher to maintain seizure control until morning (RITTER 1992).

III. Pharmacodynamics

The antiepileptic profile of ethotoin resembles more closely that of mephenytoin than that of phenytoin. The ED_{50}, administered intraperitoneally, against electrically induced seizures was 85 mg/kg and that against seizures elicited with pentylenetetrazole was 48 mg/kg. The duration of the protective effects was shorter than that of mephenytoin (KUPFERBERG 1982).

IV. Pharmacokinetics

1. Absorption and Disposition

The absorption of ethotoin is adequate at lower oral doses of the drug but with higher single doses the plasma levels of the drug have been lower than expected. The time to peak plasma level following ingestion of 250 mg was 1–

2h, while following 2500mg the peak was reached in 4–6h (Meyer et al. 1983). About 50% of the ethotoin in plasma is protein bound (Troupin et al. 1979). The plasma half-life of ethotoin generally is short (4–7h), but longer half-lives have been observed following higher single doses of the drug. In volunteers Hooper et al. (1992) found that after a 1000mg test-dose the AUCs and half-lives of the S(+)- and R(–)-enantiomers were about equal, but the half-life of the de-ethylated metabolite was 30% longer than that of the parent compound. Non-linear ethotoin kinetics have been observed in several studies, and these may explain disproportionate changes in plasma ethotoin levels relative to the size of dosage changes (Naestroft et al. 1976; Meyer et al. 1983; Carter et al. 1984). In a group of patients receiving 15–40mg/kg ethotoin daily, the K_m ranged from 9 to 43mm/l and the V_{max} from 50 to 90mg/kg/day (Carter et al. 1984). Plasma ethotoin levels may stabilize after a few days of intake at stable dosage, but may then decline, which suggests that autoinduction of ethotoin metabolism occurs (Troupin et al. 1979).

2. Metabolism

A portion of the ethotoin dose, like that of mephenytoin, undergoes arene oxidation while another portion is N-dealkylated. Over ten metabolites of ethotoin have been identified (Naestroft and Larsen 1977; Bius et al. 1980; Kupferberg 1982). The arene oxide pathway yields mainly parahydroxy-ethotoin, in amounts of 14%–32% of the dose, along with small amounts (5%) of dihydrodiol and catechol metabolites (Naestroft and Larsen 1977). The hypothetical transient epoxide intermediates are likely to be formed in this pathway, and subjects deficient in epoxide hydrolase may be at risk of toxicity.

In the dealkylation pathway, the ethyl group is removed to yield 5-phenylhydantoin, which is then hydroxylated at the 5 position of the hydantoin ring to form 5-hydroxy-5-phenylhydantoin which is the major product of metabolism, accounting for about 30% of the dose (Naestroft and Larsen 1977). A portion of the 5-phenylhydantoin undergoes opening of the hydantoin ring and appears in the urine as R(–)-2-phenylhydantoic acid, which accounts for about 10% of the dose (Kupferberg 1982). Thus there is stereoselectivity of the biotransformation of the drug in that only the R(–)-enantiomers appear in the dealkylation pathway. Less than 10% of the dose appears in urine as unchanged ethotoin.

3. Clinical Pharmacokinetics

a) Dose-Plasma Level Relationships

With a given dose of ethotoin, the plasma level of the drug stabilizes within 2–5 days, the delay being longer if higher drug doses are used. The dose and plasma level relationships are less predictable than in the case of phenytoin and are subject to fluctuation with variation in the time between the last dose and the plasma sampling time. Stable doses of about 30mg/kg have produced levels from 15 to 20mg/l, whilst doses of 40mg/kg have yielded levels of 20–

30 mg/l in samples collected 2 h following the last dose. Samples taken 6 h after dosing (20–30 mg/kg) contained 3–13 mg/l ethotoin (CARTER et al. 1984).

b) Plasma Level-Effects Relationships

α) Beneficial Effects

Improved seizure control has been seen with plasma ethotoin levels between 6 and 59 mg/l (BITON et al. 1990) and between 14 and 34 ml/l (CARTER et al. 1984).

β) Acute Toxic Effects

Drowsiness and ataxia, together with nausea and vomiting, occur predictably in the majority of patients at relatively low plasma ethotoin levels during attempts to build up the levels quickly by using high loading doses of the drug. On the other hand, patients receiving chronic medication with ethotoin may feel well yet have plasma ethotoin levels above 50 mg/l. In general, ethotoin levels have been found to be of little clinical usefulness in dosage adjustment or in the evaluation of the side effects of the drug (RITTER 1992).

V. Interactions

Ethotoin intake reduces plasma carbamazepine levels and increases plasma phenytoin levels (BITON et al. 1990). Ethotoin plasma levels were lower in patients also receiving barbiturates or carbamazepine than in those taking ethotoin monotherapy (CARTER et al. 1984).

VI. Adverse Effects

Signs and symptoms related to high ethotoin doses and concentrations include drowsiness, ataxia, gastrointestinal upsets and photophobia. Adverse cosmetic effects of the drug are rare. Remarkably, gum hypertrophy has been observed to resolve when phenytoin was replaced with ethotoin. Skin rashes occur in 5% of cases, but haematological complications and lymphadenopathies are quite rare (LIVINGSTON 1972; TROUPIN et al. 1979).

No specific adverse effects of the drug on pregnant women have been described. In teratogenic potential ethotoin resembles phenytoin. Dysmorphic features of the foetal hydantoin syndrome were observed in three children (FINNELL et al. 1983) and one baby had a cleft lip (ZAHLEN and BRAND 1977) in the offspring of mothers who took the drug during pregnancy.

E. Phenacetamide

I. Introduction

The synthesis of phenacemide was first described by BASTERFIELD et al. in 1933 (MERCK INDEX 1974) and also reported by SPIELMAN et al. (1948). The antiepileptic activity of phenacemide in animals was described by EVERETT and SCHWAB (1949). In clinical trials phenacemide was found to be effective, most notably against partial complex seizures even in patients who did not respond to phenytoin and barbiturates (GIBBS et al. 1949; LIVINGSTON and PAULI 1957). Toxic effects of the drug were frequent, however, and included numerous fatalities from liver damage, so that the drug was recommended and used infrequently. Renewed interest developed when COKER et al. (1987) reported the successful use of phenacemide monotherapy in children, without serious complications. SPIELBERG et al. (1981) have shown that phenacemide metabolites cause cell damage in vitro.

II. Chemistry and Use

1. Chemistry

Phenacemide (phenylacetylurea) is a white crystalline material with a molecular weight of 178.19. Its solubility in water is no more than fair but it dissolves in polar organic solvents. The molecule has been considered a hydantoin ring broken between the 5-C and the N atoms. In three-dimensional crystal X-ray diffraction views of the substance, the straight chain assumes a pseudo-cyclic hydantoin-like formation (CAMERMAN and CAMERMAN 1977). The conversion factor for converting its concentrations from mg/l to μmol/l is 5.6.

2. Indications and Use

Phenacemide has proved effective against complex partial and generalized tonic-clonic seizures; absence seizures have responded in some patients. It is available as 500 mg, and in some countries also as 300 and 250 mg, tablets. The effective doses have ranged from 1000 to 2000 mg daily in children and from 1500 to 3000 mg daily in adults. The recommended starting dose in children is 30 mg/kg, which is increased to 50 mg/kg or more if needed. Adults can start treatment with 1500 mg in divided doses followed by a gradual increase, as necessary. It is important to monitor the plasma biochemistry profile, including liver function tests and haematological parameters (LIVINGSTON 1972; COKER 1992). The occasionally observed elevation of serum creatinine level when the drug is used does not indicate renal insufficiency (RICHARDS et al. 1978); it is thought to be caused by inhibition of creatinine transport and a decrease in its volume of distribution (CAHEN et al. 1994).

III. Pharmacodynamics

Phenacemide is effective against electrically induced seizures in animals and also protects against pentylenetetrazole and picrotoxin seizures with a relatively high protective index (EVERETT and RICHARDS 1952).

IV. Pharmacokinetics

1. Absorption and Disposition

Phenacemide is reasonably well absorbed, peak plasma levels occurring within 1–2 h of ingestion. The plasma half-life has ranged from 22 to 25 h. Following a 1000 mg test-dose the apparent volume of distribution was 1.5 l/kg, the plasma clearance 41 ml/h/kg and the elimination rate constant 0.0027/h (COKER et al. 1987). The extent of binding of phenacemide to plasma proteins ranged from 28% to 36% (KUTT 1992).

2. Metabolism

Information about phenacemide's biotransformation in man is scarce. Several additional "drug" peaks have been observed in chromatographic assays of phenacemide plasma levels. Some of these peaks appear to be more polar than the parent compound, suggesting the possibility of hydroxylated metabolites (KUTT 1992). In rabbits TATSUMI et al. (1967) found that the major pathway of biotransformation seemed to be parahydroxylation of the phenol ring followed by methylation; the ureide group may also be removed. Only a small portion of the drug was recovered unchanged. In this hydroxylation (arene oxide) pathway, generation of toxic epoxide intermediaries is likely to occur. This might be relevant in view of toxic metabolites of phenacemide generated in vitro, which caused destruction of lymphocytes; the damage was enhanced by adding epoxide hydrolase inhibitors (SPIELBERG et al. 1981).

3. Clinical Pharmacokinetics

a) Dose, Plasma Level and Effect Relationships

In phenacemide monotherapy, following stabilization of dosage, steady-state plasma levels are reached in 5–10 days. Phenacemide doses of 30–40 mg/kg have produced plasma phenacemide levels of 30–50 mg/l, and 50–90 mg/kg daily doses levels of 50–70 mg/l. Beneficial effects may be seen with plasma levels over 40 mg/l, whilst for good seizure control levels over 50 mg/l usually are needed. High concentration-related symptoms and signs begin to occur with plasma phenacetamide levels over 70 mg/l (COKER et al. 1987; COKER 1992). Polytherapy, particularly if enzyme inducing drugs are used, may increase the incidence of cell-toxic reactions.

V. Interactions

No reports of pharmacokinetic interactions of phenacemide are available but its ethylated derivative, pheneturide, has caused elevation of phenytoin levels. Microsomal oxidation-inducing drugs would be expected to reduce phenacemide level-to-dose ratios. A pharmacodynamic interaction in the form of a severe psychotic reaction occurred in a patient receiving phenacemide with ethotoin (LIVINGSTON 1972).

VI. Adverse Effects

Manifestations related to high phenacemide concentrations include drowsiness, ataxia and nystagmus. Personality changes such as irritability and aggression, as well as depression, suicidal tendencies and paranoid and delusional reactions have been observed (LIVINGSTON 1972).

The most serious complication of phenacemide therapy is liver damage. If the drug is stopped in time, the patient may recover, although some have developed residual cirrhosis. The clinical incidence of hepatitis has been about 6%; ten fatalities have been reported (LIVINGSTON 1972; COKER et al. 1987). Aplastic anaemia has also been of concern, as several fatalities have been reported. Leucopenia has been observed in up to 6% of patients (ROBINS 1962). Skin rashes may occur in 5%–8% of patients, usually appearing soon after the onset of therapy. They will subside when the drug is discontinued (LIVINGSTON and PAULI 1957). Insufficient data are available concerning the effects of phenacemide in pregnancy.

F. Albutoin

I. Introduction

The synthesis of albutoin was reported by Oba et al. in 1952 (MERCK INDEX 1974). DAVIS and SCHWADE (1959) first described its successful use in the treatment of patients with various types of seizure. Subsequent reports emphasized its low toxicity, but it had a variable effectiveness seen mostly in generalized tonic-clonic and partial seizures (GREEN et al. 1969; MILLICHAP and ORTIZ 1969; CARTER 1971). Since the mid 1970s, interest in albutoin has waned.

II. Chemistry and Use

Albutoin, 3-allyl-5-isobutyl-2-thiohydantoin, is a crystalline material with a molecular weight of 212.33 and a melting point of 210–211°C (MERCK INDEX 1974). The factor to convert its concentrations from mg/l to μmol/l is 4.7. Albutoin was available in 50, 100, and 200 mg tablets.

III. Pharmacology

1. Animal Pharmacology

In mice the ED_{50} of albutoin given intraperitoneally against electrically induced seizures was 50–60 mg/kg and that against pentylenetetrazole seizures was 11 mg/kg (GESLER et al. 1961).

2. Human Use

In a random series of patients, Millichap and Ortiz used 5 mg/kg albutoin as a starting dose to be increased slowly to 7.5 mg/kg. They found that in equal doses albutoin and phenytoin were equally effective but that there were fewer side effects with albutoin in the higher dosage range. In drug-resistant institutionalized patients, 1200 mg/day albutoin compared poorly with 300 mg phenytoin or 750 mg primidone as an anticonvulsant. Albutoin plasma levels up to 4 mg/l were recorded in these patients (Cereghino et al. 1972). Even 1600 mg/day albutoin was not particularly successful (Green et al. 1969). Nausea, vomiting and anorexia were the common side effects in all studies, while one instance of skin rash was observed. No characteristic laboratory abnormalities occurred.

References

Aarli JA (1976) Phenytoin-induced depression of salivary IgA and gingival hyperplasia. Epilepsia 17:283–291

Abbott JA, Schwab RS (1954) Mesantoin in the treatment of epilepsy: a study of its effects on the leucocyte count in seventy-nine cases. New Engl J Med 250:197–199

Andersson T, Miners JO, Veronese ME, Birkett DJ (1994) Diazepam metabolism by human microsomes is mediated by both (S)-mephenytoin hydroxylase and CYP3 A isoforms. Br J Clin Pharmacol 38:131–137

Aweeka F, Alldredge B, Boyer T, Warnock D, Gambertoglio J (1989) Conversion of ACC-9653 to phenytoin in patients with renal or hepatic diseases. Clin Pharmacol Ther 45:152

Bennett GD, Lau F, Calvin JA, Finnel RH (1997) Phenytoin-induced teratogenesis: a molecular basis for the observed developmental delay during neurulation. Epilepsia 38:415–423

Bertilsson L (1995) Geographical/interracial differences of polymorphic drug oxidation. Current state of knowledge of cytochromes P450 (CYP) 26D and 2C19. Clin Pharmacokinet 23:192–209

Bertilsson L, Lou YQ, Du YL et al. (1992) Pronounced differences between native Chinese and Swedish population in the polymorphic hydroxylation of debrisoquin and S-mephenytoin. J Chromatogr 51:388–397

Biltz H (1908) Uber die Konstitution der Einwirkungsprodukte von substituierten Harnstoffen auf Benzil und einige neue Methoden zur Darstellung der 5,5-Diphenylhydantoine. Ber Dtsch Chem Ges 41:1379–1393

Biton V, Gates JR, Ritter FJ, Loewenson RB (1990) Adjunctive therapy for intractable epilepsy with ethotoin. Epilepsia 31:433–337

Bius DL, Yonekawa WD, Kupferberg HJ, Cantor F, Dudley KH (1980) Gas chromatographic-mass spectrometric studies on the metabolic fate of ethtoin in man. Drug Metab Dispos 8:223–229

Browne TR, Le Duc B (1995) Phenytoin. Chemistry and biotransformation. In: Levy RH, Mattson RH, Meldrum BS (eds) Antiepileptic drugs, 4th edn. Raven Press, New York, pp. 283–300

Browne TR, Davoudi H, Donn Khet et al. (1989) Bioavailability of ACC-9653 (phenytoin prodrug). Epilepsia 30 [Suppl 2]:S27–S32

Browne TR, Kugler AR, Eldon MA (1996) Pharmacology and pharmacokinetics of fosphenytoin. Neurology 46 [Suppl 1]:S3–S7

Browne TR, Szabo GK, McEntagert C et al. (1993) Bioavailability studies of drugs with nonlinear pharmacokinetics. II. Absolute bioavailability of intravenous phenytoin

prodrug at therapeutic phenytoin serum concentration determined by double stable phenytoin isotope technique. J Clin Pharmacol 33:89–94
Brunius G, Yucel-Lindberg T, Shinoda K, Modeer T (1996) Effect of phenytoin on interleukin-1 beta production in human gingival fibroblasts challenged to tumor necrosis factor alpha in vitro. Eur J Oral Sci 104:27–33
Buehler BA, Delimont D, van Waes M, Finnell RH (1990) Prenatal prediction of risk of the fetal hydantoin syndrome. N Engl J Med 322:1567–1572
Burgeois BFD, Kupfer A, Wad N, Egli M (1986) Pharmacokinetics of R-enantiomeric normephenytoin during chronic administration in epileptic patients. Epilepsia 27:412–418
Butler TC, Dudley KH, Johnson D, Roberts SB (1976) Studies of the metabolism of 5,5-diphenylhydantoin relating principally to the stereoselectivity of the hydroxylation reaction in man and the dog. J Pharmacol Exp Ther 199:82–92
Cahen R, Martin A, Francois B, Baltassat P, Loisot P (1994) Creatinine metabolism impairment by an anticonvulsant drug, phenacemide. Ann Pharmacother 28:49–51
Camerman A, Camerman N (1977) Ethyl-phenacemide and phenacemide conformational similarities to diphenyl-hydantoin and stereochemical basis of anticonvulsant activity. Proc Natl Acad Sci 74:1264–1266
Carter AC, Helms RA, Boehm R (1984) Ethotoin in seizures of childhood and adolescence. Neurology 34:791–795
Carter CH (1971) Albutoin in treatment of epilepsy. Clin Med 78:33–35
Cerebyx (fosphenytoin sodium injection) (1996) Package insert. Parke-Davis, Morris Plains, NJ
Cereghino JJ, Brock JT, Penry JK (1972) Other hydantoins. Albutoin. In: Woodbury DM, Penry JK, Schmidt RP (eds) Antiepileptic drugs. Raven Press, New York, pp. 283–291
Chang M, Dahl ML, Tybring G, Gotharson E, Bertilsson L (1995) Use of omeprazole as a probe for CYP2C19 phenotype in Swedish Caucasians: comparison with S-mephenytoin hydroxylation phenotype and CYP2C19 genotype. Pharmacogenetics 5:358–363
Coker SB (1986) The use of phenacemide for intractable partial complex epilepsy in children. Pediatr Neurol 2:230–232
Coker SB (1992) Phenacemide. In: Resor SR, Kutt H (eds) The medical treatment of epilepsy. Marcel Dekker, New York, pp. 389–392
Coker SB, Holmes EW, Egel RT (1981) Phenacemide therapy of complex partial epilepsy in children: determination of plasma drug concentration. Neurology 37:1861–1866
Courtney KR, Etter EF (1983) Modulated anticonvulsant block of sodium channels in nerve and muscle. Eur J Pharmacol 88:1–9
Dansky LV, Rosenblatt DS, Andermann E (1992) Mechanisms of teratogenesis: folic acid and antiepileptic therapy. Neurology 42 [Suppl 5]:S8–S16
Davis JP, Schwade ED (1959) Anticonvusant effects of 3-allyl-5-isobutyl-2-thiohydantoin (Bax 422Z). Fed Proc 18:380
De Moraise SMF, Wilkinson GR, Blaisdell J, Meyer UA, Nakamura K, Goldstein JA (1994) Identification of a new genetic defect responsible for the polymorphism of (S)-mephenytoin metabolism in Japanese. Mol Pharmacol 46:594–598
DeLorenzo RJ (1995) Phenytoin. Mechanism of action. In: Levy RH, Mattson RH, Meldrum BS (eds) Antiepileptic drugs. 4th edn. Raven Press, New York, pp. 271–282
Eadie MJ (1984) Anticonvulsant drugs. An update. Drugs 27:328–363
Eadie MJ, Tyrer JH (1980) Anticonvulsant therapy. Pharmacological basis and practice. Edinburgh, London and New York, Churchill Livingstone
Edeki TI, Brase DA 1995 Phenytoin disposition and toxicity: role of pharmacogenetic and interethnic factors. Drug Metabol Rev 27:449–469
Eldon MA, Loewen GR, Voightman RE et al. (1993) Safety, tolerance and pharmacokinetics of intravenous fosphenytoin. Clin Pharmacol Ther 53:212

England NJ, McEachern D (1949) Aplastic anaemia during Mesantoin therapy Can Med Assoc J 60:173–175
Esplin D (1957) Effect of diphenylhydantoin on synaptic transmission in the cat spinal cord and stellate ganglion. J Pharmacol Exp Ther 120:301–323
Everett GM, Richards RK (1952) Pharmacological studies of phenylacetylurea (Phenurone), an anticonvulsant drug. J Pharmacol Exp Ther 106:303–313
Finnell RD, DiLiberti JH (1983) Hydantoin-induced teratogenesis: are arene oxide intermediaries really responsible? Helv Paediatr Acta 38:171–177
Finnell RH, Buehler BA, Kerr BM, Ager PL, Levy RH (1992) Clinical and experimental studies linking oxidative metabolism to phenytoin-induced teratogenesis. Neurology 42 [Suppl 5]:S25–S31
Finnell RH, Nau H, Yerby MS (1995) Teratogenicity of antiepileptic drugs. In: Levy RH, Mattson RH, Meldrum BS (eds) Antiepileptic drugs. 4th edn, Raven Press, New York, pp. 209–230
Fritz S, Lindner W, Roots I, Frey BM Kupfer A (1987) Stereochemistry of aromatic phenytoin hydroxylation in various drug hydroxylation phenotypes in humans. J Pharmacol Exp Ther 241:615–622
Garcia-Suarez J, Dominguez-Franjo P, Del Campo J, Herrero B, Munoz MA, Piris MA, Pardo A (1996) EBV-positive non-Hodgkin's lymphoma developing after phenytoin therapy. Br J Haematol 95:376–379
Gesler RM, Lints CE, Swinyard EA (1961) Pharmacology of some substituted 2-thiohydantoin with particular reference to anticonvulsant properties. Toxicol Appl Pharmacol 3:107–121
Gibbs FA, Everett GM, Richards RK (1949) Phenurone in epilepsy. Dis Nerv Syst 10:47–49
Goldstein JA, Faletto MB, Romkes-Sparks M et al. (1994) Evidence that CYP2C19 is the major (S)-mephenytoin 4′-hydroxylase in humans. Biochemistry 33:1743–1752
Green JR, Miller LH, Burnett PD, Wasch AA Jr (1969) Clinical evaluation of albutoin. Neurology 19:1207–1211
Haidi HF, Irshaid YM, Woolsey RL, Idle JR, Flockhart DA (1995) S-Mephenytoin hydroxylation phenotype in a Jordanian population. Clin Pharmacol Ther 56:542–547
Hartsfield JK Jr, Benford SA, Hibelink DR (1995) Induction of microsomal epoxide hydrolase activity in inbred mice by chronic phenytoin exposure. Biochem Molec Medicine 56:144–151
Hashimoto Y, Otsuki Y, Odani A, Tanako M, Hattori E, Furusho K, Iui K (1996) Effect of CYP2 C polymorphism on the pharmacokinetics of phenytoin in Japanese patients with epilepsy. Biol Pharm Bull 19:1103–1105
Hauck JC, Cheng RF, Waters MD (1972) Diphenylhydantoin. Effects on connective tissue and wound repair. In: Woodbury DM, Penry JK, Schmidt RP (eds) Antiepileptic drugs. 1st edn, Raven Press, New York, pp. 267–274
Ieiri I, Mamiya K, Urae A et al. (1997) Stereoselective 4′-hydroxylation of phenytoin: a relationship to (S)-mephenytoin polymorphism in Japanese. Brit J Clin Pharmacol 43:441–445
Inaba T (1990) Phenytoin: pharmacogenetic polymorphism of 4′-hydroxylation. Pharmac Ther 46:341–347
Jacqz E, Dulac H, Mathieu H (1988) Phenotyping polymorphic drug metabolism in French Caucasian population. Eur J Clin Pharmacol 35:167–171
Jones JD, Jacobs JL (1932) The treatment of obstinate chorea with Nirvanol with notes on its mode of action. J Amer Med Assoc 99:18–21
Kiivet RA, Svensson JO, Bertilsson L, Sjoqvist F (1993) Polymorphism of debrisoquine and mephenytoin hydroxylation among Estonians. Pharmacol Toxicol 72:113–115
Kim PM, Wells PG (1995) Phenytoin-initiated hydroxyl radical formation: characterization by enhanced salicylate hydroxylation. Mol Pharmacol 49:172–181
Kozol HL (1950) Mesantoin in treatment of epilepsy. Arch Neurol Psychiatr 63:235–248

Kugler AR, Knapp LE, Eldon MA (1996) Rapid attainment of therapeutic phenytoin concentrations following administration of loading doses of fosphenytoin: a meta-analysis. Neurology 46 [Suppl]:A176
Kupfer A, Branch RA (1985) Stereoselective mephobarbital hydroxylation cosegregates with mephenytoin hydroxylation. Clin Pharm Ther 38:414–418
Kupfer A, Preisig R (1984) Pharmacogenetics of mephenytoin: a new drug hydroxylation polymorphism in man. Eur J Clin Pharmacol 26:753–759
Kupfer A, Desmond PV, Schenker S, Branch RA (1982) Stereoselective metabolism and disposition of the enantiomers of mephenytoin during oral administration of the racemic drug in man. J Pharmacol Exp Ther 221:590–597
Kupfer A, Desmond P, Patwardhan R, Schenker S, Branch RA (1984a) Mephenytoin hydroxylation deficiency: kinetics after repeated doses. Clin Pharmacol Ther 35:33–39
Kupfer A, Lawson J, Branch RA (1984b) Stereoselectivity in the arene oxide pathway of mephenytoin hydroxylation in man. Epilepsia 25:1–7
Kupferberg HJ (1982) Other hydantoins. Mephenytoin and ethotoin. In: Woodbury DM, Penry JK, Pippenger C (eds) Antiepileptic drugs. 2nd edn, Raven Press, New York, pp. 282–295
Kuruvilla T, Bharucah NE (1997) Cerebellar atrophy after acute phenytoin intoxication. Epilepsia 38:500–502
Kutt H (1990) Hydantoins. In: Dam M, Gram L (eds) Comprehensive epileptology. Raven Press, New York, pp. 563–577
Kutt H (1995) Phenytoin. Interactions with other drugs: clinical aspects. In: Levy RH, Mattson RH, Meldrum BS (eds) Antiepileptic drugs. 4th edn. Raven Press, New York, pp. 315–328
Kutt H, McDowell F (1968) Management of epilepsy with diphenylhydantoin. J Amer Med Assoc 203:969–972
Kutt H, Penry JK (1974) Usefulness of blood levels of antiepileptic drugs. Arch Neurol 31:283–288
Kutt H, Wolk M, Scherman R, McDowell F (1964) Insufficient parahydroxylation as cause of diphenylhydantoin toxicity. Neurology 14:542–548
Le Duc BW, Szabo GK, Browne TR (1997) Phenytoin metabolism: pharmacogenetic differences and lack of inhibition by carbamazepine, carbamazepine epoxide and carbamazepine diol. Neurology 48 [Suppl 5]:A110
Leeder JS, Riley RJ, Cook VA, Spielberg SP (1992) Human anti-cytochrome P450 antibodies in aromatic anticonvulsant induced hypersensitivity. J Pharmacol Exper Ther 263:360–367
Levy RH (1995) Cytochrome P450 izoenzymes and antiepileptic drug interactions. Epilepsia 36 [Suppl] 5:S8–13
Levy RH, Bajpai M (1995) Phenytoin. Interactions with other drugs: mechanistic aspects. In: Levy RH, Mattson RH, Meldrum BS (eds) Antiepileptic drugs. 4th edn, Raven Press, New York, pp. 329–338
Lindhout D (1992) Pharmacogenetics and drug interactions: role in antiepileptic-drug-induced teratogenesis. Neurology 42 [Suppl 5]:S43–S47
Liu L, Wells PG (1995) DNA oxidation as a potential molecular mechanism mediating drug-induced birth defects: phenytoin and structurally related teratogens initiate the formation of 8-hydroxy-2′-deoxyguanosine in vitro in murine maternal hepatic and embryonic tissues. Free Radic Biol Med 19:639–648
Livingston S (1956) The use of peganone (AC–695) in the treatment of epilepsy. J Pediatr 49:728–733
Livingston S (1972) Comprehensive management of epilepsy in infancy, childhood and adolescence. Charles C Thomas, Springfield
Livingston S, Pauli LL (1957) Phenacemide in the treatment of epilepsy. New Eng J Med 256:588–592
Loscalzo AE (1945) Treatment of epileptic patients with a combination of 3-methyl 5-5-phenylethyl hydantoin and phenobarbital. J Nerv Ment Dis 101:537–544

Loscalzo A (1952) Mesantoin in the control of epilepsy. Neurology 2:403–411
Louis S, Kutt H, McDowell F (1967) The cardiocirculatory changes caused by intravenous Dilantin and its solvent. Am Heart J 74:523–529
Louis S, Kutt H, McDowell F (1968) Intravenous diphenylhydantoin in experimental seizures. II. Effect on penicillin-induced seizures in the cat. Arch Neurol 18:472–477
Lund L (1974) Anticonvulsant effect of diphenylhydantoin relative to plasma level. A prospective three year study in ambulant patients with generalized epileptic seizures. Arch Neurol 31:289–294
Macdonald RL (1989) Antiepileptic drug actions. Epilepsia 30 [Suppl 1]:S19–S28
Maguire JH, Wettrell C, Rane A (1987) Apparently normal phenytoin metabolism in a patient with phenytoin-induced rash and lymphadenopathy. Br J Clin Pharmac 24:554–557
Masimirembwa C, Bertilsson L, Johansson I, Hasler JA, Ingelman-Sudberg M (1995) Phenotyping and genotyping of S-mephenytoin hydroxylase (cytochrome P450 2C19) in a Shona population in Zimbabwe. Clin Pharmacol Ther 57:656–661
Mays DC, Pawluk LJ, Apseloff G, Davis WB, She ZW, Sagone AL, Gerber N (1995) Metabolism of phenytoin and covalent binding of reactive intermediates in activated human neutrophils. Biochem Pharmacol 50:367–380
McLanahan JS, Maguire JH (1986) High-performance liquid chromatographic determination of the enantiomeric composition of urinary metabolites of phenytoin. J Chromat 381:438–446
Merck Index (1974) Piscattaway, NJ. Merck Publications
Meyer MC, Holocombe BJ, Burckart GJ, Raghow G, Yau MK (1983) Nonlinear ethotoin kinetics. Clin Pharmacol Ther 33:329–334
Millichap JG, Ortiz WR (1967) Albutoin, a new thiohydantoin derivative for grand mal epilepsies. Comparison with diphenylhydantoin in a double-blind study. Neurology 17:163–165
Miranda AF, Wiley MJ, Wells PG (1994) Evidence for embryonic peroxidase-catalyzed bioactivation and glutathione-dependent cytoprotection in phenytoin teratogenecity: modulation by eicosatetraynoic acid and buthionine sulphoximidine in murine embryo culture. Toxicol Applied Pharmacol 124:230–241
Murray M (1992) P450 enzymes. Inhibition mechanisms, genetic regulation and effects of liver disease. Clin Pharmacokinet 23:123–146
Naestroft J, Larsen NE (1977) Mass fragmentographic quantitation of ethotoin and some of its metabolites in human urine. J Chromatogr 143:161–169
Naestroft J, Hvidberg EF, Sjo O (1976) Saturable metabolic pathway for ethotoin in man. Clin Pharmacol Physiol 3:453–459
Nation RL, Evans AM, Milne RW (1990a) Pharmacokinetic drug interaction with phenytoin (Part I). Clin Pharmacokinet 18:37–60
Nation RL, Evans AM, Milne (1990b) Pharmacokinetic drug interactions with phenytoin (Part II) Clin Pharmacokinet 18:131–150
Osborne HH, Zisfein J, Sparano R (1987) Single-dose oral phenytoin loading. Ann Emerg Med 16:407–12
Pollock BG, Perel JM, Kirshner M, Altieri LP, Yaeger AL (1991) Mephenytoin 4-hydroxylation in older Americans. Br J Clin Pharmacol 31:689–692
Puttnam TJ, Rothenberg SF (1953) Results of intensive (narcosis) and standard medical treatment of epilepsy. J Amer Med Assoc 152:1400–1406
Quon CY, Stampfli HE (1987) In vitro hydrolysis of ACC–0653 (phosphate ester prodrug of phenytoin) by human, dog, rat, blood and tissues. Pharm Res 3 [Suppl 5]:1349
Raines A, Standaert FR (1966) Pre- and post-junctional effects of DPH at the cat soleus neuromuscular junction. J Pharmacol Exp Ther 153:361–366
Ramsay RE, Barkley GL, Garnett WR et al (1995) Safety and tolerance of intramuscular fosphenytoin (Cerebyx) in patients requiring a loading dose of phenytoin. Neurology 45 [Suppl 4]:A249

Rapport RL, Shaw CM (1977) Phenytoin-related cerebellar degeneration without seizures. Ann Neurol 2:437–439
Reviriego J, Bertilsson L, Carillo JA, Llerena A, Valdivielso MJ, Benitez J (1993) Frequency of S-mephenytoin hydroxylation deficiency in 373 Spanish subjects compared to other Caucasian populations. Eur J Clin Pharmacol 44:593–595
Richards RK, Bjornsson TD, Waterbury LD (1978) Rise in serum and urine creatinine after phenacemide. Clin Pharmacol Ther 23: 430–437
Robins MM (1962) Aplastic anaemia secondary to anticonvulsant medication. Amer J Dis Child 104:614–624
Schick B, Sobotka H, Peck S (1933) Chemical allergy and Nirvanol sickness. Amer J Dis Child 45:1216–1220
Schwade ED, Richards RK, Everett GM (1956) Peganone, a new antiepileptic drug. Dis Nerv Syst 17:155–158
Skjelbo E, Mutabingwa TK, Bygbjerg IB, Nielsen KK, Gram LF, Broosen K (1996) Chloroguanide metabolism in relation to the efficacy in malaria prophylaxis and the S-mephenytoin oxidation in Tanzanians. Clin Pharmacol Ther 59:304–311
Smith RD, Brown BS, Maher RW, Matier WL (1989) Pharmacology of ACC-9653 (Phenytoin Prodrug). Epilepsia 30 [Suppl 2]:S15–S21
Spielberg SP, Gordon GB, Blake DA, Mellitis ED, Bross DS (1981) Anticonvulsant toxicity in vitro : possible role of arene oxides. J Exp Ther 217:386–389
Spielman MA, Geiszler AO, Close WJ (1948) Anticonvulsant drugs, II. Some acetylureas. J Amer Chem Soc 70:4189–4191
Stella V, Higuchi T (1973) Esters of hydantoic acid as prodrugs of hydantoins. J Pharm Sci 62:962
Tainter ML, Tainter EG, Sherwood Lawrence W et al. (1943) Influence of various drugs on the threshold for electrical convulsions. J Pharmacol Exp Ther 79:42–54
Tatsumi K, Yoshimura H, Tsukamoto (1967) Metabolism of drugs – the fate of phenylacetylurea. Biochem Pharmacol 16:1941–1951
Theodore WH, Newmark ME, Desai BT, Kupferberg HJ, Penry JK, Porter RJ, Yonekawa WD (1984) Disposition of mephenytoin and its metabolite, Nirvanol, in epileptic patients. Neurology 34:1100–1102
Troupin AS (1992) Mephenytoin. In: Resor SR, Kutt H (eds) The medical treatment of epilepsy. Marcel Dekker, New York, pp. 399–404
Troupin AS, Ojeman LM, Dodrill CB (1976) Mephenytoin: a reappraisal. Epilepsia 17:403–414
Troupin AS, Friel P, Lovely MP, Wilensky AJ (1979) Clinical pharmacology of mephenytoin and ethotoin. Ann Neurol 34:410–414
Tunnicliff G (1996) Basis of the anticonvulsive action of phenytoin. Gen Pharmacol 27:1092–1097
Tybring G, Bertilsson L (1992) A methodological investigation on the estimation of the S-mephenytoin hydroxylation phenotype using urinary S/R ratio. Pharmacogenetics 2:241–243
Veronese ME, Mackenzie PI, Doecke CJ, McManus ME, Miners JO, Birket DJ (1991) Tolbutamide and phenytoin hydroxylations by cDNA-expressed human liver cytochrome P4502C9. Biochem Biophys Res Commun 175:1112–1118
Veronese ME, Mackenzie PI, McManus ME et al. (1993) Site-directed mutation studies of human liver cytochrome P-450 isoenzymes in the GYP2 C subfamily. Biochem J 289:533–538
Vesell ES, Page JG (1969) Genetic control of phenobarbital induced shortening of plasma antipyrine half-lives in man. J Clin Invest 48:2202–2209
Wallis W, Kutt H, McDowell F (1968) Intravenous diphenylhydantoin in treatment of acute repetitive seizures. Neurology 18:513–525
Ward SA, Goto F, Nakamura K, Jacqz E, Wilkinson GR, Branch RA (1987) S-mephenytoin 4-hydroxylase is inherited as an autosomal recessive trait in Japanese families. Clin Pharmacol Ther 36:96–99

Wedlund PJ, Aslanian WS, McAllister CB, Wilkinson GB, Branch RA (1984) Mephenytoin hydroxylation deficiency in Caucasians: frequency of a new oxidative drug metabolism polymorphism. Clin Pharmacol Ther 36:773–788
Wilensky AJ, Lowden JA (1973) Inadequate serum levels after intramuscular administration of diphenylhydantoin. Neurology 23:318–324
Woodbury DM (1955) Effect of diphenylhydantion on electrolytes and radiosodium turnover in brain and other tissues of normal, hyponatremic and postictal rats. J Pharmacol Exp Ther 115:74–95
Woodbury DM (1980) Phenytoin: proposed mechanism of action. Adv Neurol 27:447–471
Woodbury DM (1989) Phenytoin. Absorption, distribution, and excretion. In: Levy RH, Mattson RH, Meldrum BS, Penry JK, Dreifuss FE (eds) Antiepileptic drugs. 3rd edn, Raven Press, New York, pp. 177–195
Wrighton SA, Stevens JC, Becker GW, van den Branden M (1993) Isolation and characterization of human liver cytochrome P450 2C19: correlation between 2C19 and S-mephenytoin 4′-hydroxylation Arch Biochem Biophys 306:240–245
Yerby MS, Leavitt A, Erickson DM, McCormick KB, Loewenson RB, Sells CJ, Benedetti TJ (1992) Antiepileptics and the development of congenital anomalies. Neurology 42 [Suppl 5]:S132–S140
Zahlen M, Brand N (1977) Cleft lip and palate with the anticonvulsant ethotoin. New Engl J Med 297:1404

CHAPTER 10

Carbamazepine

R.G. Dickinson, M.J. Eadie and F.J.E. Vajda

A. Introduction

The history of the development of carbamazepine was outlined in an earlier volume in this series (Schmutz 1985). By that time, the drug had already been in clinical use for two decades and was a well established antiepileptic agent, with certain other uses in human medicine. Its animal pharmacology and toxicology were reasonably adequately documented and some information on its human pharmacokinetics was available, though the drug's essential mechanism of action at the molecular level was unclear. The latter has now been elucidated, and considerable additional information has become available concerning the disposition, interactions and toxicity of the drug, mainly in humans, whilst its range of therapeutic uses has expanded. The present chapter deals chiefly with this newer information.

B. Chemistry and Use

I. Chemistry

Carbamazepine (5*H*-dibenz[*b,f*]azepine-5-carboxamide) is a white neutral lipophilic material (MW 236.3) which is virtually insoluble in water, though more easily dissolved in certain organic solvents. For human use the drug is supplied either in tablet form (some preparations having modified release characteristics) or as a syrup. No parenteral preparation has been marketed, though one has been used in experimental studies (Löscher et al. 1995; Löscher and Hönack 1997), and the drug has been administered rectally in solution in certain pharmacokinetic investigations (Graves et al. 1985; Neuvonen and Tokola 1987; Arvidsson et al. 1995).

Carbamazepine is biotransformed to a biologically active metabolite, carbamazepine-10,11-epoxide, whose pharmacological properties have undergone some study in their own right (Kerr and Levy 1995). These properties will be mentioned in the following account, where appropriate. At concentrations likely to be encountered in human therapeutics, no other known metabolite of the drug appears to possess significant pharmacological activity.

II. Use

In clinical practice, carbamazepine is used mainly in the treatment of epilepsy. It is effective in preventing simple and complex partial seizures, and in preventing their generalization into secondarily generalized seizures. It is also effective in preventing the bilateral tonic, clonic and tonic-clonic seizures of generalized epilepsy, but is not useful in treating absence, atonic and myoclonic seizures or juvenile myoclonic epilepsy (Johnsen et al. 1984). Recently it has been shown effective in managing neonatal seizures (Singh et al. 1996). It is ineffective in the prophylaxis of simple febrile seizures in infancy (Antony and Hawke 1983).

The first reported successful clinical use of carbamazepine was in preventing attacks of trigeminal neuralgia (Blom 1962), and it remains the treatment of choice for this disorder (Green and Selman 1991; Sidebottom and Maxwell 1995). The drug will also prevent attacks of glossopharyngeal neuralgia (King 1987). It decreases the severity of symptoms in certain painful peripheral neuropathies, including those of diabetes (Calissi and Jaber 1995) and Fabry's disease (Filling et al. 1989) and it relieves the lightning pains of tabes (Ekbom 1972). The drug is of little value in postherpetic neuralgia (Killian and Fromm 1968). It has been reported useful in managing various involuntary movement disorders, e.g. chorea (Roig et al. 1988), paroxysmal choreoathetosis (Jan et al. 1995; Wein et al. 1996), dystonia (Fahn 1987), restless legs (Zucconi et al. 1989; O'Keefe 1996), diaphragmatic flutter (Vantrappen et al. 1992), palatal myoclonus (Lapresle 1986), and myotonia (Sechi et al. 1983; Topaloglu et al. 1993; Squires and Prangley 1996) and neuromyotonia, both generalized (Kukowski and Feldmann 1992) and ocular (Ezra et al. 1996; Yee et al. 1996), as well as Isaac's syndrome of continuous muscle fibre activity (Thomas et al. 1994), myokymia (Auger et al. 1984), and superior oblique myokymia (Brazis et al. 1994). However, in the latter disorder the response may be temporary (Rosenberg and Glaser 1983). Cerebellar tremor (Sechi et al. 1989 a,b), familial rectal pain (Schuberet and Cracco 1992) and cataplexy (Vaughn and D'Cruz 1996) have also been reported to benefit from use of the drug.

In psychiatry, carbamazepine has found a major use in the prophylaxis of bipolar affective disorder (manic-depressive psychosis) (Denicoff et al. 1994; Emilien et al. 1996), where it is sometimes used in combination with lithium. In clinical trials it has proved useful in managing benzodiazepine (Galpern et al. 1991; Garcia-Borreguero et al. 1991) and alcohol withdrawal (Butler and Messiha 1986).

The drug is also used to manage milder degrees of neurogenic diabetes insipidus, though not more severe instances of the disorder (Wales 1975).

C. Pharmacodynamics

In the following account, particular attention has been paid to studies carried out at carbamazepine concentrations similar to those encountered in human therapeutics.

I. Biochemical Effects

1. Ion Channels and Receptors

a) Na^+ Channels

The molecular basis of the antiepileptic action of carbamazepine is now widely accepted to be the blockade of voltage-gated (voltage-dependent, frequency-dependent and use-dependent) Na^+ channels in cell membranes. This effect occurs in a concentration-dependent manner at therapeutically relevant drug concentrations and in a variety of experimental preparations (WILLOW et al. 1984, 1985; SCHWARTZ and GRIGAT 1989; LANG et al. 1993). Carbamazepine binds selectively to the inactive form of nerve and skeletal muscle cell membranes Na^+ channels whilst they are closed after depolarization (COURTNEY and ETTER 1983). The drug interacts with the site on the Na^+ channel to which lignocaine (ZIMANYI et al. 1989) and batrachotoxin (WORLEY and BARABAN 1987) bind. Carbamazepine has a mechanism of action on Na^+ channels in common with those of phenytoin, lamotrigine (WORLEY and BARABAN 1987: MACDONALD and KELLY 1995) and probably valproate (MACDONALD and KELLY 1995). The action of carbamazepine on Na^+ channels described above will tend to selectively impede the passage along axons of higher frequency impulse traffic, such as occurs during an epileptic seizure, but will leave axon traffic at more physiological frequency largely unaltered.

Several other receptor or ion channel actions of carbamazepine, as described immediately below, are known to occur at drug concentrations similar to those which apply in humans when the drug is used in therapeutics. However, the extent to which these particular actions contribute to the pharmacological effects of the drug is unclear.

b) Benzodiazepine Receptors

Carbamazepine inhibits benzodiazepine binding to, and displaces bound benzodiazepines from, the peripheral type of benzodiazepine receptor (BENDER and HERTZ 1988; WEISS and POST 1991) present on astrocytes and human lymphocytes (FERRARESE et al. 1995). An experimental agent which blocks the peripheral type of benzodiazepine receptor antagonizes the antiepileptic effect of carbamazepine against amygdaloid-kindled seizures (WEISS et al. 1985), suggesting that this class of receptor may be involved in the anticonvulsant actions of the drug. Carbamazepine binds to $GABA_A$ receptors to potentiate Cl^- currents (GRANGER et al. 1995) and also prevents upregulation of cortical and hypothalamic $GABA_A$ receptors (GALPERN et al. 1991). SPECT studies in a patient with temporal lobe epilepsy showed that numbers of central nervous system benzodiazepine receptors were increased after 2 months intake of the drug (STAEDT et al. 1995).

c) Ca^{2+} Channels

Carbamazepine acts as an antagonist at cell membrane Ca^{2+} channels. It appears to block Ca^{2+} currents in rat dorsal root ganglion neurons, probably by acting at "L" type channels (SCHIRRMACHER et al. 1993, 1995). However, in therapeutic concentrations it fails to alter Ca^{2+} currents in acutely isolated human neocortical neurons (SAYER et al. 1993) but, at therapeutic concentrations, it blocks Ca^{2+} entry into rat cerebellar granule cells which have been activated by *N*-methyl-D-aspartate (HOUGH et al. 1996). Carbamazepine also blocks "N" type voltage dependent Ca^{2+} channels in cultured bovine adrenal medullary cells (YOSHIMURA et al. 1995). It has little effect on Ca^{2+} conductance in thalamic neurons (COULTER et al. 1989).

d) Adenosine Receptors

Carbamazepine is an antagonist at A_1 type adenosine receptors (MARANGOS et al. 1987; GASSER et al. 1988; BIBER et al. 1996), and its binding to this class of receptor leads to receptor upregulation (WEIR et al. 1990; VAN CALKER et al. 1991). Experimental studies suggest that carbamazepine binding to A_1 receptors is not responsible for the antiepileptic actions of the drug (WEISS et al. 1985a; CZUCZWAR et al. 1991). At least one study has shown that carbamazepine also binds to A_2 receptors (FUJIWARA et al. 1986).

Chronic exposure to carbamazepine also leads to decreased sensitivity of rat brain presynaptic dopamine receptors (ELPHICK 1989).

2. Effects on Neurotransmitters

a) GABA

Contrary to the findings of some earlier studies (LUST et al. 1978), chronic exposure to carbamazepine appears to lead to a dose-related increase in GABA concentrations, in the rat substantia nigra (MITSUSHIO et al. 1988), in the temporal cortex (HIGUCHI et al. 1986), and in the brain more generally (BATTISTIN et al. 1984), though there is decreased GABA release in the preoptic areas (WOLF et al. 1993).

b) Catecholamines

Following exposure to carbamazepine, dopamine concentrations were raised in the intact rat brain (KOWALIK et al. 1984) and in the hippocampus (SUDHA et al. 1995), but were reduced in the motor cortex and cerebellum. In contrast, noradrenaline concentrations were increased in the latter two brain regions (BAF et al. 1994). Brain catecholamine turnover was decreased in the presence of the drug (WALDMEIER et al. 1984).

c) Serotonin

Carbamazepine intake results in increased serotonin concentrations in the mouse brain (PRATT et al. 1985) and in the hippocampus (SUDHA et al. 1995), striatum-accumbens area and brainstem of rats but not in the motor cortex or hypothalamus (BAF et al. 1994).

d) Acetylcholine

In rats carbamazepine causes increased acetylcholine concentrations in the striatum (CONSOLO et al. 1976).

e) Substance P

Increased substance P concentrations were found in the striatum and substantia nigra of rats treated with carbamazepine (MITSUSHIO et al. 1988).

f) Glutamate

Glutamate release in brain slices is reduced in the presence of carbamazepine (WALDMEIER et al. 1995).

g) Somatostatin

Carbamazepine exposure did not alter rat brain somatostatin concentrations (WEISS et al. 1987), but produced a dose-dependent inhibition in the release of this substance from cultured neurons of rats (REICHLIN and MOTHON 1991; RICHARDSON and TWENTE 1992).

3. Other Biochemical Changes

Carbamazepine has been reported to cause some rather diverse biochemical changes, e.g. decreased brain glucose metabolisn in humans, demonstrated in PET studies (THEODORE et al. 1989), inhibited Ca^{2+} calmodulin regulated protein phosphorylation (DE LORENZO 1984) and decreased generation of cyclic AMP in the cerebral cortex of rats (CHEN et al. 1996), release of cGMP from human lymphocytes (SCHUBERT et al. 1991), and of corticotrophin-releasing hormone from cultured hypothalamic neurons (WEISS et al. 1992), and increased plasma aspirin esterase activity in patients (PUCHE et al. 1989), prolactin release after tryptophan injection and growth hormone release after apomorphine administration in humans (ELPHICK et al. 1990). It is unclear whether any of these biochemical changes plays a role in the therapeutic or toxic effects of the drug, but the decreased arginine vasopressin response to osmotic stimulation together with an increased renal responsiveness to available arginine vasopressin which has been found to develop in the presence of carbamazepine (GOLD et al. 1983) may be relevant to the drug's effect in non-nephrogenic diabetes insipidus.

II. Electrophysiological Effects

1. Effects at the Cellular Level

Earlier investigations, outlined in JURNA (1985), showed relatively few clear-cut effects of clinically relevant concentrations of carbamazepine on aspects of axon conduction. More recent studies have demonstrated that carbamazepine stabilizes nerve cell membranes (Löscher 1987), reduces the amplitude of Ca^{2+} spikes in neurons (Crowder and Bradford 1987; Elliott 1990), diminishes spontaneous discharging of saphenous neuromas (Burchiel 1988), decreases the ability of mouse cultured neurons to sustain high frequency repetitive action potential firing (McLean and Macdonald 1986; Macdonald 1989) and, in a dose-dependent fashion, blocks *N*-methyl-D-aspartate activated currents in cultured spinal cord neurons (Lampe and Bigalke 1990). The spontaneous burst firing of neurons in the CA_1 region of rat hypothalamic slices maintained in a low Ca^{2+}, high Mg^{2+} environment is lessened in the presence of 1–15 μM carbamazepine (Heinemann et al. 1985).

2. Effects on Neuronal Pools

Julien and Hollister (1975) showed that carbamazepine concentrations of 3.5–10 mg/l did not alter post-tetanic potentiation. At a concentration of 5 mg/l, the drug facilitated previously induced long-term potentiation of population spikes (with enhanced synaptic inhibition) and also postsynaptic excitatory potentials in rabbit hippocampal neurons; at a concentration of 15 mg/l (at which some mild clinically apparent toxicity might be expected in humans), it inhibited the long-term potentiation (Kubota et al. 1992). Carbamazepine blocked long-term potentiation in the perforant path-dentate gyrus pathway in a chronic rabbit preparation (Kubota et al. 1994), suppressed thalamic relay mechanisms in cats (Shouse et al. 1988) and blocked spontaneous complex thalamo-cortical rhythms in rodents (Zhang and Coulter 1996). In the trigeminal nuclear complex it decreased afferent excitation and facilitated segmental inhibition (Fromm 1985). In the rat cerebral cortex the drug failed to suppress the afterdischarges which develop following stimulation of the sensorimotor cortex (Kubova et al. 1996), though it suppressed penicillin-induced afterdischarging in the immature rat hippocampus (Smith and Swann 1987). It did not suppress spiking in penicillin induced cortical foci in cats (Julien and Hollister 1975) or in an amygdala-kindled rat preparation (Gigli and Gotman 1991). In this preparation the drug seemed to accelerate the development of kindling as assessed by the rate at which afterdischarges developed (Schmutz et al. 1988).

Earlier Hernandez-Peon (1964) had shown in cats that carbamazepine suppressed electrically evoked afterdischarges in the amygdala and hippocampus. However, the drug failed to suppress focal seizure activity evoked by stimulating the amygdaloid with locally applied alumina, though it did inhibit the propagation of spike activity from an alumina-induced focus in the sensorimotor cortex in the rhesus monkey (David and Grewal 1976), and diminished seizure activity at a penicillin-induced focus in the rat cerebral cortex (Julien and Hollister 1975).

Whilst in a general way the electrophysiological actions of carbamazepine on single neurons can be regarded as being potentially antiepileptic, those effects demonstrated in neuronal collections sometimes appear more ambiguous in relation to the drug's action in preventing epileptic seizures. However, the effects of the drug within the trigeminal nuclear complex do seem relevant to the drug's efficacy in reducing the severity of trigeminal neuralgia.

III. Effects in Animal Models of Epilepsy

1. Models of Generalized Epilepsy

The efficacy of carbamazepine in preventing maximum electroshock seizures in rodents was well established at a relatively early, stage of the drugs development (SCHMUTZ 1985), and has been confirmed since (PALMER et al. 1992). By 1985, it was also known that the drug possessed some efficacy against pentylenetetrazole-induced seizures in mice. It was later found that the drug was more effective in this seizure model than in bicuculline-induced seizures (DE FEO et al. 1991) and that it was the tonic but not the clonic phase of the pentylenetetrazole seizure that was inhibited (KUBOVA and MARES 1993). SCHMUTZ (1985) also described studies done carried out in certain other animal models of epilepsy, including the photosensitive baboon *Papio papio,* in which species carbamazepine at clinically relevant concentrations was of equivocal efficacy.

2. Models of Partial Epilepsy

Carbamazepine proved effective against hippocampal (e.g. SCHMUTZ et al. 1981) and cortical epileptogenesis (e.g. HERNANDEZ-PEON 1964) in experimental animals and against cortical and limbic kindled seizures in cats, baboons and rabbits, but not rats (SCHMUTZ 1985). Subsequently there have been further reports of the ability of carbamazepine to suppress seizures and afterdischarges, or to shorten their duration, in kindled (usually amygdaloid-kindled) experimental animals (MAJKOWSKI et al. 1994; VOITS and FREY 1994; EBERT et al. 1995). Unlike the situation for other antiepileptic drugs, the protective effect of carbamazepine against kindled seizures is lost after bilateral destruction of the substantia nigra, though protection against maximum electroshock seizures persists (WAHNSCHAFFE and LÖSCHER 1990). If carbamazepine intake is begun before kindling is commenced, tolerance to that phenomenon occurs (WEISS et al. 1993).

In recent years, the drug has been investigated in numerous additional animal models of epilepsy, though the emphasis in these studies has been rather more on the ability of the models studied to predict therapeutic responsiveness of human epilepsies to new agents than simply to know the efficacy of carbamazepine in these models. It has been shown that carbamazepine protects against, or reduces, the severity of seizures initiated by: hyperoxia in rats (RESHEF et al. 1991); 4-aminopyridine (FUETA and AVOLI 1992); intraventricular administration of the K^+ blocking agent dendrotoxin (COLEMAN et al. 1992); the glutamate agonist ATPA (α-amino-3-hydroxy-5-terbutyl-4-isoxazolepropionate), but not by the glutamate agonists kainate and *N*-methyl-D-aspartate

(Steppuhn and Turski 1993); cobalt, in rats (Craig and Colasanti 1992); direct electrical stimulation of the rat cerebral cortex (Hoogerkamp et al. 1994), in which preparation the drug raised the threshold for evoking a generalized seizure, but probably not the threshold for initiating the preliminary partial seizure; tetanus toxoid, which induced chronic limbic epilepsy (Hawkins et al. 1985); and seizures in the rat genetic epilepsy model (Dailey and Jobe 1985). However, carbamazepine has failed to protect against pilocarpine induced limbic seizures in rats (Leite and Cavalheiro 1995) and against seizures induced by an "L" type Ca^{2+} channel agonist in a mouse strain with genetic epilepsy (De Sarro et al. 1992). It also failed to prevent seizures in a Wistar mouse line with spontaneous petit mal-like seizures (Micheletti et al. 1985).

Carbamazepine-10,11-epoxide has been proven effective against amygdaloid kindled seizures in rodents (Albright and Bruni 1984).

It thus appears that carbamazepine is effective in many animal models of human partial epilepsy, in particular limiting the propagation and generalization of seizure discharges, and in models of generalized epilepsy with bilateral tonic-clonic seizures. It is inactive in models of generalized epilepsy with absence seizures. In these regards, the therapeutic response in the animal models correlates with responsiveness in human epilepsies. However, carbamazepine may have efficacy in a model which seems to resemble human myoclonic epilepsy clinically, even though the drug is not regarded as particularly useful in this situation in patients.

IV. Human Studies

The patterns of usefulness in human epilepsies mentioned immediately above have been derived from accumulated clinical experience and are now fairly widely accepted. In one large clinical trial in adult patients with partial epilepsies and generalized epilepsy resulting in bilateral tonic-clonic seizures, carbamazepine was as effective as phenytoin and phenobarbitone, and was less toxic than the latter (Mattson et al. 1985), and in another trial proved as effective as valproate for secondarily generalized seizures and more effective for partial seizures (Mattson et al. 1992). It was also as effective as phenobarbitone, phenytoin and valproate in newly diagnosed childhood partial and generalized epilepsy with convulsive seizures (de Silva et al. 1996). In other studies it was as effective as vigabatrin (Tanganelli and Regesta 1996) and lamotrigine (Brodie et al. 1995). A meta-analysis of all recently published large scale trials suggested that carbamazepine probably has an efficacy similar to those of gabapentin, topiramate and tiagabine (Marson et al. 1997).

D. Pharmacokinetics

The pharmacokinetics of carbamazepine have been reviewed by Bertilsson (1978), Pynnonen (1979), Bertilsson and Tomson (1986) and Morselli (1995).

I. Absorption

Carbamazepine is marketed only for oral use, in various solid dosage forms and as a syrup. In retrospect, it appears possible that drug preparations with different absorption rates (perhaps dependent on different drug particle sizes in different preparations – DAM et al. 1981), and sometimes with incomplete oral bioavailabilities, may have been used in earlier pharmacokinetic studies on the drug. As well, the bioavailability of a given manufacturer's carbamazepine preparation may not have always remained constant over the years (EADIE and HOOPER 1987). At one stage NEUVONEN et al. (1985) studied five generic carbamazepine preparations that were available in Europe. Whilst the overall extent of carbamazepine absorption from these preparations did not differ, there was a 50% difference in the peak plasma drug concentration which they produced after a single oral dose. In another study the oral bioavailability range of the drug was 60%–113% (MEYER et al. 1992). There have been reports of loss of seizure control when one brand of carbamazepine was substituted for another (WELTY et al. 1992).

Peak plasma carbamazepine concentrations have been found to occur around 4h (MACPHEE et al. 1987), between 6 and 8h (MORSELLI et al. 1975), or between 4 and 24h (POPOVIC et al. 1995) after administration of a single oral dose of the drug given in tablet form. However, under steady-state conditions the T_{max} should occur earlier, because of consequences of the autoinduction of the drug's metabolism which will have occurred by then (see "Elimination"), and because of the effects on the drug's elimination rate from the higher plasma drug concentrations which are then present. Values for the absorption half-time of the drug are likely to vary with the absorption characteristics of the drug preparation studied. Carbamazepine is absorbed more rapidly from an oral solution than from tablets (COTTER et al. 1977).

Because of the lack of a suitable intravenous preparation, there appear to be no published data for the absolute oral bioavailability of carbamazepine in solid dosage form, though the absolute bioavailability of a carbamazepine suspension was said to be 1.0 (GERARDIN et al. 1990), and did not differ from the bioavailability of the drug in tablet form (GRAVES et al. 1985; HOOPER et al. 1985). The bioavailability of the drug from a rectal suppository was 0.8 (ARVIDSSON et al. 1995), or around 1.0 (GRAVES et al. 1985; NEUVONEN and TOKOLA 1987), providing it could be retained in the rectum for at least 2h.

In recent years several carbamazepine solid dose preparations with modified release profiles have been marketed for use in humans, to try to avert the occurrence of toxic effects that may occur at the time of peak plasma concentrations of the drug when certain conventional tablet forms of the drug are used, and to reduce plasma carbamazepine concentration fluctuations across the dosage interval (WOLF et al. 1992). Some of these modified release preparations have similar oral bioavailabilities to conventional tablets of the drug (THAKKER et al. 1992), but others differ in the extent of the amount of drug absorbed by up to a mean of 22% (CANGER et al. 1990; EEG-OLOFSSON et al. 1990; REUNANEN et al. 1992). It seems that it is difficult to manufacture a carbamazepine solid dosage form which can achieve full oral bioavailability for the drug without simultaneously producing a preparation which may sometimes yield clinically troublesome fluctuations in its steady-state plasma concentrations.

Carbamazepine-10,11-epoxide has been administered orally to humans. Since it is unstable in an acid environment it must be given together with antacids, or in an enteric coated preparation (TOMSON et al. 1983).

II. Distribution

1. Apparent Volume of Distribution

Values of the apparent volume of distribution of carbamazepine in humans have been around 0.74–1.3 l/kg (EADIE and TYRER 1989). However, these figures are really the value of the parameter V/F. Under steady-state conditions carbamazepine is probably distributed fairly uniformly throughout body water, with little differential regional concentration. This is in keeping with the results of radioautographic studies in experimental animals (MORSELLI et al. 1971).

The apparent volume of distribution of carbamazepine-10,11-epoxide is 0.74 l/kg (BERTILSSON and TOMSON 1986).

2. Plasma Protein Binding

In human plasma both carbamazepine and its 10,11-epoxide are bound to α_1-acid glycoprotein and to albumin. Some 72.1 ± 1.2% (RAWLINS et al. 1975) to 81 ± 3% (ELYAS et al. 1986) of the carbamazepine in plasma is protein bound, a typical figure for the free fraction of the drug being 0.255 (BACKMAN et al. 1987). The binding is concentration independent, at least up to carbamazepine concentrations of 50 mg/l. About 50% of the carbamazepine-10,11-epoxide in plasma is protein bound (VREE et al. 1986), though a figure for this parameter as high as 63 ± 9% has been published (ELYAS et al. 1986). Some 70% of the carbamazepine-10,11-*trans*-diol in plasma is protein bound (VREE et al. 1986). Published values for the apparent association constants for carbamazepine binding to α_1-acid glycoprotein include: 0.053, 0.071 and 0.096 l/μmol of the drug, the latter value applying to children, and for carbamazepine-10,11-epoxide binding 0.013, 0.016 and 0.023 l/μmol (KODAMA et al. 1993a,b, 1994). In human neonatal plasma, a mean of 29.8% of carbamazepine, at low drug concentrations, and of 30.6% at high concentrations, is unbound; the corresponding figures for the epoxide are 47.5% and 52.0%, respectively (GROCE et al. 1985). The unbound fractions of carbamazepine and carbamazepine-10,11-epoxide increase slightly throughout pregnancy (YERBY et al. 1990).

3. Body Fluid and Tissue Distribution

a) Blood

Red blood cell carbamazepine concentrations are 38.3 ± 17.9% of whole plasma ones (Hooper et al. 1975).

b) Cerebrospinal Fluid

The carbamazepine concentration in CSF is similar to that in plasma water, e.g. 19%–25% (Morselli et al. 1975) or 31% (Post et al. 1983) of the whole plasma concentration. In anaesthetized dogs, the drug's mean entry time into CSF was 12–18 min (Löscher and Frey 1984).

c) Saliva

Salivary carbamazepine concentrations in humans are similar to simultaneous plasma water ones, e.g. 27% of whole plasma carbamazepine concentrations (Knott and Reynolds 1984). Some authors have reported wide fluctuations in salivary carbamazepine concentrations (Paxton et al. 1983), or quite deviant values (Paxton 1983). However, Dickinson et al. (1985) noted that, for 2h after swallowing a carbamazepine tablet, detectable amounts of drug remained in the mouth and could invalidate salivary carbamazepine concentration measurements carried out during this period. Lack of attention to this factor may explain some of the aberrant values recorded.

d) Milk

The human milk to whole plasma carbamazepine concentration ratio is 0.433 ± 0.017 (Kaneko et al. 1984), 0.32–0.80 (Meyer et al. 1988), 0.364 (Froescher et al. 1984) or 0.39 ± 0.22 [1902/1983] Kuhnz et al. 1983). The last-mentioned workers showed that the corresponding figure for carbamazepine-10,11-epoxide was 0.49 ± 0.28.

e) Foetal Blood and Amniotic Fluid

Carbamazepine concentrations in human umbilical cord serum averaged 0.73 (Takeda et al. 1992), 0.845 (Froscher et al. 1991) or 0.60–0.76 (Meyer et al. 1988) of simultaneous whole maternal plasma ones. Carbamazepine and carbamazepine-10,11-epoxide concentrations in amniotic fluid also correlated with those in maternal plasma (Omtzigt et al. 1993), though they were higher than the simultaneous plasma water concentrations of these substances.

f) Body Tissues

Carbamazepine concentrations in postmortem human cerebral cortex have averaged 1.1 (Morselli et al. 1977), 1.4 (Rambeck et al. 1993) or 1.4–1.6 times (Friis et al. 1978) those simultaneously present in serum. Carbamazepine concentrations between 1.2 and 57.4 mg/kg were found in hair from patients taking the drug (Kintz et al. 1995).

III. Elimination

Carbamazepine is eliminated mainly by biotransformation.

1. Metabolism

Most carbamazepine metabolic studies in humans have been carried out under steady-state conditions, and therefore describe the situation in which the drug's metabolism has already been autoinduced. Carbamazepine metabolism appears to occur mainly in the liver, though in rats it has been calculated that 5% of a carbamazepine dose is biotransformed in the lungs (Wedlund et al. 1983). Only 1%–2% of an oral carbamazepine dose in humans is excreted in urine as the intact molecule (Faigle and Feldmann 1975), and at least half the dose cannot be accounted for as identified excretion products (Faigle and Feldmann 1995). The outstanding portion of the dose is probably either excreted in the form of as yet unidentified, probably polar, biotransformation products in urine, or is lost in the faeces, in which Faigle and Feldmann (1995) could trace 28% of a dose of radioactive drug.

The main pathway of carbamazepine biotransformation (Faigle and Feldmann 1995) is the so-called epoxide-diol one, in which the drug is first oxidized to the chemically stable carbamazepine-10,11-epoxide in a reaction catalysed by the microsomal cytochrome P450 isoenzymes CYP3A4 and, to a lesser extent, CYP2C8 (Kerr et al. 1994). Except for a small portion excreted in urine, the epoxide undergoes hydration catalysed by microsomal epoxide hydrolase (Kitteringham et al. 1996) to form carbamazepine-10,11-*trans*-diol (10,11-dihydro-10,11-dihydroxycarbamazepine). The *trans*-diol, which is present in human plasma mainly as its S,S-enantiomer (Eto et al. 1996), is then conjugated to form a 10-hydroxy-*O*-glucuronide (Beyer and Spiteller 1992) in a reaction catalysed by UDP-glucuronosyl transferase. The diol and its conjugate are then excreted in urine where they account for some 35% of a carbamazepine dose (Bourgeois and Wad 1984).

Phenolic excretion products of the drug, arising from oxidations at the 2- and 3-positions (equivalent to the 7- and 8-positions) of the molecule, possibly via transient arene oxide intermediate stages (Lillibridge et al. 1996; Madden et al. 1996), and their *O*-glucuronide and *O*-sulphate conjugates, have been identified in urine. The microsomal P450 isoenzymes involved in these aromatic oxidations are not those responsible for the formation of carbamazepine-10,11-epoxide (Faigle and Feldmann 1995). Evidence for the excretion of other monohydroxy (phenol) and dihydroxy (catechol) metabolites has been presented, though these pathways appear to be quantitatively minor (Lynn et al. 1978; Lertratanangkoon and Horning 1982; Maggs et al. 1997). The azepine moiety of the carbamazepine molecule may undergo a condensation reaction to form 9-hydroxymethyl-10-carbamoyl acridan, which occurs in measurable quantity in plasma (ETO et al. 1995) and is excreted in urine mainly as its glucuronide conjugate. In humans, this acridan appears to be formed mainly from carbamazepine itself, rather than from carbamazepine-10,11-epoxide (EICHELBAUM et al. 1985; FAIGLE and FELDMANN 1995). A 9-acridine carboxaldehyde derivative, formed as result of oxidation by the myeloperoxidase system in leucocytes, has also been identified (FURST and UETRECHT 1993). Indeed, there has been considerable recent interest in ascertaining whether and which reactive metabolites of carbamazepine are responsible for idiosyncratic responses to the drug (FURST et al. 1995; MADDEN et al. 1996). A direct *N*-glucuronide conjugate of the drug also forms. It accounts for some 10% of a carbamazepine dose (FAIGLE and FELDMANN 1995) and is generally regarded as the third most important pathway (quantitatively) of the drug's metabolism. In the rat, however, *N*-glucuronidation of carbamazepine (and of its 10,11-epoxide metabolite) is the major pathway of metabolism (MADDEN et al. 1996). Pathway details are shown in Fig. 1.

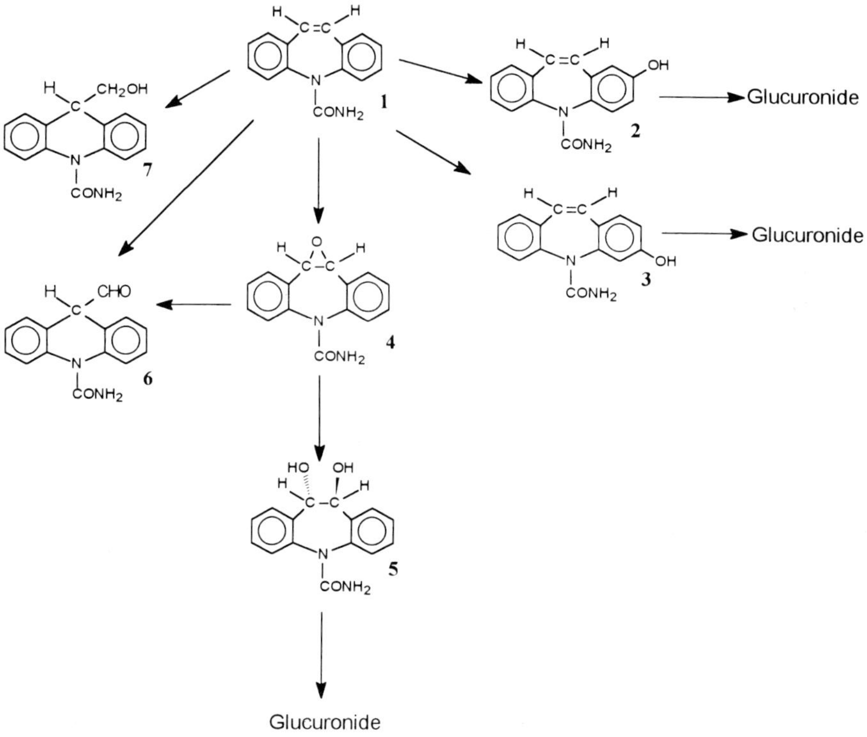

Fig. 1. Carbamazepine metabolic pathways. *1,* carbamazepine; *2,3,* phenolic metabolites; *4,* carbamazepine-10,11-epoxide; *5,* carbamazepine-10-11-*trans*-diol; *6,* 9-acridine carboxaldehyde; *7,* 9-hydroxymethyl-10-carbamoyl acridan

As already mentioned, the metabolism of carbamazepine is autoinducible in humans and in certain animal species (FREY and LÖSCHER 1980). This autoinduction chiefly involves the epoxide-diol pathway at the consecutive stages of epoxide and diol formation (EICHELBAUM et al. 1985). The subsequent glucuronidation of the diol does not appear to be autoinducible (BERNUS et al. 1996) in humans, though RIVA et al. (1996) stated that carbamazepine was a potent inducer of UDP glucuronosyl transferase. EICHELBAUM et al. (1985) found some evidence in humans that formation of 9-hydroxymethyl-10-carbamoyl acridan also underwent autoinduction, but BERNUS et al. (1994, 1996) failed to confirm this, though they showed some autoinduction of the formation of the phenolic derivatives of the drug. There is evidence that the process of autoinduction is complete within 1 week of initial exposure to the drug (KUDRIAKOVA et al. 1992) or within 1 month (BERTILSSON et al. 1986) of a dosage increase. There is also evidence that the process of autoinduction commences within 24h of first exposure to the drug (BERNUS et al. 1994). At least in rats, autoinduction seems to have a finite capacity, reaching its maximum at a carbamazepine dose of 60mg/kg in this species (REGNAUD et al. 1988).

2. Elimination Parameters

The values of the elimination parameters of carbamazepine depend on whether the drug has been studied after its first dose, or after there has been time for autoinduction to occur, and on whether any co-administered drug which interacts pharmacokinetically is present, a situation to be considered in the following section of this chapter.

a) *Half-life*

Carbamazepine is much more rapidly eliminated in most experimental animal species than in humans (FAIGLE and FELDMANN 1995). The first dose half-life of the drug in humans averages around 36h. POPOVIC et al. (1997) cited a half-life range of 22.19–39.61 h. The half-life is shorter in young children (BATTINO et al. 1995; LEPPIK 1992) than in adults. GERARDIN et al. (1976) and COTTER et al. (1977) noted that the elimination rate constant of carbamazepine appeared to increase when increasing doses of the drug were given on separate occasions.

Relatively few measurements of the half-life at steady state are available, though it appears to be in the range 12–18h (e.g. 14.5 ± 5.3h – WESTENBERG et al. 1978; 12.3 ± 0.8h – EICHELBAUM et al. 1982). EICHELBAUM et al. (1975) found that a first dose carbamazepine half-life of 35.6 ± 15.3h fell to 20.9 ± 5.0h after continued intake of the drug. PITLICK et al. (1976) showed a similar shortening from 33.9 ± 3.5h to 19.8 ± 4.0h after 3 weeks of use of the drug. It is the autoinduced half-life value which will determine the time to achieve new steady-state conditions after a carbamazepine dosage increase.

Interactions with co-administered drugs may result in alterations in carbamazepine's half-life and clearance (see "Interactions", below).

b) Clearance

Because no intravenous preparation of carbamazepine has been available, published clearance values for carbamazepine are necessarily those for the parameter CL/F. Published values for this parameter after an initial dose of carbamazepine have been in the range 0.011–0.026 l/h (MORSELLI 1975), 0.0156 ± 0.006 l/kg/h (COTTER et al. 1977) or 1.05–2.06 l/h (POPOVIC et al. 1995). In the study of EICHELBAUM et al. (1985) the first dose clearance of the drug averaged 0.0198 l/kg/h while, after chronic intake, the clearance rose to 0.0546 l/kg/h. In children, the mean first dose clearance (0.028 ± 0.003 l/kg/h) doubled to 0.056 ± 0.011 l/kg/h after 17–32 days of carbamazepine use (BERTILSSON et al. 1980). The value of CL/F is higher in males than females, though not to a statistically significant extent (SUMMERS and SUMMERS 1989). It diminishes with increasing body weight (LIU and DELGADO 1994a) and with age in childhood (ALBANI et al. 1992; YUKAWA et al. 1992; LIU and DELGARDO 1994b). The value of CL/F increases with increasing dosage of carbamazepine (SUMMERS and SUMMERS 1989; HARTLEY et al. 1990; BERNUS et al. 1996), and does so in a nonlinear fashion (YUKAWA and AOYAMA 1996).

The renal clearances of carbamazepine, carbamazepine-10,11-epoxide and carbamazepine-10,11-*trans*-diol are, respectively, 0.001, 0.008 and 0.160–0.350 l/h, the values being urine flow dependent (VREE et al. 1986).

c) Carbamazepine-10,11-epoxide

In humans, carbamazepine-10,11-epoxide has a half-life of 6.1 ± 0.9 h (TOMSON et al. 1983), 7.4 ± 1.8 h (SPINA et al. 1988) or 6.9 ± 2.7 h (HOOPER et al. 1985), a plasma clearance of 0.105 ± 0.017 l/kg/h (SPINA et al. 1988) or 0.089 l/kg/h (TOMSON et al. 1983) and an apparent volume of distribution (V/F) of 1.1 ± 0.2 l/kg (SPINA et al. 1988). Some 90% of a carbamazepine-10,11-epoxide dose is excreted in urine as carbamazepine-10,11-*trans*-diol and its *O*-glucuronide conjugate (TOMSON et al. 1983).

IV. Clinical Pharmacokinetics

Under conditions of continuing carbamazepine intake, a new steady state should exist within 3 or 4 days of a carbamazepine dosage change. Steady-state plasma carbamazepine concentrations may show considerable interdosage fluctuations, e.g. by 79 ± 29% with twice daily administration (TOMSON 1984). The fluctuation is probably mainly due to the absorption characteristics of the carbamazepine dosage form in use. When carbamazepine is used as monotherapy, plasma carbamazepine-10,11-epoxide concentrations average 18.9% (in children – SCHOEMAN et al. 1984), 19.6 ± 2.4% (ALTAFULLAH et al. 1989) or 20%–25% (MCKAUGE et al. 1981) of simultaneous plasma carbamazepine ones, though the ratio between metabolite and parent substance increased with increasing plasma carbamazepine concentrations (FROSCHER et al. 1988;

THEODORE et al. 1989b) and was higher in adults than in children (MCKAUGE et al. 1981).

In individual patients receiving carbamazepine monotherapy, steady-state plasma carbamazepine concentrations rise less than proportionately in relation to the magnitude of drug dosage increases (COTTER et al. 1977; TOMSON et al. 1989; BERNUS et al. 1996). This non-linearity is due to the ongoing dose-dependent autoinduction which involves the drug's major elimination mechanism (see above). In populations of treated patients there has been a wide scatter of steady-state carbamazepine concentrations relative to drug dose, so that in various studies there has (LANDER et al. 1977; KUMPS 1981) or has not (MORSELLI 1975; BOURGEOIS and WAD 1984) been a statistically significant correlation between the two. The dose-dependent clearance of carbamazepine contributes to this relative lack of correlation.

The therapeutic range of plasma carbamazepine concentrations for treating epilepsy in humans is generally regarded as 4–6 to 10–12 mg/l when the drug is used in monotherapy (e.g. BERTILSSON and TOMSON 1986). SCHMIDT et al. (1986) found that plasma carbamazepine concentrations above 5.5 mg/l were required to prevent bilateral tonic-clonic seizures, but concentrations above 7 mg/l were needed to control partial seizures. EADIE (1994) noted that carbamazepine concentrations above 5 mg/l were needed to have a reasonable chance of achieving seizure control in epileptic patients under his care. No clear information is available regarding the contribution to the overall antiepileptic and toxic effect made by the carbamazepine-10,11-epoxide that is also present. When carbamazepine is used in combination with other microsomal P450 inducing anticonvulsants, or with valproate, plasma carbamazepine concentrations tend to fall relative to plasma carbamazepine-10,11-epoxide levels (also see "Interactions"). In such circumstances the limits of the therapeutic range for carbamazepine prove to be lower than when the drug is used as the sole antiepileptic agent prescribed. These limits cannot be defined accurately, partly because the magnitude of the interaction probably varies with the dosage of the interacting drug from case to case, and there do not appear to be good data relating the sum of simultaneous carbamazepine and metabolite concentrations to the biological effects that are present. In treating neuralgia, plasma carbamazepine concentrations in the range 2–7 mg/l were associated with a 25%–75% decrease in pain (MOOSA et al. 1993), while TOMSON et al. (1980) quoted a plasma carbamazepine concentration range of 5.7–10.1 mg/l as associated with control of trigeminal neuralgia.

Epilepsy may worsen with plasma carbamazepine concentrations above 20 mg/l (TROUPIN and OJEMANN 1976). In carbamazepine overdosage, plasma drug concentrations above 40 mg/l have been associated with an increased risk of coma, seizures, respiratory failure and cardiac conduction defects (HOJER et al. 1993). In the study of TIBBALLS (1992), patients in moderate coma after carbamazepine overdosage had a mean serum drug concentration of 28 mg/l (112 μM) while those with mildly depressed or normal levels of consciousness had a mean plasma carbamazepine level of 18 mg/l (73 μM), though 53% of the latter subjects had ataxia, 38% had nystagmus and 17% experienced vomiting. During recovery from carbamazepine overdosage, plasma carbamazepine concentrations above 24 mg/l were associated with seizures and coma, levels of 15–25 mg/l with combativeness, hallucinations and choreiform dyskinesis, and levels in the range 11–15 mg/l with ataxia and drowsiness (Weaver et al. 1988).

a) Pregnancy

There is some inconsistency in the literature as to whether plasma carbamazepine concentrations fall relative to drug dose as pregnancy progresses, and whether the value of CL/F inceases. Plasma unbound concentrations of carbamazepine and carbamazepine-10,11-epoxide averaged 25% and 50%, respectively, of whole plasma concentrations of these substances during pregnancy, but 22% and 43% postpartum in the same women (Yerby et al. 1985). Battino et al. (1985) and Yerby et al. (1992) found that, during pregnancy, plasma carbamazepine concentrations fell relative to drug dose but plasma unbound concentrations of the drug did not. In contrast, Bardy et al. (1982), Levy and Yerby (1985) and Tomson et al. (1994) found no significant change in whole plasma carbamazepine concentrations during pregnancy, though the last mentioned authors showed that the value of CL/F for both the unbound drug and the total drug in plasma did increase in the final trimester. Lander and Eadie (1991) noted that it had been necessary to increase carbamazepine dose in 70% of pregnancies in which the drug was used to maintain plasma carbamazepine concentrations throughout pregnancy at prepregnancy or early pregnancy values. However, they also noted that the dose increases were necessary mainly in women who took carbamazepine with antiepileptic comedications. Subsequently, Bernus et al. (1995), in metabolic balance studies, showed that the oxidation of carbamazepine to carbamazepine-10,11-epoxide increased during pregnancy, though to a greater extent in women taking carbamazepine with phenytoin or phenobarbitone; conversion of the epoxide to the subsequent *trans*-diol derivative was less increased, and formation of 9-hydroxymethyl acridan and probably 2-hydroxy carbamazepine was also increased. Glucuronidation of all the phase I metabolites of the drug was unaltered. In the co-medicated women, the greater increase in epoxide formation caused an increase in the overall plasma clearance of the drug, whereas in the women receiving carbamazepine in monotherapy the lesser increase in flux through the earlier stage of the epoxide-diol pathway resulted in relatively little change in carbamazepine clearance. When this situation was recognized and previous reports were reviewed, it became apparent that earlier workers who had found increased carbamazepine clearances in pregnancy had studied mainly co-medicated women, and those who had not found increased clearances had studied mainly women receiving carbamazepine as monotherapy.

b) Disease States

Plasma carbamazepine concentrations show a temporary rise following epilepsy surgery, without change in the unbound fraction of the drug in plasma

(GIDAL et al. 1996). The value of V_{area}/F after a first dose of carbamazepine is higher (98.4 ± 26.9 vs. 60.7 ± 8.51), and the half-life longer (59.4 ± 14.7 vs. 31.0 ± 5.0 h), in the obese than in the lean (CARACO et al. 1995). Following myocardial infarction, plasma α_1-acid glycoprotein and total carbamazepine and carbamazepine-10,11-epoxide concentrations rise (CLOYD 1991), while in various disease states the carbamazepine unbound fraction in plasma is inversely related to the plasma concentration of this particular circulating protein. Plasma protein binding capacity for carbamazepine was unaltered in renal disease, but slightly increased in liver disease, in the study of HOOPER et al. (1975). The oral bioavailability of carbamazepine is decreased in children with protein-energy malnutrition (BANO et al. 1986).

E. Interactions

I. Pharmacodynamic Interactions

Carbamazepine is sometimes prescribed with other antiepileptic drugs in the hope of achieving better control of epileptic seizures, and there is some evidence that this aim is sometimes realized (CEREGHINO et al. 1975). The question of rational combinations of antiepileptic drugs, in particular agents with different and therefore potentially additive mechanisms of antiepileptic action, has attracted some recent interest (EADIE 1997). However, pharmacokinetic interactions between the agents involved may confound the interpretation of the situation with such drug combinations.

If carbamazepine is used together with other drugs which also have sedative properties, or with alcohol, increased overall sedation may occur.

II. Pharmacokinetic Interactions

The pharmacokinetic interactions in which carbamazepine is involved have been reviewed by LEVY and WURDEN (1995), RIVA et al. (1996) and SPINA et al. (1996).

1. Interactions Which Lower Plasma Carbamazepine Concentrations

Activated charcoal (NEUVONEN and OLKKOLA 1988; NEUVONEN et al. 1988; MONTOYA-CABRERA et al. 1996) and enteral feeding (BASS et al. 1989) lower plasma carbamazepine concentrations by interfering with the absorption of the drug from the alimentary tract. Salicylates displace carbamazepine from plasma proteins, thus lowering whole plasma carbamazepine concentrations rather than plasma water ones (DASGUPTA and THOMPSON 1995; DASGUPTA and VOLK 1996).

Apart from these displacement type processes, the interactions which result in lowered plasma carbamazepine concentrations appear due to increased clearance of the drug, probably arising from hetero-induction of its metabolism. The agents responsible for such interactions include antipyrine (WEITHOLTZ et al. 1989); cyclosporin A (PICHARD et al. 1990); felbamate (FUERST et al. 1988; GRAVES et al. 1989; ALBANI et al. 1991), though simultaneous carbamazepine-10,11-epoxide concentrations may rise (RAMBECK et al. 1996); fluoxetine and fluvoxamine (NEMEROFF et al. 1996); nefazodone (NEMEROFF et al. 1996); phenobarbitone (LIU and DELGARDO 1995; YUKAWA and AOYAMA 1996); associated with a decreased clearance of carbamazepine-10,11-epoxide (SPINA et al. 1991); phenytoin (ZIELINSKI and HAIDUKEWYCH 1987; RAMSAY et al. 1990; DUNCAN et al. 1991; LIU and DELGARDO 1994c, 1995); primidone (BENETELLO and FERLANUT 1987; LIU and DELGADO 1994c); progabide (GRAVES et al. 1988); sertraline (NEMEROFF et al. 1996); topiramate (BOURGEOIS 1996; SACHEDO et al. 1996); zonisamide (MINAMI et al. 1994) and zopiclone (FERNANDEZ et al. 1995), in this case associated with reduced plasma carbamazepine-10,11-epoxide concentrations (KUITUNEN et al. 1990).

When valnoctamide is administered together with carbamazepine, plasma concentrations of the latter are unaltered but concentrations of carbamazepine-10,11-epoxide fall (PISANI et al. 1993).

2. Interactions Which Raise Plasma Carbamazepine Concentrations

Interactions between carbamazepine and other drugs which lead to raised plasma carbamazepine concentrations (probably by inhibition of carbamazepine metabolism) have been described, involving: alcohol, after a debauch (STERNEBRING et al. 1992); certain Ca^{2+} channel antagonists, viz. diltiazem (MAOZ et al. 1992) and verapamil (MACPHEE et al. 1986; BEATTIE et al. 1988; BAHLS et al. 1991), but not nifedipine (CHEYMOL and ENGEL 1989; BAHLS et al. 1991); cimetidine, but only at the commencement of therapy with the drug (DALTON et al. 1985); danazol (ZIELIKSKI et al. 1987): dextropropoxyphene (OLES et al. 1989; ALLEN 1994); fluvoxamine (PERUCCA et al. 1994; COTTENCIN et al. 1995; VAN HARTEN 1995); fluoxetine (NEMEROFF et al. 1996); imipramine (DANIEL and NETTER 1988); influenza vaccine (JANN and FIDONE 1986); isoniazid (GARCIA et al. 1992); lithium (CHAUDRY and WATERS 1983); some macrolide antibiotics, including clarithromycin (ALBANI et al. 1993; O'CONNOR and FRIS 1994), erythromycin (MILES and TENNISON 1989), josamycin (VINCON et al. 1987); troleandeomycin (VON ROSENSTEIL and ADAM 1995) but not azithromycin and spiramycin (VON ROSENSTEIL and ADAM 1995); nafimidone (TREIMAN and BEN-MENACHEM 1987); naproxen (DASGUPTA and VOLK 1996); nicotinamide (BOURGEOIS et al. 1982); quinine (AMABEOKU et al. 1993); remacemide (LEACH et al. 1996); stiripentol (KERR et al. 1991; TRAN et al. 1996); valproamide [399/1983] (MACPHEE et al. 1988); viloxazine (PISANI et al. 1984, 1986) and zonisamide (MACPHEE et al. 1988).

Co-administration of lamotrigine does not alter plasma carbamazepine concentrations but raises plasma carbamazepine-10,11-epoxide concentrations (RAMBECK and WOLF 1993). Combining carbamazepine with valproate leads to increased concentrations of plasma unbound carbamazepine and carbamazepine-10,11-epoxide, and either to unaltered total plasma carbamazepine and raised total plasma carbamazepine-10,11-epoxide concentrations (McKauge et al. 1981; Robbins et al. 1990; McKee et al. 1992) or to raised concentrations of both (LIU and Delgado 1994d; Liu et al. 1995; Svinarov and Pippenger 1995; Bernus et al. 1997). Metabolic balance studies (Bernus et al. 1997) suggest that valproate inhibits both epoxide hydrolase and UDP-glucuronosyl transferase activity. The drug loxepine also appears to inhibit carbamazepine-10,11-epoxide metabolism (Collins et al. 1993).

3. Interactions in Which Carbamazepine Lowers the Plasma Concentrations, or Increases the Clearances, of Other Drugs

Carbamazepine not only induces cartain CYP450 isoforms involved in its own metabolism. It also probably induces other P450 isoforms and thus enhances the biological oxidations of numerous co-administered drugs. It also increases epoxide hydrolase and UDP-glucuronosyl transferase activities. In rats it induces certain cytochrome P450 isoenzymes, principally CYP2B1 and CYP2B2 and, to a lesser extent CYP3 (Panesar et al. 1996). Drugs whose clearances are increased by carbamazepine administration include: alprazolam (Arana et al. 1988); antipyrine (Patsalos et al. 1988); bupropion (Ketter et al. 1995); clobazam, but with a decreased clearance of desmethylclobazam (Sennoune et al. 1992); clozapine (Jerling et al. 1994; Tiihonen et al. 1995); various "conazoles" e.g. fluconazole, itraconazole and ketoconazole (Tucker et al. 1992); coumarins (Harder and Thurmann 1996); cyclosporin A (Cooney et al. 1995; Campana et al. 1996), desipramine (Spina et al. 1995); dexamethasone (Guthrie 1991); doxepin (Leinonen et al. 1991); doxycycline (Neuvonen et al. 1975); erythromycin (Warren et al. 1980); ethinyloestradiol and levonorgesterol (Crawford et al. 1990); ethosuximide (Duncan et al. 1991); felbamate (Wagner et al. 1993; Rambeck et al. 1996); haloperidol (Jann et al. 1985; Kahn et al. 1990); hydroxycarbazepine (McKee et al. 1994); imipramine (Brown et al. 1990); lamotrigine (Brodie 1996); merbendazole (Luder et al. 1986); midazolam (Backman et al. 1996); nimodipine (Muck et al. 1995); nortriptyline (Brosen and Kragh-Sorensen 1993); opiates (Maurer and Bartkowski 1993); praziquantel (Bittencourt et al. 1992); prednisolone (Olivesi 1986); primidone (Battino et al. 1983); remacemide (Leach et al. 1996); rifampicin (Bachmann and Jauregui 1993); trazodone (Otani et al. 1996); theophylline (Jonkman and Upton 1984); thioridazine (Tiihonen et al. 1995); valproate (Duncan et al. 1991; Suzuki et al. 1991; Battino et al. 1992), with increased plasma concentrations of 4-en-valproate (Kondo et al. 1990; Levy et al. 1990), vecuronium (Alloul et al. 1996) and warfarin (Wells et al. 1994).

4. Interactions Leading to Raised Concentrations of Other Drugs

Although earlier studies suggested that carbamazepine administration caused plasma phenytoin concentrations to fall (Richens and Houghton 1975;

WINDORFER and SAUER 1977), more recent data indicate that the drug causes raised plasma phenytoin concentrations (ZIELINSKI et al. 1985; ZIELINSKI and HAIDUKEWYCH 1987; BROWNE et al. 1988; DUNCAN et al. 1991). In human foetal liver microsomes, carbamazepine inhibited the 2-hydroxylation of desipramine (SPINA et al. 1986), and in rats decreased imipramine demethylation (DANIEL and NETTER 1988).

F. Adverse Effects

The unwanted effects of carbamazepine were reviewed by SHAHAR and BEN ZE'EV (1989). They are dealt with below under the categories of (1) isolated (typically asymptomatic) biochemical abnormalities, (2) dose-determined abnormalities, (3) idiosyncratic abnormalities, and (4) foetal abnormalities.

I. Biochemical Abnormalities

Such abnormalities associated with carbamazepine intake include: raised serum concentrations of: alkaline phosphatase (OKESINA et al. 1991), occurring in 14% of treated subjects (ALDENHOVEL 1988); apolipoprotein A (CALANDRE et al. 1991); total, HDL and LDL cholesterol (FRANZONI et al. 1992; ISOJARVI et al. 1993; EIRIS et al. 1995); copper (SOZUER et al. 1995); γ-glutamyl transpeptidase (in 64% of treated subjects – ALDENHOVEL 1988); sex hormone binding globulin in females (ISOJARVI et al. 1995a) and males (ISOJARVI et al. 1995b), and reduced serum or plasma levels of: bilirubin (GOUGH et al. 1989); carnitine (HUG et al. 1991); cortisol (PERINI et al. 1992); folate (REIZENSTEIN and LUND 1973), though BENTSEN et al. (1983) obtained a contrary result; immunoglobulin G2 but not G1, G3 or G4 (GILHUS and LEA 1988); free luteinizing hormone, testosterone and dehydroepiandrosterone sulphate in females (ISOJARVI 1990); 17β-oestradiol (ISOJARVI et al. 1995a); thyroxine and tri-iodothyronine (ISOJARVI et al. 1990); tryptophan (PRATT et al. 1984); uric acid (RING et al. 1991; FICHSEL et al. 1993) and 24-hydroxy-vitamin D (LAMBERG et al. 1990).

Red blood cell folate concentrations may be reduced by carbamazepine intake (AL MUSAED et al. 1992; FROSCHER et al. 1995), whilst interleukin 2 production by peripheral blood mononuclear cells is increased (PACIFICI et al. 1995). There are increased excretion of α_1-microglobin in urine (KORINTHENBERG et al. 1994), increased levels of thyrotropin releasing hormone in affectively ill patients (MARANGELL et al. 1994) and decreased concentrations of somatostatin in CSF (RICHARDSON and TWENTE 1992).

II. Dose-Determined Adverse Effects

Within the range of plasma carbamazepine concentrations which is usually considered "therapeutic" in treating epilepsy, the drug can cause measurable effects on aspects of cognitive function, including memory and on behaviour (Forsythe et al. 1991; Ronnberg et al. 1992), together with a selective measurable decline in psychomotor performance (Gillham et al. 1990). These changes are usually mild enough to be regarded as acceptable by patients and their families: if not, carbamazepine dosage will probably be reduced. A number of studies have suggested that, when carbamazepine and phenytoin are compared, the latter drug has a less favourable neuropsychological profile (Dodrill and Troupin 1991), but more recent work has not confirmed this (Meador et al. 1991; Verma et al. 1993; Aldenkamp and Vermeulen 1995; Devinsky 1995; Pulliainen and Jokelainen 1995).

At higher plasma carbamazepine concentrations there may be a phase of temporary drug toxicity coinciding with the expected time of peak plasma drug concentration after each drug dose (Haefeli et al. 1994; Riva et al. 1984), particularly when rapidly absorbed carbamazepine preparations are used. The usual symptoms are sensations of dysequilibrium, ataxia of gait, nystagmus and sometimes diplopia. At still higher plasma carbamazepine concentrations such manifestations occupy increasing proportions of the dosage interval until they are present continuously. Fatigue and drowsiness develop as the drug concentration rises further, consciousness becomes impaired, and coma and ultimately death may follow. Prior to this stage seizures, dystonia and cardiac conduction defects may appear (Bridge et al. 1994; Schmidt and Schmidt-Buhl 1995; Stremski et al. 1995). Hyponatraemia was noted in 12% of the carbamazepine overdosage cases described by Seymour (1993).

1. Hyponatraemia

Serum Na^+ concentrations tend to be reduced in patients taking long term carbamazepine therapy, and actual hyponatraemia sometimes develops (Glandelman 1994; Van Amelsvoort et al. 1994). This is usually asymptomatic, but it can produce symptoms and, uncommonly, may worsen the epilepsy for which the drug has been prescribed (Ballardie and Mucklow 1984). The severity of the disturbance appears to some extent related to the carbamazepine dose and the duration of therapy with the drug. The electrolyte disturbance is usually attributed to inappropriate antidiuretic hormone secretion induced by the drug, but the detailed mechanisms involved are not fully elucidated (see "Other Biochemical Effects").

III. Idiosyncratic Adverse Effects

Many of the reported unwanted effects of carbamazepine appear to be idiosyncratic in nature. Their severity is not dose-proportional and they may affect various bodily organs and systems. Their pathogenesis is often poorly understood, with the exception of a pattern of hypersensitivity reaction which is described below, and which typically affects multiple tissues soon after carbamazepine intake commences.

1. Aromatic Anticonvulsant Hypersensitivity Syndrome

In its fully developed form, this syndrome (De Vriese et al. 1995) may affect multiple bodily organs and tissues. Shear and Spielberg (1988) found that fever occurred in 94% of cases, skin rashes in 87%, hepatitis in 51% and haematological abnormalities (often eosinophilia) in 51%. The kidneys, lymphoid tissue (sometimes a pseudolymphoma reaction – De Vriese et al. 1995) and lungs are involved less frequently. Manifestations usually first appear in the 2nd or 3rd week of exposure to carbamazepine. If death occurs, it is usually due to liver failure. The syndrome occurs in 1:1000 to 1:10000 persons who receive carbamazepine (Vittorio and Muglia 1995). Some affected individuals show a similar pattern of adverse reaction after intake of other antiepileptic drugs which contain an aromatic moiety in their chemical structure. A good deal of work has been done on the pathogenesis of the syndrome (Davis et al. 1995). There is some evidence that a reactive metabolite of carbamazepine may be responsible, possibly 9-acridine carboxyaldehyde (Furst and Uetrecht 1995; Furst et al. 1995) or an arene oxide derivative (Pirmohamed et al. 1992; Gaedigk et al. 1994), but not carbamazepine-10,11-epoxide. Altered immunological reactivity is present (Horneff et al. 1992; Mauri-Hellweg et al. 1995), with production of antibodies against carbamazepine (Leeder et al. 1992). The skin lesions have shown histological changes consistent with delayed-type allergy (Gall et al. 1994) and an imune complex drug reaction (Scerri et al. 1993).

It seems feasible that a number of idiosyncratic toxic reactions to the drug described below which involve single organs or tissues may depend on similar mechanisms, so that they are really formes fruste of the full syndrome which may not have had time to develop before carbamazepine intake was terminated.

2. Skin

A degree of alopecia occurs in 6% of persons taking carbamazepine (McKinney et al. 1996), and skin rashes in 12% (Kramlinger et al. 1994) or 16.6% (Chadwick et al. 1984). The usual pattern of rash begins as an erythematous macular one, which disappears if carbamazepine intake is ceased. Other patterns of skin reaction are known, e.g. erythroderma (Okuywama et al. 1996), a psoriatiform (Brenner et al. 1994) or lichenoid eruption (Yasuda et al. 1988; Atkin et al. 1990), a nodular cutaneous lymphoproliferative disorder (Sigal-Nahum et al. 1992), a mycosis fungoides-like dermatosis (Rijlaarsdam et al. 1991; Fitzpatrick 1992) and toxic epidermal necrolysis (Sakellariou et al. 1991; Friedmann et al. 1994; Roujeau et al. 1995).

3. Nervous System

Various uncommon, presumably idiosyncratic neurological complications of carbamazepine intake have been described, including: increased seizures (Snead and Hosey 1985; Horn et al. 1986; Neufeld 1993; Miyamoto et al.

1995); tics (Neglia et al. 1984; Robertson et al. 1993); asterixis (Ng et al. 1991; Rittmannsberger et al. 1991); dyskinesis (Schwartzman and Leppik 1990); non-epileptic myoclonus (Aguglia et al. 1987); external ophthalmoplegia (Schwartzman and Leppik 1990; Rittmannsberger et al. 1991); the neuroleptic malignant syndrome (O'Griofa and Voris 1991); encephalomyelopathy (Vestermark and Vestermark 1991); oculogyric crisis (Gorman and Barkley 1995); psychosis (Schmitz and Trimble 1995), sometimes following carbamazepine withdrawal (Darbar et al. 1996); aseptic meningitis (Simon et al. 1990; Maignen et al. 1992) and (almost always asymptomatic) slowed peripheral nerve conduction velocities (Geraldini et al. 1984; Krause and Berlit 1990).

4. Haematological

Leucopenia occurred in 2.1% of 977 persons taking carbamazepine (Tohen et al. 1995), though Sobotka et al. (1990) had earlier reported this abnormality in 12% of children and 7% of adults. Other reported abnormalities include: agranulocytosis (Olcay et al. 1995; Spickett et al. 1996; Kaufman et al. 1996); aplastic anaemia (Gerson et al. 1983; Franceschi et al. 1988; Betticher et al. 1991; Kaufman et al. 1996); pure red cell aplasia (Buitendag 1990); haemolytic anaemia (Stroink et al. 1984); and thrombocytopenia (Kaneko et al. 1993; Shechter et al. 1993; Kimura et al. 1995).

There have also been reports of systemic lupus erythematosus due to carbamazepine (Boon et al. 1992; Schmidt et al. 1992; Dvory and Korczyn 1993).

5. Cardiovascular

Reported cardiovascular toxic effects of carbamazepine include: eosinophilic myocarditis (Salzman et al. 1997); arrhythmias (Kenneback et al. 1991); cardiac conduction abnormalities (Benassi et al. 1987; Hantson et al. 1993); bradycardia (Kenneback et al. 1992), which nearly always occurs in the elderly (Kasarskis et al. 1992); tachycardia in the overdosed (Kasarskis et al. 1992); syncope (Stone and Lange 1986; Jacome 1987); vasculitis (Harats and Shalit 1987); and granulomatous angiitis (Imai et al. 1989).

6. Respiratory

Carbamazepine has been reported to cause pneumonitis (Takahashi et al. 1993; King et al. 1994) and pulmonary eosinophilia (Tolmie et al. 1983).

7. Alimentary Tract

Carbamazepine may cause intractable diarrhoea (Iyer et al. 1992) and eosinophilic colitis (Anttila and Valtonen 1992), whilst excessive appetite and weight gain have been reported (Lampl et al. 1991; Pijl and Meinders 1996).

8. Liver

As well as being part of the aromatic anticonvulsant hypersensitivity syndrome, hepatitis may occur as a seemingly isolated and usually reversible manifestation of carbamazepine toxicity (HOROWITZ et al. 1988; MARTINEZ et al. 1993). Cholangitis (LA SPINA et al. 1994) and the vanishing bile duct syndrome (DE GALOSEY et al. 1994) have also been reported.

9. Pancreas

Pancreatitis may complicate carbamazepine use (SOMAN and SWENSON 1985; TSAO and WRIGHT 1993).

10. Kidneys

Carbamazepine has caused interstitial nephritis (LAMBERT and FOURNIER 1992; EIJGENRAAM et al. 1997).

11. Bone

Used in continuing monotherapy, carbamazepine appears to produce no significant adverse effects on bone (TJELLERSEN et al. 1983). In confirmation of this, SHETH et al. (1995) found no changes in bone mineral density in children after at least 6 months intake of the drug.

12. Porphyria

Carbamazepine may precipitate attacks of porphyria (YEUNG-LAIWAH et al. 1983), by inducing 5-aminolaevulinate synthase, secondary to an increased utilization of heme by tryprophan pyrrolase (MORGAN and BADAWY 1992).

13. Thyroid

Although carbamazepine intake is associated with measured alterations in concentration of circulating thyroid hormones (see above – "Biochemical Abnormalities"), there is no clinical evidence of associated thyroid disease. Some evidence exists that the abnormal biochemical findings may be consequences of carbamazepine displacing thyroid hormones from plasma protein binding sites (SURKS and DE FESI 1996) so that thyroid stimulating hormone concentrations (which are unaltered) provide more reliable measures of thyroid function in the presence of the drug.

IV. Foetal Toxicity

For some years, carbamazepine was regarded as the least foeto-toxic of the commonly used antiepileptic drugs in humans (STARREVELD-ZIMMERMAN et al. 1973), but its use in pregnancy is now believed to be associated with a foetal carbamazepine syndrome (JONES et al. 1989; ORNOY and COHEN 1996; NULMAN et al. 1997) comprising minor cranio-facial defects, fingernail hypoplasia and developmental delay, and with decreased foetal growth (Bertollini et al. 1987). More importantly, carbamazepine intake during pregnancy is associated with an increased incidence of spinal dysraphism in the offspring (Kallen et al. 1989; Rosa 1991; Lindhout and Omtzigt 1992; Kallen 1994; Shurtleff and Lemire 1995). Hypospadias may also occur (Lindhout and Omtzigt 1992). Hansen et al. (1996) have shown that carbamazepine, but not carbamazepine-10,11-epoxide, is embryotoxic to rodents, though of course the foetal tissue injury could depend on carbamazepine metabolites apart from the epoxide (Finnell et al. 1995).

The mutagenicity of carbamazepine in humans has been studied by Sinues et al. (1995). There was an increase in sister chromatid exchange frequencies and in proliferation indices, but not in other measures of mutagenic potential.

References

Aguglia U, Zappia M, Quattrone A (1987) Carbamazepine-induced nonepileptic myoclonus in a child with benign epilepsy. Epilepsia 28:515–518

Albani F, Theodore WH, Washington P, Devinsky O, Bromfield E, Porter RJ, Nice FJ (1991) Effects of felbamate on plasma levels of carbamazepine and its metabolites. Epilepsia 32:130–132

Albani F, Riva R, Contin M, Baruzzi A (1992) A within-subject analysis of carbamazepine disposition related to development in children with epilepsy. Ther Drug Monit 14:457–460

Albani F, Riva R, Baruzzi A (1993) Clarithromycin-carbamazepine interaction: a case report. Epilepsia 34:161–162

Albright PS, Bruni J (1984) Effects of carbamazepine and its epoxide metabolite on amygdala-kindled seizures in rats. Neurology 34:1383–1386

Aldenhovel HG (1988) The influence of long-term anticonvulsant therapy with diphenylhydantoin and carbamazepine on serum gamma-glutamyltransferase, aspartate aminotransferase and alkaline phosphatase. Eur Arch Psychiatry Neurol Sci 237:312–316

Aldenkamp AP, Vermeulen J (1995) Phenytoin and carbamazepine: differential effects on cognitive function. Seizure 4:95–104

Lamberg-Allardt C, Saraste KL, Gronlund T (1990) Vitamin D status of ambulatory and nonambulatory mentally retarded children with and without carbamazepine treatment. Ann Nutr Metab 34:216–220

Allen S (1994) Cerebellar dysfunction following dextropropoxyphene-induced carbamazepine toxicity. Postgrad Med J 70:764

Alloul K, Whalley DG, Shutway F, Ebrahim F, Varin F (1996) Pharmacokinetic origin of carbamazepine-induced resistance to vecuronium blockade in anesthetized patients. Anesthesiology 84:330–339

al Musaed AA, Zakrzewska JM, Bain BJ (1992) Carbamazepine and folic acid in trigeminal neuralgia patients. J Roy Soc Med 85:19–22

Altafullah I, Talwar D, Loewenson R, Olson K, Lockman LA (1989) Factors influencing serum levels of carbamazepine and carbamazepine-10,11-epoxide in children. Epilepsy Res 4:71–80

Amabeoku GJ, Chikuni O, Akino C, Mutetwa S (1993) Pharmacokinetic interaction of single doses of quinine and carbamazepine, phenobarbitone and phenytoin in healthy volunteers. East Afr Med J 70:90–93

Antony JH, Hawke SH (1983) Phenobarbital compared with phenobarbital in prevention of recurrent febrile convulsions. A double-blind study. Amer J Dis Child 137:892–895

Anttila VJ, Valtonen M (1992) Carbamazepine-induced eosinophilic colitis. Epilepsia 33:119–121

Arana GW, Epstein S, Molloy M, Greenblatt DJ (1988) Carbamazepine-induced reduction of plasma alprazolam concentrations: a clinical case report. J Clin Psychiatry 49:448–449

Arvidsson J, Nilsson HL, Sandstedt P, Steinwall G, Tonnby B, Flesch G (1995) Replacing carbamazepine slow-release tablets with carbamazepine suppositories: a pharmacokinetic and clinical study in children with epilepsy. J Child Neurol 10:114–117

Atkin SL, McKenzie TM, Stevenson CJ (1990) Carbamazepine-induced lichenoid eruptions. Clin Exp Dermatol 15:382–383

Auger RG, Daube JR, Gomez MR, Lambert EH (1984) Hereditary form of sustained muscular activity of peripheral nerve origin causing generalized myokymia and muscle stiffness. Ann Neurol 15:13–21

Bachmann KA, Jauregui L (1993) Use of single sample clearance estimates of cytochrome P450 substrates to characterize human hepatic CYP status in vivo. Xenobiotica 23:307–315

Backman E, Dahlstron G, Eeg-Olofsson O, Bertler A (1987) The 24 hour variation of salivary carbamazepine and carbamazepine-10,11-epoxide concentrations in children with epilepsy. Pediatr Neurol 3:327–330

Backman JT, Olkkola KT, Ojala M, Laaksovirta H, Neuvonen PL (1996) Concentration and effects of oral midazolam are greatly reduced in patients treated with carbamazepine or phenytoin. Epilepsia 37:253–257

Baf MH, Subhash MN, Lakesmana KM, Rao BS (1994) Alterations in monoamine levels in discrete regions of rat brain after chronic administration of carbamazepine. Neurochem Res 19:1139–1143

Bahls FH, Ozuna J, Ritchie DE (1991) Interactions between calcium channel blockers and the anticonvulsants carbamazepine and phenytoin. Neurology 41:740–742

Ballardie F, Mucklow JC (1984) Partial reversal of carbamazepine-induced water intolerance by demeclocycline. Brit Med J 17:763–765

Bano G, Raina RK, Sharma DB (1986) Pharmacokinetics of carbamazepine in protein energy malnutrition. Pharmacology 32:232–236

Bardy AH, Teramo K, Hiilesmaa VK (1982) Apparent clearances of phenytoin, phenobarbitone, primidone and carbamazepine during pregnancy: results of the prospective Helsinski study. In: Janz D, Bossi L, Helge H, Richens A, Schmidt D (eds) Epilepsy, pregnancy, and the child. Raven Press, New York, pp. 141–145

Bass J, Miles MV, Tennison MB, Holcombe BJ, Thorn MD (1989) Effects of enteral tube feeding on the absorption and pharmacokinetic profile of carbamazepine suspension. Epilepsia 30:364–369

Battino D, Avanzini G, Bossi L, Croci D, Cusi C, Gomeni C, Moise A (1983) Plasma levels of primidone and its metabolite phenobarbital: effects of age and associated therapy. Ther Drug Monit 5:73–79

Battino D, Binelli S, Bossi L et al. (1985) Plasma concentrations of carbamazepine and carbamazepine-10,11-epoxide during pregnancy and after delivery. Clin Pharmacokinet 10:279–284

Battino D, Croci D, Granata T, Bernardi G, Monza G (1992) Changes in unbound and total valproic acid concentrations after replacement of carbamazepine with oxcarbazepine. Ther Drug Monit 14:376–379

Battino D, Estienne M, Avanzini G (1995) Clinical pharmacokinetics of antiepileptic drugs in paediatric patients. Part II. Phenytoin, carbamazepine, sulthiame, lamotrigine, vigabatrin, oxcarbazepine and felbamate. Clin Pharmacokinet 29:341–369

Battistin L, Varotto M, Berlese G, Roman G (1984) Effects of some anticonvulsant drugs on brain GABA level and GAD and GABA-T activities. Neurochem Res 9:225–231
Beattie B, Biller J, Mehlhaus B, Murray M (1988) Verapamil-induced carbamazepine neurotoxicity. A report of two cases. Eur Neurol 28:104–105
Benassi E, Bo GP, Cocito L, Maffini M, Loeb C (1987) Carbamazepine and cardiac conduction disturbances. Ann Neurol 22:280–281
Bender AS, Hertz L (1988) Evidence for involvement of the astrocytic benzodiazepine receptor in the mechanism of action of convulsant and anticonvulsant drugs. Life Sci 43:477–484
Benetello P, Ferlanut M (1987) Primidone-carbamazepine interaction: clinical consequences. Int J Clin Pharmacol Res 7:165–168
Bentsen KD, Gram L, Veje A (1983) Serum thyroid hormones and blood folic acid during monotherapy with carbamazepine or valproate. Acta Neurol Scand 67:235–241
Bernus I, Dickinson RG, Hooper WD, Eadie MJ (1994) Early stage autoinduction of carbamazepine metabolism in humans. Europ J Clin Pharmacol 47:355–360
Bernus I, Hooper WD, Dickinson RG, Eadie MJ (1995) Metabolism of carbamazepine and co-administered anticonvulsants during pregnancy. Epilepsy Res 21:65–75
Bernus I, Dickinson RG, Hooper WG, Eadie MJ (1996) Dose-dependent metabolism of carbamazepine in humans. Epilepsy Res 24:163–172
Bernus I, Dickinson RG, Hooper WD, Eadie MJ (1997) The mechanism of the carbamazepine-valproate interaction in humans. Br J Clin Pharmac 44:21–27
Bertilsson L (1978) Clinical pharmacokinetics of carbamazepine. Clin Pharmacokinet 3:128–143
Bertilsson L, Tomson T (1986) Clinical pharmacokinetics and pharmacological effects of carbamazepine and carbamazepine-10,11-epoxide: an update. Clin Pharmacokinet 11:177–198
Bertilsson L, Hojer B, Tybring G, Osterloh J, Rane A (1980) Autoinduction of carbamazepine metabolism in children by a stable isotope technique. Clin Pharmacol Ther 27:83–88
Bertilsson L, Tomson T, Tybring G (1986) Pharmacokinetics: time-dependent changes – autoinduction of carbamazepine epoxidation. J Clin Pharmacol 26:459–462
Bertollini R, Kallen B, Mastroiacorvo P, Robert E (1987) Anticonvulsant drugs in monotherapy. Effect on the fetus. Eur J Epidemiol 3:164–171
Betticher DC, Wolfisberg HP, Krapf R (1991) Aplastic anemia in carbamazepine therapy. Schweitz Med Wochenschr 121:583–588
Beyer C, Spiteller G (1992) A new carbamazepine metabolite in uraemic filtrate. Xenobiotica 22:1029–1035
Biber K, Walden J, Gebicke-Harter P, Berger M, van Calker D (1996) Carbamazepine inhibits the potentiation by adenosine analogues of agonist induced inositolphosphate formation in hippocampal astrocyte cultures. Biol Psychiatry 40:563–567
Bittencourt PR, Gracia CM, Martins R, Fernandes AG, Dickmann HW, Jung W (1992) Phenytoin and carbamazepine decreased oral bioavailability of praziquantel. Neurology 42:492–496
Blom S (1962) Trigeminal neuralgia: its treatment with a new anticonvulsant drug (G32883). Lancet 1:839–840
Boon DM, van Parys JA, Swaak AJ (1992) Disseminated lupus erythematosus induced by carbamazepine (Tegretol). Ned tijdschr Geneeskd 136:2085–2087
Bourgeois B (1996) Drug interaction profile of topiramate. Epilepsia 37[Suppl 2]:S14–S17
Bourgeois B, Wad N (1984) Carbamazepine-10,11-diol steady-state serum levels and renal excretion during carbamazepine therapy in adults and children. Ther Drug Monit 6:259–265
Bourgeois BFD, Dodson WE, Ferrendelli JA (1982) Interactions between primidone, carbamazepine, and nicotinamide. Neurology 32:1122–1126

Brazis PW, Niller NR, Henderer JD, Lee AG (1994) The natural history and results of treatment of superior oblique myokymia. Arch Ophthalmol 112:1063–1067
Brenner S, Wolf R, Landau M, Politi Y (1994) Psoriasiform eruption induced by anticonvulsants. Isr J Med Sci 30:283–286
Bridge TA, Norton RL, Robertson WO (1994) Pediatric carbamazepine overdoses. Pediatr Emerg Care 10:260–263
Brodie MJ (1996) Lamotrigine – an update. Can J Neurol Sci 23:S6–S9
Brodie MJ, Richens A, Yuen AWC (1995) Double-blind comparison of lamotrigine and carbamazepine in newly diagnosed epilepsy. Lancet 345:476–479
Brosen K, Kragh-Sorensen P (1993) Concomitant intake of nortriptyline and carbamazepine. Ther Drug Monit 15:258–260
Brown CS, Wells BG, Cold JA, Froemming JH, Self TH, Jabbour JT (1990) Possible influence of carbamazepine on plasma imipramine concentrations in children with attention deficit disorder. J Clin Psychopharmacol 10:359–362
Browne TR, Szabo GK, Evans JE, Evans BA, Greenblatt DJ, Mikati MA (1988) Carbamazepine increases phenytoin serum concentration and reduces phenytoin clearance. Neurology 38:1146–1150
Buitendag DJ (1990) Pure red cell aplasia associated with carbamazepine. S Afr Med J 78:214–215
Burchiel KJ (1988) Carbamazepine inhibits spontaneous activity in experimental neuromas. Exp Neurol 102:249–253
Butler D, Messiha PS (1986) Alcohol withdrawal and carbamazepine. Alcohol 3:113–129
Calandre EP, Rodriquez-Lopez C, Blazquez A, Cano D (1991) Serum lipids, lipoproteins and apolipoproteins A and B in epileptic patients treated with valproic acid, carbamazepine or phenobarbital. Acta Neurol Scand 83:250–253
Calissi PT, Jaber LA (1995) Peripheral diabetic neuropathy: current concepts in treatment. Ann Pharmacother 29:769–777
Campana C, Regazzi MB, Buggia I, Molinaro M (1996) Clinically significant drug interactions with cyclosporin. An update. Clin Pharmacokinet 30:141–179
Canger R, Altamura AC, Belvedere O, Monaco F, Monza GC, Muscas GC, Mutani R, Panetta B, Pisani F, Zaccara G et al (1990) Conventional vs. controlled release carbamazepine: a multicentre, double-blind, cross-over study. Acta Neurol Scand 82:9–13
Caraco Y, Zylber-Katz E, Berry EM, Levy M (1995) Carbamazepine pharmacokinetics in obese and lean subjects. Ann Pharmacother 29:843–847
Cereghino JJ, Brock JT, Van Meter JC, Penry JK, Smith LD, White BG (1975) The efficacy of carbamazepine combinations in epilepsy. Clin Pharmacol Ther 18:733–741
Chadwick D, Shaw MDM, Foy P, Rawlins MD, Turnbull DM (1984) Serum anticonvulsant concentrations and the risk of drug induced skin eruptions. J Neurol Neurosurg Psychiat 47:642–644
Chaudry RP, Waters BGH (1983) Lithium and carbamazepine interaction: possible neurotoxicity. J Clin Psychiatry 44:30–31
Chen G, Pan B, Hawver DB, Wright CB, Potter WZ, Manji HK (1996) Attenuation of cyclic AMP production by carbamazepine. J Neurochem 67:2079–2086
Cheymol G, Engel F (1989) Drug interactions with calcium inhibitors in man. Therapie 44:189–196
Cloyd J (1991) Pharmacokinetic pitfalls of present antiepileptic medications. Epilepsia 32 [Suppl 5]:S53–S65
Coleman MH, Yamaguchi S, Rogawski MA (1992) Protection against dendrotoxin-induced clonic seizures in mice by anticonvulsant drugs. Brain Res 575:138–142
Collins DM, Gidal BE, Pitterle ME (1993) Potential interaction between carbamazepine and loxapine: case report and retrospective review. Ann Pharmacother 27:1180–1187

Consolo S, Bianchi S, Ladinsky H (1976) Effect of carbamazepine on cholinergic parameters in rat brain areas. Neuropharmacology 15:653–657
Cooney GF, Mochon M, Kaiser B, Dunn SP, Goldsmith B (1995) Effects of carbamazepine on cyclosporine metabolism in pediatric renal transplant recipients. Pharmacotherapy 15:353–356
Cottencin O, Regnaut N, Thevenon-Gignac C, Goudemand M, Debruille C, Robert H (1995) [Carbamazepine-fluvoxamine interaction. Consequences for the carbamazepine plasma level]. Encephale 21:141–145
Cotter LM, Eadie MJ, Hooper WD, Lander CM, Smith GA, Tyrer JH (1977) The pharmacokinetics of carbamazepine. Europ J Clin Pharmacol 12:451–456
Coulter DA, Huguenard JR, Prince DA (1989) Specific petit mal anticonvulsants reduce calcium currents in thalamic neurons. Neurosci Lett 98:74–78
Courtney KR, Etter EF (1983) Modulated anticonvulsant block of sodium channels in nerve and muscle. Eur J Pharmacol 88:1–9
Craig CR, Colasanti BK (1992) Reduction of frequency of seizures by carbamazepine during cobalt experimental epilepsy in the rat. Pharmacol Biochem Behav 41:813–816
Crawford P, Chadwick DJ, Martin C, Tjia J, Black DJ, Orme M (1990) The interaction of phenytoin and carbamazepine with combined oral contraceptive steroids. Br J Clin Pharmac 30:892–896
Crowder JM, Bradford HF (1987) Common anticonvulsants inhibit Ca^{2+} uptake and amino acid neurotransmitter release in vitro. Epilepsia 28:378–382
Czuczwar SJ, Janusz W, Szezepanik B, Kleinrok Z (1991) Influence of CGS15943 A (a non-xanthine adenosine antagonist) on the protection offered by a variety of antiepileptic drugs against maximum electroshock induced seizures in mice. J Neural Transm Gen Sect 86:127–134
Dailey JW, Jobe PC (1985) Anticonvulsant drugs and the genetically epilepsy-prone rat. Federation Proc 44:2640–2644
Dalton MJ, Powell JR, Messenheimer JAJ (1985) The influence of cimetidine on single-dose carbamazepine pharmacokinetics. Epilepsia 26:127–130
Dam M, Christiansen J, Kristensen CB, Helles A, Jaegerskou A, Schmiegelow M (1981) Carbamazepine: a clinical biopharmaceutical study. Europ J Clin Pharmacol 20:59–64
Daniel W, Netter KJ (1988) Metabolic interaction between imipramine and carbamazepine in vivo and in vitro in rats. Naunyn-Schmiedebergs Arch Pharmacol 337:105–110
Darbar D, Connachie AM, Jones AM, Newton RW (1996) Acute psychosis associated with abrupt withdrawal of carbamazepine following intoxication. Br J Clin Pract 50:350–351
Dasgupta A, Thompson WC (1995) Carbamazepine-salicylate interaction in normal and uremic sera: reduced interaction in uremic sera. Ther Drug Monit 17:217–220
Dasgupta A, Volk A (1996) Displacement of valproic acid and carbamazepine from protein binding in normal and uremic sera by tolmetin, ibuprofen and naproxen: presence of inhibitor in uremic serum that blocks valproic acid-naproxen interactions. Ther Drug Monit 18:284–287
David J, Grewal RS (1976) Effect of carbamazepine (Tegretol) on seizure and EEG patterns in monkeys with alumina-induced focal motor and hippocampal foci. Epilepsia 17:415–422
Davis CD, Pirmohamed M, Kitteringham NR, Allott RL, Smith D, Park BK (1995) Kinetic parameters of lymphocyte microsomal epoxide hydrolase in carbamazepine hypersensitive patients. Assessment by radiometric HPLC. Biochem Pharmacol 50:1361–1366
de Feo MR, Mecarelli O, Ricci G, Rina MF (1991) Effects of carbamazepine on bicuculline- and pentylenetetrazole-induced seizures in developing rats. Brain Develop 13:343–347

de Galosey C, Horsmans Y, Rahier J, Geubel AP (1994) Vanishing bile duct syndrome occurring after carbamazepine administration: a second case report. J Clin Gastroenterol 19:269–271
DeLorenzo RJ (1984) Calmodulin systems in neuronal excitability: a molecular approach to epilepsy. Ann Neurol 16 [Suppl]:S104–S114
Denicoff KD, Meglathery SB, Post RM, Tandeciarz SI (1994) Efficacy of carbamazepine compared with other agents: a clinical practice survey. J Clin Psychiatry 55:70–76
De Sarro G, Ascioti C, di Paola ED, Vidal MJ, De Sarro A (1992) Effect of antiepileptic drugs, calcium channel blockers and other compounds on seizures induced by activation of voltage-dependent L calcium channels in DBA/2 mice. Gen Pharmacol 23:1205–1216
de Silva M, MacArdle B, McGowan B, Hughes E, Stewart J, Neville BG, Johnson AL, Reynolds EH (1996) Randomised comparative monotherapy trial of phenobarbitone, phenytoin, carbamazepine, or sodium valproate for newly diagnosed childhood epilepsy. Lancet 347:709–713
Devinsky O (1995) Cognitive and behavioural effects of antiepileptic drugs. Epilepsia 36 [Suppl 2]:S46–S65
DeVriese AS, Phillipe J, Van Reterghem DM, De Cuyper CA, Hindryckx PH, Matthys EG, Louagie A (1995) Carbamazepine hypersensitivity syndrome: report of 4 cases and review of the literature. Medicine Baltimore 74:144–151
Dickinson RG, Hooper WD, King AR, Eadie MJ (1985) Fallacious results from measuring salivary carbamazepine concentrations. Ther Drug Monit 7:41–45
Dodrill CB, Troupin AS (1991) Neuropsychological effects of carbamazepine and phenytoin: a reanalysis. Neurology 41:141–143
Drory VE, Korczyn AD (1993) Hypersensitivity vasculitis and systemic lupus erythematosus induced by anticonvulsants. Clin Neuropharmac 16:19–29
Duncan JS, Patsalos PN, Shorvon SD (1991) Effects of discontinuation of phenytoin, carbamazepine, and valproate on concomitant antiepileptic medication. Epilepsia 32:101–115
Eadie MJ (1994) Plasma antiepileptic drug monitoring in a neurological practice: a 25-year experience. Ther Drug Monit 16:458–468
Eadie MJ (1997) The place of antiepileptic drug combinations. J Clin Neurosci 4
Eadie MJ, Hooper WD (1987) Intermittent carbamazepine intoxication possibly related to altered absorption characteristics of the drug. M J Australia 146:313–316
Eadie MJ, Tyrer JH (1989) Anticonvulsant therapy: pharmacological basis and practice, 3rd edn. Churchill-Livingstone, Edinburgh
Ebert U, Rundfeldt C, Löscher W (1995) Development and pharmacological suppression of secondary afterdischarges in the hippocampus of amygdaloid kindled rats. Eur J Neurosci 7:732–741
Eeg-Olofsson O, Nilsson HL, Tonnby B, Arvidsson J, Grahn PA, Gylje H, Larsson C, Noren L (1990) Diurnal variation of carbamazepine and carbamazepine-10,11-epoxide in plasma and saliva in children with epilepsy: a comparison between conventional and slow-release formulations. J Child Neurol 5:159–165
Eichelbaum M, Ekbom K, Bertilsson L, Ringberger VA, Rane A (1975) Plasma kinetics of carbamazepine and its epoxide metabolite in man after single and multiple doses. Europ J Clin Pharmacol 8:337–341
Eichelbaum M, Kothe KW, Hoffman F, Von Uruth GE (1982) Use of stable labelled carbamazepine to study its kinetics during chronic carbamazepine treatment. Europ J Clin Pharmacol 23:241–244
Eichelbaum M, Tomson T, Tybring G, Bertilsson L (1985) Carbamazepine metabolism in man. Induction and pharmacogenetic aspects. Clin Pharmacokinet 10:80–90
Eijgenraam JW, Buurke EJ, van der Laan JS (1997) Carbamazepine-associated acute tubulointerstitial nephritis. Neth J Med 50:25–28
Eiris JM, Lojo S, Del Rio MC, Novo I, Bravo M, Pavon P, Castro-Gago M (1995) Effect of long-term treatment with antiepileptic drugs on serum lipid levels in children with epilepsy. Neurology 45:1155–1157

Ekbom KA (1972) Carbamazepine in the treatment of tabetic lightning pains. Arch Neurol 26:374–378

Elliott P (1990) Action of antiepileptic and anaesthetic drugs on Na- and Ca-spikes in mammalian non-myelinated axons. Eur J Pharmacol 175:155–163

Elphick M (1989) Effects of carbamazepine on dopamine function in rodents. Psychopharmacology Berl 99:532–536

Elphick M, Yang JD, Cowen PJ (1990) Effects of carbamazepine on dopamine- and serotonin-mediated neuroendocrine responses. Arch Gen Psychiatry 47:135–140

Elyas AA, Patsalos PN, Agbato OA, Brett EM, Lascelles PT (1986) Factors influencing simultaneous concentrations of total and free carbamazepine and carbamazepine-10,11-epoxide in serum of children with epilepsy. Ther Drug Monit 8:288–292

Emilien G, Maloteaux JM, Seghers A, Charles G (1996) Lithium compared to valproic acid and carbamazepine in the treatment of mania: a statistical meta-analysis. Eur Neuropsychopharmacol 6:245–252

Eto S, Tanaka N, Noda H, Noda A (1995) 9-Hydroxymethyl-10-carbamoylacridan in human serum is one of the major metabolites of carbamazepine. Biol Pharm Bull 18:926–928

Eto S, Tanaka N, Noda H, Noda A (1996) Chiral separation of 10,11-dihydro-10,11-trans-dihydroxycarbamazepine, a metabolite of carbamazepine with two asymmetric carbons, in human serum. J Chromatog B Biomed Appl 677:325–330

Ezra E, Spalton D, Sanders MD, Graham EM, Plant GT (1996) Ocular neuromyotonia. Br J Ophthalmol 80:350–355

Fahn S (1987) Systemic therapy of dystonia. Can J Neurol Sci 14 (Suppl 3):528–532

Faigle JW, Feldmann KF (1975) Pharmacokinetic data of carbamazepine and its major metabolites in man. In: Schneider H, Janz D, Gardner-Thorpe C, Meinardi H, Sherwin AL (eds) Clinical pharmacology of antiepileptic drugs. Springer-Verlag, Berlin, pp. 159–165

Faigle JW, Feldmann KF (1995) Carbamazepine. Chemistry and biotransformation. In: Levy RH, Mattson RH, Meldrum BH (eds) Antiepileptic drugs, 4th edn. Raven, New York, pp. 499–513

Fernandez C, Martin C, Gimenez F, Farinotti R (1995) Clinical pharmacokinetics of zopiclone. Clin Pharmacokinet 29:431–441

Ferrarese C, Marzorati C, Perego M, Bianchi G, Cavarretta R, Pierpaoli C, Moretti G, Frattola L (1995) Effect of anticonvulsant drugs on peripheral benzodiazepine receptors of human lymphocytes. Neuropharmacology 34:427–431

Fichsel G, Fichsel H, Liappis N (1993) Harnsaureserumkonzentration und antiepileptische Therapie im Kindesalter [serum uric acid concentration and anticonvulsant therapy in childhood]. Klin Pediatr 205:429–431

Filling-Katz MR, Merrick HF, Fink JK, Miles RB, Sokol J, Barton NW (1989) Carbamazepine in Fabry's disease: effective analgesia with dose-dependent exacerbation of autonomic dysfunction. Neurology 39:598–600

Finnell RH, Bennett GD, Slattery JT, Amore BM, Bajpai M, Levy RH (1995) Effect of treatment with phenobarbital and stiripentol on carbamazepine-induced teratogenicity and reactive metabolite formation. Teratology 52:324–332

Fitzpatrick JE (1992) New histopathologic findings in drug eruptions. Dermatol Clin 10:19–36

Forsythe I, Butler R, Berg I, McGuire R (1991) Cognitive impairment in new cases of epilepsy randomly assigned to carbamazepine, phenytoin and sodium valproate. Develop Med Child Neurol 33:524–534

Franceschi M, Ciboddo G, Truci G, Borri A, Canal N (1988) Fatal aplastic anemia in a patient treated with carbamazepine. Epilepsia 29:582–583

Franzoni E, Govoni M, D'Addato S, Gualandi S, Sangiorgi Z, Descovich GC, Salvioli GP (1992) Total cholesterol, high-density lipoprotein cholesterol, and trigylcerides in children receiving antiepileptic drugs. Epilepsia 33:932–935

Frey H-H, Löscher W (1980) Pharmacokinetics of carbamazepine in the dog. Arch Internat Pharmacodyn Therap 243:180–190

Friedmann PS, Strickland I, Pirmohamed M, Park BK (1994) Investigation of mechanisms of toxic epidermal necrolysis induced by carbamazepine. Arch Dermatol 130:598–604
Friis ML, Christiansen J, Hvidberg EF (1978) Brain concentrations of carbamazepine and carbamazepine-10,11-epoxide in epileptic patients. Europ J Clin Pharmacol 14:47–51
Froescher W, Eichelbaum M, Niesen M, Dietrich K, Rausch P (1984) Carbamazepine levels in breast milk. Ther Drug Monit 6:266–271
Fromm GH (1985) Effects of different classes of antiepileptic drugs on brain-stem pathways. Federation Proc 44:2432–2435
Froscher W, Stoll KD, Hildenbrand G, Eichelbaum M (1988) Investigations on the intraindividual constancy of the ratio of carbamazepine to carbamazepine-10,11-epoxide in man. Arzneimittelforschung 38:724–726
Froscher W, Herrmann R, Niesen M, Bulau P, Penin H, Hildenbrand G (1991) The course of pregnancy and teratogenicity of antiepileptic agents in 66 patients with epilepsy. Schweitz Arch Neurol Psychiatr 142:389–407
Froscher W, Maier V, Laage M, Wolfersdorf M, Straub R, Rothmeier J, Steinert T, Fiaux A, Frank U, Grupp D (1995) Folate deficiency, anticonvulsant drugs, and psychiatric morbidity. Clin Neuropharmac 18:165–182
Fuerst RH, Graves NM, Leppik IE, Brundage RC, Holmes GB, Remmel RP (1988) Felbamate increases phenytoin but decreases carbamazepine concentrations. Epilepsia 29:488–491
Fueta Y, Avoli M (1992) Effects of antiepileptic drugs on 4-aminopyridine-induced epileptiform activity in young and adult rat hippocampus. Epilepsy Res 12:207–215
Fujiwara Y, Sato M, Otsuki S (1986) Interaction of carbamazepine and other drugs with adenosine (A_1 and A_2) receptors. Psychopharmacology Berl 90:332–335
Furst SM, Uetrecht JP (1993) Carbamazepine metabolism to a reactive intermediate by the myeloperoxidase system of activated neutrophils. Biochem Pharmacol 45:1267–1275
Furst SM, Uetrecht JP (1995) The effect of carbamazepine and its reactive metabolite, 9-acridine carboxaldehyde, on immune cell function in vitro. Int J Immunopharmacol 17:445–452
Furst SM, Sukhai P, McClelland RA, Uetrecht JP (1995) Covalent binding of carbamazepine oxidative metabolites to neutrophils. Drug Metabol Disposit 23:590–594
Gaedigk A, Spielberg SP, Grant DM (1994) Characterization of the microsomal epoxide hydrolase gene in patients with adverse drug reactions. Pharmacogenetics 4:142–153
Gall H, Merk H, Scherb W, Sterry W (1994) [Anticonvulsant hypersensitivity syndrome to carbamazepine]. Hautarzt 45:494–498
Galpern WR, Miller LG, Greenblatt DJ, Szabo GK, Browne TR, Shader RJ (1991) Chronic benzodiazepine administration. IX. Attenuation of alprazolam discontinuation effects by carbamazepine. Biochem Pharmacol 42 [Suppl]:S99–S104
Garcia B, Zaborras E, Areas V, Obeso G, Jiminez I, de Juana P, Bermejo T (1992) Interaction between isoniazid and carbamazepine potentiated by cimetidine. Ann Pharmacother 26:841–842
Garcia-Borreguero D, Bronisch T, Apelt S, Yassouridis A, Emrich HM (1991) Treatment of benzodiazepine withdrawal symptoms with carbamazepine. Eur Arch Psychiatry Clin Neurosci 241:145–150
Gasser T, Reddington M, Schubert P (1988) Effects of carbamazepine on stimulus-evoked Ca^{2+} fluxes in rat hippocampal slices and its interaction with A_1 adenosine receptors. Neurosci Lett 91:189–193
Geraldini C, Faedda MT, Sideri G (1984) Anticonvulsant therapy and its possible consequences on peripheral nervous system: a neurographic study. Epilepsia 25:502–505

Gerardin AP, Abadie FV, Campestrini JA (1976) Pharmacokinetics of carbamazepine in normal humans after single and repeated oral doses. J Pharmacokin Biopharm 4:521–535

Gerardin A, Dubois JP, Moppert J, Geller L (1990) Absolute bioavailability of carbamazepine after oral administration of a 2% syrup. Epilepsia 31:334–338

Gerson WT, Fine DG, Spielberg SP, Sensenbrenner LL (1983) Anticonvulsant-induced aplastic anemia: increased susceptibility to toxic drug metabolites in vitro. Blood 61:889–893

Gidal BE, Spencer NW, Maly MM, Pitterie ME (1996) Evaluation of carbamazepine and carbamazepine-epoxide protein binding in patients undergoing epilepsy surgery. Epilepsia 37:381–385

Gigli GL, Gotman J (1991) Effect of seizures and carbamazepine on interictal spiking in amygdala kindled cats. Epilepsy Res 8:204–212

Gilhus NE, Lea T (1988) Carbamazepine: effect on IgG subclasses in epileptic patients. Epilepsia 29:317–320

Gillham RA, Williams N, Wiedmann KD, Butler E, Larkin JG, Brodie MJ (1990) Cognitive function in adult epileptic patients established on anticonvulsant monotherapy. Epilepsy Res 7:219–225

Glandelman MS (1994) Review of carbamazepine-induced hyponatremia. Prog Neuropsychopharmacol Biol Psychiatry 18:211–233

Gold PW, Robertson GL, Ballenger JC, Kaye W, Chen J, Rubinow DR, Goodwin FK, Post RM (1983) Carbamazepine diminishes the sensitivity of the plasma arginine vasopressin response to osmotic stimulation. J Clin Endocrinol Metab 57:952–957

Gorman M, Barkley GL (1995) Oculogyric crisis induced by carbamazepine. Epilepsia 36:1158–1160

Gough H, Goggin T, Crowley M, Callaghan N (1989) Serum bilirubin levels with antiepileptic drugs. Epilepsia 30:597–602

Granger P, Biton B, Faure C, Vige X, Depoortere H, Graham D, Langer SZ, Scatton B, Avenet P (1995) Modulation of the gamma-aminobutyric acid type A receptor by the antiepileptic drugs carbamazepine and phenytoin. Mol Pharmacol 47:1189–1196

Graves NM, Kriel RL, Jones-Saete C, Cloyd JC (1985) Relative bioavailability of rectally administered carbamazepine suspension in humans. Epilepsia 26:429–433

Graves NM, Fuerst RH, Cloyd JC, Brundage RC, Welty TE, Leppik IE (1988) Progabide-induced changes in carbamazepine metabolism. Epilepsia 29:775–780

Graves NM, Holmes GB, Fuerst RH, Leppik IE (1989) Effect of felbamate on phenytoin and carbamazepine serum concentrations. Epilepsia 30:225–229

Green MW, Selman JE (1991) Review article: the medical management of trigeminal neuralgia. Headache 31:588–592

Groce JB III, Casto DT, Gal P (1985) Carbamazepine and carbamazepine-epoxide serum protein binding in newborn infants. Ther Drug Monit 7:274–276

Guthrie S (1991) The impact of dexamethasone pharmacokinetics on the DST: a review. Psychopharmacol Bull 27:565–576

Haefeli WE, Meyer PG, Luscher TF (1994) Circadian carbamazepine toxicity. Epilepsia 35:400–402

Hansen DK, Dial SL, Terry KK, Grafton TF (1996) In vitro embryotoxicity of carbamazepine and carbamazepine-10,11-epoxide. Teratology 54:45–51

Hanston P, Ilunga K, Martin N, Ziade D, Evenepoel M, Cojocaru M, Mahieu P (1993) Cardiac conduction abnormalities during carbamazepine therapy for neuralgias following Guillain-Barre syndrome. Acta Neurol Belg 93:40–43

Harats N, Shalit M (1987) Carbamazepine indued vasculitis. J Neurol Neurosurg Psychiat 50:1241–1243

Harder S, Thurmann P (1996) Clinically important drug interactions with anticoagulants. An update. Clin Pharmacokinet 30:416–444

Hartley R, Lucock MD, Ng PC, Forsythe WI, McLain B, Bowmer CJ (1990) Factors influencing plasma level/dose ratios of carbamazepine and its major metabolites in epileptic children. Ther Drug Monit 12:438–444
Hawkins CA, Mellanby J, Brown J (1985) Antiepileptic and antiamnesic effect of carbamazepine in experimental limbic epilepsy. J Neurol Neurosurg Psychiat 48: 459–468
Heinemann U, Franceschetti S, Hamon B, Konnerth A, Yaari Y (1985) Effects of anticonvulsants on spontaneous epileptiform activity which develops in the absence of chemical synaptic transmission in hippocampal slices. Brain Res 325:349–352
Hernandez-Peon R (1962) Anticonvulsive action of G32883. Proceedings of the Third Meeting of CINP:303–311
Higuchi T, Yamazaki O, Takazawa A, Kato N, Watanabe N, Minatogawa Y, Yamazaki J, Ohshima H, Nagaki S, Igarashi Y et al. (1986) Effects of carbamazepine and valproic acid on brain immunoreactive somatostatin and gamma-aminobutyric acid in amygdaloid-kindled rats. Eur J Pharmacol 125:169–175
Hojer J, Malmlund HO, Berg A (1993) Clinical features of 28 consecutive cases of laboratory confirmed massive poisoning with carbamazepine alone. J Toxicol Clin Toxicol 31:449–458
Hoogerkamp A, Vis PW, Danhof M, Voskuyl RA (1994) Characterization of the pharmacodynamics of several antiepileptic drugs in a direct cortical stimulation model of anticonvulsant effect in the rat. J Pharmacol Exp Therap 269:521–528
Hooper WD, Du Betz DK, Bochner F, Cotter LM, Smith GA, Eadie MJ, Tyrer JH (1975) Plasma protein binding of carbamazepine. Clin Pharmacol Ther 17:433–440
Hooper WD, King AR, Patterson M, Dickinson RG, Eadie MJ (1985) Simultaneous plasma carbamazepine and carbamazepine epoxide concentrations in pharmacokinetic and bioavailability studies. Ther Drug Monit 7:36–40
Horn CS, Ater SB, Hurst DL (1986) Carbamazepine-exacerbated epilepsy in children and adolescents. Pediatr Neurol 2:340–345
Horneff G, Lenard HG, Wahn V (1992) Severe adverse reactions to carbamazepine: significance of humoral and cellular reactions to the drug. Neuropediat 23:272–275
Horowitz S, Patwardhan R, Marcus E (1988) Hepatotoxic reactions associated with carbamazepine therapy. Epilepsia 29:149–154
Hough CJ, Irwin RP, Gao XM, Rogawaski MA, Chuang DM (1996) Carbamazepine inhibition of N-methyl-D-aspartate-evoked calcium influx in rat cerebellar granule cells. J Pharmacol Exp Therap 276:143–149
Hug G, McGraw CA, Bates SR, Landrigan EA (1991) Reduction of serum carnitine concentrations during anticonvulsant therapy with phenobarbital, valproic acid, phenytoin, and carbamazepine in children. J Pediat 119:799–802
Imai H, Nakamoto Y, Hirokawa M, Akihama T, Miura AB (1989) Carbamazepine-induced granulomatous necrotizing angiitis with acute renal failure. Nephron 51:405–408
Isojarvi JI (1990) Serum steroid hormones and pituitary function in female epileptic patients during carbamazepine therapy. Epilepsia 31:438–445
Isojarvi JI, Pakarinen AJ, Ylipalosaari PJ, Myllyla VV (1990) Serum hormones in male epileptic patients receiving anticonvulsant medication. Arch Neurol 47:670–676
Isojarvi JI, Pakarinen AJ, Myllyla VV (1993) Serum lipid levels during carbamazepine medication. A prospective study. Arch Neurol 50:590–593
Isojarvi JI, Laatikainen TJ, Pakarinen AJ, Juntunen KT, Myllyla VV (1995a) Menstrual disorders in women with epilepsy receiving carbamazepine. Epilepsia 36:676–681
Isojarvi JI, Repo M, Pakarinen AL, Lukkarinen O, Myllyla VV (1995b) Carbamazepine, phenytoin, sex hormones, and sexual function in men with epilepsy. Epilepsia 36:366–370
Iyer V, Holmes JW, Richardson RL (1992) Intractable diarrhoea from carbamazepine. Epilepsia 33:149–153
Jacome DE (1987) Syncope and sudden death attributed to carbamazepine. J Neurol Neurosurg Psychiat 50:1245

Jan JE, Freeman RD, Good WV (1995) Familial paroxysmal kinesigenic choreoathetosis in a child with visual hallucinations and obsessive-compulsive behaviour. Develop Med Child Neurol 37:366–369

Jann MW, Fidone GS (1986) Effect of influenza vaccine on anticonvulsant concentrations. Clin Pharm 5:817–820

Jann MW, Ereshefsky L, Saklad SR, Seidel DR, Davis CM, Burch NR, Bowde CL (1985) Effects of carbamazepine on plasma haloperidol levels. J Clin Psychopharmacol 5:106–109

Jerling M, Lindstrom L, Bondesson U, Bertilsson L (1994) Fluvoxamine inhibition and carbamazepine induction of the metabolism of clozapine: evidence from a therapeutic drug monitoring service. Ther Drug Monit 16:368–374

Johnson SD, Tarby TJ, Sidell AD (1984) Carbamazepine-induced seizures. Neurology 16:392–393

Jones KL, Lacro RV, Johnson KA, Adams J (1989) Pattern of malformations in children of women treated with carbamazepine during pregnancy. New Eng J Med 320:1661–1666

Jonkman JH, Upton RA (1984) Pharmacokinetic drug interactions with theophylline. Clin Pharmacokinet 9:309–334

Julien RM, Hollister RP (1975) Carbamazepine: mechanism of action. Adv Neurol 11:263–276

Jurna I (1985) Electrophysiological effects of antiepileptic drugs. In: Frey H-H, Janz D (eds) Antiepileptic drugs. Springer-Verlag, Berlin, pp. 611–658

Kahn EM, Schulz SC, Perel JM, Alexander JE (1990) Changes in haloperidol level due to carbamazepine – a complicating factor in combined medication for schizophrenia. J Clin Psychopharmacol 10:54–57

Kallen AJ (1994) Maternal carbamazepine and infant spina bifida. Reprod Toxicol 8:203–205

Kallen B, Robert E, Mastroiacovo P, Martinez-Frias ML, Castilla EE, Cocchi G (1989) Anticonvulsant drugs and malformations: is there a drug specificity? Eur J Epidemiol 5:31–36

Kaneko S, Fukushima Y, Sato T, Ogaea Y, Nomura Y, Shinagawa S (1984) Breast feeding in epileptic mothers. In: Sato T, Shinagawa S (eds) Antiepileptic drugs and pregnancy. Excerpta Medica, Amsterdam 38–45

Kaneko K, Igarashi J, Suzuki Y, Niijima S, Ishimoto K, Yabuta K (1993) Carbamazepine-induced thrombocytopenia and leucopenia complicated by Henoch-Schonlein purpura syndrome. Eur J Pediatr 152:769–770

Kasarskis EJ, Kuo CS, Berger R, Nelson KR (1992) Carbamazepine-induced cardiac dysfunction. Chaaracterization of two distinct clinical syndromes. Arch Intern Med 152:186–191

Kaufman DW, Kelly JP, Jurgelon JM, Anderson T, Issaragrisil S, Wiholm BE, Young NS, Leaverton P, Levy M, Shapiro S (1996) Drugs in the aetiology of agranulocytosis and aplastic anaemia. Eur J Haematol 60 [Suppl]:23–30

Kenneback G, Bergfeldt L, Vallin H, Tomson T, Edhag O (1991) Electrophysiologic effects and clinical hazards of carbamazepine treatment for neurologic disorders in patients with abnormalities of the cardiac conduction system. Am Heart J 121:1421–1429

Kenneback G, Bergfeldt L, Tomson T, Spina E, Edhag O (1992) Carbamazepine induced bradycardia – a problem in general or only in susceptible persons? A 24-h long-term electrocardiogram study. Epilepsy Res 13:141–145

Kerr BM, Levy RH (1995) Carbamazepine. Carbamazepine epoxide. In: Levy RH, Mattson RH, Meldrum BS (eds) Antiepileptic drugs, 4th edn. Raven Press, New York, pp. 529–541

Kerr BM, Martinez-Lage JM, Viteri C, Tor J, Eddy AC, Levy RH (1991) Carbamazepine dose requirements during stiripentol therapy: influence of cytochrome P-450 inhibition by stiripentol. Epilepsia 32:267–274

Kerr BM, Thummel KE, Wurden CJ, Klein SM, Kroetz DL, Gonzales FJ, Levy RH (1994) Human liver carbamazepine metabolism. Role of CYP3A4 and CYP2C8 in 10,11-epoxide formation. Biochem Pharmacol 47:1969–1979

Ketter TA, Jenkins JB, Schroeder DH, Pazzaglia PJ, Marangell LB, George MS, Callahan AM, Hinton ML, Chao J, Post RM (1995) Carbamazepine but not valproate induces bupropion metabolism. J Clin Psychopharmacol 15:327–333

Killian JM, Fromm GH (1968) Carbamazepine in the treatment of neuralgia. Arch Neurol 19:129–136

Kimura M, Yoshino K, Maeoka Y, Suzuki N (1995) Carbamazepine-induced thrombocytopenia and carbamazepine-10,11-epoxide: a case report. Psychiatry Clin Neurosci 49:69–70

King GG, Barnes DJ, Hayes MJ (1994) Carbamazepine-induced pneumonitis. M J Australia 160:126–127

King J (1987) Glossopharyngeal neuralgia. Clin Exptl Neurol 24:113–121

Kintz P, Marescaux C, Mangin P (1995) Testing human hair for carbamazepine in epileptic patients: is hair investigation suitable for drug monitoring? Hum Exp Toxicol 14:812–815

Kitteringham NR, Davis C, Howard N, Pirmohamed M, Park BK (1996) Interindividual and interspecies variation in hepatic microsomal epoxide hydrolase activity: studies with cis-stilbene oxide, carbamazepine-10,11-epoxide and naphthalene. J Pharmacol Exp Therap 278:1018–1027

Knott C, Reynolds F (1984) The place of saliva in antiepileptic drug monitoring. Ther Drug Monit 6:35–41

Kodama Y, Tsutsumi K, Kuranari M, Kodama H, Fujii I, Takeyama M (1993) In vivo binding characteristics of carbamazepine and carbamazepine-10,11-epoxide to serum proteins in pediatric patients with epilepsy. Europ J Clin Pharmacol 44:291–293

Kodama Y, Kuranari M, Tsutsumi K, Okamoto T, Kodama H, Yasunaga F, Fujii I, Takeyama M (1994) In vivo binding characteristics of carbamazepine and carbamazepine-10,11-epoxide to serum proteins in monotherapy adult patients. Int J Clin Pharmac Ther Toxicol 32:618–621

Kondo T, Otani K, Hirano T, Kaneko S, Fukushima Y (1990) The effect of phenytoin and carbamazepine on serum concentrations of mono-unsaturated metabolites of valproic acid. Br J Clin Pharmac 29:116–119

Korinthenberg R, Wehrle L, Zimmerhackl LB (1994) Renal tubular dysfunction following treatment with anti-epileptic drugs. Eur J Pediatr 153:855–858

Kowalik S, Levitt M, Barkai AI (1984) Effect of carbamazepine and anti-depressant drugs on endogenous catecholamine levels in the cerebroventricular compartment of the rat. Psychopharmacology Berl 83:169–171

Kramlinger KG, Phillips KA, Post RM (1994) Rash complicating carbamazepine treatment. J Clin Psychopharmacol 14:408–413

Krause KH, Berlit P (1990) Nerve conduction velocity in patients under long term treatment with antiepileptic drugs. Electromyogr Clin Neurophysiol 30:61–64

Kubota T, Jibiki I, Fujimoto K, Yamaguchi N (1992) Facilitative effect of carbamazepine on previously induced hippocampal long-term potentiation. Pharmacol Biochem Behav 42:843–847

Kubota T, Jibiki I, Fukushima T, Kurokawa K, Yamaguchi N (1994) Carbamazepine-induced blockade of induction of long-term potentiation in the perforant path-dentate gyrus pathway in chronically prepared rabbits. Neurosci Lett 28:171–174

Kubova H, Mares P (1993) Anticonvulsant action of oxcarbazepine, hydroxycarbamazepine, and carbamazepine against metrazol-induced motor seizures in developing rats. Epilepsia 34:188–192

Kubova H, Lanstiakova M, Mockova M, Mares P, Vorlicek J (1996) Pharmacology of cortical afterdischarges in rats. Epilepsia 37:336–341

Kudriakova TB, Sirota LA, Ruzova GI, Gorkov VA (1992) Autoinduction and steady-state pharmacokinetics of carbamazepine and its major metabolites. Br J Clin Pharmac 33:611–615

Kuhnz W, Jager-Roman E, Rating D, Deichl A, Kunze J, Helge H, Nau H (1983) Carbamazepine and carbamazepine-10,11-epoxide during pregnancy and postnatal period in epileptic mothers and their nursed infants: pharmacokinetics and clinical effects. Pediatr Pharmacol New York 3:199–208

Kuitunen T, Mattila MJ, Seppala T, Aranko K, Mattila ME (1990) Actions of zopiclone and carbamazepine, alone and in combination, on human skilled performance in laboratory and clinical tests. Br J Clin Pharmac 30:453–461

Kukowski B, Feldmann M (1992) Neuromyotonia: report of a case. Clin Investig 70:517–519

Kumps AH (1981) Dose-dependency of the ratio between carbamazepine serum levels and dosage in patients with epilepsy. Ther Drug Monit 3:271–274

Lambert M, Fournier A (1992) [Acute renal failure complicating carbamazepine hypersensitivity]. Rev Neurol Paris 148:574–576

Lampe H, Bigalke H (1990) Carbamazepine blocks NMDA-activated currents in cultured spinal cord neurons. Neuroreport 1:26–28

Lampl Y, Eshel Y, Rapaport A, Sarova-Pinhas I (1991) Weight gain, increased appetite, and excessive food intake induced by carbamazepine. Clin Neuropharmac 14:251–255

Lander CM, Eadie MJ (1991) Plasma antiepileptic drug concentrations during pregnancy. Epilepsia 32:257–266

Lander CM, Eadie MJ, Tyrer JH (1977) Factors influencing plasma carbamazepine concentrations. Proc Austn Assoc Neurol 12:111–116

Lang DG, Wang CM, Cooper BR (1993) Lamotrigine, phenytoin and carbamazepine interactions on the sodium current present in N4TG1 mouse neuroblastoma cells. J Pharmacol Exp Therap 266:829–835

Lapresle J (1986) Palatal myoclonus. Adv Neurol 43:265–273

LaSpina I, Secchi P, Grampa G, Uccellini D, Porazzi D (1994) Acute cholangitis induced by carbamazepine. Epilepsia 35:1029–1031

Leach JP, Blacklaw J, Jamieson V, Jones T, Richens A, Brodie MJ (1996) Mutual interaction between remacemide hydrochloride and carbamazepine: two drugs with active metabolites. Epilepsia 37:1100–1106

Leeder JS, Riley RJ, Cook VA, Spielberg SP (1992) Human anti-cytochrome P450 antibodies in aromatic anticonvulsant-induced hypersensitivity reactions. J Pharmacol Exp Therap 263:360–367

Leinonen E, Lillsunde P, Laukkanen V, Ylitalo P (1991) Effect of carbamazepine on serum antidepressant concentrations in psychiatric patients. J Clin Psychopharmacol 11:313–318

Leite JP, Cavalheiro EA (1995) Effects of conventional antiepileptic drugs in a model of spontaneous recurrent seizures in rats. Epilepsy Res 20:93–104

Leppik IE (1992) Metabolism of antiepileptic medication: newborn to elderly. Epilepsia 33 [Suppl 4]:S32–S40

Lertratanangkoon K, Horning MG (1982) Metabolism of carbamazepine. Drug Metab Disposit 10:1–10

Levy RH, Wurden CJ (1995) Carbamazepine. Interactions with other drugs. In: Levy RH, Mattson RH, Meldrum BS (eds) Antiepileptic drugs, 4th edn. Raven Press, New York, pp. 543–554

Levy RH, Yerby MS (1985) Effects of pregnancy on antiepileptic drug utilization. Epilepsia 26 [Suppl 1]:S52–S57

Levy RH, Rettenmeier AW, Anderson GD, Wilensky AJ, Friel PN, Baillie TA, Acheampong A, Tor J, Guyot M, Loiseau P (1990) Effects of polytherapy with phenytoin, carbamazepine, and stiripentol in formation of 4-ene-valproate, a hepatotoxic metabolite of valproic acid. Clin Pharmacol Ther 48:225–235

Lillibridge JH, Amore BM, Slattery JT, Kalhorn TF, Nelson SD, Finnell RH, Bennett GD (1996) Protein-reactive metabolites of carbamazepine in mouse liver microsomes. Drug Metabol Disposit 24:509–514
Lindhout D, Omtzigt JG (1992) Pregnancy and the risk of teratogenicity. Epilepsia 33 [Suppl 4]:S41–S48
Liu H, Delgardo MR (1994a) A comprehensive study of the relation between serum concentrations, concentration ratios, and level/dose ratios of carbamazepine and its metabolites with age, weight, dose, and clearances in epileptic children. Epilepsia 35:1221–1229
Liu H, Delgardo MR (1994b) Improved therapeutic monitoring of drug interactions in epileptic children using carbamazepine polytherapy. Ther Drug Monit 16:132–138
Liu H, Delgardo MR (1994c) The influence of polytherapy on the relationships between serum carbamazepine and its metabolites in epileptic children. Epilepsy Res 17:257–269
Liu H, Delgardo MR (1994d) Influence of sex, age, weight, and carbamazepine dose on serum concentrations, concentration ratios, and level/dose ratios of carbamazepine and its metabolites. Ther Drug Monit 16:469–476
Liu H, Delgado MR (1995) Interactions of phenobarbital and phenytoin with carbamazepine and its metabolites' concentrations, concentration ratios, and level/dose ratios in epileptic patients. Epilepsia 36:249–254
Liu H, Delgado MR, Browne RH (1995) Interactions of valproic acid with carbamazepine and its metabolites' concentrations, concentration ratios, and level/dose ratios in epileptic children. Clin Neuropharmac 18:1–12
Löscher W (1987) [Neurophysiologic and neurochemical principles of the effect of anticonvulsants]. Fortschr Neurol Psychiatr 55:145–157
Löscher W, Frey HH (1984) Kinetics of penetration of common antiepileptic drugs into cerebrospinal fluid. Epilepsia 25:346–352
Löscher W, Hönack D (1997) Intravenous carbamazepine: comparison of different parenteral formulations in a mouse model of convulsive status epilepticus. Epilepsia 38:106–113
Löscher W, Hönack D, Richter A, Schulz HU, Schurer M, Dusing R, Brewster ME (1995) New injectable aqueous carbamazepine solution through complexing with 2-hydroxypropyl-beta-cyclodextrin: tolerability and pharmacokinetics after intravenous injection in comparison to a glycofurol-based formulation. Epilepsia 36:255–261
Luder PJ, Siffert B, Witassek F, Meister F, Bircher J (1986) Treatment of hydatid disease with high doses of mebendazole. Long-term follow-up of plasma mebendazole levels and drug interactions. Europ J Clin Pharmacol 31:443–448
Lust WD, Kupferberg HJ, Yonekawa WD, Penry JK, Passonneau JV, Wheaton AB (1978) Changes in brain metabolites induced by convulsants or electroshock: effects of anticonvulsant agents. Mol Pharmacol 14:347–356
Lynn RK, Smith RG, Thompson RM, Deinzer ML, Griffin D, Gerber N (1978) Characterization of glucuronide metabolites of carbamazepine in human urine by gas chromatography and mass spectrometry. Drug Metab Disposit 6:494–501
Macdonald RL (1989) Antiepileptic drug actions. Epilepsia 30 [Suppl 1]:S19–S28
Macdonald RL, Kelly KM (1995) Antiepileptic drug mechanisms of action. Epilepsia 36 [Suppl 2]:S2–S12
Macphee GJ, McInnes GT, Thompson GG, Brodie MJ (1986) Verapamil potentiates carbamazepine neurotoxicity: a clinically important inhibitory interaction. Lancet 1:700–703
Macphee GJ, Butler E, Brodie MJ (1987) Intradose and circadian variation in circulating carbamazepine and its epoxide in epileptic patients: a consequence of autoinduction of metabolism. Epilepsia 28:286–294

Macphee GJ, Mitchell JR, Wiseman L, McLennan AR, Park BK, McInnes GT, Brodie MJ (1988) Effect of sodium valproate on carbamazepine disposition and psychomotor profile in man. Br J Clin Pharmac 25:59–66
Madden S, Maggs JL, Park BK (1996) Bioactivation of carbamazepine in the rat in vivo. Evidence for the formation of reactive arene oxide(s). Drug Metabol Disposit 24:469–479
Maggs JL, Pirmohamed M, Kitteringham NR, Park BK (1997) Characterization of the metabolites of carbamazepine in patient urine by liquid chromatography/mass spectrometry. Drug Metabol Disposit 25:275–280
Maignen F, Castot A, Falcy M, Efthymiou ML (1992) [Drug induced aseptic meningitis]. Therapie 47:399–402
Majkowski J, Diawichowska E, Sobieszek A (1994) Carbamazepine effects on afterdischarges, memory retrieval, and conditioned avoidance response latency in hippocampally kindled cats. Epilepsia 35:209–215
Maoz E, Grossman E, Thaler M, Rosenthal T (1992) Carbamazepine neurotoxic reactions after administration of diltiazem. Arch Intern Med 152:2503–2504
Marangell LB, George MS, Bissette G, Pazzaglia P, Huggins T, Post RM (1994) Carbamazepine increases cerbrospinal fluid thyrotropin-releasing hormone levels in affectively ill patients. Arch Gen Psychiatry 51:625–628
Marangos PJ, Patel J, Smith KD, Post RM (1987) Adenosine antagonist properties of carbamazepine. Epilepsia 28:387–394
Marson AG, Kadir ZA, Hutton JL, Chadwick DW (1997) The new antiepileptic drugs: a systematic review of their efficacy and tolerability. Epilepsia 38:859–880
Martinez P, Gonzalez de Etxabarri S, Ereno C, Lopez G, Hinojal C, Teira R (1993) [Acute severe hepatic insufficiency caused by carbamazepine]. Rev Esp Enferm Dig 84:124–126
Mattson RH, Cramer JA, Collins JF, Smith DB, Delgardo-Escueta AV, Browne TR, Williamson PD, Treiman DM, McNamara JO, McCutchen CB, Homan R, Crill WE, Lubozynski MF, Rosenthal NP, Mayersdorf A (1985) Comparison of carbamazepine, phenobarbital, phenytoin, and primidone in partial and secondarily generalized tonic-clonic seizures. New Eng J Med 313:145–151
Mattson RH, Cramer JA, Collins JF, and the Department of Veterans Affairs Epilepsy Cooperative Study Group (1992) A comparison of valproate with carbamazepine for the treatment of complex partial seizures and secondarily generalized tonic-clonic seizures in adults. New Eng J Med 327:765–771
Maurer PM, Bartkowski RR (1993) Drug interactions of clinical significance with opioid analgesics. Drug Safety 8:30–48
Mauri-Hellweg D, Bettens F, Mauri D, Brander C, Hunziker T, Pichler WJ (1995) Activation of drug-specific CD4+ and CD8+ cells in individuals allergic to sulfonamides, phenytoin, and carbamazepine. J Immunol 155:462–472
McKauge L, Tyrer JH, Eadie MJ (1981) Factors influencing simultaneous concentrations of carbamazepine and its epoxide in plasma. Ther Drug Monit 3:63–70
McKee PJ, Blacklaw J, Butler E, Gillham RA, Brodie MJ (1992) Variability and clinical relevance of the interaction between sodium valproate and carbamazepine in epileptic patients. Epilepsy Res 11:193–198
McKee PW, Blacklaw J, Forrest G, Gillham RA, Walker SM, Connelly D, Brodie MJ (1994) A double-blind, placebo-controlled interaction study between oxcarbazepine and carbamazepine, sodium valproate and phenytoin in epileptic patients. Br J Clin Pharmac 37:27–32
McKinney PA, Finkenbine RD, DeVane CL (1996) Alopecia and mood stabiliser therapy. Ann Clin Psychiatry 8:183–185
McLean MJ, Macdonald RL (1986) Carbamazepine and 10,11-epoxycarbamazepine produce use- and voltage-dependent limitation of rapidly firing action potentials of mouse central neurons in cell culture. J Pharmacol Exp Therap 238:727–738

Meador KJ, Loring DW, Allen ME, Zamrini EY, Moore EE, Abney OL, King DW (1991) Comparative cognitive effects of carbamazepine and phenytoin in healthy adults. Neurology 41:1537–1540
Meyer FP, Quednow B, Potrafki A, Walther H (1988) Pharmacokinetics of anticonvulsants in the perinatal period. Zentralbl Gynakol 110:1195–1205
Meyer MC, Straughn AB, Jarvi EJ, Wood GC, Pelsor FR, Shah VP (1992) The bioinequivalence of carbamazepine tablets with a history of clinical failures. Pharm Res 9:1612–1616
Micheletti G, Vergnes M, Marescaux C, Reis J, Depaulis A, Rumbach L, Warter JM (1985) Antiepileptic drug evaluation in a new animal model: spontaneous petit mal epilepsy in the rat. Arzneimittelforschung 35:483–485
Miles MV, Tennison MB (1989) Erythromycin effects on multiple-dose carbamazepine kinetics. Ther Drug Monit 11:47–52
Minami T, Ieiri I, Ohtsubo K, Hirakawa Y, Ueda K, Higuchi S, Aoyama T (1994) Influence of additional therapy with zonisamide (Excegran) on protein binding and metabolism of carbamazepine. Epilepsia 35:1023–1025
Mitsushio H, Takashima M, Mataga N, Toru M (1988) Effects of chronic treatment with trihexyphenidyl and carbamazepine alone or in combination with haloperidol on substance P in rat brain: a possible implication of substance P in affective disorders. J Pharmacol Exp Therap 245:982–989
Miyamoto A, Takahashi S, Oki J, Itoh J, Cho K (1995) [Exacerbation of seizures by carbamazepine in four children with symptomatic localization related epilepsy]. No To Hattatsu 27:23–28
Montoya-Cabrera MA, Sauceda-Garcia JM, Escalante-Galindo P, Flores-Alvarez E, Ruiz-Gomez A (1996) Carbamazepine poisoning in adolescent suicide attempters. Effectiveness of multiple-dose activated charcoal in enhancing carbamazepine elimination. Arch Med Res 27:485–489
Moosa RS, McFadyen ML, Miller R, Rubin J (1993) Carbamazepine and its metabolites in neuralgias: concentration-effect relations. Europ J Clin Pharmacol 45:297–301
Morgan CJ, Badawy AA (1992) Effects of acute carbamazepine administration on haem metabolism in rat liver. Biochem Pharmacol 43:1473–1477
Morselli PL (1975) Carbamazepine: absorption, distribution and excretion. Adv Neurol 11:279–293
Morselli PL (1995) Carbamazepine. Absorption, distribution, and excretion. In: Levy RH, Mattson RH, Meldrum BS (eds) Antiepileptic drugs, 4th edn. Raven, New York, pp. 515–528
Morselli PL, Gerna M, Garattini S (1971) Carbamazepine plasma and tissue levels in the rat. Biochem Pharmacol 19:1846–1847
Morselli PL, Gerna M, DeMaio D, Zanda G, Viani F, Garattini S (1975) Pharmacokinetic studies on carbamazepine in volunteers and in epileptic patients. In: Schneider H, Janz D, Gardner-Thorpe C, Meinardi H, Sherwin AL (eds) Clinical pharmacology of antiepileptic drugs. Springer-Verlag, Berlin, pp. 166–179
Morselli PL, Baruzzi A, Gerna M, Bossi L, Porta M (1977) Carbamazepine and carbamazepine-10,11-epoxide concentrations in human brain. Br J Clin Pharmac 4:535–540
Muck W, Ahr G, Kuhlmann J (1995) Nimodipine. Potential for drug-drug interactions in the elderly. Drugs Aging 6:229–242
Neglia JP, Glaze DG, Zion TE (1984) Tics and vocalizations in children treated with carbamazepine. Pediatrics 73:841–844
Nemeroff CB, DeVane CL, Pollock BG (1996) Newer antidepressants and the cytochrome P450 system. Am J Psychiatry 153:311–320
Neufeld MY (1993) Exacerbation of focal seizures due to carbamazepine treatment in an adult patient. Clin Neuropharmac 16:359–361
Neuvonen PJ (1985) Bioavailability and central side effects of different carbamazepine tablets. Int J Clin Pharmacol Ther Toxico; 23:226–232

Neuvonen PJ, Olkkola KT (1988) Oral activated charcoal in the treatment of intoxications. Role of single and repeated doses. Med Toxicol Adverse Drug Exp 3:33–58
Neuvonen PJ, Tokola O (1987) Bioavailability of rectally administered carbamazepine mixture. Br J Clin Pharmac 24:839–841
Neuvonen PJ, Pentilla O, Lehtovarrq R, Aho K (1975) Effects of antiepileptic drugs on the elimination of various tetracycline derivatives. Europ J Clin Pharmacol 9:147–154
Neuvonen PJ, Kivisto K, Hirvisalo EL (1988) Effects of resins and activated charcoal on the absorption of digoxin, carbamazepine and frusemide. Br J Clin Pharmac 25:229–233
Ng K, Silbert PL, Edis RH (1991) Complete external ophthalmoplegia and asterixis with carbamazepine toxicity. Aust N Z J Med 21:886–887
Nulman I, Scolnik D, Chitayat D, Farkas LD, Koren G (1997) Findings in children exposed in utero to phenytoin and carbamazepine monotherapy: independent effects of epilepsy and medications. Am J Med Genet 68:18–24
O'Connor MK, Fris J (1994) Clarithromycin-carbamazepine interaction in a clinical setting. J Am Board Fam Pract 7:489–492
O'Griofa FM, Voris JC (1991) Neuroleptic malignant syndrome associated with carbamazepine. South Med J 84:1378–1380
O'Keefe ST (1996) Restless legs syndrome. A review. Arch Intern Med 156:243–248
Okesina AB, Donaldson D, Lascelles PT (1991) Isoenzymes of alkaline phosphatase in epileptic patients receiving carbamazepine monotherapy. J Clin Pathol 44:480–482
Okuyama R, Ichinohasama R, Tagami H (1996) Carbamazepine induced erythroderma with systemic lymphadenopathy. J Dermatol 23:489–494
Olcay L, Pekcan S, Yalnizoglu D, Buyukpamukcu M, Yalaz K (1995) Fatal agranulocytosis developed in the course of carbamazepine therapy. A case report and review of the literature. Turk J Pediatr 37:73–77
Oles KS, Mirza W, Penry JK (1989) Catastrophic neurologic signs due to drug interaction: Tegretol and Darvon. Surg Neurol 32:144–151
Olivesi A (1986) Modified elimination of prednisolone in epileptic patients on carbamazepine monotherapy, and in women using low-dose oral contraceptives. Biochem Pharmacol 40:301–308
Omtzigt JGC, Los FJ, Meijer JWA, Lindhout D (1993) The 10,11-epoxide-diol pathway of carbamazepine in early pregnancy in maternal serum, urine, and amniotic fluid: effect of dose, comedication, and relation to outcome of pregnancy. Ther Drug Monit 15:1–10
Ornoy A, Cohen E (1996) Outcome of children born to epileptic mothers treated with carbamazepine during pregnancy. Arch Dis Childh 75:517–520
Otani K, Ishida M, Kaneko S, Mihara K, Ohkubo T, Osanai T, Sugawara K (1996) Effects of carbamazepine coadministration on plasma concentrations of trazodone and its active metabolite, m-chlorophenylpiperazine. Ther Drug Monit 18:164–167
Pacifici R, Paris L, DiCarlo S, Bacosi A, Pichini S, Zuccaro P (1995) Cytokine production in blood mononuclear cells from epileptic patients. Epilepsia 36:384–387
Palmer GC, Harris EW, Ray R, Stagnitto ML, Schmiesing RJ (1992) Classification of compounds for prevention of NMLDA-induced seizures/mortality, or maximum electroshock and pentylenetetrazol seizures in mice and antagonism of MK801 binding in vitro. Arch Internat Pharmacodyn Therap 317:16–34
Panesar SK, Bandiera SM, Abbott FS (1996) Comparative effects of carbamazepine and carbamazepine-10,11-epoxide on hepatic cytochromes P450 in the rat. Drug Metabol Disposit 24:619–627
Patsalos PN, Duncan JS, Shorvon SD (1988) Effect of the removal of individual antiepileptic drugs on antipyrine kinetics, in patients taking polytherapy. Br J Clin Pharmac 26:253–259
Paxton JW (1983) Salivary and serum concentrations, and protein binding of carbamazepine in young epileptic patients. Methods Find Exp Clin Pharmacol 5:397–401

Paxton JW, Aman MG, Werry JS (1983) Fluctuations in salivary carbamazepine and carbamazepine-10,11-epoxide concentrations during the day in epileptic children. Epilepsia 24:716–724

Perini GI, Devinsky O, Hauser P, Gallucci WT, Theodore WH, Chrousos GP, Gold PW, Kling MA (1992) Effects of carbamazepine on pituitary-adrenal function in healthy volunteers. J Clin Endocrinol Metab 74:406–412

Perucca E, Gatti G, Spina E (1994) Clinical pharmacokinetics of fluvoxamine. Clin Pharmacokinet 27:175–190

Pichard L, Fabre I, Fabre G, Domergue J, Saint-Aubert B, Mourad G, Maurel P (1990) Cyclosporin A drug interactions. Screening for inducers and inhibitors of cytochrome P450 (cyclosporin A oxidase) in primary cultures of human hepatocytes and in liver microsomes. Drug Metabol Disposit 18:595–606

Pijl H, Meinders AE (1996) Bodyweight changes as an adverse effect of drug treatment. Mechanism and management. Drug Safety 14:329–342

Pirohamed M, Kitteringham NR, Guenthner TM, Breckenridge AM, Park BK (1992) An investigation of the formation of cytotoxic, protein-reactive and stable metabolites from carbamazepine in vitro. Biochem Pharmacol 43:1675–1682

Pisani F, Narbone MC, Fazio A, Crisafulli P, Primerano G, D'Agostino AA, Oteri G, Di Perri R (1984) Effects of viloxazine on serum carbamazepine levels in epileptic patients. Epilepsia 25:482–485

Pisani F, Fazio A, Oteri G, Perucca E, Russo M, Trio R, Pisani B, Di-Perri R (1986) Carbamazepine-viloxazine interaction in patients with epilepsy. J Neurol Neurosurg Psychiat 49:1142–1145

Pisani F, Haj-Yehia A, Fazio A et al. (1993) Carbamazepine-valnoctamide interaction in epileptic patients: in vitro/in vivo correlation. Epilepsia 34:954–959

Pitlick WH, Levy RH, Troupin AS, Green JR (1976) Pharmacokinetic model to describe self-induced decreases in steady-state concentrations of carbamazepine. J Pharm Sci 65:462–463

Popovic J, Mikov M, Jakovljevic V (1995) Pharmacokinetics of carbamazepine derived from a new tablet formulation. Eur J Drug Metab Pharmacokinet 20: 297–300

Post RM, Uhde TW, Ballenger JC, Chatterji DC, Greene RF, Bunney WEJ (1983) Carbamazepine and its -10,11-epoxide metabolite in plasma and CSF. Relationship to antidepressant response. Arch Gen Psychiatry 40:673–676

Pratt JA, Jenner P, Johnson AL, Shorvon SD, Reynolds EH (1984) Anticonvulsant drugs alter plasma tryptophan concentrations in epileptic patients: implications for antiepileptic action and mental function. J Neurol Neurosurg Psychiat 47:1131–1133

Pratt JA, Jenner P, Marsden CD (1985) Comparison of the effects of benzodiazepines and other anticonvulsant drugs on synthesis and utilization of 5-HT in mouse brain. Neuropharmacology 24:59–68

Puche E, Garcia-Morillas M, Garcia de la Serrana H, Mota C (1989) Probable pseudocholinesterase induction by valproic acid, carbamazepine and phenytoin leading to increased serum aspirin-esterase activity in epileptics. Int J Clin Pharmacol Res 9:309–311

Pullainen V, Jokelainen M (1995) Comparing the cognitive effects of phenytoin and carbamazepine in long-term monotherapy: a two year follow-up. Epilepsia 36:1195–1202

Pynnonen S (1979) Pharmacokinetics of carbamazepine in man: a review. Ther Drug Monit 1:409–431

Rambeck B, Wolf P (1993) Lamotrigine: clinical pharmacokinetics. Clin Pharmacokinet 25:433–443

Rambeck B, Schnabel R, May T, Jurgens U, Villagran R (1993) Postmortem concentrations of phenobarbital, carbamazepine, and its metabolite carbamazepine-10,11-epoxide in different regions of the brain and in the serum: analysis of autopic specimens from 51 epileptic patients. Ther Drug Monit 15:91–98

Rambeck B, Specht U, Wolf P (1996) Pharmacokinetic interactions of the new antiepileptic drugs. Clin Pharmacokinet 31:309–324
Ramsay RE, McManus DQ, Guterman A, Briggle TV, Vazquez D, Perschalski R, Yost RA, Wong P (1990) Carbamazepine metabolism in humans: effect of concurrent anticonvulsant therapy. Ther Drug Monit 12:235–241
Rawlins MD, Collste P, Bertilsson L, Palmer L (1975) Distribution and elimination kinetics of carbamazepine in man. Europ J Clin Pharmacol 8:91–96
Regnaud L, Sirois G, Chakrabarti S (1988) Effect of four-day treatment with carbamazepine at different dose levels on microsomal enzyme induction, drug metabolism and drug toxicity. Pharmacol Toxicol 62:3–6
Reichlin S, Mothon S (1991) Carbamazepine and phenytoin inhibit somastatin release from dispersed cerebral cells in culture. Ann Neurol 29:413–417
Reizenstein P, Lund L (1973) Effect of anticonvulsive drugs on folate absorption and the cerebrospinal fluid folate pump. Scand J Haematol 11:158–165
Reshef A, Bitterman N, Kerem D (1991) The effect of carbamazepine and ethosuximide on hyperoxic seizures. Epilepsy Res 8:117–121
Reunanen M, Heinonen EH, Nyman L, Anttila M (1992) Comparative bioavailability of carbamazepine from two slow-release preparations. Epilepsy Res 11:61–66
Richans A, Houghton GW (1975) Effect of drug therapy on the metabolism of phenytoin. In: Schneider H, Janz D, Gardner-Thorpe C, Meinardi H, Sherwin AL (eds) Clinical pharmacology of antiepileptic drugs. Springer-Verlag, Berlin, pp. 87–95
Richardson SB, Twente S (1992) Anticonvulsants inhibit rat neuronal somatostatin release. Brain Res 571:230–234
Richens A, Houghton GW (1975) Effect of drug therapy on the metabolism of phenytoin. In: Schneider H, Janz D, Gardner-Thorpe C, Meinardi H, Sherwin AL (eds) Clinical pharmacology of antiepileptic drugs. Springer, Berlin, pp. 87–95
Rijlaarsdam U, Scheffer E, Meijer CJ, Kruyswijk MR, Willemze R (1991) Mycosis fungoides-like lesions associated with phenytoin and carbamazepine therapy. J Am Acad Dermatol 24:216–220
Ring HA, Heller AJ, Marshall WJ, Johnson AL, Reynolds EH (1991) Plasma uric acid in patients receiving anticonvulsant monotherapy. Epilepsy Res 8:241–244
Rittmannsberger H, Leblhuber F, Sommer R (1991) Asterixis as a side effect of carbamazepine therapy. Klin Wochenschr 69:279–281
Riva R, Contin M, Albani F et al. (1984) Free and total plasma concentrations of carbamazepine and carbamazepine-10,11-epoxide in epileptic patients: diurnal fluctuations and relationship with side effects. Ther Drug Monit 6:408–413
Riva R, Albani F, Contin M, Baruzzi A (1996) Pharmacokinetic interactions between antiepileptic drugs. Clinical considerations. Clin Pharmacokinet 31:470–493
Robbins DK, Wedlund PJ, Kuhn R, Baumann RJ, Levy RH, Chang SL (1990) Inhibition of epoxide hydrolase by valproic acid in epileptic patients receiving carbamazepine. Br J Clin Pharmac 29:759–762
Robertson PL, Garofalo EA, Silverstein FS, Komarynski MA (1993) Carbamazepine-induced tics. Epilepsia 34:965–968
Roig M, Montserrat L, Gallart A (1988) Carbamazepine: an alternative drug for the treatment of nonhereditary chorea. Pediatrics 82:492–495
Ronnberg J, Samuelsson S, Soderfeldt B (1992) Memory effects following carbamazepine monotherapy in patients with complex partial epilepsy. Seizure 1:247–253
Rosa FW (1991) Spina bifida in infants of women treated with carbamazepine during pregnancy. New Eng J Med 324:674–677
Rosenberg ML, Glaser JS (1983) Superior oblique myokymia. Ann Neurol 13:667–669
Roujeau JC, Kelly JP, Naldi L, Rzany B, Stern RS, Anderson T, Auquier A, Bastuji-Garin S, Correia O, Locati F (1995) Medication use and the risk of Stevens-Johnson syndrome or toxic epidermal necrolysis. New Eng J Med 333:1600–1607

Sachedo RC, Sachedo SK, Walker SA, Kramer LD, Nayak RK, Doose DR (1996) Steady-state pharmacokinetics of topiramate and carbamazepine in patients with epilepsy during monotherapy and concomitant therapy. Epilepsia 37:769–773

Sakellariou G, Koukoudis P, Karpouzas J, Alexopoulos E, Papadopoulos D, Chrisomalis F, Skenteris N, Tsakaris D, Papadimitriou M (1991) Plasma exchange (PE) treatment in drug-induced toxic epidermal necrolysis (TEN). Int J Artif Organs 14:634–638

Salzman MB, Valderrama E, Sood SK (1997) Carbamazepine and fatal eosinophilic myocarditis. New Eng J Med 336:878–879

Sayer RJ, Brown AM, Schwindt PC, Crill WE (1993) Calcium currents in acutely isolated neocortical neurons. J Neurophysiol 69:1596–1606

Scerri L, Shall L, Zaki I (1993) Carbamazepine-induced anticonvulsant hypersensitivity syndrome – pathogenic and diagnostic considerations. Clin Exp Dermatol 18:540–542

Schirrmacher K, Mayer A, Walden J, Dusing R, Bingmann D (1993) Effects of carbamazepine on action potentials and calcium currents in rat spinal ganglion cells in vitro. Neuropsychobiology 27:176–179

Schirrmacher K, Mayer A, Walden J, Dusing R, Bingmann D (1995) Effect of carbamazepine on membrane properties of rat sensory spinal ganglion cells in vitro. Eur Neuropsychopharmacol 5:501–507

Schmidt D, Einicke I, Haenel F (1986) The influence of seizure type on the efficacy of plasma concentrations of phenytoin, phenobarbital, and carbamazepine. Arch Neurol 43:263–265

Schmidt S, Schmitz-Buhl M (1995) Signs and symptoms of carbamazepine overdose. J Neurol 242:169–173

Schmidt S, Welcker M, Greil W, Schatterkirchner M (1992) Carbamazepine-induced systemic lupus erythematosus. Brit J Psychiatry 161:560–561

Schmitz B, Trimble MR (1995) Carbamazepine and PIP-syndrome in temporal lobe epilepsy. Epilepsy Res 22:215–220

Schmutz M (1985) Carbamazepine. In: Frey H-H, Janz D (eds) Antiepileptic drugs, Springer-Verlag, Berlin, pp. 479–506

Schmutz M, Buerki H, Koella WP (1981) Electrically induced hippocampal afterdischarges in the freely moving cat: an animal model of focal (possibly temporal lobe) epilepsy. In: Dam M, Gram L, Penry JK (eds) Advances in epileptology – 12th epilepsy international symposium. Raven Press, New York, pp. 59–65

Schmutz M, Klebs K, Baltzer V (1988) Inhibition or enhancement of kindling evolution by antiepileptics. J Neural Transm 72:245–257

Schoeman JF, Elyans AA, Brett EM, Lascelles PT (1984) Correlation between plasma carbamazepine-10,11-epoxide concentration and drug side-effects in children with epilepsy. Develop Med Child Neurol 26:756–764

Schubert R, Cracco JB (1992) Familial rectal pain: a type of reflex epilepsy? Ann Neurol 32:824–826

Schubert T, Stoll L, Muller WE (1991) Therapeutic concentrations of lithium and carbamazepine inhibit cGMP accumulation in human lymphocytes. A clinical model for a possible common mechanism of action. Psychopharmacology Berl 104:45–50

Schwartzman MJ, Leppik IE (1990) Carbamazepine-induced dyskinesia and ophthalmoplegia. Cleve Clin J Med 57:367–372

Schwarz JR, Grigat G (1989) Phenytoin and carbamazepine: potential- and frequency-dependent block of Na currents in mammalian myelinated nerve fibres. Epilepsia 30:286–294

Sechi GP, Traccis S, Durelli L, Monaco F, Mutani R (1983) Carbamazepine versus diphenylhydantoin in the treatment of myotonia. Eur Neurol 22:113–118

Sechi GP, Pirisi A, Agnetti V, Piredda M, Zuddas M, Tanca S, Piras ML, Aiello I, Deserra F, Rosati G (1989a) Efficacy of carbamazepine on cerebellar tremors in patients with superior cerebellar artery syndrome. J Neurol 236:461–463

Sechi GP, Zuddas M, Piredda M, Agnetti V, Sau G, Piras ML, Tranca S, Rosati G (1989b) Treatment of cerebellar tremors with carbamazepine: a controlled trial with long-term follow-up. Neurology 39:1113–1115

Sennoune S, Mesdjian E, Bonneton J, Genton P, Dravet C, Roger J (1992) Interactions between clobazam and standard antiepileptic drugs in patients with epilepsy. Ther Drug Monit 14:269–274

Seymour JF (1993) Carbamazepine overdose. Features of 33 cases. Drug Safety 8:81–88

Shahar E, Ben-Zeev B (1989) Adverse effects of carbamazepine. Current Opin Neurol Neurosurg 2:367–370

Shear NH, Spielberg SP (1988) Anticonvulsant hypersensitivity syndrome. In vitro assessment of risk. J Clin Invest 82:1826–1832

Shechter Y, Brenner B, Klein E, Tatarsky I (1993) Carbamazepine (Tegretol)-induced thrombocytopenia. Vox Sang 65:328–330

Sheth RD, Wesolowski C, Jacob JC, Penney S, Hobbs GR, Riggs JE, Bodensteiner JB (1995) Effect of carbamazepine and valproate on bone mineral density. J Pediat 127:256–262

Shouse MN, Stroh PJ, Vreeken T (1988) Temporal lobe and petit mal antiepileptics differentially affect ventral lateral thalamic and motor cortex excitability. Brain Res 473:372–379

Shurtleff DB, Lemire RJ (1995) Epidemiology, etiologic factors, and prenatal diagnosis of open spinal dysraphism. Neurosurg Clin N Am 6:183–193

Sidebottom A, Maxwell S (1995) The medical and surgical management of trigeminal neuralgia. J Clin Pharm Ther 20:31–35

Sigal-Nahum M, Petit A, Gaulier A, Torrent J, Mourier C, Karmochkine M (1992) A nodular cutaneous lymphoproliferative disorder during carbamazepine administration. Br J Dermat 127:545–547

Simon LT, Hsu B, Adornato BT (1990) Carbamazepine-induced aseptic meningitis. Ann Intern Med 112:627–628

Singh B, Singh P, al Hifzi I, Khan M, Majeed-Saidan M (1996) Treatment of neonatal seizures with carbamazepine. J Child Neurol 11:378–382

Sinues B, Gazulla J, Bernal ML, Lanuza J, Fanlo A, Saenz MA, Barolome M (1995) Six mutagenicity assays in exposure biomonitoring of patients receiving carbamazepine for epilepsy or trigeminal neuralgia. Mutat Res 334:259–265

Smith KL, Swann JW (1987) Carbamazepine suppresses synchronized afterdischarging in disinhibited immature rat hippocampus. Brain Res 400:371–376

Snead OC III, Hosey LC (1985) Exacerbation of seizures in children by carbamazepine. New Eng J Med 313:916–921

Sobotka JL, Alexander B, Cook BL (1990) A review of carbamazepine's hematologic reactions and monitoring recommendations. DICP 24:1214–1219

Soman M, Swenson C (1985) A possible case of carbamazepine-induced pancreatitis. Drug Intell Clin Pharm 19:925–927

Sozuer DT, Barutcu UB, Karakoc Y, Yalcin E, Onen S (1995) The effect of antiepileptic drugs on serum zinc and copper levels in children. J Basic Clin Physiol Pharmacol 6:265–269

Spickett GP, Gompels MM, Saunders PW (1996) Hypogammaglobulinaemia with absent B lymphocytes and agranulocytosis after carbamazepine treatment. J Neurol Neurosurg Psychiat 60:459

Spina E, Pacifici GM, von Bahr C, Rane A (1986) Characterization of desmethylimipramine 2-hydroxylation in human foetal and adult liver microsomes. Acta Pharmacol Toxicol 58:277–281

Spina E, Tomson T, Svensson JO, Faigle JW, Bertilsson L (1988) Single-dose kinetics of an enteric-coated formulation of carbamazepine-10,11-epoxide, an active metabolite of carbamazepine. Ther Drug Monit 10:382–385

Spina E, Martines C, Fazio A, Trio R, Pisani F, Tomson T (1991) Effect of phenobarbital on the pharmacokinetics of carbamazepine-10,11-epoxide, an active metabolite of carbamazepine. Ther Drug Monit 13:109–112

Spina E, Avenoso A, Campo GM, Caputi AP, Perucca E (1995) The effect of carbamazepine on the 2-hydroxylation of desipramine. Psychopharmacology Berl 117: 413–416
Spina E, Pisani F, Perucca E (1996) Clinically significant pharmacokinetic drug interactions with carbamazepine. An update. Clin Pharmacokinet 31:198–214
Squires LA, Prangley J (1996) Neonatal diagnosis of Schwartz-Jampel syndrome and dramatic response to carbamazepine. Pediatr Neurol 15:172–174
Staedt J, Stoppe G, Kogler A, Steinhoff BJ (1995) Changes of central receptor density in the course of anticonvulsant treatment in temporal lobe epilepsy. Seizure 4:49–52
Starreveld-Zimmerman AAE, Van Der Kolk WJ, Meinardi H, Elshove J (1973) Are anticonvulsants teratogenic? Lancet 2:48–49
Steppuhn KG, Turski L (1993) Modulation of the seizure threshold for excitatory amino acids in mice by antiepileptic drugs and chemoconvulsants. J Pharmacol Exp Therap 265:1063–1070
Sternebring B, Liden A, Andersson A, Melander A (1992) Carbamazepine kinetics and adverse effects during and after ethanol exposure in alcoholics and in healthy volunteers. Europ J Clin Pharmacol 43:393–397
Stone S, Lange LS (1986) Syncope and sudden unexpected death attributed to carbamazepine in a 20-year-old epileptic. J Neurol Neurosurg Psychiat 49:1460–1461
Stremski ES, Brady WB, Prasad K, Hennes HA (1995) Pediatric carbamazepine intoxication. Ann Emerg Med 25:624–630
Stroink AR, Skillrud DM, Kiely JM, Sundt TMJ (1984) Carbamazepine-induced hemolytic anemia. Acta Haematol 72:346–348
Sudha S, Lakshmana MK, Pradhan N (1995) Changes in learning and memory, acetylcholinesterase activity and monoamines in brain after chronic carbamazepine administration in rats. Epilepsia 36:416–422
Summers B, Summers RS (1989) Carbamazepine clearance in paediatric epilepsy patients. Influence of body mass, dose, sex and co-medication. Clin Pharmacokinet 17:208–216
Surks MI, DeFesi CR (1996) Normal serum free thyroid hormone concentrations in patients treated with phenytoin or carbamazepine. A paradox resolved. J Amer Med Assoc 275:1495–1498
Suzuki Y, Cox S, Hayes J, Watson PD (1991) Valproic acid dosages necessary to maintain therapeutic concentrations in children. Ther Drug Monit 13:314–317
Svinarov DA, Pippenger CE (1995) Valproic acid-carbamazepine interaction: is valproic acid a selective inhibitor of epoxide hydrolase? Ther Drug Monit 17:217–220
Takahashi N, Aizawa H, Takata S, Matsumoto K, Koto H, Inoue H, Hara N (1993) Acute interstitial pneumonitis induced by carbamazepine. Nippon Rinsho 6:1409–1411
Takeda A, Okada H, Tanaka H, Izumi M, Ishikawa S, Noro T (1992) Protein binding of four antiepileptic drugs in maternal and umbilical cord serum. Epilepsy Res 13:147–151
Tanganelli P, Regesta G (1996) Vigabatrin vs. carbamazepine monotherapy in newly diagnosed focal epilepsy: a randomized response conditional cross-over study. Epilepsy Res 25:257–262
Thakker KM, Magnat S, Garnett WR, Levy RH, Kochak GM (1992) Comparative bioavailability and steady state fluctuations of Tegretol commercial and carbamazepine OROS tablets. Biopharm Drug Dispos 13:559–569
Theodore WH, Bromfield E, Onorati L (1989a) The effect of carbamazepine on cerebral glucose metabolism. Ann Neurol 25:516–520
Theodore WH, Narang PK, Holmes M, Reeves P, Nice FJ (1989b) Carbamazepine and its epoxide: relation of plasma levels to toxicity and seizure control. Ann Neurol 25:194–196
Thomas NH, Heckmatt JZ, Rodillo E, Ransley YF, Dubowitz V (1994) Continuous muscle fibre activity (Isaacs' syndrome) in infancy: a report of two cases. Neuromusc Disord 4:147–151

Tibballs J (1992) Acute toxic reaction to carbamazepine: clinical effects and serum concentrations. J Pediat 121:295–299
Tiihonen J, Vartiainen H, Hakola P (1995) Carbamazepine-induced changes in plasma levels of neuroleptics. Pharmacopsychiatry 28:26–28
Tjellersen L, Gotfredsen A, Christensen C (1983) Effect of vitamins D2 and D3 on bone-mineral content in carbamazepine-treated epileptic patients. Acta Neurol Scand 68:424–428
Tohen M, Castillo J, Baldessarini RJ, Zarate CJ, Kando JC (1995) Blood dyscrasias with carbamazepine and valproate: a pharmacoepidemiological study of 2228 patients at risk. Am J Psychiatry 152:413–418
Tolmie J, Steer CR, Edmunds AT (1983) Pulmonary eosinophilia associated with carbamazepine. Arch Dis Childh 58:833–834
Tomson T (1984) Interdosage fluctuations in plasma carbamazepine concentration determine intermittent side effects. Arch Neurol 41:830–834
Tomson T, Tybring G, Bertilsson L, Ekbom K, Rane A (1980) Carbamazepine therapy in trigeminal neuralgia. Clinical effects in relation to plasma concentration. Arch Neurol 37:699–703
Tomson T, Tybring G, Bertilsson L (1983) Single-dose kinetics and metabolism of carbamazepine-10,11-epoxide. Clin Pharmacol Ther 33:58–65
Tomson T, Svensson JO, Hilton-Brown P (1989) Relationship of intraindividual dose to plasma concentration of carbamazepine: indication of dose-dependent induction of metabolism. Ther Drug Monit 11:533–539
Tomson T, Lindbom U, Ekqvist B, Sundqvist A (1994) Disposition of carbamazepine and phenytoin in pregnancy. Epilepsia 35:131–135
Topaloglu H, Serdaroglu A, Okan M, Gucuyener K, Topcu M (1993) Improvement of myotonia with carbamazepine in three cases with the Schwartz-Jampel syndrome. Neuropediat 24:232–234
Tran A, Vauzelle-Kervroedan F, Rey E, Pous G, d'Athis P, Chiron C, Dulac O, Renard F, Olive G (1996) Effect of stiripentol on carbamazepine plasma concentration and metabolism in epileptic children. Europ J Clin Pharmacol 50:497–500
Treiman DM, Ben-Menachem E (1987) Inhibition of carbamazepine and phenytoin metabolism by nafimidone, a new antiepileptic drug. Epilepsia 28:699–705
Troupin AS, Ojemann LM (1976) Paradoxical intoxication – a complication of anticonvulsant intoxication. Epilepsia 16:753–758
Tsao CY, Wright FS (1993) Acute chemical pancreatitis associated with carbamazepine intoxication. Epilepsia 34:174–176
Tucker RM, Denning DW, Hanson LH, Rinaldi MG, Graybill JR, Sharkey PK, Pappagianis D, Stevens DA (1992) Interaction of azoles with rifampin, phenytoin, and carbamazepine: in vitro and clinical observations. Clin Infect Dis 14:165–174
Van Amelsvoort T, Bakshi R, Devaux CB, Schwabe S (1994) Hyponatremia associated with carbamazepine and oxcarbazepine therapy: a review. Epilepsia 35:181–188
Van Calker D, Steber R, Klotz KN, Greil W (1991) Carbamazepine distinguishes between adenosine receptors that mediate different second messenger responses. Eur J Pharmacol 206:285–290
van Harten J (1995) Overview of the pharmacokinetics of fluvoxamine. Clin Pharmacokinet 29 [Suppl 1]:1–9
Vantrappen G, Decramer M, Harlet R (1992) High-frequency diaphragmatic flutter: symptoms and treatment by carbamazepine. Lancet 339:265–267
Vaughn BV, D'Cruz OF (1996) Carbamazepine as a treatment for cataplexy. Sleep 19:101–103
Verma NP, Yusko MJ, Greiffenstein MF (1993) Carbamazepine offers no psychotropic advantage over phenytoin in adult epileptic subjects. Seizure 2:53–56
Vestermark V, Vestermark S (1991) Teratogenesis after carbamazepine. Arch Dis Childh 66:641–642
Vincon G, Albin H, Demotes-Mainard F, Guyot M, Bistue C, Loiseau P (1987) Effect of josamycin on carbamazepine kinetics. Europ J Clin Pharmacol 32:297–301

Vittorio CC, Muglia JJ (1995) Anticonvulsant hypersensitivity syndrome. Arch Intern Med 155:2285–2290
Voits M, Frey HH (1994) Stimulation-dependent effect of antiepileptic drugs in amygdala kindled rats on both seizure score and duration of afterdischarges. Pharmacol Toxicol 75:54–61
von Rosensteil NA, Adam D (1995) Macrolide antibacterials. Drug interactions of clinical significance. Drug Safety 13:105–122
Vree TB, Janssen TH, Hekster YA, Termond EF, van de Dries AC, Wijnards WJ (1986) Clinical pharmacokinetics of carbamazepine and its epoxy and hydroxy metabolites in humans after an overdose. Ther Drug Monit 8:297–304
Wagner ML, Rommel RP, Graves NM, Leppik IE (1993) Effect of felbamate on carbamazepine and its metabolites. Clin Pharmacol Ther 53:536–543
Wahnschaffe U, Löscher W (1990) Effect of selective bilateral destruction of the substantia nigra on antiepileptic drug actions in kindled rats. Eur J Pharmacol 186:157–167
Wain T, Andermann F, Silver K, Dubeau F, Andermann E, Rourke-Frew F, Keene D (1996) Exquisite sensitivity of paroxysmal kinesigenic choreoathetosis to carbamazepine. Neurology 47:1104–1106
Waldmeier PC, Baumann PA, Fehr B, De Herdt P, Maitre L (1984) Carbamazepine decreases catecholamine turnover in the rat brain. J Pharmacol Exp Therap 231:166–172
Waldmeier PC, Baumann P, Wicki P, Feldtrauer JJ, Stierlin C, Schmutz M (1995) Similar potency of carbamazepine, oxcarbazepine, and lamotrigine in inhibiting the release of glutamate and other neurotransmitters. Neurology 45:1907–1913
Wales JK (1975) Treatment of diabetes insipidus with carbamazepine. Lancet 4:948–951
Warren JWJ, Bennaman JD, Wannamaker BB, Levy RH (1980) Kinetics of a carbamazepine-ethosuximide interaction. Clin Pharmacol Ther 28:646–651
Weaver DF, Camfield P, Fraser A (1988) Massive carbamazepine overdose: clinical and pharmacologic observations in five episodes. Neurology 38:755–759
Wedlund PL, Chang SL, Levy RH (1983) Steady-state determination of the contribution of lung metabolism to the total body clearance of drugs: application to carbamazepine. J Pharm Sci 72:860–862
Weir RL, Anderson SM, Daly JW (1990) Inhibition of N6-[^{3}H]cyclohexyladenosine binding by carbamazepine. Epilepsia 31:503–512
Weiss SR, Post RM (1991) Contingent tolerance to carbamazepine: a peripheral-type benzodiazepine mechanism. Eur J Pharmacol 193:150–163
Weiss SR, Post RM, Marangos PJ, Patel J (1985a) Adenosine antagonists. Lack of effect on the inhibition of kindled seizures in rats by carbamazepine. Neuropharmacology 24:635–638
Weiss SR, Post RM, Patel J, Marangos PJ (1985b) Differential mediation of the anticonvulsant effects of carbamazepine and diazepam. Life Sci 36:2413–2419
Weiss SR, Nguyen T, Rubinow DR, Helke CJ, Narang PK, Post RM, Jacobowitz DM (1987) Lack of effect of chronic carbamazepine on brain somatostatin in the rat. J Neural Transm 68:325–333
Weiss SR, Nirenberg J, Lewis R, Post RM (1992) Corticotropin-releasing hormone: potentiation of cocaine-kindled seziures and lethality. Epilepsia 33:248–254
Weiss SR, Post RM, Sohn E, Berger A, Lewis R (1993) Cross-tolerance between carbamazepine and valproate on amygdaloid-kindled seizures. Epilepsy Res 16:37–44
Weitholtz H, Zysset T, Kreiten K, Kohl D, Buchsel R, Matern S (1989) Effects of phenytoin, carbamazepine, and valproic acid on caffeine metabolism. Europ J Clin Pharmacol 36:401–406
Wells PS, Holbrook AM, Crowther NR, Hirsh J (1994) Interactions of warfarin with drugs and food. Ann Intern Med 121:676–683
Welty TE, Pickering PR, Hale BC, Arazi R (1992) Loss of seizure control associated with generic substitution of carbamazepine. Ann Pharmacother 26:775–777

Westerberg HGM, Van Der Kleijn E, Oei TT, DeZeeuw RA (1978) Kinetics of carbamazepine and carbamazepine-epoxide determined by use of plasma and saliva. Clin Pharmacol Ther 23:320–328
Willow M, Kuenzel EA, Catterall WA (1984) Inhibition of voltage-sensitive sodium channels in neuroblastoma cells and synaptosomes by the anticonvulsant drugs diphenylhydantoin and carbamazepine. Mol Pharmacol 25:228–234
Willow M, Gonoi T, Catterall WA (1985) Voltage clamp analysis of the inhibitory actions of diphenylhydantoin and carbamazepine on voltage-sensitive sodium channels in neuroblastoma cells. Mol Pharmacol 27:549–558
Windorfer AJ, Sauer W (1977) Drug interactions during anticonvulsant therapy in childhood: diphenylhydantoin, primidone, phenobarbitone, clonazepam, nitrazepam, carbamazepine and dipropylacetate. Neuropediatrie 8:29–41
Wolf P, May T, Tiska G, Schreiber G (1992) Steady state concentrations and diurnal fluctuations of carbamazepine in patients after different slow release formulations. Arzneimittelforschung 42:284–288
Wolf R, Strehle F, Emrich HM (1993) Carbamazepine effects on preoptic GABA release and pituitary luteinizing hormone secretion in rats. Epilepsia 34:1110–1116
Worley PF, Baraban JM (1987) Site of anticonvulsant action on sodium channels: autoradiographic and electrophysiological studies in rat brain. Proc Natl Acad Sci USA 84:3051–3055
Yasuda S, Mizuno N, Kawabe Y, Sakakibara S (1988) Photosensitive lichenoid reaction acompanied by nonphotosensitive subacute prurigo caused by carbamazepine. Photodermatol 5:206–210
Yee RD, Purvin VA, Azzarelli B, Nelson PB (1996) Intermittent diplopia and strabismus caused by ocular neuromyotonia. Trans Am Ophthalmol Soc 94: 207–223
Yerby MS, Friel P, Miller DQ (1985) Carbamazepine protein binding and disposition in pregnancy. Ther Drug Monit 7:269–273
Yerby MS, Friel PN, McCormick K, Koerner M, Van Allen M, Leavitt AM, Sells CJ, Yerby JA (1990) Pharmacokinetics of anticonvulsants in pregnancy: alterations in plasma protein binding. Epilepsy Res 5:223–228
Yerby MS, Friel PN, McCormick K (1992) Antiepileptic drug disposition during pregnancy. Neurology 42 [Suppl 5]:132–140
Yeung-Laiwah AA, Rapeport WG, Thompson GG et al. (1983) Carbamazepine-induced non-hereditary porphyria. Lancet 1:790–792
Yoshimura Y, Yanagihara N, Terao T, Minami K, Abe K, Izumi F (1995) Inhibition by carbamazepine of various ion channels-mediated catecholamine secretion in cultures bovine adrenal medullary cells. Naunyn-Schmiedebergs Arch Pharmacol 352:297–303
Yukawa E, Aoyama T (1996) Detection of carbamazepine drug interaction by multiple peak approach screening using routine clinical pharmacokinetic data. J Clin Pharmacol 36:752–759
Yukawa E, Suzuki A, Higuchi S, Aoyama T (1992) Influence of age and co-medication on steady-state carbamazepine serum levels-dose ratios in Japanese pediatric patients. J Clin Pharm Ther 17:65–69
Zhang YF, Coulter DA (1996) Anticonvulsant drug effects on spontaneous thalamocortical rhythms in vitro: phenytoin, carbamazepine, and phenobarbital. Epilepsy Res 23:55–70
Zielinski JJ, Haidukewych D (1987) Dual effects of carbamazepine-phenytoin interaction. Ther Drug Monit 9:21–23
Zielinski JJ, Haidukewych D, Leheta BJ (1985) Carbamazepine-phenytoin interaction: elevation of plasma phenytoin concentrations due to carbamazepine comedication. Ther Drug Monit 7:51–53
Zielinski JJ, Lichten EM, Haidukewych D (1987) Clinically significant danazol-carbamazepine interaction. Ther Drug Monit 9:24–27

Zimanyi I, Weiss SR, Lajtha A, Post RM, Reith ME (1989) Evidence for a common site of action of lidocaine and carbamazepine in voltage-dependent sodium channels. Eur J Pharmacol 167:419–422

Zucconi M, Goggin T, Crowley M, Callaghan N (1989) Nocturnal myoclonus in restless legs syndrome effect of carbamazepine treatment. Funct Neurol 4:263–271

CHAPTER 11

Oxcarbazepine

S.C. SCHACHTER

A. Introduction

Oxcarbazepine (OXC) was first introduced in 1990, in Denmark, and is now registered in 31 countries worldwide for use as monotherapy and as add-on treatment for partial seizures, whether or not they became secondarily generalized, and for primary generalized tonic-clonic seizures. The estimated patient exposure to the drug currently exceeds 50,000 patient years. Oxcarbazepine is under active investigation in the United States.

This chapter will discuss the mechanisms of action, metabolism, and pharmacokinetics of both oxcarbazepine and its pharmacologically active metabolite mono-hydroxycarbazepine, as well as the efficacy, safety, and tolerability profiles of the drug. Unless otherwise referenced, all study-related data are on file at Novartis Pharmaceuticals Corporation, Basel, Switzerland.

B. Chemistry and Use

Oxcarbazepine (10,11-dihydro-10-oxo-carbamazepine) is a neutral lipophilic compound (MW 252.28) with a very low solubility in water. Although oxcarbazepine is chemically and structurally similar to carbamazepine (CBZ), its biotransformation pattern is completely different. Oxcarbazepine is rapidly metabolized by reduction to an active monohydroxy derivative (10-hydroxycarbazepine), which is thought to be responsible for the antiepileptic effect of the drug (Fig. 1).

C. Pharmacodynamics

I. Biochemical Pharmacology

Oxcarbazepine and mono-hydroxycarbazepine have demonstrable effects on neuronal ion channels. Firstly, at therapeutically relevant concentrations, both oxcarbazepine and mono-hydroxycarbazepine limit high-frequency, repetitive firing of cultured mouse spinal cord neurons by an effect on voltage-dependent Na^+ channels (WAMIL et al. 1991; SCHMUTZ et al. 1994). Secondly, in the in vitro hippocampal slice model, mono-hydroxycarbazepine reduces the frequency of penicillin-induced epileptiform spike discharges as recorded

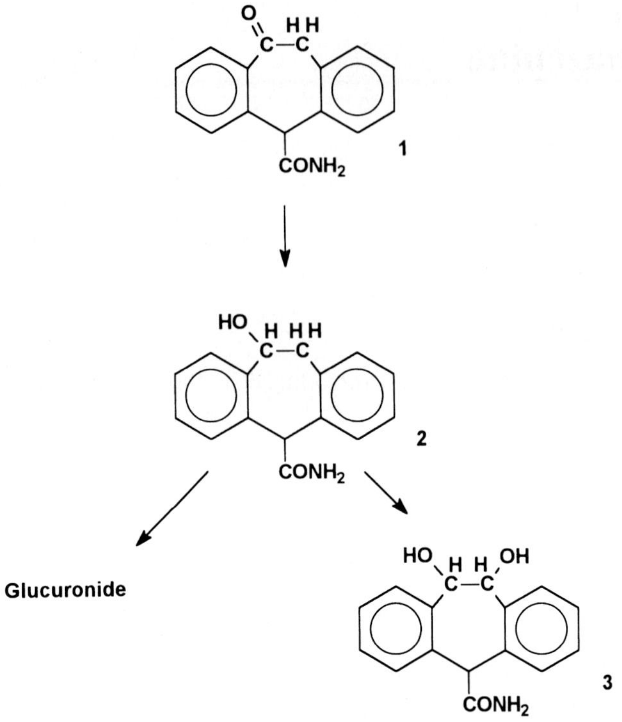

Fig. 1. The main metabolic pathway of oxcarbazepine. Oxcarbazepine (*1*) is rapidly reduced to the pharmacologically active metabolite MHD (*2*), which is then glucuronidated (*3*)

extracellularly over the CA3 area. This effect is reversed by the K^+-channel blocker 4-aminopyridine, suggesting an effect on K^+ channels (McLean et al. 1994; Schmutz et al. 1994). Thirdly, mono-hydroxycarbazepine produces a reversible, dose-dependent decrease in high-voltage-activated Ca^{2+} currents evoked by membrane depolarization in isolated striatal and cortical pyramidal cells. This effect is not antagonized by nifedipine (Stefani et al. 1995).

Neither oxcarbazepine nor mono-hydroxycarbazepine has an effect at γ-aminobutyrate or other neurotransmitter receptor binding sites.

II. Animal Models of Epilepsy

In general, oxcarbazepine, mono-hydroxycarbazepine, and carbamazepine have similar spectra of anticonvulsant activity in animal models (McLean et al. 1994; Schmutz et al. 1994; Wamil et al. 1994). Mono-hydroxycarbazepine has therapeutic indices of more than 6 for sedation and 10 for motor impairment. There has been no evidence of tolerance or withdrawal seizures with either oxcarbazepine or mono-hydroxycarbazepine in monkeys or rats.

III. Human Epilepsies

1. Monotherapy Trials

a) Controlled Monotherapy Trials in Newly Diagnosed or Previously Untreated Patients

Oxcarbazepine and carbamazepine were compared in a blinded study of 235 patients with newly diagnosed partial-onset or primary generalized seizures and were found to be equivalent in efficacy (DAM et al. 1989). Three other international, double-blind, monotherapy trials of oxcarbazepine in patients with newly diagnosed or previously untreated partial-onset or primary generalized seizures have been published and are described in detail below. One study compared oxcarbazepine with valproate (CHRISTE et al. 1997) and the other two, one in adults (BILL et al. 1997) and one in children and adolescents (GUERREIRO et al. 1997), compared oxcarbazepine with phenytoin.

α) Study Designs

Each of these studies was a multicentre, randomized, double-blind, parallel group trial with a retrospective baseline period. Equal numbers were randomized to each group. Blinded treatment was titrated over 8 weeks, based on the clinical response; antiepileptic drugs were administered 3 times daily. Their efficacy and tolerability were recorded during a 48-week maintenance period. The patients had to have at least two seizures separated by more than 48 h in the preceding 6 months to qualify for entry to the trial.

In the oxcarbazepine versus valproate study, the therapy of randomized patients was titrated to doses of between 900 and 2400 mg daily for both antiepileptic drugs. In the other two studies, the oxcarbazepine and phenytoin dosages were 450–2400 mg daily and 150–800 mg daily, respectively.

β) Enrolment Information

In the oxcarbazepine versus valproate study, 249 patients aged 15–65 years were randomized to the drugs. The groups were well matched with respect to age, gender, seizure type, and duration of epilepsy. Nearly 62% of the patients had partial seizures as their predominant seizure type; the others had generalized seizures without a focal onset. Though this was a study of newly diagnosed patients, the mean duration of epilepsy in the subjects was approximately 180 weeks.

In the adult oxcarbazepine versus phenytoin study, 287 patients aged 15–91 years were randomized to the therapies studied. The treatment groups were well matched. A majority of patients (63%) had partial seizures as their main seizure type (59% of the oxcarbazepine- and 68% of the phenytoin-treated patients); the rest had generalized seizures without partial onset. The mean durations of epilepsy were 95 and 89 weeks for the oxcarbazepine- and phenytoin-treated patients, respectively. The patients' seizures were previously untreated.

In the paediatric oxcarbazepine versus phenytoin study, 193 patients aged 5–17 years were randomized to the two groups, which proved to be well matched. A majority of the patients (78%) had partial seizures as their main seizure type; the rest had generalized seizures without a partial onset. The mean durations of epilepsy were 30 and 38 weeks for the oxcarbazepine- and phenytoin-treated patients, respectively. The patients' seizures were previously untreated.

γ) Results

In each study, the primary efficacy variable was the proportion of seizure-free patients who had at least one seizure assessment during the maintenance period.

In the oxcarbazepine versus valproate study, 212 patients (85% of those randomized) were included in the efficacy analysis. Slightly more than half of the patients in each treatment group remained seizure-free during the maintenance period; there was no statistically significant treatment difference. Similarly, there was no treatment difference in the percentage of patients with partial-onset seizures who were seizure-free (46% and 48% for oxcarbazepine and valproate, respectively) or in the percentage of patients with primary generalized seizures who were seizure-free (72% and 62%, respectively). A greater proportion of the valproate-treated patients with secondarily generalized seizures as their main seizure type were seizure-free compared with the oxcarbazepine-treated patients, though the number of patients in each treatment arm was low. Six patients in each treatment group discontinued treatment prematurely because of its lack of efficacy.

In the adult oxcarbazepine versus phenytoin study, 237 patients (83% of those randomized) were included in the efficacy analysis. Overall, nearly 60% of the patients in each treatment group were seizure-free during the maintenance period; there was no statistically significant difference between the treatments. Similarly, there was no treatment difference in the percentages of patients with partial-onset seizures who were seizure-free (56% and 53% for oxcarbazepine and phenytoin, respectively) or in the percentages of patients with primary generalized seizures who were seizure-free (64% and 68%, respectively). One patient in each treatment group discontinued treatment prematurely, because of its lack of efficacy.

In the paediatric oxcarbazepine versus phenytoin study, 158 patients (82% of those randomized) were included in the efficacy analysis. Nearly 60% of patients in each treatment group were seizure-free during the maintenance period; there was no statistically significant difference between the treatments. Similarly, there was no difference in the percentages of patients with partial-onset seizures who were seizure-free (60% and 62% for oxcarbazepine and phenytoin, respectively) or in the percentages of patients with primary generalized seizures who were seizure-free (59% and 54%, respectively). Four oxcarbazepine- and three phenytoin-treated patients discontinued treatment prematurely, because of a lack of efficacy of the therapy.

δ) Conclusions

These comparative trials showed that oxcarbazepine had an efficacy in partial-onset and generalized tonic-clonic seizures similar to that of valproate in adults and to that of phenytoin in both children and adults. The comparative tolerability and safety of the drug will be discussed below.

b) Pre-surgery Trials

An impressive degree of seizure protection was seen in an open-label pilot trial of oxcarbazepine in pre-surgical patients (Fisher et al. 1996). To confirm these results, the first and only placebo-controlled trial of oxcarbazepine performed to date – a multicentre, double-blind, randomized, two-arm parallel monotherapy trial – compared oxcarbazepine 1200 mg twice daily with placebo in inpatients with refractory partial seizures who were undergoing pre-surgical evaluations (Schachter et al. 1999). Patients exited the trial after completing the 10-day treatment period or after experiencing four partial seizures, two new-onset secondarily generalized seizures, serial seizures, or status epilepticus, whichever came first. The primary efficacy variable, the time to meeting one of the exit criteria, was statistically significant in favour of oxcarbazepine ($p = 0.0001$). The secondary efficacy variables, the percentage of patients who met one of the exit criteria and the total partial seizure frequency from the 2nd to the 10th day of double-blind treatment, were also statistically significantly in favour of oxcarbazepine. Thirteen of the 51 oxcarbazepine-treated patients (25%) remained seizure-free throughout the entire 10-day treatment period, compared with only one placebo-treated patient (2%).

2. Add-on and Open-label, Long-term Trials

A double-blind, randomized, cross-over study compared oxcarbazepine to carbamazepine as add-on therapy in 48 patients with refractory epilepsy (Houtkooper et al. 1987). The mean daily doses of oxcarbazepine and carbamazepine were 2628 mg and 1302 mg, respectively. Patients with tonic-clonic or clonic seizures had significantly fewer seizures when treated with oxcarbazepine as compared with carbamazepine; no significant treatment differences were seen in the frequencies of partial or myoclonic seizures.

Van Parys and Meinardi (1994) treated 260 patients with open-label oxcarbazepine for a total exposure of 935 patient-years. In 89 patients, the treatment was changed to oxcarbazepine because carbamazepine therapy had been ineffective. Eight patients (9%) became seizure-free and 36 others (40%) showed substantial improvements in seizure frequency.

D. Pharmacokinetics

I. Absorption, Bioavailability, and Distribution

Oxcarbazepine is quickly and nearly completely absorbed after oral administration. When oxcarbazepine is taken with food, the area under the concentration-time curve (AUC) is increased by 16% (DEGEN et al. 1994). In plasma, and at therapeutically meaningful concentrations, mono-hydroxycarbazepine is approximately 40% protein-bound.

Oxcarbazepine and mono-hydroxycarbazepine cross the placenta and are excreted in breast milk, with a milk:plasma concentration ratio of 0.5 (CIBA-GEIGY LIMITED 1996).

II. Elimination

Oxcarbazepine is eliminated almost entirely by metabolism.

1. Metabolism

Whereas carbamazepine initially undergoes hepatic oxidation to its 10,11-epoxide (which then undergoes hydrolysis to form a diol derivative, followed by glucuronidation of this diol), oxcarbazepine is reduced to yield 10-hydroxycarbazepine as its initial biotransformation product. This reduction is catalyzed by a cytosolic, non-microsomal, and non-inducible keto-reductase. The mono-hydroxy-carbazepine subsequently is either glucuronidated or oxidized to the same carbamazepine-10,11-*trans*-diol metabolite that is formed from carbamazepine. While UDP-glucuronosyltransferase (the enzyme which glucuronidates mono-hydroxycarbazepine) is inducible, this induction is less pronounced than the carbamazepine-associated induction of the cytochrome P450 family of enzymes. Thus the metabolism of oxcarbazepine is independent of the cytochrome P450 system; induction or inhibition of this system by the presence of other antiepileptic drugs will have little effect on the metabolism of oxcarbazepine and mono-hydroxycarbazepine.

The metabolites of oxcarbazepine are excreted predominantly by the kidneys.

2. Elimination Parameters

The plasma elimination half-life of oxcarbazepine is 1–2.5 h due to its rapid and almost complete conversion to mono-hydroxycarbazepine. The elimination kinetics of mono-hydroxycarbazepine are first order. The plasma half-life of mono-hydroxycarbazepine averages 9 h and is stable over time.

III. Clinical Pharmacokinetics

Studies in volunteers and in patients with epilepsy show a linear, proportional relationship between daily dosages of oxcarbazepine and serum mono-hydroxycarbazepine concentrations (AUGUSTEIJN and VAN PARYS 1990).

1. Special Patient Groups

a) Hepatic and Renal Impairment

Hepatic impairment has no apparent effect on the pharmacokinetics of oxcarbazepine or mono-hydroxycarbazepine. However, because oxcarbazepine metabolites are cleared renally, mono-hydroxycarbazepine levels are significantly increased in patients with creatinine clearances under 30 ml/min; oxcarbazepine dosages in this group of patients should be reduced by 50% and the dosage titration phase should be prolonged (ROUAN et al. 1994).

b) The Elderly and Children

In volunteers aged 60–82 years, peak plasma mono-hydroxycarbazepine concentrations and the AUC for mono-hydroxycarbazepine were significantly higher than in younger adults, probably due to the diminished creatinine clearance in older persons (VAN HEININGEN et al. 1991).

Mono-hydroxycarbazepine concentrations in children aged from 6 to 18 years are similar to those observed in adults (HOUTKOOPER et al. 1987), but those reported in children aged 2–5 years have been lower.

E. Interactions

I. Effects on Other Drugs

Drug interaction trials showed that there was no auto-induction following oxcarbazepine use, and little or no hetero-induction of the metabolism of common co-medications such as cimetidine, erythromycin, and warfarin (KERANEN et al. 1992; KRÄMER et al. 1992). These results permit the prediction that oxcarbazepine at clinically relevant doses should not interact pharmacokinetically with other drugs that are metabolized by any of the eight isoforms of the P450 system.

Oxcarbazepine does not alter sex hormone binding globulin or androgen levels in men (ISOJARVI et al. 1994) but, like carbamazepine, does reduce ethinyloestradiol and levonorgestrel concentrations in non-epileptic women taking oral contraceptives (KLOSTERSKOV JENSEN et al. 1992). Breakthrough bleeding has been reported in patients with epilepsy taking oxcarbazepine and 30 μg ethinyloestradiol daily (SONNEN 1990).

II. Effects of Other Drugs on Oxcarbazepine

Although they inhibit the metabolism of carbamazepine, erythromycin, cimetidine and propoxyphene have no effects on the pharmacokinetics of oxcarbazepine (KERÄNEN et al. 1992a,b; MOGENSEN et al. 1992). In one study, verapamil slightly reduced mono-hydroxycarbazepine plasma concentrations (KRÄMER et al. 1991).

F. Adverse Effects

I. Animal Studies

1. Acute Exposure

The LD_{50} for a single oral administration of oxcarbazepine or mono-hydroxycarbazepine ranged between 1240 mg/kg and greater than 6000 mg/kg, depending on the species studied.

2. Teratogenicity/Carcinogenicity/Mutagenicity

Oxcarbazepine doses of up to 150 mg/kg had no effect on male and female rat fertility, or on the course of gestation in female rats. No teratogenicity was observed in mice and rabbits; one of two studies in rats showed dose-related teratogenicity at daily oxcarbazepine doses of 300 and 1000 mg/kg. Mono-hydroxycarbazepine showed no teratogenic potential in rats and rabbits.

Studies of long-term exposure to oxcarbazepine in rodents showed no evidence of carcinogenicity; no evidence of mutagenicity was found in any of the studies performed with oxcarbazepine or mono-hydroxycarbazepine.

II. Human Studies

1. Add-on, Open-label Trials

In an open-label, retrospective study of 947 oxcarbazepine-treated patients, FRIIS et al. (1993) found that 33% of patients reported adverse events. Most of the adverse effects involved the central nervous system (dizziness 6%, sedation 6%, fatigue 6%). Rashes occurred in 6% of the patients, half of whom had experienced a rash previously when receiving carbamazepine. Because of their adverse effects, 18% of the patients discontinued oxcarbazepine therapy.

VAN PARYS and MEINARDI (1994) used open-label oxcarbazepine to treat 164 patients who had previously had adverse effects from, and/or intolerability to, carbamazepine. Thirty patients (18%) became free of adverse effects, and in 99 others (60%) the symptoms became tolerable. In addition to the improved tolerability of the therapy, the seizure control improved in 45 patients, and 13 became seizure-free.

2. Monotherapy Trials in Newly Diagnosed or Previously Untreated Patients

In the three controlled monotherapy trials discussed above, the primary tolerability criterion was the result of the log-rank test on the time to the premature discontinuation of oxcarbazepine because of adverse experiences.

In the oxcarbazepine versus valproate study, there was no difference in tolerability between the treatment groups (CHRISTE et al. 1997). Fifteen oxcarbazepine-treated patients withdrew prematurely because of adverse effects, compared with ten valproate-treated patients (a difference that was not statistically significant). The most frequent adverse effect from oxcarbazepine, which led to premature discontinuation of therapy, was skin allergy, which occurred in 5% of patients; in the study, hair loss was the most frequent reason for the premature discontinuation of valproate (3%). Two oxcarbazepine-treated patients had plasma sodium concentrations of 130 mmol/l or less; both were asymptomatic.

In the adult oxcarbazepine versus phenytoin study, the primary tolerability variable showed a statistically significant difference in favour of oxcarbazepine: 5 oxcarbazepine-treated patients, compared with 16 phenytoin-treated patients ($p = 0.02$), withdrew prematurely from the study because of adverse effects (Bill et al. 1997). The most frequent adverse effects from phenytoin leading to premature discontinuation of therapy were rash (ten patients) and hirsutism/gum hypertrophy (five patients). One oxcarbazepine-treated patient withdrew because of a rash. No oxcarbazepine-treated patient became hyponatraemic.

In the paediatric oxcarbazepine versus phenytoin study, the primary tolerability variable showed a statistically significant difference ($p = 0.002$) in favour of oxcarbazepine: 2 oxcarbazepine-treated patients withdrew prematurely because of adverse effects, compared with 14 phenytoin-treated patients (Guerreiro et al. 1997). The most frequent adverse effects from phenytoin which led to premature discontinuation of therapy were hypertrichosis and/or gingival hypertrophy (ten patients), and rash (four patients). Two oxcarbazepine-treated patients withdrew due to rashes. No oxcarbazepine-treated patient became hyponatraemic.

III. Particular Adverse Effects in Humans

1. Rashes

Allergy in the form of skin reactions appears to occur less frequently with oxcarbazepine than with carbamazepine.

In the study of Dam et al. (1989), 10% of oxcarbazepine-treated patients discontinued therapy prematurely because of allergic reactions, compared with 16% of carbamazepine-treated patients. Similarly, in the Novartis safety database for oxcarbazepine, which includes data on 2436 patients treated with the drug and 277 treated with carbamazepine, only 2.8% of oxcarbazepine-treated patients had hypersensitivity reactions, compared with 6.5% of those who received carbamazepine.

In the study of Van Parys and Meinardi (1994), 46 of 55 patients (84%) whose treatment was switched from carbamazepine to oxcarbazepine because of skin reactions of undetermined nature or 'evidently allergic reactions' did not experience a recurrence whilst taking oxcarbazepine. In an unpublished study, 51 patients with previous cutaneous hypersensitivity reactions to carbamazepine were treated with oxcarbazepine. In 37 patients (73%), no rash reappeared (Jensen 1983). In 11 of the remaining 14 patients, a rash reoccurred within the 1st month of treatment.

2. Overdosage

According to the international product information brochure, patients who take an overdose of oxcarbazepine should be treated symptomatically, and the drug removed by gastric lavage and/or inactivated by administering activated charcoal (Ciba-Geigy Limited 1996). Admission to an intensive care unit is advisable, with careful monitoring for cardiac conduction disturbances, electrolyte abnormalities, and respiratory difficulties.

IV. Laboratory Abnormalities

Hyponatraemia occurs more commonly with oxcarbazepine than with carbamazepine, but is rarely of clinical significance (Van Amelsvoort et al. 1994). In a cross-sectional study of 41 oxcarbazepine-treated patients, 50% had a serum sodium concentration below 135 mmol/l, but in no case was discontinuation of oxcarbazepine clinically necessary (Nielsen et al. 1988). Patients treated with oxcarbazepine dosages above 30 mg/kg/day had a significantly higher risk of becoming hyponatraemic than those taking lower dosages. In a retrospective study, plasma sodium concentration values before and during oxcarbazepine treatment were available for 350 patients (Friis et al. 1993). Two-thirds of the patients had normal sodium concentrations before and during treatment. Approximately one-quarter of the patients had a shift to low sodium values with oxcarbazepine treatment, though only four patients (1%) were withdrawn from oxcarbazepine because of hyponatraemia.

No clinically relevant fluctuations of the white blood cell count have been observed in clinical studies of oxcarbazepine and clinically relevant elevations of liver function tests appear to occur less often than with carbamazepine. In a retrospective study, liver and bone marrow function tests became abnormal in 2% or fewer patients who received the drug (Friis et al. 1993).

V. Pregnancy

In the presence of the developing foetus, the relative safety of oxcarbazepine and mono-hydroxycarbazepine, compared with that of other antiepileptic drugs, is unknown.

References

Augusteijn R, van Parys JAP (1990) Oxcarbazepine (Tripetal, OXC) – dose-concentration relationship in patients with epilepsy. Acta Neurol Scand 82 [Suppl 133]:37

Bill PA, Vigonius U, Pohlmann H, Guerrio CAM, Kochen S, Saffer D, Moore A (1997) A double-blind controlled clinical trial of oxcarbazepine versus phenytoin in adults with previously untreated epilepsy. Epilepsy Res 27:195–204

Christe W, Krämer G, Vigonius U, Pohlmann H, Steinhoff BJ, Brodie MJ, Moore A (1997) A double-blind controlled clinical trial: oxcarbazepine versus sodium valproate in adults with newly diagnosed epilepsy. Epilepsy Res 26:451–460

Ciba-Geigy Limited (1996). International product information. Ciba, Basel
Dam M, Ekberg R, Loyning Y, Waltimo O, Jakoben K (1989) A double-blind study comparing oxcarbazepine and carbamazepine in patients with newly diagnosed, previously untreated epilepsy. Epilepsy Res 3:70–76
Degen PH, Flesch G, Cardot JM, Czendlik C, Dieterle W (1994) The influence of food on the disposition of the antiepileptic oxcarbazepine and its major metabolites in healthy volunteers. Biopharm Drug Dispos 15:519–526
Fisher RS, Eskola J, et al. (1996) Open-label, pilot study of oxcarbazepine for inpatients under evaluation for epilepsy surgery. Drug Dev Res 38:43–49
Friis ML, Kristensen O, Boas J et al. (1993) Therapeutic experiences with 947 epileptic out-patients in oxcarbazepine treatment. Acta Neurol Scand 87:224–227
Guerreiro MM, Vigonius U, Pohlmann H, de Manreza MLG, Fejerman N, Antonick SA, Moore A (1997) A double-blind controlled clinical trial of oxcarbazepine versus phenytoin in children and adolescents with epilepsy. Epilepsy Res 27:205–213
Houtkooper MA, Lammertsma A, Meyer JW et al. (1987) Oxcarbazepine (GP 47680) – a possible alternative to carbamazepine? Epilepsia 28:693–698
Isojarvi JIT, Pakarinen AJ, Rautio A, Pelkonen O, Mykyla W (1994) Serum sex hormone levels after replacing carbamazepine with oxcarbazepine. Pharmokinet Disposit:461–464
Jensen NO (1983) Oxcarbazepine in patients hypersensitive to carbamazepine. 16th Epilepsy International Congress, Hamburg
Keranen T, Jolkkonen J, Jensen P, Menge GP, Anderson P (1992) Absence of interaction between oxcarbazepine and erythromycin. Acta Neurol Scand 86:120–123
Keränen T, Jolkkonen J, Klosterskov-Jensen P, Menge GP (1992) Oxcarbazepine does not interact with cimetidine in healthy volunteers. Acta Neurol Scand 85:239–242
Klosterskov Jensen P, Saano V, Saano V, Haring P, Svenstrup B, Menge GP (1992) Possible interaction between oxcarbazepine and an oral contraceptive. Epilepsia 33:1149–1152
Krämer G, Tettenborn B, Flesch G (1991) Oxcarbazepine-verapamil drug interaction in healthy volunteers. Epilepsia 32 [Suppl 1]:70–71
Krämer G, Tettenborn B, Klosterskov-Jensen P, Menge GP, Stoll KD (1992) Oxcarbazepine does not affect the anticoagulant activity of warfarin. Epilepsia 33:1145–1148
McLean MJ, Schmutz M, Wamil AW, Olpe HR, Portet C, Feldmann KF (1994) Oxcarbazepine: mechanisms of action. Epilepsia 35 [Suppl 3]:S5–S9
Mogensen PH, Jorgensen L, Boas J, Dam M, Vesterager A, Flesch G, Jensen PK (1992) Effects of dextropropoxyphene on the steady-state kinetics of oxcarbazepine and its metabolites. Acta Neurol Scand 85:14–17
Nielsen OA, Johannessen AC, Bardrum B (1988) Oxcarbazepine-induced hyponatremia, a cross-sectional study. Epilepsy Res 2:269–271
Rouan MC, Lecaillon JB, Godbillon J et al. (1994) The effect of renal impairment on the pharmacokinetics of oxcarbazepine and its metabolites. Eur J Clin Pharmacol 47:161–167
Schachter SC, Vazquez B et al. (1999) Oxcarbazepine: double-blind, randomised placebocontrol, monotherapy trial for partial seizures. Neurology (in press)
Schmutz M, Brugger F, Gentsch C, McLean MJ, Olbe HR (1994) Oxcarbazepine: preclinical anticonvulsant profile and putative mechanisms of action. Epilepsia 35 [Suppl 5]:S47–S50
Sonnen AEH (1990) Oxcarbazepine and oral contraceptives. Acta Neurol Scand 82 [Suppl 133]:37
Stefani A, Pisani A, DeMurtas M, Mercuri NB, Marciana MG, Calabresi P (1995) Action of GP 47779, the active metabolite of oxcarbazepine, on the corticostriatal system. II. Modulation of high-voltage-activated calcium currents. Epilepsia 36:997–1002

Van Amelsvoort T, Bakshi R, Devauz CB, Schwabe S (1994) Hyponatremia associated with carbamazepine and oxcarbazepine therapy: a review. Epilepsia 35:181–188

van Heiningen PN, Eve MD, Oosterhuis B et al. (1991) The influence of age on the pharmacokinetics of the antiepileptic agent oxcarbazepine. Clin Pharmacol Ther 50:410–419

Van Parys JAP, Meinardi H (1994) Survey of 260 epileptic patients treated with oxcarbazepine (Trileptal) on a named-patient basis. Epilepsy Res 19:79–85

Wamil AW, Portet CH, Jensen PK et al. (1991) Oxcarbazepine and its monohydroxy metabolite limit action potential firing by mouse central neurons in cell culture. Epilepsia 32 [Suppl 3]:65–66

Wamil AW, Schmutz M, Portet C, Feldmann KF, McLean MJ (1994) Effects of oxcarbazepine and 10-hydroxycarbamazepine on action potential firing and generalized seizures. Eur J Pharmacol 271:301–308

CHAPTER 12

Lamotrigine

M.C. WALKER and J.W.A.S. SANDER

A. Introduction

In 1966, REYNOLDS et al. proposed that the antiepileptic actions of the then available antiepileptic drugs might be partially mediated through their antifolate effects. This idea gained further credence when it was discovered that folate and its derivatives were proconvulsant when given in large doses systemically or applied directly onto the cortex (FISHER 1989). The hypothesis resulted in the development of a number of antifolate agents and their testing in animal models of epilepsy. These experiments revealed a poor correlation between antifolate properties and anticonvulsant effects, but a group of phenyltriazine compounds, which had weak antifolate properties, proved to be potent anticonvulsants. Lamotrigine was developed from these compounds, though neither short-term nor chronic lamotrigine therapy appears to be associated with significant changes in serum or red cell folate concentrations (SANDER and PATSALOS 1992).

B. Chemistry and Use

I. Chemistry

Lamotrigine [3,5-diamino-6-(2,3-dichlorophenyl)-1,2,4-triazine] is structurally distinct from the other antiepileptic drugs. The molecule consists of a phenyl group with two chloride substituents joined to a triazine structure with two amino substitutions. It is synthesized from thionyl chloride and 2,3-dichlorobenzoic acid. These form the acid chloride which when reacted with cuprous cyanide is converted to the alpha-ketonitrile; this added to aminoguanidine in nitric acid gives the imine, which readily cyclizes in base to yield lamotrigine (MILLER et al. 1986a). Lamotrigine has a molecular weight of 256.09 and is a weak base with a pK_a of 5.5 (MILLER et al. 1986a). It is poorly soluble in water, and is therefore either given parenterally as a suspension or as an isothionate or mesylate salt.

1. Analytical Methods

Methods using high performance liquid chromatography (HPLC), gas chromatography, radioimmunoassay, immunofluorescence or spectroscopy have

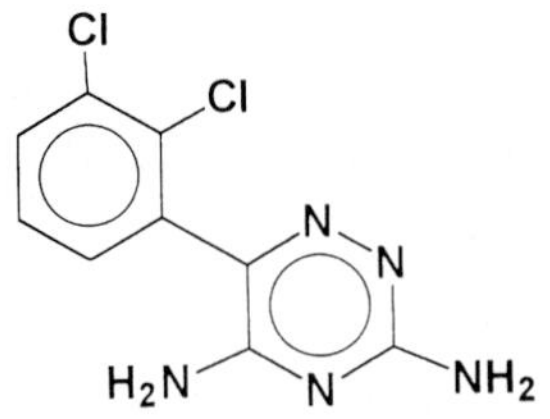

been described for the determination of lamotrigine concentrations. Both reverse phase and normal HPLC have been used successfully and can distinguish lamotrigine from other antiepileptic drugs with a lower limit of detection of 0.1 to 0.5 μg/ml on a serum sample of 100–200 μl (COCIGLIO et al. 1991; FAZIO et al. 1992; RAMACHANDRAN et al. 1994; FRASER et al. 1995; GEORGE et al. 1995; YAMASHITA et al. 1995; BARTOLI et al. 1997b; HART et al. 1997; LENSMEYER et al. 1997; LONDERO and LO GRECO 1997; SALLUSTIO and MORRIS 1997). A gas chromatographic technique using nitrogen phosphorus detection was similarly sensitive and precise (WATELLE et al. 1997), and techniques using gas chromatography-mass spectroscopy have also been successful, with the reference spectrum for pure lamotrigine now being published (DASGUPTA and HART 1997; HALLBACH et al. 1997). The use of thermospray liquid chromatography-mass spectrometry has permitted the structural elucidation of a number of urinary metabolites of lamotrigine, formed after administering the drug in man and in a number of laboratory animal species (DOIG and CLARE 1991b). A precise and sensitive radioimmunoassay technique to determine human plasma lamotrigine concentrations has also been described (BIDDLECOMBE et al. 1990). The method is a direct double antibody procedure employing a rabbit polyclonal antibody raised against a bovine serum albumin conjugate of lamotrigine. The method was specific and showed a reasonable correlation with the results of HPLC. An immunofluorometric assay has also been developed for lamotrigine (SAILSTAD and FINDLAY 1991). This assay involves competition for a limited amount of polyclonal lamotrigine antiserum between lamotrigine free in solution and bound to a bovine thyroglobulin conjugate. There was, however, some cross-reactivity with the drug's metabolites in both humans and rats. No significant interference was demonstrated in the analysis of plasma samples from clinical trials when comparing sample analysis by the immunofluorometric assay and HPLC.

II. Use

In clinical trials, lamotrigine has been shown to be an effective add-on therapy in partial seizures, generalized tonic-clonic seizures, absences and the Lennox-Gastaut syndrome (GOA et al. 1993). It has also been found to be effective as monotherapy in patients with newly diagnosed epilepsy (BRODIE et al. 1995).

C. Pharmacodynamics

I. Anticonvulsant Effects

1. Animal Models of Epilepsy

a) Maximal Electroshock Seizures

In the maximal electroshock test, the animals received a supramaximal stimulus via corneal electrodes; this induced a tonic extension, and the ED_{50} for the suppression of the hindlimb extension phase was determined in mice and rats (MILLER et al. 1986b). This model is useful for detecting drugs that are likely to be effective against tonic-clonic seizures. To evaluate the latency of onset and the duration of action, drug-to-shock intervals from 0.25 to 24 h were used, and the ED_{50} values of oral lamotrigine were compared with those of standard antiepileptic drugs given orally (MILLER et al. 1986b). Lamotrigine was the most potent drug tested, having a similar peak ED_{50} to diazepam and phenytoin in mice (2.6 mg/kg), and to carbamazepine in rats (1.9 mg/kg). Lamotrigine had the longest duration of action with a similar ED_{50} between 1 and 8 h, whilst at 25 h the ED_{50} was only 3–4 times the peak ED_{50} (MILLER et al. 1986b).

No tolerance was noted to the anticonvulsant action of oral lamotrigine in the maximal electroshock model over 28 days in both mice and rats, and lamotrigine was equally effective given subcutaneously, intraperitoneally or intravenously (MILLER et al. 1986a).

b) Chemoconvulsant Tests

Lamotrigine was tested in mice given pentylenetetrazole via a tail vein (MILLER et al. 1986b). In this model, the abolition of hindlimb extension is equivalent to the maximal electroshock test, and the latency to facial or forelimb clonus has been useful in detecting drugs that are effective against absence seizures. Lamotrigine abolished the hindlimb extension with an ED_{50} of 7.2 mg/kg; this was a similar potency to that of phenytoin and phenobarbitone, but lamotrigine was less potent than diazepam (MILLER et al. 1986b). The clonus latency was not increased by carbamazepine, lamotrigine or phenytoin at many times their maximal electroshock ED_{50} doses. Indeed, at very high doses, both lamotrigine (160 mg/kg) and phenytoin (640 mg/kg) reduced the clonus latency, indicating a proconvulsant action (MILLER et al. 1986b). In a study in rats aged 7–90 days (STANKOVA et al. 1992), lamotrigine 2.5–20 mg/kg showed the same anticonvulsant activity in pentylenetetrazole-induced seizures regardless of the animals' ages (i.e. there was no effect of ontogenesis on lamotrigine's anticonvulsant activity in this model); this study confirmed the efficacy of lamotrigine against hindlimb extension, but not against clonic (minimal) seizures in this model. This finding would seem to imply that lamotrigine would be ineffective in absence seizures, but this prediction has proved incorrect as the drug has been shown to be effective against absences in humans and in other animal models of seizure disorders (see below).

c) *Afterdischarge Tests*

Lamotrigine has been tested against electrically evoked and visually evoked afterdischarges (MILLER et al. 1986a; WHEATLEY and MILLER 1989). Electrically evoked discharges in the limbic system have been used as a model for complex partial seizures. Intravenous lamotrigine, phenytoin and phenobarbitone were compared for their action on the durations of electrically induced afterdischarges in the hippocampus in halothane-anaesthetized beagle dogs and rats. Lamotrigine reduced the afterdischarge duration in a dose-dependent manner and was approximately twofold more potent than phenytoin in the dog and three- to fourfold more potent than phenobarbitone in both the dog and the rat, in which species the intravenous lamotrigine ED_{50} values were 4.5 and 11.7 mg/kg, respectively (WHEATLEY and MILLER 1989). Phenytoin was ineffective in the rat at sublethal doses. In limited studies in electrically induced cortical afterdischarges in marmosets, intravenous administration of both lamotrigine and phenytoin (both 5–15 mg/kg) reduced or abolished the afterdischarges (WHEATLEY and MILLER 1989).

Visually evoked afterdischarges were elicited in conscious rats, and were dose dependently inhibited by lamotrigine with an ED_{50} of 5.6 mg/kg (MILLER et al. 1986a). Phenobarbitone, diazepam and ethosuximide were also effective against visually evoked afterdischarges; phenytoin and carbamazepine were ineffective.

d) *Electrically Induced Kindling*

Kindling involves the repetitive application of stimuli (usually electrical ones) to a specific area of an animal's brain. The procedure initially evokes discharges but not seizures (MCNAMARA et al. 1993). Repetition of the same stimuli results in a gradual lengthening of the afterdischarges and eventually leads to progressively more severe seizures. Once an animal has been kindled, the heightened response to the stimulus seems to be permanent, and spontaneous seizures may occur (MCNAMARA et al. 1993). A fully kindled animal is an animal with partial seizures, and is used as a model of partial seizures in which prospective antiepileptic compounds can be tested. The kindling process itself has been argued to represent the development of epilepsy, and it has therefore been proposed that compounds that inhibit the kindling process may also inhibit epileptogenesis (LÖSCHER and SCHMIDT 1993; MCNAMARA et al. 1993). In electrically induced cortical kindling in rats, lamotrigine (3–18 mg/kg orally) was administered 2 h before each stimulation (O'DONNELL and MILLER 1991). Lamotrigine failed to prevent the kindling process, but 12 and 18 mg/kg of the drug did reduce the number of kindled responses and their duration. Lamotrigine at all doses tested increased the number of nil responses (where stimulation failed to evoke a behavioural clonus or afterdischarge) in a dose-dependent manner (O'Donnell and Miller 1991).

e) Genetic Seizure Models

Lamotrigine has been tested in the genetically epilepsy-prone rat, and in DBA/2 mice (Smith et al. 1993; Dalby and Nielsen 1997). Both species have seizures that can be induced by a sound stimulus. Lamotrigine was similarly effective in the two models, with an ED_{50} in the genetically epilepsy-prone rat of 4.8 μmol/kg (1.2 mg/kg), and in the DBA/2 mice one of 6 μmol/kg (1.5 mg/kg). The relationship of these results to effectiveness in human epilepsy is unknown. Lamotrigine at intraperitoneal doses of 0.5 and 1.25 mg/kg, which did not significantly affect the occurrence of audiogenic seizures in DBA/2 mice markedly potentiated the anticonvulsant activity of carbamazepine, diazepam, phenytoin, phenobarbitone and valproate against sound-induced seizures in DBA/2 mice (De Sarro et al. 1996). The potentiation by lamotrigine was greatest for diazepam and valproate, less for phenobarbitone, and least for phenytoin and carbamazepine. This interaction did not appear to be a pharmacokinetic one as lamotrigine did not significantly affect the plasma levels of the other antiepileptic drugs studied. This does not, however, exclude an effect of the drug on protein binding or brain penetration.

Lamotrigine has also been tested in the lethargic (lh/lh) mouse, a genetic model of absence seizures (Hosford and Wang 1997). This model has correctly predicted the efficacy of ethosuximide, valproate and benzodiazepines, and the lack of efficacy of carbamazepine and phenytoin, in absence seizures (Hosford and Wang 1997). In this model, lamotrigine decreased absence seizures; this effect was not seen with vigabatrin, tiagabine, gabapentin and topiramate (Hosford and Wang 1997).

f) Models of Status Epilepticus

Because of the anticonvulsant properties it shares with phenytoin, and the widespread use of the latter in the treatment of status epilepticus, there has been interest in the possible use of lamotrigine in this situation. This possibility has been explored in an animal model in which status epilepticus is induced in rats with epileptogenic cortical cobalt lesions through the administration of homocysteine thiolactone (Walton et al. 1996). In this model, phenytoin given after the second generalized tonic-clonic seizure prevented convulsive status epilepticus with an ED_{50} of 100.5 mg/kg; when given 30 min prior to the homocysteine thiolactone, phenytoin (50 mg/kg) prevented the onset of status epilepticus in half the animals. In contrast, lamotrigine, 10–100 mg/kg, had no effect given after the second generalized tonic-clonic seizure, whilst lamotrigine, 10–20 mg/kg, had no effect given 0–120 min prior to the homocysteine thiolactone (Walton et al. 1996). In a model of refractory status epilepticus induced in rats by constant stimulation of the perforant path for 2 h, neither phenytoin (50 mg/kg) nor lamotrigine(20 mg/kg), given during the status epilepticus, had any effect on the seizure or on the consequent neuronal damage (WALKER et al. 1996b).

2. Mechanism of Action

a) Neurochemical Actions

Glutamate, being the major excitatory transmitter in the central nervous system, is proposed to play a critical role in the generation of epileptic seizures. Indeed, glutamate antagonists at a variety of glutamate receptors have antiepileptic properties. The effect of lamotrigine on the release of glutamate (and other neurotransmitters) is of great interest. This matter was initially explored in cortical slices in which neurotransmitter release was stimulated through depolarization either via the application of high extracellular potassium concentrations (55 mM) or by veratrine (10 μg/ml) which specifically opens Na^+ channels (LEACH et al. 1986). The veratrine-evoked neurotransmitter release was very sensitive to blockade by tetrodotoxin, a Na^+ channel blocker. The K^+-evoked glutamate release showed a marked Ca^{2+} dependence, suggesting that it was mainly vesicular release. Lamotrigine had no effect on K^+-evoked neurotransmitter release at concentrations up to 300 μM. In contrast, lamotrigine inhibited the veratrine-evoked release of glutamate, GABA, aspartate and acetylcholine with ED_{50} values of 21, 44, 21 and 100 μM, respectively. These results strongly suggest that lamotrigine inhibits neurotransmitter release through its action on Na^+ channels (see below). In the same study, the effects of phenytoin were investigated with similar results except that phenytoin was equipotent in inhibiting GABA and glutamate release (lamotrigine was approximately twice as potent as an inhibitor of glutamate release). The selectivity of lamotrigine in inhibiting glutamate release led to its being considered as a neuroprotectant (see below). The relevance of lamotrigine's effect on veratrine-evoked glutamate release has been explored in rat brain slices in a comparison of the effects of carbamazepine, oxcarbazepine and lamotrigine on the release of neurotransmitters elicited by veratrine or electrical stimulation. The three antiepileptic drugs inhibited veratrine-evoked release of endogenous glutamate, [^{3}H]GABA, and [^{3}H]dopamine, with IC_{50} values between 23 and 150 μM, there being little difference between the compounds (WALDMEIER et al. 1995). They were, however, 5–7 times less potent in inhibiting electrically evoked as compared with veratrine-evoked release of neurotransmitters. Therefore it is uncertain whether lamotrigine's inhibition of glutamate release has any significance in relation to the treatment of epilepsy (WALDMEIER et al. 1995). Further evidence that these effects may not be relevant has come from in vivo experiments with veratrine-evoked glutamate release in rats (WALDMEIER et al. 1996). Microdialysis measurements of extracellular glutamate and aspartate concentrations were carried out in conscious rats, veratrine being applied via the perfusion medium to the cortex and the corpus striatum in the presence of the glutamate uptake inhibitor L-

trans-pyrrolidine-2,4-dicarboxylic acid. Maximally effective anticonvulsant doses of carbamazepine (30 mg/kg), oxcarbazepine (60 mg/kg) and lamotrigine (15 mg/kg) were given orally. None of the anticonvulsant compounds affected the veratrine-evoked increases in extracellular glutamate or aspartate in the striatum or affected the rises in glutamate concentrations caused by the glutamate uptake inhibitor (WALDMEIER et al. 1996). In the cortex, these drugs reduced the veratrine-evoked increase in extracellular glutamate concentrations only by about 50% (WALDMEIER et al. 1996).

The effects of lamotrigine on other neurotransmitter systems have also yielded results that are difficult to interpret. Local injection of lamotrigine (600 μM) into the hippocampus of freely moving rats prevented pilocarpine-induced seizures and resulted in a simultaneous rise in hippocampal extracellular dopamine concentrations (SMOLDERS et al. 1997). The local concentration of lamotrigine was much higher than that achieved after oral ingestion of clinically relevant doses of the drug, and indeed, in the same publication, it was found that lamotrigine (10 mg/kg) had no effect on seizures or dopamine concentrations (SMOLDERS et al. 1997). Furthermore, it has been demonstrated in mice that, at a dose that abolishes audiogenic seizures, lamotrigine inhibited the synthesis of dopamine in the striatum (VRIEND and ALEXIUK 1997).

b) Ionic Conductances

α) Na^+ Channels

The work on neurotransmitter release suggested that lamotrigine has an action upon Na^+ channels (LEACH et al. 1986). Using cultures of fetal mouse spinal neurons, CHEUNG et al. (1992) investigated the effect of lamotrigine on the sustained repetitive firing of Na^+-dependent action potentials, and on [^{3}H]batrachotoxin binding to rat synaptosomes. In a similar fashion to carbamazepine and phenytoin, lamotrigine blocked sustained repetitive firing in a concentration-, voltage- and use-dependent manner (CHEUNG et al. 1992). Lamotrigine had no effect on the first action potential elicited by a depolarizing step, but it caused limitation of the firing of subsequent action potentials. The effect of lamotrigine could be reversed by hyperpolarization (CHEUNG et al. 1992). The estimated IC_{50} for lamotrigine was 20 μM. Lamotrigine inhibited the binding of [^{3}H]batrachotoxin (which binds specifically to receptor site 2 on Na^+ channels) to rat synaptosomes with a K_D of 114 μM (CHEUNG et al. 1992). The relatively high K_D value represents a tonic blockade of Na^+ channels, and not a frequency-dependent blockade (Na^+ channels cannot be activated repetitively during binding experiments – CHEUNG et al. 1992). In further studies on the action of lamotrigine (10 or 100 μM) using primary rat neuroglial cultures, LEES and LEACH (1993) demonstrated that the drug did not significantly attenuate fast Na^+ spikes when these were evoked at low frequencies, but attenuated (at 10 μM) or abolished (at 100 μM) spike bursts induced by iontophoretic application of glutamate or potassium. To characterize further the mechanism of action of lamotrigine, its effect on voltage-sensitive Na^+ channels present in

N4TG1 mouse neuroblastoma clonal cells was compared with those of phenytoin and carbamazepine (LANG et al. 1993). Lamotrigine, phenytoin and carbamazepine produced a tonic inhibition of Na^+ channels with IC_{50} values of 91, 58 and 140 μM, respectively. At a concentration of 100 μM, all compounds shifted the voltage-dependency of steady-state inactivation toward the more negative, slowed the rate of recovery from inactivation and produced a use-dependent inhibition of Na^+ channels (LANG et al. 1993). This demonstrated that lamotrigine, phenytoin and carbamazepine had similar effects on Na^+ channels, and that they had an action on the inactive state of the Na^+ channel. Furthermore, it demonstrated that at high concentrations lamotrigine can exhibit tonic inhibition of Na^+ channels even at low frequencies; this is in contrast to the findings of LEES and LEACH (1993). This discrepancy may be due to differing pharmacologies of Na^+ channels in different cell types or to different experimental techniques used. These findings have been confirmed in rat cerebellar granule cell cultures in which lamotrigine reduced the amplitude of the voltage-gated Na^+ inward current and induced a negative shift of the steady-state inactivation curve (ZONA and AVOLI 1997).

The effect of lamotrigine on the Na^+ channel was characterized using recombinant rat brain type IIA Na^+ channels expressed in hamster ovary cells and native Na^+ channels in rat hippocampal pyramidal neurons, using whole-cell recording and intracellular recording techniques (XIE et al. 1995). The IC_{50} of lamotrigine in inhibiting Na^+ currents was approximately 500 μM at a holding potential of –90 mV, compared with an IC_{50} of 100 μM at a holding potential of –60 mV. Lamotrigine caused a negative shift in the slow, steady-state inactivation curve and delayed considerably the recovery from inactivation. Lamotrigine had no significant effects on the voltage dependence of activation or fast inactivation. The authors suggested that lamotrigine thus acts mainly on the slow inactivated state of the Na^+ channels. An alternative interpretation is that lamotrigine binds only slowly to the fast inactivated state of the Na^+ channel. In the study discussed immediately above, the affinity for the inactivated channels was estimated at 12 μM. The tonic inhibition was augmented by a use-dependent action in which further inhibition by the drug could be induced by rapid repetitive stimulation. The differentiation between slow binding of lamotrigine to the fast inactivated state and selective binding of the drug to the slow inactivated state of Na^+ channels was investigated by determining the affinity and kinetics of lamotrigine binding to the Na^+ channels in acutely dissociated hippocampal neurons of the rat (KUO and LU 1997). The apparent dissociation constant for lamotrigine was approximately 7 μM for binding to the inactivated channels, and was more than 200 times larger for binding to the resting channels, thus confirming previous studies. The recovery of lamotrigine-bound inactivated Na^+ channels was faster than the recovery of slow inactivated channels, and the binding kinetics of lamotrigine onto the inactivated channels were faster than the development of the slow inactivated state (KUO and LU 1997). These data suggest that lamotrigine in therapeutic concentrations binds slowly to the fast inactivated state, rather than to the slow inactivated state (KUO and LU 1997). Thus the inactivated Na^+

channel is one of the primary targets for the action of lamotrigine at therapeutic concentrations and the slow binding rates explain why lamotrigine inhibits seizure discharges, yet spares most normal neuronal activities.

β) Ca^{2+} Channels

Calcium channels provide a second potential target for the action of lamotrigine. LEES and LEACH (1993), using nystatin-perforated patches in the presence of Na^+ and K^+ channel blockers, were able to demonstrate an inhibitory effect of lamotrigine (100 μM) on presumptive inward Ca^{2+} currents. In these experiments, the holding potential was cycled between –80 and –40 mV, as the Ca^{2+} currents showed a progressive tendency to fade with repeated pulsing which could be reversed by a brief period of hyperpolarization. From these experiments, it was difficult to determine whether the effect of lamotrigine as a Ca^{2+} channel blocker was a genuine phenomenon or promoted the physiological fade through interference with Ca^{2+} sequestration or binding (LEES and LEACH 1993). Lamotrigine had no effect on the nystatin-induced cation channels. There has been further characterization of the effect of lamotrigine on Ca^{2+} channels (STEFANI et al. 1996; WANG et al. 1996). The effects of lamotrigine on Ca^{2+} channels were studied in rat amygdaloid slices using intracellular recording and whole-cell patch clamp techniques (WANG et al. 1996). Lamotrigine (50 μM) reversibly suppressed stimulation-evoked excitatory postsynaptic potentials and currents, and this inhibition was characteristic of a presynaptic effect of the drug (WANG et al. 1996). The L-type Ca^{2+} channel blocker nifedipine had no effect on lamotrigine-induced presynaptic inhibition. The inhibitory effect of lamotrigine was, however, markedly reduced by the N-type Ca^{2+} channel blocker, omega-conotoxin-GVIA, and the broad spectrum Ca^{2+} channel blocker, omega-conotoxin-MVIIC (WANG et al. 1996). Furthermore, in rat cortical neurons, lamotrigine inhibited high-voltage activated Ca^{2+} channels with an IC_{50} of 12.3 μM (STEFANI et al. 1996). Using specific Ca^{2+} channel blockers, it was determined that this effect occurred at N- and P-type Ca^{2+} channels (STEFANI et al. 1996). Thus lamotrigine at therapeutic concentrations significantly inhibits presynaptic N-type and P-type Ca^{2+} channels, resulting in decreased glutamate release. The potency of lamotrigine against high-voltage activated Ca^{2+} channels is in contrast to the relative ineffectiveness of phenytoin (STEFANI et al. 1997), and presents one of the major differences between the action of lamotrigine and phenytoin.

γ) K^+ Channels

Lamotrigine exhibited no effect on K^+ channels (LEES and LEACH 1993).

c) Ligand Binding to Receptors

From the above, it is apparent that lamotrigine exhibits binding to some Ca^{2+} channels, and predominantly to inactivated Na^+ channels. Using a variety of ligands, lamotrigine has been shown not to bind significantly to A_1 adenosine,

$GABA_B$ or K-opioid receptors, all of which have a role in antiepileptic activity. Furthermore, lamotrigine was found not to bind significantly to adrenergic, dopaminergic, adenosine A_2, histamine H_1, muscarinic, AMPA or NMDA receptors. Lamotrigine did, however, inhibit [^{3}H]BRL23694 binding to 5-HT3 receptors ($pK_i = 4.75$) and [^{3}H]ditoylguanidine to sigma receptors ($pK_i = 3.86$). The significance of these findings is as yet unknown.

II. Other Central Nervous System Effects

1. Effects on the EEG and Sleep

Lamotrigine's lack of effect on background EEG activity in healthy adults and in adults with epilepsy is in keeping with its effect upon sustained repetitive neuronal firing but not on physiological processes (VAN WIERINGEN et al. 1989; MARCIANI et al. 1996). Furthermore, in healthy adults, central conduction as studied in cortical (visual) and brainstem (auditory) event-related potentials was not influenced either by lamotrigine or by phenytoin; peripheral nerve conduction of the brainstem event-related potential (latency of wave I in the brainstem auditory-evoked response) was delayed by phenytoin, but not by lamotrigine (VAN WIERINGEN et al. 1989). Using EEG activity to stage sleep and wakefulness in rats for 6h after dosage, lamotrigine (3–30mg/kg) increased wakefulness in the light phase (BERTORELLI et al. 1996), and during the dark phase, at 30mg/kg, reduced REM sleep, but had no effect on the total amount of sleep. These effects were similar to those of carbamazepine, but contrasted with the effects of phenobarbitone, which increased the total amount of sleep (BERTORELLI et al. 1996).

2. Memory and Long-Term Potentiation

NMDA antagonists are known to inhibit memory (LEACH et al. 1991) and long-term potentiation (a neurophysiological correlate). Lamotrigine, despite its modulatory effect upon the glutamatergic system, in oral doses up to 160mg/kg which produced signs of ataxia and sedation, caused no impairment of memory in rats, as assessed using the T-maze test (LEACH et al. 1991). Similarly, lamotrigine at this dose had no effects on memory in rats trained to discriminate phencyclidine from saline (LEACH et al. 1991).

Long-term potentiation has been proposed as a mechanism involved in synaptic memory. Lamotrigine (15mg/kg given intraperitoneally) had no effect upon the induction of long-term potentiation induced by tetanic stimulation in the hippocampus of urethane-anaesthetized rats (XIONG and STRINGER 1997). Long-term potentiation in rat amygdala brain slices resulting from the application of tetraethylammonium, a K^+ antagonist, was, however, inhibited by perfusion with 50μM lamotrigine (WANG et al. 1997). This potentiation is dissimilar to tetanic potentiation, in that it is not NMDA receptor mediated, and its applicability to physiological processes is unknown (WANG et al. 1997). It is dependent upon postsynaptic voltage-dependent Ca^{2+} channel activation; lamotrigine's effect upon this process thus provides further evidence for the action of the drug on these channels.

3. Excitotoxic and Ischaemic Neuronal Injury

Lamotrigine has been shown to be neuroprotective in a variety of models of excitotoxicity and ischaemia. Pretreatment of rats with lamotrigine (8–16 mg/kg) protected against lesions produced by microinjections of kainate into the rat striatum (McGeer and Zhu 1990). Lamotrigine, however, did not protect against the toxicity of intrastriatal injections of quinolinic acid, an NMDA agonist (McGeer and Zhu 1990), even at doses as high as 50 mg/kg (Mary et al. 1995). Similar results have been obtained in hippocampal slices in which lamotrigine (100 μM) protected against amplitude reduction of CA_1 synaptic responses caused by kainic acid, but did not protect against amplitude reduction of CA_1 synaptic responses caused by NMDA or AMPA (Longo et al. 1995). These results suggest that lamotrigine specifically inhibits neurotoxicity induced by kainic acid, perhaps by an effect on glutamate release, but has no direct effect on inhibiting neurotoxicity resulting from direct stimulation of glutamate receptors.

Excessive glutamate release has been proposed as one of the mechanisms of neurotoxicity resulting from ischaemia, and thus lamotrigine has been suggested as a potential neuroprotectant in this condition. Lamotrigine at 20 mg/kg given intravenously before, and 1 h after, or lamotrigine at 50 mg/kg given intraperitoneally 0.5 and 24.5 h after middle cerebral artery occlusion, reduced the volume of cortical infarcts (Rataud et al. 1994; Smith and Meldrum 1995). Similarly, lamotrigine had neuroprotective effects in a gerbil model of global cerebral ischaemia involving bilateral occlusion of the common carotid arteries when given orally 2 h before and again immediately after reperfusion (2◊30 mg/kg or 2◊50 mg/kg doses) or as a single oral dose (100 mg/kg) given immediately after reperfusion (Wiard et al. 1995). Lamotrigine protected gerbils against behavioural deficits resulting from 15 min of carotid occlusion and also prevented histological damage resulting from 5 and 15 min of global cerebral ischaemia (Wiard et al. 1995). Lamotrigine has also been tested in cardiac arrest-induced global cerebral ischaemia with reperfusion in rats (Crumrine et al. 1997). Lamotrigine (100 mg/kg) was administered orally before the induction of ischaemia, or 10 mg/kg was given intravenously 15 min after ischaemia and a second intravenous dose (also 10 mg/kg) was given 5 h later. Both these treatment protocols were significantly neuroprotective (Crumrine et al. 1997). Thus lamotrigine may be effective in preventing brain damage after recovery from cardiac arrest.

The mechanism underlying the neuroprotective properties of lamotrigine in ischaemia is unknown, but may involve (1) maintenance of cellular ATP levels, (2) effects on calcium homeostasis, (3) effects on hypoxic depolarization, and (4) reduced ischaemic glutamate release (Taylor and Meldrum 1995). The effects of lamotrigine on extracellular glutamate were studied by

Bacher and Zornow (1997). These workers used microdialysis techniques in rabbits with cerebral ischaemia induced by two inflations of a neck tourniquet (each of 10 min duration with 90 min between the inflations) and gave 20 or 50 mg/kg lamotrigine intravenously 90 min prior to the insult. During the first ischaemic period, the glutamate concentration increased only slightly from its baseline value. A significant increase was observed during the second ischaemic period, sixfold for the control and threefold for the intravenous lamotrigine (20 mg/kg) groups. Glutamate concentrations in the lamotrigine (50 mg/kg) group were significantly lower than in the other two groups and remained at the baseline level during the entire experiment. How these findings related to neuronal damage was not studied (Bacher and Zornow 1997). In a further microdialysis study of glutamate release during ischaemia, lamotrigine (50 mg/kg) was administered to gerbils 30 min before the ischaemic insult (Shuaib et al. 1995). Histology and behavioural testing demonstrated the neuroprotective effect of the drug. Lamotrigine significantly attenuated the ischaemia-induced glutamate surge when compared with saline-treated animals. In the same experiments, lamotrigine given 30 min after the insult still resulted in significant neuroprotection, even though it would not have prevented the glutamate surge (Shuaib et al. 1995). Mechanisms other than inhibition of glutamate release thus have to be invoked to explain neuroprotection produced by postischaemic lamotrigine administration.

In addition to the mechanisms mentioned above, in rat forebrain slices lamotrigine also attenuates rises in nitric oxide and cGMP concentrations without inhibiting nitric oxide synthase activity in veratrine-induced neurotransmitter release (Lizasoain et al. 1995), and similarly inhibits rises in nitric oxide and cGMP concentrations in focal cerebral ischaemia in rats (Balkan et al. 1997).

Lamotrigine has been shown to be neuroprotective in a number of other circumstances. The drug rescued motoneurons from cell death induced by axotomy of the neonatal rat facial nerve (Casanovas et al. 1996). Local infusions of malonate, an inhibitor of mitochondrial function, into the nucleus basalis magnocellularis result in a dose-related depletion in ipsilateral cortical and amygdaloid choline acetyltransferase activity (Connop et al. 1997). This depletion was attenuated by pretreatment with lamotrigine (Connop et al. 1997). Other studies have confirmed the existence of a neuroprotective role for lamotrigine pretreatment in lesions created by mitochondrial toxins (Schulz et al. 1996). Lamotrigine (25 mg/kg) given 20 min after brain irradiation (2.5 Gy) has been shown to be neuroprotective in rats (Alaoui et al. 1995).

4. Effects on Involuntary Movement Disorders

Glutamatergic pathways are integral to the physiology of the basal ganglia, and indeed, both NMDA and non-NMDA antagonists have had anti-Parkinsonian effects in a variety of animal models. Excitotoxicity has been proposed as a mechanism by which depletion of dopaminergic neurons occurs within the basal ganglia in Parkinson's disease; excitotoxicity has also been proposed as the mechanism underlying Huntington's disease. Thus there has been interest in drugs that affect glutamatergic transmission, not only from the point of view of the symptomatic treatment of such disorders, but also in terms of neuroprotection and the possible prevention of these disease processes.

Lamotrigine failed to exert anti-Parkinsonian activity in reserpinized rats when administered alone or in combination with the dopamine receptor agonist apomorphine (LOSCHMANN et al. 1995). In rats with 6-hydroxydopamine lesions of the substantia nigra, lamotrigine did not induce rotations when given alone, and did not modify rotations induced by apomorphine or the preferential dopamine D_2 receptor agonist lisuride (LOSCHMANN et al. 1995). Lamotrigine, however, did appear to potentiate the prokinetic effects of a D_2 receptor agonist and L-dopa in reserpinized mice, but was ineffective alone and did not potentiate the effects of a D_1 receptor agonist (KAUR and STARR 1996). Furthermore, lamotrigine appears to decrease striatal dopamine synthesis by decreasing the activity of tyrosine hydroxylase (VRIEND and ALEXIUK 1997).

From the neuroprotective viewpoint, lamotrigine prevented MPTP-induced dopamine depletion in mice (JONES-HUMBLE et al. 1994), but was ineffective (albeit at much smaller doses) in methamphetamine-induced dopamine depletion in mice.

Certain conclusions can be drawn from these studies; lamotrigine appears likely to be ineffective as a lone agent in the symptomatic treatment of Parkinson's disease; it does have an effect upon potentiating D_2 agonists in some models of the disease, but has no activity in potentiating D_1 agonists, so that its overall effects in potentiating other agents are difficult to predict. In addition, its neuroprotective effect in preventing dopamine depletion is possibly model-related, and requires high doses of the drug.

In a further study, the effects of lamotrigine on generalized dystonia were examined in a genetic hamster model (RICHTER et al. 1994). Despite the effectiveness of glutamate antagonists in inhibiting dystonia in this model, lamotrigine (5–30 mg/kg) had a prodystonic effect at all doses tested (RICHTER et al. 1994).

5. Morphine Withdrawal

The effects of lamotrigine on naloxone-precipitated morphine withdrawal were studied in mice (LIZASOAIN et al. 1996). This withdrawal is manifested by micturition, diarrhoea, stereotypical movements, tremor, jumping off and shaking. Pretreatment with subcutaneous lamotrigine (5–100 mg/kg) reduced the number of escape jumps and at the higher doses also reduced the diarrhoea, stereotypical movements and tremor (LIZASOAIN et al. 1996). The drug reversed the increase in cerebellar calcium-dependent nitric oxide synthase activity during morphine withdrawal, which is proposed to be one of the mechanisms underlying the withdrawal syndrome (LIZASOAIN et al. 1996). The actions of lamotrigine on the effects of morphine withdrawal were dose dependent; this contrasted with the lack of dose dependence of the effects of MK 801, an NMDA antagonist, the use of which was also associated with greater side effects.

6. Increased Atmospheric Pressure

Exposure to increased atmospheric pressure results in a syndrome characterized by tremor, myoclonus and seizures in rats, primates and humans (PEARCE et al. 1994). This syndrome responds poorly to antiepileptic drugs, but does respond to glutamate receptor antagonists. In a study in baboons and rats, lamotrigine had minimal effects upon the high pressure neurological syndrome resulting from the effects of increasing the atmospheric pressure achieved by the addition of helium (PEARCE et al. 1994).

7. Anxiolytic Effects

In the Vogel conflict model of anxiety in rats, oral lamotrigine (20–40 mg/kg) produced a dose-dependent increase in punished drinking responses (CRITCHLEY 1994). This effect of lamotrigine was not prevented by the benzodiazepine antagonist flumazenil, suggesting that this effect is not due to an action of the drug on benzodiazepine receptors (CRITCHLEY 1994).

III. Effects Outside the Central Nervous System

1. Effects on Peripheral Nerves and Analgesic Effects

Glutamate is a potent hyperalgesic, and drugs that affect the glutamatergic system have been proposed as analgesics. Similar to its effects in the central nervous system, lamotrigine has been shown to decrease electrically evoked glutamate release from isolated rat spine dorsal horn slices twice as potently as it inhibits GABA release (TEOH et al. 1995). Indeed lamotrigine, given intravenously or applied iontophoretically to dorsal horn neurons, selectively decreases the activation of these neurons by noxious as compared with innocuous stimuli (BLACKBURN-MUNRO and FLEETWOOD-WALKER 1997). Lamotrigine had analgesic effects in a rat acute model of prostaglandin E_2 (PGE_2)-induced hyperalgesia when given before or after the subplantar injection of PGE_2 in the rat (NAKAMURA-CRAIG and FOLLENFANT 1995). The drug also inhibited the development of sustained hyperalgesia induced by multiple subplantar injections of PGE_2 (NAKAMURA-CRAIG and FOLLENFANT 1995). Furthermore, lamotrigine had an analgesic effect in a rat model of diabetic neuropathic pain (NAKAMURA-CRAIG and FOLLENFANT 1995). HUNTER et al. (1997) showed that lamotrigine also reversed cold allodynia in a rat experimental model (with an ED_{50} of 28 mg/kg when given subcutaneously), but had no effect on tactile allodynia (modelled by spinal nerve ligation) at subcutaneous doses of up to

100 mg/kg. Phenytoin and carbamazepine had no effect in either of these models (Hunter et al. 1997). Lamotrigine's analgesic effect was studied in a separate model using stimulation of C-fibres (pain carrying fibres) to assess acute effects of the drug, and also its effects upon "wind up", the phenomenon of repeat stimulations leading to enhanced C-fibre evoked responses in dorsal horn neurones (Chapman et al. 1997). Lamotrigine given spinally (50–1000 μg/μl) was ineffective on both the acute C-fibre evoked responses and on "wind up"; this contrasted with the effectiveness of spinal bupivicaine (Chapman et al. 1997). Such a result may be due to the mode of administration of lamotrigine. Additionally, the authors hypothesized that lamotrigine may have specific effectiveness in different pain states, depending upon the role of GABA in their pathogenesis. Thus pain states with high levels of GABA release, such as chronic inflammatory conditions, may be exacerbated by lamotrigine (which inhibits GABA release), whilst pain states in which GABA release is reduced, such as neuropathic pain, may be relieved by the drug (Chapman et al. 1997).

2. Other Effects

Lamotrigine is a weak inhibitor of dihydrofolate reductase. No haematological consequences of this inhibition have been observed in humans, and serum and red blood cell folate concentrations were unaffected by lamotrigine both in the short-term and in patients observed for up to 5 years (Sander and Patsalos 1992).

Lamotrigine has been found to have no effects on cardiovascular parameters in anaesthetized dogs in doses up to 10 mg/kg (Miller et al. 1986a). At higher doses (30–100 mg/kg), however, there was a dose-dependent depression of cardiac function. Lamotrigine at high concentrations (greater than 100 μM) reduced intestinal smooth muscle tone and peristaltic reflexes in in vivo and in vitro guinea-pig ileum studies (Miller et al. 1986a).

D. Pharmacokinetics

I. Absorption

In all animals tested, lamotrigine has been well absorbed (Parsons et al. 1995). However, in rats at high doses, there is a suggestion that there is a rodent-specific delay in absorption, with the gastric emptying half-life increasing up to 22.6 h after oral administration of 50 mg/kg lamotrigine (Parsons et al. 1995). This effect is also seen in mice, but not in other species or with lower doses (less than 25 mg/kg). Following oral, single dose administration to patients and healthy volunteers, maximum plasma concentrations of lamotrigine were achieved after 1–3 h (Cohen et al. 1987; Ramsay et al. 1991). A second peak, however, was evident 4–6 h after an oral dose in patients (Mikati et al. 1989). Similarly, after intravenous administration, multiple peaks were apparent (YUEN and PECK 1988). This phenomenon may be due to salivary excretion of the drug, and subsequent reabsorption of the drug from the stomach.

Both the maximum plasma concentration and the plasma AUC increase linearly with dose over the dosage range of 30–240 mg in healthy volunteers (COHEN et al. 1987), and over the range of 100–300 mg in patients (RAMSAY et al. 1991). This linearity has been reported with doses up to 450 mg in healthy volunteers, and up to 700 mg in patients (PECK 1991).

In eight healthy volunteers the oral bioavailability of 75 mg lamotrigine was approximately 98% (YUEN and PECK 1988). The absorption of lamotrigine is unaffected by food (RICHENS 1992).

II. Distribution

As expected, because of its high lipophilicity, lamotrigine is well distributed throughout all tissues in all test animals (PARSONS et al. 1995). It has a particular affinity for melanin in both the retina and, to a lesser extent, in the skin (PARSONS et al. 1995). In addition, in male rats, there is considerable binding of the drug to the kidneys (kidney to plasma ratios of over 300 are seen); this may be due to the unique handling of α_2-microglobulin by the kidneys of male rats (PARSONS et al. 1995).

The volume of distribution of the drug varies from species to species. Mice have the highest volume of distribution, at 6.69 l/kg (PARSONS et al. 1995). In adult humans the volume of distribution is approximately 1.0–1.3 l/kg (COHEN et al. 1987; RAMSAY et al. 1991). Approximately 56% of the drug in human plasma is bound to plasma proteins, as calculated from in vitro equilibrium dialysis, and the protein-bound fraction is unaffected by the drug's concentration or the concomitant presence of other antiepileptic drugs (MILLER et al. 1986a). In laboratory animals, values for the proportion protein bound in plasma were similar, varying from 40 to 62%. Salivary lamotrigine concentrations are approximately 46% of the total plasma concentration of the drug, and are directly correlated with its total plasma concentration in patients (COHEN et al. 1987; TRNAVSKA et al. 1991).

Following intravenous or intraperitoneal administration of 50 mg/kg to rats, the brain to serum concentration ratio rose over a period of approximately 30 min to a value of approximately 2 (WALTON et al. 1996). Similar ratios have been found in a variety of laboratory animals at a variety of lamotrigine doses. In one human postsurgical specimen, the total brain concentration of lamotrigine (4.2 μg/g) was higher than the unbound plasma concentration of 2.64 μg/ml (REMMEL et al. 1992). A comparison of the CSF and blood kinetics of the drug has been performed in the rat. Lamotrigine entered the CSF rapidly, with a time course similar to that seen for its entry into brain (WALKER et al. 1996a; WALTON et al. 1996). At steady state, the ratio of the CSF concentration to the serum concentration was consistent with the free lamotrigine concentration in serum (WALKER et al. 1996a). Interestingly, there was a rise in the CSF to serum concentration ratio for the drug during the period of the initial fall in serum concentration, which may be due to delay in the passage of lamotrigine from the CSF compartment to the vascular compartment (WALKER et al. 1996a). Another explanation may be that during the acute phase the hypothesis is incorrect that the free serum drug concentration reflects the tissue exchangeable drug concentration.

In studies in rats, lamotrigine was found to cross the placenta and its concentrations in the foetus and placenta were comparable to those in maternal plasma (PARSONS et al. 1995). There is a low level of transfer of the drug to maternal milk in rats. In humans, RAMBECK et al. (1997) have studied the transfer of lamotrigine from a mother to her child in pregnancy and during lactation. Lamotrigine concentrations were measured in umbilical cord serum, and maternal serum and milk. There was significant transfer of the drug from the mother to the child, not only after birth, but also during lactation. In the child, lamotrigine serum concentrations of up to 2.8 μg/ml occurred, but no adverse effects were seen.

III. Elimination

Lamotrigine is eliminated mainly by being metabolized.

1. Elimination Parameters

Because of variability in the metabolism of lamotrigine, there is a wide interspecies range of plasma elimination half-lives, ranging from 3 h in the beagle dog to over 20 h in certain monkeys. In healthy human volunteers, the half-life lay between 23 and 36 h after a single dose (COHEN et al. 1987; POSNER et al. 1989, 1991; DEPOT et al. 1990). The pharmacokinetics for multiple dose regimens in humans are consistent with those predicted from the single dose data (COHEN et al. 1987). The kinetics of lamotrigine are linear, with doses up to 450 mg in volunteers (PECK 1991). Autoinduction has been reported during the early stages of treatment (RICHENS 1992). In patients the kinetics are dependent on the intake of any co-medication (see below), but are linear and adequately described by a one compartment pharmacokinetic model (RAMSAY et al. 1991). The population pharmacokinetics of lamotrigine monotherapy have been determined in 163 patients with newly diagnosed epilepsy (HUSSEIN and POSNER 1997); this study confirmed the phase I results. There was no significant effect of body weight, age (>14 years), gender or dose on the oral clearance of lamotrigine (HUSSEIN and POSNER 1997). There was some auto-induction over the first 2 weeks of therapy that increased the clearance of the drug by 17%, which is not clinically significant in view of the wide therapeutic margin of lamotrigine and the large interindividual variability of 32% (HUSSEIN and POSNER 1997). Autoinduction reduced the mean half-life of lamotrigine amongst Caucasians from 27.6 h to 23.5 h (HUSSEIN and POSNER 1997). There was also a small effect of race, Asians having a lower clearance, which again probably would not be clinically significant (HUSSEIN and POSNER 1997).

2. Metabolism

The metabolism of lamotrigine occurs primarily by an attack at the *N*-2 nitrogen atom of the molecule either by glucuronidation (in most species), oxidation (predominant in the hamster and some rats) or methylation (predominant in beagle dogs). In humans, lamotrigine is eliminated in the urine mainly as the 2-*N*-glucuronide metabolite (SINZ and REMMEL 1991), with the 5-*N*-glucuronide accounting for about 10% of the urinary recovery, and the parent drug for about 7%–30% (DOIG and CLARE 1991a). The 2-*N*-glucuronide metabolite also predominates in the guinea pig (REMMEL and SINZ 1991). This provides a rare example of the efficient formation of a quaternary ammonium glucuronide in a lower animal species (this route of metabolism is usually confined to humans and some monkeys). In healthy volunteers, the total urinary recovery of the drug over 144 h was 70% of the dose, approximately 90% of the material recovered being in the form of the glucuronide conjugate (COHEN et al. 1987). In patients, 43%–87% of the dose was recovered in the urine mainly as the glucuronide metabolite (MIKATI et al. 1989).

The metabolism of the antiepileptic drug lamotrigine was further characterized in human liver microsomes (MAGDALOU et al. 1992). The reaction had an apparent V_{max} of 0.65 nmol/min/mg protein and a K_m of 2.56 mM (MAGDALOU et al. 1992). The average value of lamotrigine glucuronidation in four human samples of transplantable liver demonstrated a large interindividual variation (MAGDALOU et al. 1992). An interspecies comparison of hepatic lamotrigine glucuronidation in liver microsomes (human, rabbit, rat, monkey) confirmed the in vivo work (MAGDALOU et al. 1992). Humans glucuronidated the drug to the greatest extent, at a rate that was approximately twice that observed in rabbit liver microsomes (MAGDALOU et al. 1992). The rate was very slow in rhesus monkey liver microsomes (20-fold lower than humans), and the process was barely detectable in rat liver microsomes (MAGDALOU et al. 1992). Guinea pig liver microsomes metabolized lamotrigine at a rate similar to human liver microsomes with similar K_m and V_{max} values (REMMEL and SINZ 1991).

IV. Clinical Pharmacokinetics

Although the study of HUSSEIN and POSNER (1997) found no effect of increasing age on the pharmacokinetics of lamotrigine, this was not the case in a comparative formal phase I study of the drug's pharmacokinetics in elderly and young healthy volunteers. In the elderly healthy volunteers, the clearance was lower and the C_{max}, AUC and half-life were increased by approximately 27%, 55% and 26% respectively (POSNER et al. 1991). This reduction in clearance is perhaps due to decreased glucuronidation in the elderly, secondary to changes in liver blood flow. The differences, however, are probably not clinically relevant.

In children (aged 0.5–4.5 years) with epilepsy either receiving no comedication or taking comedication that does not affect the pharmacokinetics of lamotrigine, the mean half-life was 21.9 ± 6.8h and thus was comparable to that in adults (VAUZELLE-KERVROEDAN et al. 1996). In children taking comedication which does affect the pharmacokinetics of lamotrigine the quantitative effects of the comedication were different from those in adults (VAUZELLE-KERVROEDAN et al. 1996; BARTOLI et al. 1997a; BATTINO et al. 1997).

Diseases that affect liver glucuronidation will affect lamotrigine metabolism. Patients with Gilbert's syndrome (unconjugated hyperbilirubinaemia) have lamotrigine clearances more than 30% lower and half-lives longer than those of healthy volunteers (POSNER et al. 1989). The differences, however, are probably of little clinical consequence.

In chronic renal failure, there is a large interpatient variability in the pharmacokinetics of lamotrigine (FILLASTRE et al. 1993; WOOTTON et al. 1997). The half-life of lamotrigine tends to be increased by 50%–100% in patients with chronic renal failure (FILLASTRE et al. 1993; WOOTTON et al. 1997). The pharmacokinetics of the 2-*N*-glucuronide metabolite seem to be more significantly affected, as the clearance of this substance was reduced by a factor of 9 (WOOTTON et al. 1997). In those patients undergoing dialysis, however, the half-life appeared to be reduced to about 12h (FILLASTRE et al. 1993).

E. Interactions

I. Pharmacodynamic Interactions

Adding lamotrigine to the therapy of patients who are already receiving other drugs with sedative properties, or adding such drugs to the treatment of patients taking lamotrigine, may sometimes increase the patient's overall level of sedation, without evidence that a pharmacokinetic interaction is involved.

II. Pharmacokinetic Interactions

The effects of drugs that undergo quaternary ammonium glucuronidation on the metabolism of lamotrigine were studied in vitro, in human liver microsomes (MAGDALOU et al. 1992). Chlorpromazine, but not to any extent imipramine, amitriptyline and cyproheptadine, inhibited the glucuronidation of lamotrigine (IC_{50} of 5.0×10^{-4} M – MAGDALOU et al. 1992). Testosterone, ethynyl oestradiol and norethindrone were even more potent inhibitors (IC_{50} values of 6.3×10^{-5} M to 3.1×10^{-4} M – MAGDALOU et al. 1992).

In humans, co-medication with antiepileptic drugs has a profound effect on the metabolism of lamotrigine. Enzyme-inducing antiepileptic drugs (phenytoin, phenobarbitone and carbamazepine) reduce the half-life of lamotrigine to 13–15h (BINNIE et al. 1986; JAWAD et al. 1987; RAMSAY et al. 1991).

Co-medication with valproate prolonged the half-life of lamotrigine to 59h (BINNIE et al. 1986). The mechanism of the interaction with valproate is thought to be that valproate competes with lamotrigine for glucuronidation, rather than that there is an effect on renal clearance or on absorption (YUEN et al. 1992; ANDERSON et al. 1996). These interactions are quantitatively different in children (BATTINO et al. 1997). In children, enzyme inducers reduce the half-life by a greater degree to 7.7 ± 1.8h (VAUZELLE-KERVROEDAN et al. 1996). Valproate increased the half-life to 44.7 ± 10.2h in children (VAUZELLE-KERVROEDAN et al. 1996). Lamotrigine concentration to dose ratios at steady state are lower in children taking enzyme inducers than in adults receiving enzyme inducers (BARTOLI et al. 1997a; BATTINO et al. 1997). The concentration to dose ratio is probably also lower for children taking valproate than for adults receiving this drug (BARTOLI et al. 1997a; BATTINO et al. 1997).

Lamotrigine itself has no clinically significant effect on the plasma concentrations of other antiepileptic drugs. The addition of lamotrigine to therapy was associated with a 25% decrease in steady-state valproate plasma concentrations with an increase in oral clearance of valproate (ANDERSON et al. 1996). However, the formation and clearance of the hepatotoxic valproate metabolites were unaffected by lamotrigine administration (ANDERSON et al. 1996).

Paracetamol (acetaminophen) would be expected to inhibit the metabolism of lamotrigine. Paradoxically it decreases the half-life and AUC by an undetermined mechanism (DEPOT et al. 1990). With intermittent use of paracetamol, this interaction is of no clinical importance.

In healthy volunteers, lamotrigine has no effect on the metabolism of the combined oral contraceptive pill (DEPOT et al. 1990).

It has been suggested that there is an interaction of lamotrigine with carbamazepine in which the incidence of carbamazepine toxicity appears to be increased. It has been proposed that this is either due to increased concentrations of carbamazepine-epoxide (WARNER et al. 1992) or to a pharmacodynamic interaction (WOLF 1992). Further studies in both adults and children have failed to find an increase in carbamazepine-epoxide concentrations or any other change in carbamazepine pharmacokinetics with the addition of lamotrigine (ERIKSSON and BOREUS 1997; GIDAL et al. 1997). Indeed, a comparison of the single dose pharmacokinetic of carbamazepine-epoxide in patients on lamotrigine, and in healthy volunteers, failed to detect an effect of lamotrigine on carbamazepine-epoxide disposition (PISANI et al. 1994). It is thus likely that lamotrigine does not have an effect upon the pharmacokinetics of carbamazepine or of carbamazepine-epoxide, and that the original anecdotal report may have misrepresented the matter (WARNER et al. 1992).

F. Adverse Effects

I. Animal Toxicity

The acute toxicity of intravenous and oral lamotrigine has been studied in rats and mice (MILLER et al. 1986a). The LD_{50} was 40–100 times the ED_{50} for maximal electroshock 2h postdosing, and was of the order of 100–300mg/kg (MILLER et al. 1986a).

The acute behavioural toxic effects of lamotrigine have also been studied in mice and in genetically epilepsy-prone rats. The mice were observed for the grip reflex, ataxia and jitteriness (MILLER et al. 1986b). No important effects were seen following the administration of 80mg/kg (28 times the ED_{50} for maximal electro-shock). Higher lamotrigine doses did result in significant behavioural toxicity. In genetically epilepsy-prone rats, locomotor performance was assessed using a rotarod (SMITH et al. 1993). The peak ED_{50} for a locomotor deficit was approximately 20 times that of the peak ED_{50} for antagonism of clonic seizures (SMITH et al. 1993). The peak motor deficit occurred 0.5h after intraperitoneal injection, at a lamotrigine concentration of 24 μg/ml.

Subacute and chronic toxicity studies on the drug have also been undertaken (MILLER et al. 1986a). In rats and primates 30 day studies with oral doses up to 50mg/kg/day, and 3-, 6- and 12-month studies in rats (oral doses up to 25mg/kg/day) and primates (doses up to 20mg/kg/day), demonstrated no significant toxic effects (MILLER et al. 1986a).

Lamotrigine was not teratogenic when given orally during the period of organogenesis to rats (doses up to 25mg/kg/day), mice (doses up to 125mg/kg/day) and rabbits (doses up to 30mg/kg/day) (MILLER et al. 1986a). The drug was non-mutagenic in both the Ames *Salmonella* test and in an in vitro study in cultured peripheral human lymphocytes (MILLER et al. 1986a).

II. Human Toxicity

The safety of lamotrigine in animal studies has been confirmed in humans. In healthy volunteers, carbamazepine (600mg) impaired adaptive tracking, body sway, smooth pursuit movements and saccadic velocity, whilst lamotrigine (150mg, 300mg) had no adverse effect at mean plasma concentrations up to 3.16 μg/ml (HAMILTON et al. 1993). In a study comparing lamotrigine (120mg, 240mg) with phenytoin (0.5g, 1g) and diazepam (10mg), diazepam impaired eye movements, adaptive tracking and body sway, phenytoin impaired adaptive tracking, increased body sway and impaired smooth pursuit eye movement, whilst lamotrigine produced only a possible increase in body sway (COHEN et al. 1985). This last effect was possibly spurious, and resulted from multiple comparisons.

In clinical practice, neurological side-effects of lamotrigine are infrequent and mild. In four randomized, double-blind, placebo-controlled crossover trials of lamotrigine (50–400mg/day) as add-on therapy in refractory epilepsy (n = 92), the incidence of adverse experiences did not differ significantly between lamotrigine and placebo (BETTS et al. 1991). In pooled data from open studies of 572 patients analysed in the same paper, the most commonly reported adverse experiences were dizziness, diplopia, somnolence, headache, ataxia, and asthenia (10%–14% incidence).

Rash is the most common of the hypersensitivity reactions to lamotrigine, and occurs in about 10% of adult patients (YUEN 1992). The rash usually is mild and rarely requires withdrawal of treatment (YUEN 1992). Stevens-Johnson syndromes and toxic epidermal necrolysis have, however, both been described in association with lamotrigine treatment (DOOLEY et al. 1996; CHAFFIN and DAVIS 1997; SACHS et al. 1997). In one patient with a Stevens-Johnson syndrome which developed 5 weeks after adding low-dose lamotrigine co-medication to sodium valproate therapy, there was a positive lymphocyte transformation test to lamotrigine which confirmed the role of this drug in the aetiology of the syndrome (SACHS et al. 1997). Other serious possible reactions to the drug have included isolated reports of leucopenia, disseminated intravascular coagulation and hepatic failure (MAKIN et al. 1995; NICHOLSON et al. 1995; CHATTERGOON et al. 1997).

References

Alaoui F, Pratt J, Trocherie S, Court L, Stutzmann JM (1995) Acute effects of irradiation on the rat brain: protection by glutamate blockade. Eur J Pharmacol 276:55–60

Anderson GD, Yau MK, Gidal BE et al. (1996) Bidirectional interaction of valproate and lamotrigine in healthy subjects. Clin Pharmacol Therap 60:145–156

Bacher A, Zornow MH (1997) Lamotrigine inhibits extracellular glutamate accumulation during transient global cerebral ischemia in rabbits. Anesthesiology 86:459–463

Balkan S, Ozben T, Balkan E, Oguz N, Serteser M, Gumuslu S (1997) Effects of Lamotrigine on brain nitrite and cGMP levels during focal cerebral ischemia in rats. Acta Neurol Scandinav 95:140–146

Bartoli A, Guerrini R, Belmonte A, Alessandri MG, Gatti G, Perucca E (1997a) The influence of dosage, age, and comedication on steady state plasma lamotrigine concentrations in epileptic children: a prospective study with preliminary assessment of correlations with clinical response. Ther Drug Monit 19:252–260

Bartoli A, Marchiselli R, Gatti G (1997b) A rapid and specific assay for the determination of lamotrigine in human plasma by normal-phase HPLC. Ther Drug Monit 19:100–107

Battino D, Croci D, Granata T, Estienne M, Pisani F, Avanzini G (1997) Lamotrigine plasma concentrations in children and adults: influence of age and associated therapy. Ther Drug Monit 19:620–627

Bertorelli R, Ferri N, Adami M, Ongini E (1996) Effects of four antiepileptic drugs on sleep and waking in the rat under both light and dark phases. Pharmacol Biochem Behavior 53:559–565

Betts T, Goodwin G, Withers RM, Yuen AW (1991) Human safety of lamotrigine. Epilepsia 32 [Suppl 2]:S17–S21

Biddlecombe RA, Dean KL, Smith CD, Jeal SC (1990) Validation of a radioimmunoassay for the determination of human plasma concentrations of lamotrigine. J Pharm Biomed Analysis 8:691–694

Binnie CD, van Emde Boas W, Kasteleijn Nolste Trenite DG et al. (1986) Acute effects of lamotrigine (BW430 C) in persons with epilepsy. Epilepsia 27:248–254

Blackburn-Munro G, Fleetwood-Walker SM (1997) The effects of Na^+ channel blockers on somatosensory processing by rat dorsal horn neurones. Neuroreport 8:1549–1554

Brodie MJ, Richens A, Yuen AWC (1995) Double-blind comparison of lamotrigine and carbamazepine in newly diagnosed epilepsy. Lancet 345:476–479

Casanovas A, Ribera J, Hukkanen M, Riveros-Moreno V, Esquerda JE (1996) Prevention by lamotrigine, MK-801 and N-omega-nitro-L-arginine methyl ester of motoneuron cell death after neonatal axotomy. Neuroscience 71:313–325

Chaffin JJ, Davis SM (1997) Suspected lamotrigine-induced toxic epidermal necrolysis. Ann Pharmacother 31:720–723
Chapman V, Wildman MA, Dickenson AH (1997) Distinct electrophysiological effects of two spinally administered membrane stabilising drugs, bupivacaine and lamotrigine. Pain 71:285–295
Chattergoon DS, McGuigan MA, Koren G, Hwang P, Ito S (1997) Multiorgan dysfunction and disseminated intravascular coagulation in children receiving lamotrigine and valproic acid. Neurology 49:1442–1444
Cheung H, Kamp D, Harris E (1992) An in vitro investigation of the action of lamotrigine on neuronal voltage-activated sodium channels. Epilepsy Res 13:107–112
Cociglio M, Alric R, Bouvier O (1991) Performance analysis of a reversed-phase liquid chromatographic assay of lamotrigine in plasma using solvent-demixing extraction. J Chromatogr 572:269–276
Cohen AF, Ashby L, Crowley D, Land G, Peck AW, Miller AA (1985) Lamotrigine (BW430 C), a potential anticonvulsant. Effects on the central nervous system in comparison with phenytoin and diazepam. Br J Clin Pharmacol 20:619–629
Cohen AF, Land GS, Breimer DD, Yuen WC, Winton C, Peck AW (1987) Lamotrigine, a new anticonvulsant: pharmacokinetics in normal humans. Clin Pharmacol Ther 42:535–541
Connop BP, Boegman RJ, Beninger RJ, Jhamandas K (1997) Malonate-induced degeneration of basal forebrain cholinergic neurons: attenuation by lamotrigine, MK-801, and 7-nitroindazole. J Neurochem 68:1191–1199
Critchley MAE (1994) Effects of lamotrigine (lamictal) in an animal model of anxiety. Br J Pharmacol 111 [Suppl]:205P
Crumrine RC, Bergstrand K, Cooper AT, Faison WL, Cooper BR (1997) Lamotrigine protects hippocampal CA1 neurons from ischemic damage after cardiac arrest. Stroke 28:2230–2236
Dalby NO, Nielsen EB (1997) Comparison of the preclinical anticonvulsant profiles of tiagabine, lamotrigine, gabapentin and vigabatrin. Epilepsy Res 28:63–72
Dasgupta A, Hart AP (1997) Lamotrigine analysis in plasma by gas chromatography-mass spectrometry after conversion to a tert-butyldimethylsilyl derivative. J Chromatogr B, Biomedical Sc:101–107
De Sarro G, Nava F, Aguglia U, De Sarro A (1996) Lamotrigine potentiates the antiseizure activity of some anticonvulsants in DBA/2 mice. Neuropharmacology 35:153–158
Depot M, Powell JR, Messenheimer Jr JA, Cloutier G, Dalton MJ (1990) Kinetic effects of multiple oral doses of acetaminophen on a single oral dose of lamotrigine. Clin Pharmacol Ther 48:346–355
Doig MV, Clare RA (1991) Use of thermospray liquid chromatography-mass spectrometry to aid in the identification of urinary metabolites of a novel antiepileptic drug, lamotrigine. J Chromatogr 554:181–189
Dooley J, Camfield P, Gordon K, Camfield C, Wirrell Z, Smith E (1996) Lamotrigine-induced rash in children. Neurology 46:240–242
Eriksson AS, Boreus LO (1997) No increase in carbamazepine-10,11-epoxide during addition of lamotrigine treatment in children. Ther Drug Monit 19:499–501
Fazio A, Artesi C, Russo M, Trio R, Oteri G, Pisani F (1992) A liquid chromatographic assay using a high-speed column for the determination of lamotrigine, a new antiepileptic drug, in human plasma. Ther Drug Monit 14:509–512
Fillastre JP, Taburet AM, Fialaire A, Etienne I, Bidault R, Singlas E (1993) Pharmacokinetics of lamotrigine in patients with renal impairment: influence of haemodialysis. Drugs Exp Clin Res 19:25–32
Fisher RS (1989) Animal models of the epilepsies. Brain Res Rev 14:245–278
Fraser AD, MacNeil W, Isner AF, Camfield PR (1995) Lamotrigine analysis in serum by high-performance liquid chromatography. Ther Drug Monit 17:174–178

George S, Wood AJ, Braithwaite RA (1995) Routine therapeutic monitoring of lamotrigine in epileptic patients using a simple and rapid high performance liquid chromatographic technique. Ann Clin Biochem 32:584–588

Gidal BE, Rutecki P, Shaw R, Maly MM, Collins DM, Pitterle ME (1997) Effect of lamotrigine on carbamazepine epoxide/carbamazepine serum concentration ratios in adult patients with epilepsy. Epilepsy Res 28:207–211

Goa KL, Ross SR, Chrisp P (1993) Lamotrigine. A review of its pharmacological properties and clinical efficacy in epilepsy. Drugs 46:152–176

Hallbach J, Vogel H, Guder WG (1997) Determination of lamotrigine, carbamazepine and carbamazepine epoxide in human serum by gas chromatography mass spectrometry. Europ J Clin Chem Clin Biochem 35:755–759

Hamilton MJ, Cohen AF, Yuen AW, Harkin N, Land G, Weatherley BC, Peck AW (1993) Carbamazepine and lamotrigine in healthy volunteers: relevance to early tolerance and clinical trial dosage. Epilepsia 34:166–173

Hart AP, Mazarr-Proo S, Blackwell W, Dasgupta A (1997) A rapid cost-effective high-performance liquid chromatographic (HPLC) assay of serum lamotrigine after liquid-liquid extraction and using HPLC conditions routinely used for analysis of barbiturates. Ther Drug Monit 19:431–435

Hosford DA, Wang Y (1997) Utility of the lethargic (lh/lh) mouse model of absence seizures in predicting the effects of lamotrigine, vigabatrin, tiagabine, gabapentin, and topiramate against human absence seizures. Epilepsia 38:408–414

Hunter JC, Gogas KR, Hedley LR, Jacobson LO, Kassotakis L, Thompson J, Fontana DJ (1997) The effect of novel anti-epileptic drugs in rat experimental models of acute and chronic pain. Eur J Pharmacol 324:153–160

Hussein Z, Posner J (1997) Population pharmacokinetics of lamotrigine monotherapy in patients with epilepsy: retrospective analysis of routine monitoring data. Br J Clin Pharmacol 43:457–465

Jawad S, Yuen WC, Peck AW, Hamilton MJ, Oxley JR, Richens A (1987) Lamotrigine: single-dose pharmacokinetics and initial 1 week experience in refractory epilepsy. Epilepsy Res 1:194–201

Jones-Humble SA, Morgan PF, Cooper BR (1994) The novel anticonvulsant lamotrigine prevents dopamine depletion in C57 black mice in the MPTP animal model of Parkinson's disease. Life Sci 54:245–252

Kaur S, Starr M (1996) Motor effects of lamotrigine in naive and dopamine-depleted mice. Eur J Pharmacol 304:1–6

Kuo CC, Lu L (1997) Characterization of lamotrigine inhibition of Na^+ channels in rat hippocampal neurones. Br J Pharmacol 121:1231–1238

Lang DG, Wang CM, Cooper BR (1993) Lamotrigine, phenytoin and carbamazepine interactions on the sodium current present in N4TG1 mouse neuroblastoma cells. J Pharmacol Exp Ther 266:829–835

Leach MJ, Marden CM, Miller AA (1986) Pharmacological studies on lamotrigine, a novel potential antiepileptic drug: II. Neurochemical studies on the mechanism of action. Epilepsia 27:490–497

Leach MJ, Baxter MG, Critchley MA (1991) Neurochemical and behavioral aspects of lamotrigine. Epilepsia 32 [Suppl 2]:S4–S8

Lees G, Leach MJ (1993) Studies on the mechanism of action of the novel anticonvulsant lamotrigine (Lamictal) using primary neurological cultures from rat cortex. Brain Res 612:190–199

Lensmeyer GL, Gidal BE, Wiebe DA (1997) Optimized high-performance liquid chromatographic method for determination of lamotrigine in serum with concomitant determination of phenytoin, carbamazepine, and carbamazepine epoxide. Ther Drug Monit 19:292–300

Lizasoain I, Knowles RG, Moncada S (1995) Inhibition by lamotrigine of the generation of nitric oxide in rat forebrain slices. J Neurochem 64:636–642

Lizasoain I, Leza JC, Cuellar B, Moro MA, Lorenzo P (1996) Inhibition of morphine withdrawal by lamotrigine: involvement of nitric oxide. Eur J Pharmacol 299:41–45

Londero D, Lo Greco P (1997) New micromethod for the determination of lamotrigine in human plasma by high-performance liquid chromatography. J Chromatogr B, Biomedical Sc:139–144

Longo R, Domenici MR, Scotti de Carolis A, Sagratella S (1995) Felbamate selectively blocks in vitro hippocampal kainate-induced irreversible electrical changes. Life Sci 56:PL409–PL414

Löscher W, Schmidt D (1993) New drugs for the treatment of epilepsy. Curr Opin Invest Drugs 2:1067–1095

Loschmann PA, Eblen F, Wullner U, Wachtel H, Kockgether T (1995) Lamotrigine has no antiparkinsonian activity in rat models of Parkinson's disease. Eur J Pharmacol 284:129–134

Magdalou J, Herber R, Bidault R, Siest G (1992) In vitro N-glucuronidation of a novel antiepileptic drug, lamotrigine, by human liver microsomes. J Pharmacol Exper Therap 260:1166–1173

Makin AJ, Fitt S, Williams R, Duncan JS (1995) Fulminant hepatic failure induced by lamotrigine. Brit Med J 311:292

Marciani MG, Spanedda F, Bassetti MA, Maschio M, Gigli GL, Mattia D, Bernardi G (1996) Effect of lamotrigine on EEG paroxysmal abnormalities and background activity: a computerized analysis. Br J Clin Pharmacol 42:621–627

Mary V, Wahl F, Stutzmann JM (1995) Effect of riluzole on quinolinate-induced neuronal damage in rats: comparison with blockers of glutamatergic neurotransmission. Neurosci Lett 201:92–96

McGeer EG, Zhu SG (1990) Lamotrigine protects against kainate but not ibotenate lesions in rat striatum. Neurosci Lett 112:348–351

McNamara JO, Bonhaus W, Shin C (1993) The kindling model of epilepsy. In: Schwartzkroin PA (ed) Epilepsy: models, mechanisms, and concepts. Cambridge University Press, Cambridge, pp 27–47

Mikati MA, Schachter SC, Schomer DL et al. (1989) Long-term tolerability, pharmacokinetic and preliminary efficacy study of lamotrigine in patients with resistant partial seizures. Clin Neuropharmacol 12:312–321

Miller AA, Sawyer DA, Roth B et al. (1986a) Lamotrigine. In: Meldrum BS, Porter RJ (eds) New anticonvulsant drugs. John Libbey, London, pp 165–177

Miller AA, Wheatley P, Sawyer DA, Baxter MG, Roth B (1986b) Pharmacological studies on lamotrigine, a novel potential antiepileptic drug: I. Anticonvulsant profile in mice and rats. Epilepsia 27:483–489

Nakamura-Craig M, Follenfant RL (1995) Effect of lamotrigine in the acute and chronic hyperalgesia induced by PGE_2 and in the chronic hyperalgesia in rats with streptozotocin-induced diabetes. Pain 63:33–37

Nicholson RJ, Kelly KP, Grant IS (1995) Leucopenia associated with lamotrigine. Brit Med J 310:504

O'Donnell RA, Miller AA (1991) The effect of lamotrigine upon development of cortical kindled seizures in the rat. Neuropharmacol 30:253–258

Parsons DN, Dickens M, Morley TJ (1995) Lamotrigine: absorption, distribution and excretion. In: Levy RH, Mattson RH, Meldrum BS (eds) Antiepileptic drugs. Raven Press, New York, pp 877–881

Pearce PC, Halsey MJ, Maclean CJ, Ward EM, Shergill HK, Tindley G, Meldrum BS (1994) Lack of effect of lamotrigine against HPNS in rodent and primate models. Pharmacol Biochem Behavior 48:259–263

Peck AW (1991) Clinical pharmacology of lamotrigine. Epilepsia 32 [Suppl 2]: S9–S12

Pisani F, Xiao B, Fazio A, Spina E, Perucca E, Tomson T (1994) Single dose pharmacokinetics of carbamazepine-10,11-epoxide in patients on lamotrigine monotherapy. Epilepsy Res 19:245–248

Posner J, Cohen AF, Land G, Winton C, Peck AW (1989) The pharmacokinetics of lamotrigine (BW430 C) in healthy subjects with unconjugated hyperbilirubinaemia (Gilbert's syndrome). Br J Clin Pharmacol 28:117–120

Posner J, Holdrich T, Crome P (1991) Comparison of lamotrigine pharmacokinetics in young and elderly healthy volunteers. J Pharmaceut Med 1:121–128

Ramachandran S, Underhill S, Jones SR (1994) Measurement of lamotrigine under conditions measuring phenobarbitone, phenytoin, and carbamazepine using reversed-phase high-performance liquid chromatography at dual wavelengths. Ther Drug Monit 16:75–82

Rambeck B, Kurlemann G, Stodieck SR, May TW, Jurgens U (1997) Concentrations of lamotrigine in a mother on lamotrigine treatment and her newborn child. Eur J Clin Pharmacol 51:481–484

Ramsay RE, Pellock JM, Garnett WR et al. (1991) Pharmacokinetics and safety of lamotrigine (Lamictal) in patients with epilepsy. Epilepsy Res 10:191–200

Rataud J, Debarnot F, Mary V, Pratt J, Stutzmann JM (1994) Comparative study of voltage-sensitive sodium channel blockers in focal ischaemia and electric convulsions in rodents. Neurosci Lett 172:19–23

Remmel RP, Sinz MW (1991) A quaternary ammonium glucuronide is the major metabolite of lamotrigine in guinea pigs. In vitro and in vivo studies. Drug Metab Disposit 19:630–636

Remmel RP, Sinz MW, Graves NM, Ritter RJ (1992) Lamotrigine and lamotrigine-N-glucuronide concentrations in human blood and brain tissue. Seizure 1 [Suppl A]:P7/34

Reynolds EH, Milner G, Matthews PM, Chanarin I (1966) Anticonvulsant therapy, megaloblastic hematopoiesis and folic acid metabolism. Quart J Med 35:521–537

Richens A (1992) Pharmacokinetics of lamotrigine. In: Richens A (ed) Clinical update on lamotrigine: a novel antiepileptic agent. Wells Medical Limited, Royal Tunbridge Wells, pp 21–27

Richter A, Loschmann PA, Löscher W (1994) The novel antiepileptic drug, lamotrigine, exerts prodystonic effects in a mutant hamster model of generalized dystonia. Eur J Pharmacol 264:345–351

Sachs B, Ronnau AC, von Schmiedeberg S, Ruzicka T, Gleichmann E, Schuppe HC (1997) Lamotrigine-induced Stevens-Johnson syndrome: demonstration of specific lymphocyte reactivity in vitro. Dermatology 195:60–64

Sailstad JM, Findlay JW (1991) Immunofluorometric assay for lamotrigine (Lamictal) in human plasma. Ther Drug Monit 13:433–442

Sallustio BC, Morris RG (1997) High-performance liquid chromatography quantitation of plasma lamotrigine concentrations: application measuring trough concentrations in patients with epilepsy. Ther Drug Monit 19:688–693

Sander JW, Patsalos PN (1992) An assessment of serum and red blood cell folate concentrations in patients with epilepsy on lamotrigine therapy. Epilepsy Res 13:89–92

Schulz JB, Matthews RT, Henshaw DR, Beal MF (1996) Neuroprotective strategies for treatment of lesions produced by mitochondrial toxins: implications for neurodegenerative diseases. Neuroscience 71:1043–1048

Shuaib A, Mahmood RH, Wishart T et al. (1995) Neuroprotective effects of lamotrigine in global ischemia in gerbils. A histological, in vivo microdialysis and behavioral study. Brain Res 702:199–206

Sinz MW, Remmel RP (1991) Isolation and characterization of a novel quaternary ammonium-linked glucuronide of lamotrigine. Drug Metab Dispos 19:149–153

Smith SE, Meldrum BS (1995) Cerebroprotective effect of lamotrigine after focal ischemia in rats. Stroke 26:117–121

Smith SE, al-Zubaidy ZA, Chapman AG, Meldrum BS (1993) Excitatory amino acid antagonists, lamotrigine and BW 1003C87 as anticonvulsants in the genetically epilepsy-prone rat. Epilepsy Res 15:101–111

Smolders I, Khan GM, Manil J, Ebinger G, Michotte Y (1997) NMDA receptor-mediated pilocarpine-induced seizures: characterization in freely moving rats by microdialysis. Br J Pharmacol 121:1171–1179

Stankova L, Kubova H, Mares P (1992) Anticonvulsant action of lamotrigine during ontogenesis in rats. Epilepsy Res 13:17–22

Stefani A, Spadoni F, Bernardi G (1997) Differential inhibition by riluzole, lamotrigine, and phenytoin of sodium and calcium currents in cortical neurons: implications for neuroprotective strategies. Exp Neurol 147:115–122

Stefani A, Spadoni F, Siniscalchi A, Bernardi G (1996) Lamotrigine inhibits Ca^{2+} currents in cortical neurons: functional implications. Eur J Pharmacol 307:113–116

Taylor CP, Meldrum BS (1995) Sodium channels as targets for neuroprotective drugs. Trends Pharmacol Sci 16:309–316

Teoh H, Fowler LJ, Bowery NG (1995) Effect of lamotrigine on the electrically-evoked release of endogenous amino acids from slices of dorsal horn of the rat spinal cord. Neuropharmacology 34:1273–1278

Trnavska Z, Krejcova H, Tkaczykovam , Salcmanova Z, Elis J (1991) Pharmacokinetics of lamotrigine (Lamictal) in plasma and saliva. Eur J Drug Metab Pharmacokinet S:211–215

van Wieringen A, Binnie CD, Meijer JW, Peck AW, de Vries J (1989) Comparison of the effects of lamotrigine and phenytoin on the EEG power spectrum and cortical and brainstem-evoked responses of normal human volunteers. Neuropsychobiol 21:157–169

Vauzelle-Kervroedan F, Rey E, Cieuta C et al. (1996) Influence of concurrent antiepileptic medication on the pharmacokinetics of lamotrigine as add-on therapy in epileptic children. Br J Clin Pharmacol 41:325–330

Vriend J, Alexiuk NA (1997) Lamotrigine inhibits the in situ activity of tyrosine hydroxylase in striatum of audiogenic seizure-prone and audiogenic seizure-resistant Balb/c mice. Life Sci 61:2467–2474

Waldmeier PC, Baumann PA, Wicki P, Feldtrauer JJ, Stierlin C, Schmutz M (1995) Similar potency of carbamazepine, oxcarbazepine, and lamotrigine in inhibiting the release of glutamate and other neurotransmitters. Neurology 45:1907–1913

Waldmeier PC, Martin P, Stocklin K, Portet C, Schmutz M (1996) Effect of carbamazepine, oxcarbazepine and lamotrigine on the increase in extracellular glutamate elicited by veratridine in rat cortex and striatum. Naunyn Schmiedebergs Arch Pharmacol 354:164–172

Walker MC, Perry H, Tong X, Patsalos PN (1996a) Cerebrospinal fluid and blood kinetics of lamotrigine in rats. Epilepsia 37 [Suppl 4]:80

Walker MC, Tong X, Patsalos PN, Scaravilli F, Shorvon SD, Jefferys JGR (1996b) Late treatment in animal model of status epilepticus. Epilepsia 37 [Suppl 5]:70

Walton NY, Jaing Q, Hyun B, Treiman DM (1996) Lamotrigine vs. phenytoin for treatment of status epilepticus: comparison in an experimental model. Epilepsy Res 24:19–28

Wang SJ, Huang CC, Hsu KS, Tsai JJ, Gean PW (1996) Presynaptic inhibition of excitatory neurotransmission by lamotrigine in the rat amygdalar neurons. Synapse 24:248–255

Wang SJ, Tsai JJ, Gean PW (1997) Lamotrigine inhibits tetraethylammonium-induced synaptic plasticity in the rat amygdala. Neuroscience 81:667–671

Warner T, Patsalos PN, Prevett M, Elyas AA, Duncan JS (1992) Lamotrigine-induced carbamazepine toxicity: an interaction with carbamazepine-10,11-epoxide. Epilepsy Res 11:147–150

Watelle M, Demedts P, Franck F, De Deyn PP, Wauters A, Neels H (1997) Analysis of the antiepileptic phenyltriazine compound lamotrigine using gas chromatography with nitrogen phosphorus detection. Ther Drug Monit 19:460–464

Wheatley PL, Miller AA (1989) Effects of lamotrigine on electrically induced afterdischarge duration in anaesthetised rat, dog, and marmoset. Epilepsia 30:34–40

Wiard RP, Dickerson MC, Beek O, Norton R, Cooper BR (1995) Neuroprotective properties of the novel antiepileptic lamotrigine in a gerbil model of global cerebral ischemia. Stroke 26:466–472

Wolf P (1992) Lamotrigine: preliminary clinical observations on pharmacokinetics and interactions with traditional antiepileptic drugs. J Epilepsy 5:73–79

Wootton R, Soul-Lawton J, Rolan PE, Sheung CT, Cooper JD, Posner J (1997) Comparison of the pharmacokinetics of lamotrigine in patients with chronic renal failure and healthy volunteers. Br J Clin Pharmacol 43:23–27
Xie X, Lancaster B, Peakman T, Garthwaite J (1995) Interaction of the antiepileptic drug lamotrigine with recombinant rat brain type IIA Na^+ channels and with native Na^+ channels in rat hippocampal neurones. Pflugers Arch 430:437–446
Xiong ZQ, Stringer JL (1997) Effects of felbamate, gabapentin and lamotrigine on seizure parameters and excitability in the rat hippocampus. Epilepsy Res 27:187–194
Yamashita S, Furuno K, Kawasaki H, Gomita Y, Yoshinaga H, Yamatogi Y, Ohtahara S (1995) Simple and rapid analysis of lamotrigine, a novel antiepileptic, in human serum by high-performance liquid chromatography using a solid-phase extraction technique. J Chromatog B: Biomed Applicat 670:354–357
Yuen AWC (1992) Safety issues. In: Richens A (ed) Clinical update on lamotrigine: a novel antiepileptic agent. Wells Medical Limited, Kent, UK, pp 69–75
Yuen AWC, Peck AW (1988) Lamotrigine pharmacokinetics: oral and i.v. infusion in man. Br J Clin Pharmacol 26:242
Yuen AWC, Land G, Weatherley BC, Peck AW (1992) Sodium valproate inhibits lamotrigine metabolism. Br J Clin Pharmacol 33:511–513
Zona C, Avoli M (1997) Lamotrigine reduces voltage-gated sodium currents in rat central neurons in culture. Epilepsia 38:522–525

CHAPTER 13

Valproate

D.D. SHEN and R.H. LEVY

A. Introduction

Valproate is a major and well established antiepileptic agent which is in contemporary widespread use in the treatment of the disorder, especially the generalized variety, for which it has become the drug of first choice. It also appears to be finding new uses in the management of a more extensive range of neurological and psychiatric disorders.

B. Chemistry and Use

I. Chemistry

Valproate (*n*-propyl pentanoate; di-*n*-propyl acetate), a branched chain fatty acid, is commercially available as the corresponding free acid, the sodium salt and as divalproex sodium, which is a coordinated 1:1 complex of sodium valproate and valproic acid. Valproic acid (molecular weight 166.2, pK_a 4.95) is an oily liquid at room temperature and it and its sodium salt are quite water soluble and hygroscopic.

II. Use

Valproate is a major antiepileptic drug with a wide spectrum of activity. The major utility of valproate is in the treatment of primary generalized epilepsy syndromes with multiple seizure types. It is effective as monotherapy in the treatment of simple absences, in which it can be used in patients refractory to ethosuximide. In some patients the combination of both drugs may be more effective than either drug used in monotherapy. It is also effective in myoclonic seizures, particularly when they coexist with absence seizures or tonic-clonic seizures in the context of primary generalized epilepsy. Patients who have absence and generalized tonic-clonic seizures benefit most from valproate. The drug is also effective in complex partial seizures (but less so than carbamazepine), particularly if the seizures become secondarily generalized tonic-clonic ones. A recent study showed that divalproex sodium was effective in patients with medically refractory complex partial seizures treated with phenytoin or carbamazepine (WILLMORE et al. 1996). The efficacy of valproate in febrile seizures and in the Lennox-Gastaut syndrome is less well established.

Initial valproate doses are 15 mg/kg/day and can be increased at the rate of 5–10 mg/kg/day each week until 60 mg/kg/day is reached. Higher doses may be needed in children, particularly when they are also receiving enzyme-inducing drugs. If the desired clinical response is not obtained, plasma level monitoring can be used to evaluate possible poor compliance, lack of absorption or unusually high clearances. The usually accepted therapeutic levels are in the range of 60–100 mg/l in serum or plasma.

It is important to note that valproate has also been approved in certain countries for the treatment of manic episodes associated with bipolar disorder and for the prophylaxis of migraine. Its use in these two indications appears to be increasing.

C. Pharmacodynamics

I. Experimental Animal Studies

Valproate is highly effective in several animal species against pentylenetetrazol-induced seizures (a model of cortico-reticular epilepsy) and less so against maximal electroshock seizures (a model of generalized tonic-clonic seizures). Valproate protects against generalized seizures induced by bicuculline, glutamic acid, kainic acid, strychnine, ouabain, and nicotine (SWINYARD 1964), and is also effective against the feline model of cortico-reticular epilepsy induced by intramuscular injection of penicillin G (FARIELLO et al. 1995).

In two models of simple partial seizures, the cortical cobalt and alumina lesion models, valproate suppresses the spread of seizure activity, but does not inhibit the focal discharges (FARIELLO et al. 1995). Likewise, valproate blocked the spread of epileptiform activity, while having no effect on the focal electrical after discharges and focal seizures in kindling models (LEVEIL et al. 1977; LÖSCHER et al. 1988). Thus, the neural system involved in the generalization of seizure is particularly susceptible to valproate's action.

II. Biochemical Pharmacology

The antiepileptic action of valproate is not fully understood and is likely to involve multiple mechanisms. The current evidence supports the hypotheses discussed below (FARIELLO et al. 1995). The most commonly ascribed antiepileptic mechanism of valproate relates to its elevation of brain GABAergic activity. Valproate increases the neuronal supply of γ-aminobutyric acid (GABA) by direct inhibition of its primary degradative enzyme (GABA transaminase) or acts indirectly by inhibition of the next enzyme in the GABA degradative process, i.e. succinic semialdehyde dehydrogenase. Inhibition of the latter enzyme results in accumulation of succinic semialdehyde, which leads to product-inhibition of GABA transaminase (FARIELLO et al. 1995). Valproate treatment has also been demonstrated to enhance the in vivo activity of glutamic acid decarboxylase, the key synthetic enzyme for GABA. WIKINSKI et al. (1996) recently showed that valproate does not directly activate adult rat brain glutamic acid decarboxylase in vitro, and surmised that the in vivo increase in glutamic acid decarboxylase activity associated with the drug may be the result of an increase in the firing of GABAergic neurons. Most importantly, in the rat brain a significant elevation of synaptosomal GABA content occurs in discrete regions that are critical in sustaining generalized epileptiform activity (LÖSCHER and VETTER 1984).

Furthermore, at therapeutic levels, valproate has a modest in vitro potentiating effect on GABA-mediated postsynaptic inhibition, possibly through the drug's action on the picrotoxin site of the GABA receptor-Cl^- ionophore complex (TICKU and DAVIS 1981; FARIELLO et al. 1995).

Valproate has been shown to affect specific intracerebral circuitry important in the regulation of epileptiform activity (NOWACK et al. 1979; FARIELLO et al. 1995). Valproate decreases excitability of the cortex and hippocampus during stimulation of the caudate nucleus via its thalamo-cortical projections. There are ample data in support of the concept that valproate selectively increases tonic GABAergic inhibition of neurons in the substantia nigra pars reticulata, a region critical in the propagation of experimentally evoked seizures. This action effectively reduces the outflow of the dorsal striatum to the thalamus, colliculus and tegmentum (GALE 1988; ROHLFS et al. 1996). The increase in nigral GABAergic activity is thought to reflect an increase in input nerve terminal GABA (LÖSCHER and VETTER 1984). Recently, ZHANG et al. (1996) showed that augmentation of $GABA_A$-mediated inhibition is not involved in valproate's suppression of epileptiform activity in an in vitro rodent thalamo-cortical slice model.

Elevation of neuronal GABA concentrations cannot account fully for the anti-epileptic actions of valproate. Firstly, substantive elevation of brain GABA occurs only at relatively high doses of valproate. Secondly, enhanced GABAergic tone is known to aggravate seizures in several models of bilaterally synchronous spike-and-wave discharges. Moreover, some branched-chain valproate analogues (e.g. 2-ethylbutyric acid) showed anticonvulsant activity in the absence of a significant change in brain GABA (FARIELLO et al. 1995).

At therapeutically relevant levels, valproate has a direct action on NMDA receptors. Valproate has been reported to (1) block neuronal firing induced by NMDA receptor activation (LÖSCHER 1993), (2) suppress NMDA-evoked, transient depolarization in rat neocortical pyramidal cells (ZEISE et al. 1991), (3) decrease NMDA receptor-mediated synaptic responses in rat amygdala slices (GEAN et al. 1994), and (4) decrease NMDA-induced excitatory postsynaptic potentials in the rat hippocampus (KO et al. 1997).

As with several other anticonvulsants, valproate exerts effects on neuronal conductance when fibres and/or synapses are functioning abnormally. In vitro, valproate limits high frequency sustained repetitive firing of Na^+-dependent action potentials through blockade of voltage-dependent Na^+ channels (McLEAN and MACDONALD 1986).

Valproate also suppresses spontaneous epileptiform activity in hippocampal slices by activating Ca^{2+}-dependent K^+ conductances (FRANCESCHETTI et al. 1986).

D. Pharmacokinetics

I. Absorption

Three different chemical forms of valproate are in common use, viz. the free acid, sodium salt, and divalproex sodium, which is a coordinated 1:1 complex of sodium valproate and valproic acid. Valproate has been available in a variety of commercial dosage forms: syrup (acid), tablets (acid or sodium salt), capsules (acid), sprinkle capsules (divalproex), enteric-coated tablets (sodium salt and divalproex), and controlled-release tablets (divalproex). An intravenous formulation is also available for rapid loading of valproate.

The gastrointestinal absorption of valproate from all these formulations appears to be complete and is not significantly affected by food. On the other hand, the onset and rate of absorption depend on the formulation and differ between the fasted and fed states (LEVY and SHEN 1995).

Absorption from the syrup, conventional tablet formulations, or the soft-gelatine capsule of free acid (Depakane) is very rapid and is not affected by food; the peak plasma concentration is consistently reached in less than 2h. As expected, a time lag (~2–3h) is observed in the onset of absorption from enteric-coated tablets (Depakote, Epilim EC), and this is further delayed and becomes more variable in the presence of food (LEVY et al. 1980; FISCHER et al. 1988; CARRIGAN et al. 1990; ROBERTS et al. 1996). The peak plasma concentration after dosing with enteric-coated tablets is reached after about 3–5 h. Diurnal variation (i.e. variation between morning and evening doses) in absorption from the enteric-coated formulations has been reported (LOISEAU et al. 1982; YOSHIYAMA et al. 1989).

Depakote Sprinkle consists of coated divalproex particles in a pull-apart capsule, and is particularly suited to paediatric use. The onset of absorption from the sprinkle formulation is earlier than from the divalproex tablet (~1h), but the rate of absorption is slightly slower; as a result, the peak-to-trough difference in valproate plasma concentration is smaller during chronic dosing. To permit once daily dosing, two controlled release divalproex formulations have recently become available in Europe and the United States (ROBERTS et al. 1996; SAMARA et al. 1997a). Both formulations were able to maintain a 50% fluctuation in plasma valproate concentration over the course of 24h. Food does not appear to affect the absorption characteristics of the US controlled-release formulation (CAVANAUGH et al. 1997).

Rectal administration of valproate syrup has been shown to be effective in the treatment of refractory status epilepticus in both adults and children (VAJDA et al. 1978; SNEAD and MILES 1985). The plasma valproate concentration time course after rectal valproate syrup was comparable to that observed after the oral capsule (CLOYD and KRIEL 1981).

II. Distribution

Valproate has a relatively small apparent volume of distribution (~0.15–0.20 l/kg); its extravascular distribution is limited by its high binding affinity for plasma albumin. Another important feature of valproate binding to plasma proteins is its dependence on its concentration over the therapeutic range (50–150 μg/ml); i.e. the drug's therapeutic concentrations are within the range of valproate's equilibrium dissociation constant for albumin binding. The average plasma free fraction of valproate (slightly below 10%) remains constant up to a plasma concentration of 75 μg/ml, and increases to 15% at 100 μg/ml, 22% at 125 μg/ml, and 30% at 150 μg/ml (CRAMER et al. 1986; LEVY and SHEN 1995). This concentration-dependent behaviour in plasma protein binding of valproate leads to an apparent increase in the clearance of total valproate in plasma (see later). It also gives rise to a greater fluctuation in the free drug concentration compared to the total concentration in plasma during a steady-state dosing interval.

Diminished plasma valproate protein binding has been demonstrated in certain populations (women during late pregnancy, elderly patients) and pathophysiological states (liver disease, head trauma, end-stage renal diseases) that are characterized by significant hypoalbuminaemia (LEVY and SHEN 1995). Reduced plasma protein binding has also been observed in situations where there is elevation in plasma bilirubin (e.g. in liver disease and in jaundiced neonates), and in free fatty acids (e.g. insulin-dependent diabetes mellitus), and in the presence of drug interactions involving plasma protein binding displacements (e.g. with salicylate – LEVY and SHEN 1995). In the absence of any change in intrinsic metabolic clearance, the decrease in plasma protein binding leads to an apparent lowering of the area under the total plasma valproate concentration-time curve, but no change in the area under the free plasma valproate concentration curve. Assuming that the drug's antiepileptic effect is related to the free valproate concentration, changes in plasma protein binding alone should not alter the clinical response.

Extensive data exist on the tissue distribution of valproate in animals, mostly in rodents. Owing to its moderately high lipophilicity, valproate readily moves into its extravascular sites of action. The uptake of valproate and its unsaturated metabolites into the liver, the extent of which depends on their plasma protein bindings, has been demonstrated in rodents (CRAMER et al. 1986; LÖSCHER and NAU 1984). The teratogenicity of valproate has been attributed in part to its ease of crossing the placental barrier, and to its accumulation in the neuroepithelium of the mouse embryo due to the relatively high intracellular pH present during organogenesis (DENCKER et al. 1990).

Rapid entry of valproate into the brain was demonstrated in some of the early work in rodents and dogs (FREY and LÖSCHER 1978; POLLACK and SHEN

1985), which is entirely consistent with the prompt appearance of an anticonvulsant effect after a single administration of the drug. The problem associated with the distribution of valproate to the brain is the unexpectedly low steady-state concentrations of valproate in the central nervous system relative to the free drug concentration in plasma. This was first reported some years ago in a study of the cerebrospinal fluid concentration of valproate in monkeys during intravenous infusion (LEVY 1980), and recently was confirmed in humans by a study of valproate concentration in cortical specimens obtained from patients undergoing epilepsy surgery (SHEN et al. 1992). The mean brain-to-free serum concentration ratio of valproate is about 0.5, which suggests asymmetrical transport of valproate (i.e. its efflux rate exceeds its influx rate).

Recent animal studies have revealed that the bidirectional movement of valproate across the blood-brain barrier is mediated in part by carrier transport. The uptake of valproate from the blood into the brain is facilitated by a medium- and long-chain fatty acid selective anion exchanger at the brain capillary epithelium (ADKISON and SHEN 1996). The mechanism(s) governing the efficient transport of valproate in the reverse direction, i.e. from brain to blood, appear to involve a probenecid-sensitive, active transport system at the brain capillary endothelium (ADKISON et al. 1995; NAORA and SHEN 1995). Further, a recent brain microdialysis study in rabbits suggests that, at neural cell membranes, another set of transporters exists that shuttles valproate between the extracellular fluid and intracellular compartments within the brain parenchyma (SCISM et al. 1996). The putative parenchymal cell transport system is able to concentrate valproate within the cellular compartment, which has important implications in our understanding of the pharmacological mechanisms of action of valproate (i.e. membrane action versus intracellular mechanisms). Moreover, the efflux component is inhibited by probenecid, which provides another mechanism by which probenecid co-treatment increases the steady-state brain-to-plasma distribution ratio of the drug. A full elucidation of the brain transport mechanisms of valproate may hold the key to the design of "second generation" alkanoic acid type antiepileptics that have improved brain delivery, reduced systemic burdens, and lower risks of organ toxicities (e.g. teratogenicity and hepatotoxicity).

III. Elimination

1. Clearance Parameters

The intrinsic metabolic clearance and the plasma protein binding are the main determinants of the clearance of an extensively metabolized, low extraction ratio drug such as valproate. The following is a brief summary of how dose, age and pathophysiology modulate these two variables to jointly effect changes in the plasma clearance of valproate.

The plasma clearance of valproate is dose-dependent. In single dose studies, the plasma clearance of the drug shows a progressive increase, as the dose is incremented from 500 mg to as high as 3000 mg (BOWDLE et al. 1980; GOMEZ BELLVER 1993). The accelerated clearance at high doses is attributed to the increase in the average plasma free fraction. In contrast, clearance expressed in terms of plasma free valproate concentration, or intrinsic metabolic clearance, shows a downward trend with the increase in dose, which is consistent with the notion of saturation in β-oxidation based on urinary metabolite studies (see the following section on "Metabolism"). The magnitude of change in the plasma free fraction exceeded the partial saturation of intrinsic metabolic clearance, which explains the net increase in clearance of total drug in plasma with an increase in dose.

There is a large collection of data on the pharmacokinetics of valproate in various age groups, which has been summarized (LEVY and SHEN 1995). In all age groups, the clearance of valproate was notably higher (on average, by ~twofold) in patients receiving polytherapy that included the microsomal enzyme inducers (phenobarbitone, phenytoin and carbamazepine).

A continuous change in valproate clearance occurs over the entire period of childhood. The clearance of total plasma valproate in neonates is comparable to that in adult patients (10–14 ml/min/kg) despite a higher plasma free fraction due to elevated plasma free fatty acids and bilirubin (13% vs. <10%). This is consistent with low and immature microsomal drug-metabolizing enzyme activities. The low intrinsic clearance is reflected in a prolonged elimination half-life (>17 h). Rapid maturation in microsomal enzyme function occurs over the first 2 years of life, such that valproate clearance in pre-school children is nearly twice as high as that in adults (14–36 ml/min/kg), and the drug's elimination half-life is shortened (~6–12 h). From the pre-school years to adolescence, there is a gradual decline in total drug clearance and an increase in its elimination half-life towards adult values (9–18 ml/min/kg and 8–15 h, respectively). The clearance of total valproate in plasma appears to remain stable during the adult years. However, hypoalbuminaemia occurs commonly in elderly patients. The intrinsic clearance of valproate is lower in elderly patients, by an average of 40%, than in young control subjects, which is consistent with the commonly recognized age-related decline in hepatic drug-metabolizing function, especially oxidative metabolism and glucuronidation.

Only a small number of studies on valproate clearance in pregnant women have been reported (PLASSE et al. 1979; PHILBERT and DAM 1982). The available data suggest that valproate clearance begins to rise late in the second trimester, and continues to increase through the mid-portion of the third trimester. Much of the increase in drug clearance can be attributed to an increase in plasma free fraction as a result of elevated free fatty acid concentrations and low albumin level (NAU and KRAUER 1986).

The clearance kinetics of valproate have been investigated in liver and renal diseases. Liver diseases lead to a decrease in the plasma protein binding and intrinsic metabolic clearance of valproate; the changes tend to be equal in magnitude resulting in there being no apparent change in the clearance of total drug in plasma (KLOTZ et al. 1978). The primary effect of end-stage renal disease appears to be a decrease in plasma protein binding (free fraction >20%) due to displacement by uraemic plasma constituents. No significant change in intrinsic metabolic clearance was noted.

The pharmacokinetics of valproate have recently been investigated in head trauma patients as part of a clinical trial of valproate prophylaxis against post-traumatic seizures (ANDERSON et al. 1994, 1998). Head trauma causes an acute and remarkable drop in plasma albumin levels, which is reflected in a variable and significant increase in the plasma free fraction of valproate. This is accompanied by an increase in the intrinsic clearance of valproate, reflecting an apparent induction of the drug's oxidative pathways.

2. Metabolism

Valproic acid is extensively metabolized; its primary metabolic pathways involve both phase I (oxidative) and phase 2 (conjugative) biotransformation reactions (BAILLIE and SHEFFELS 1995).

Conjugation with D-glucuronic acid represents the major pathway of valproate biotransformation in humans, accounting for about 30%–40% of the usual clinical dose. Valproylcarnitine has also been identified as a minor conjugated metabolite in human urine.

Analogously to the oxidation of endogenous straight-chain fatty acids, valproate is activated to its coenzyme A thioester, which undergoes sequential mitochondrial β-oxidation to yield Δ^2-valproate (the E-isomer being the major form present in biological fluids), 3-hydroxy-valproate, and 3-oxo-valproate. E-Δ^2-Valproate possesses a slightly more potent anticonvulsant activity than its saturated precursor (LÖSCHER et al. 1991; SEMMES and SHEN 1991). Since the steady-state concentrations of Δ^2-valproate in serum or brain cortex of epileptic patients are, on average, less than 10% those of valproate (RETTENMEIER et al. 1985; ABBOTT et al. 1986a; ADKISON et al. 1995), the contribution of this metabolite to the antiepileptic efficacy of valproate is probably minimal. 3-Oxo-valproate appears to be a terminal metabolite of β-oxidation, and is largely excreted in urine. About 20%–35% of the valproate dose is recovered as 3-oxo-valproate in urine of patients receiving valproate monotherapy, an indication of the percentage contribution of β-oxidation to valproate metabolic clearance.

Aside from E-Δ^2-valproate, two other mono-unsaturated metabolites, Δ^3-valproate and Δ^4-valproate, are present in the serum and urine of epileptic patients. The mono-ene metabolites give rise to a series of diene metabolites, in particular (2E,3′E)-$\Delta^{2,3}$-valproate and (2E)-$\Delta^{2,4}$-valproate. (2E)-$\Delta^{2,4}$-Valproate is thought to be a precursor to a reactive epoxide metabolite that may be involved in the hepatotoxicity of valproate.

Other oxidative pathways include ω and ω-1 oxidation to form 5-hydroxy-valproate and 4-hydroxy-valproate, respectively. 4-Hydroxy-valproate, which also exists in its γ-lactone form, is further oxidized to 4-oxo-valproate. Both hydroxy-acids are eventually oxidized to their dicarboxylic acid end products.

All the products of ω and ω-1 oxidation are thought to be devoid of biological activity.

The metabolic profile of valproate changes with an increase in dose. The proportion of the dose recovered in urine and which has undergone glucuronidation increases with increasing valproate dose at the expense of the β-oxidation pathways. GRANNEMAN et al. (1984) showed that following a single oral dose of valproate the percentage of the dose excreted in urine as 3-oxo-valproate decreased from 33.7% at 250mg to 20.7% at 1000mg, while valproate glucuronide increased from 4.5% of the dose at 250mg to 35.2% at 1000mg. These data are thought to reflect saturation of mitochondrial β-oxidation, and compensatory increase in microsomal glucuronidation. In addition, a recent series of single dose studies in healthy volunteers (ANDERSON et al. 1992) and clinical studies in adult and paediatric patients (KONDO et al. 1992; SUGIMOTO et al. 1996) showed an increase in cytochrome P450-mediated formation of Δ^4-valproate and the ω and ω-1 oxidative products with an increase in dose.

SHEN et al. (1984) reported the average steady-state concentration ratio of various valproate metabolites to parent drug in 22 infants (4 months to 2 years), children (2–15 years), and 12 adult patients. These concentration ratios increased as a function of age for 3-oxo-valproate, remained constant for E-Δ^2-valproate, and decreased for Δ^4-valproate. The latter observation does suggest that young infants may be exposed to higher circulating concentrations of the potentially hepatotoxic Δ^4-metabolites.

Carbamazepine induces the metabolism of valproate. A profile of urinary metabolites of valproate from patients receiving polytherapy with carbamazepine indicated an increase in cytochrome P450-mediated ω and ω-1 oxidations (ABBOTT et al. 1986b). An increased urinary recovery of 3-oxo-valproate has also been observed, which may suggest induction of β-oxidation, although an alternative explanation may be an increased formation of 3-hydroxy-valproate and its conversion to 3-oxo-valproate.

Salicylate decreases β-oxidation of valproate by competitive inhibition in the formation of valproyl CoA (ABBOTT et al. 1986c).

Inducers (phenytoin and carbamazepine) and inhibitors (stiripentol) of oxidative microsomal enzymes have been shown to increase and decrease, respectively, the formation of the hepatotoxic olefin Δ^4-valproate (KONDO et al. 1990; LEVY et al. 1990).

Valproate is a potent competitive inhibitor of glucuronidation. A significant interaction between valproate and lamotrigine has been reported (YUEN et al. 1992; ANDERSON et al. 1996).

E. Interactions

I. Other Drugs Affecting Valproate

Knowledge of the metabolic fate of valproic acid provides a basis to rationalize interactions in which valproate metabolic clearance is affected. A relatively large fraction of the dose (40%) of valproic acid is eliminated by glucuronidation. Induction of the UDP glucuronosyltransferases involved in this pathway (UGT1A6, UGT1A8, UGT2B7) accounts primarily for the twofold increase in valproate clearance associated with co-administration of enzyme inducers such as phenytoin, phenobarbitone or carbamazepine. Valproate dosage adjustments are often required when these drugs are added to, or withdrawn from, a patient's treatment. Although enzyme inducers such as phenytoin and carbamazepine also affect the cytochrome P450-mediated pathways of valproate metabolism (LEVY et al. 1990), these oxidative pathways account for less than 10% of the dose and the impact of induction of those pathways on the total clearance is relatively minor. Another significant elimination pathway for valproate (20%–30%) is β-oxidation, which leads to the urinary 3-keto metabolite of the drug. This pathway is probably involved in the dose-dependent inhibition of valproate metabolism associated with felbamate co-administration (WAGNER et al. 1994; HOOPER et al. 1996).

II. Valproate Affecting Other Drugs

Interactions in which valproate affects the metabolic clearance of other drugs are related primarily to inhibition of four enzyme systems, viz. epoxide hydrolase, CYP2C9, UDP glucuronyltransferases and UDP glucosyltransferases. Inhibition of the enzyme epoxide hydrolase by valproate was discovered several years ago and provides an explanation for the elevations which are found in the plasma levels of the metabolite of carbamazepine, carbamazepine-10,11-epoxide, when valproate is added to carbamazepine therapy (LEVY et al. 1984; KERR et al. 1989; PISANI et al. 1990; ROBBINS et al. 1990). It is not clear whether this interaction is clinically meaningful. Recently, the inhibition spectrum of valproate toward several cytochrome P450 enzymes has been elucidated; CYP2C9 was the only enzyme inhibited at valproate concentrations consistent with therapeutic levels (HURST et al. 1997). Inhibition of CYP2C9 has been proposed to explain the elevations in phenytoin and phenobarbitone levels associated with valproate co-administration. Inhibition of the formation of phenobarbitone *N*-glucoside contributes also to the decrease in phenobarbitone clearance (BERNUS et al. 1994).

Valproate decreases the metabolism of several drugs eliminated by glucuronidation such as lorazepam (SAMARA 1997b), zidovudine (LERTORA 1994) and lamotrigine (YUEN et al. 1992). In the case of the latter, the effect is pronounced and may require dosage adjustments. In patients who are not concomitantly treated with enzyme inducers (e.g. phenytoin or carbamazepine), the half-life of lamotrigine increases from 30 to 60 h in the presence of valproate, and in patients receiving enzyme inducers, the lamotrigine half-life increases from approximately 15 h to 30 h. This interaction is due to inhibition of formation of lamotrigine *N*-glucuronide by UGT1A4 (GREEN et al. 1995), but the inhibition spectrum of valproate toward the various UDP glucuronyltransferases has not been completely characterized.

F. Adverse Effects

A variety of side effects have been associated with valproate therapy. The most common include (1) gastrointestinal distress (nausea, vomiting, abdominal pain), (2) weight gain in up to 20% of patients, (3) hair loss in approximately 10% of patients, and (4) tremor. Some of these side effects (weight gain and hair loss) may result in discontinuation of therapy. Side effects which are less frequent include sedation and drowsiness, especially at high plasma valproate concentrations, and encephalopathy and hyperammonaemia, particularly related to antiepileptic drug polytherapy.

Another category of adverse effects is more rare and is idiosyncratic in nature. Thrombocytopenia with inhibition of platelet aggregation and other haematological side effects such as fibrinogen depletion have been reported. Hepatic reactions range from alterations in serum biochemistry unrelated to clinical symptoms to severe, rarely fatal, hepatotoxicity. In the cases which have been reported, hepatic failure occurred within the first 6 months of therapy with a variety of non-specific symptoms such as weakness, lethargy, vomiting and loss of seizure control. The patients at a high risk of a fatal outcome (1 in 600) are children under 2 years old receiving antiepileptic polytherapy and who also have congenital metabolic disorders, organic brain disease or mental retardation. The risk decreases appreciably in older children (1 in 8300 in 3–10 years old) and in adults (1 in 35,000) receiving polytherapy. The risk also decreases when the drug is used in monotherapy. There have been a few reports of acute haemorrhagic pancreatitis which have been fatal.

Like all other antiepileptic drugs, valproate use in women of childbearing age has been associated with teratogenicity. In addition to craniofacial and digital anomalies, valproate use during pregnancy has been associated with neural tube defects (spina bifida) with an incidence of 1%–2%. Based on the belief that this adverse effect may be related to high peak plasma concentrations, the recommendation has been made to divide the daily dosage if valproate must be used during pregnancy. Also this risk should be weighed against the risk of substitution of another drug during the first trimester of pregnancy.

References

Abbott FS, Kassam J, Acheampong A et al. (1986a) Capillary gas chromatography-mass spectrometry of valproic acid metabolites in serum and urine using tert-butyldimethylsilyl derivatives. J Chromatogr 375:285–298

Abbott F, Panesar S, Orr J, Burton R, Farrell K (1986b) Effect of carbamazepine on valproic acid metabolism. Epilepsia 27:591

Abbott FS, Kassam J, Orr JM, Farrell K (1986c) The effect of aspirin on valproic acid metabolism. Clin Pharmacol Ther 40:94–100

Adkison KD, Shen DD (1996) Uptake of valproic acid into rat brain is mediated by a medium-chain fatty acid transporter. J Pharmacol Exp Ther 276:1189–1200

Adkison KDK, Ojemann GA, Rapport R, Dills RL, Shen DD (1995) Distribution of unsaturated metabolites of valproate in human and rat brain—pharmacologic relevance? Epilepsia 36:772–782

Anderson GD, Acheampong AA, Wilensky AJ, Levy RH (1992) Effect of valproate dose on formation of hepatotoxic metabolites. Epilepsia 33:736–742

Anderson GD, Gidal BE, Hendryx RJ, Awan AB, Temkin NR, Wilensky AJ, Winn HR (1994) Decreased plasma protein binding of valproate in patients with acute head trauma. Br J Clin Pharmacol 37:559–562

Anderson GD, Yau MK, Gidal BE et al. (1996) Bidirectional interaction of valproate and lamotrigine in healthy subjects. Clin Pharmacol Ther 60:145–156

Anderson GD, Awan AB, Adams CA, Temkin NR, Winn HR (1998) Increases in metabolism of valproate and excretion of 6beta-hydroxycortisol in patients with traumatic brain injury. Br J Clin Pharmacol 45:101–105

Baillie TA, Sheffels PR (1995) Valproic acid: chemistry and biotransformation. In: Levy RH, Mattson RH, Meldrum BS (eds) Antiepileptic drugs, 4th edn, Raven Press, New York

Bernus I, Dickinson RG, Hooper WD, Eadie MJ (1994) Inhibition of phenobarbitone *N*-glucosidation by valproate. Br J Clin Pharmacol 38:411–416

Bowdle TA, Patel IH, Levy RH, Wilensky AJ (1980) Valproic acid dosage and plasma protein binding and clearance. Clin Pharmacol Ther 28:486–492

Carrigan PJ, Brinker DR, Cavanaugh JH, Lamm JE, Cloyd JC (1990) Absorption characteristics of a new valproate formulation of divalproex sodium-coated particles in capsules (Depakote™ Sprinkle). J Clin Pharmacol 30:743–747

Cavanaugh JH, Granneman R, Lamm J, Linnen P, Chun AHC (1997) Effect of food on the bioavailability of a controlled-release formulation of depakote under multiple-dose conditions. Epilepsia 38:S54

Cloyd JC, Kriel RL (1981) Bioavailability of rectally administered valproic acid syrup. Neurology 31:1348–1352

Cramer JA, Mattson RH, Bennett DM, Swick CT (1986) Variable free and total valproic acid concentrations in sole- and multidrug therapy. Ther Drug Monit 8:411–415

Dencker L, Nau H, D'Argy R (1990) Marked accumulation of valproic acid in embryonic neuroepithelium of the mouse during early organogenesis. Teratology 41:699–706

Fariello RG, Varasi M, Smith MC (1995) Valproic acid: mechanisms of action. In: Levy RH, Mattson RH, Meldrum BS (eds) Antiepileptic drugs, 4th edn. Raven Press, New York

Fischer JH, Barr AN, Paloucek FP, Dorociak JV, Spunt AL (1988) Effect of food on the serum concentration profile of enteric-coated valproic acid. Neurology 38:1319–1322

Franceschetti S, Hamon B, Heineman U (1986) The action of valproate on spontaneous epileptiform activity in the absence of synaptic transmission on evoked changes in $[Ca^{++}]$ and $[K^{+}]$ in the hippocampal slice. Brain Res 386:1–11

Frey H-H, Löscher W (1978) Distribution of valproate across the interface between blood and cerebrospinal fluid. Neuropharmacology 17:637–642

Gale K (1988) Progression and generalization of seizure discharge: anatomical and neurochemical substrates. Epilepsia 29:S15–S34

Gean P-W, Hung C-C, Hung C-R, Tsai J-J (1994) Valproic acid suppresses the synaptic response mediated by the NMDA receptors in rat amygdalar slices. Brain Res Bull 33:333–336

Gomez Bellver MJ, Garcia Sanchez MJ, Alonso Gonzalez AC, Santo Buelga D, Dominquez-Gil A (1993) Plasma protein binding kinetics of valproic acid over a broad dosage range: therapeutic implications. J Clin Pharmacol Ther 18:191–197

Granneman GR, Marriott TB, Wang SI, Sennello LT, Hagen NS, Sonders RC (1984) Aspects of the dose-dependent metabolism of valproic acid. In: Levy RH, Pitlick WH, Eichelbaum M, Meijer J (eds) Metabolism of antiepileptic drugs. Raven Press, New York, pp 97–104

Green MD, Bishop WP, Tephley TR (1995) Expressed human UGT-1.4 protein catalyzes the formation of quaternary ammonium-linked glucuronides. Drug Metab Dispos 23:299–302

Hooper WD, Franklin ME, Glue P, Banfield CR, Radwanski E, McLaughlin DB, McIntyre ME, Dickinson RG, Eadie MJ (1996) Effect of falbamate on valproic acid disposition in healthy volunteers: Inhibition of β-oxidation. Epilepsia 37:91–97

Hurst S, Labroo R, Carlson S, Mather G, Levy R (1997) In vitro inhibition profile of valproic acid for cytochrome P450. International Society for the Study of Xenobiotics. Hilton Head, South Carolina (abstract):64

Kerr BM, Rettie AW, Eddy AC, Loiseau P, Guyot M, Wilensky AJ, Levy RH (1989) Inhibition of human liver microsomal epoxide hydrolase by valproate and valpromide: in vitro/in vivo correlation. Clin Pharmacol Ther 46:82–93

Klotz U, Rapp T, Müller WA (1978) Disposition of valproic acid in patients with liver disease. Eur J Clin Pharmacol 13:55–60

Ko GY-PL, Brown-Croyts LM, Teyler TJ (1997) The effects of anticonvulsant drugs on NMDA-EPSP, AMPA-DPSP, and GABA-IPSP in the rat hippocampus. Brain Res Bull 42:297–302

Kondo T, Otani K, Hirano T, Kaneko S, Fukushima Y (1990) The effects of phenytoin and carbamazepine on serum concentration of mono-unsaturated metabolites of valproic acid. Br J Clin Pharmacol 29:116–119

Kondo T, Kaneko S, Otani K et al. (1992) Associations between risk factors for valproate hepatotoxicity and altered valproate metabolism. Epilepsia 33:172–177

Lertora J, Rege A, Greenspan D, Akula S (1994) Pharmacokinetic interaction between zidovudine and valproic acid in patients infected with immunodeficiency virus. Clin Pharmacol Ther 56:272–278

Leveil V, Naquet R (1977) A study of the action of valproic acid on the kindling effect. Epilepsia 18:229–234

Levy RH (1980) CSF and plasma pharmacokinetics: relationship to mechanisms of action as exemplified by valproic acid in monkey. In: Lockard J, Ward A (eds) Epilepsy: a window to brain mechanisms. Raven Press, New York 11:191–200

Levy RH, Shen DD (1995) Valproic acid: absorption, distribution, and excretion. In: Levy RH, Mattson RH, Meldrum BS (eds) Antiepileptic drugs, 4th edn. Raven Press, New York

Levy RH, Cenraud B, Loiseau P et al. (1980) Meal-dependent absorption of enteric-coated sodium valproate. Epilepsia 21:273–280

Levy RH, Moreland TA, Morselli PL, Guyot M, Brachet-Liermain A, Loiseau P (1984) Carbamazepine/valproic acid interaction in man and rhesus monkey. Epilepsia 25:338–345

Levy RH, Rettenmeier AW, Anderson GD et al. (1990) Effects of polytherapy with phenytoin, carbamazepine, and stiripentol on formation of 4-ene-valproate, a hepatotoxic metabolite of valproic acid. Clin Pharmacol Ther 48:225–235

Loiseau P, Brachet-Liesmain A, Guyot M, Morselli P (1982) Diurnal variations in steady state plasma concentrations of valproic acid in epileptic patients. Clin Pharm 7:544–552

Löscher W (1993) Effects of the antieplieptic drug valproate on metabolism and function of inhibitory and excitatory amino acids in the brain. Neurochem Res 18:485–502

Löscher W, Nau H (1984) Comparative transfer of valproic acid and of an active metabolite into brain and liver: possible pharmacological and toxicological consequences. Arch Int Pharmacodyn Ther 270:192–202

Löscher W, Vetter M (1984) Drug-induced changes in GABA content of nerve endings in 11 rat brain regions: correlation to pharmacological effects. Neurosci Lett 47:325–331

Löscher W, Fisher JE, Nau H, Hönack D (1988) Marked increase in anticonvulsant activity but decrease in wet-dog shake behaviour during short-term treatment of amygdala-kindled rats with valproic acid. Eur J Pharmacol 150:221–232

Löscher W, Hönack D, Nolting B, Fassbender CP (1991) Trans-2-en-valproate: reevaluation of its anticonvulsant efficacy in standardized seizure models in mice, rats and dogs. Epilepsy Res 9:195–210

McLean MJ, MacDonald RL (1986) Sodium valproate, but not ethosuximide, produces use and voltage-dependent limitation of high frequency repetitive firing of action potentials of mouse central neurons in cell culture. J Pharmacol Exp Ther 237:1001–1011

Naora K, Shen DD (1995) Mechanism of valproic acid uptake by isolated rat brain microvessels. Epilepsy Res 22:97–106

Nau H, Krauer B (1986) Serum protein binding of valproic acid in fetus-mother pairs throughout pregnancy: correlation with oxytocin administration and albumin and free fatty acid concentrations. J Clin Pharmacol 26:215–221

Nowack WJ, Johnson RN, Englander RN, Hanna GR (1979) Effects of valproate and ethosuximide on thalamocortical excitability. Neurology 29:96–99

Philbert A, Dam M (1982) The epileptic mother and her child. Epilepsia 23:85–99

Pisani F, Caputo M, Fazio A et al (1990) Interaction of carbamazepine-10,11-epoxide, an active metabolite of carbamazepine, with valproate: a pharmacokinetic study. Epilepsia 31:339–342

Plasse J-C, Revol M, Chabert G, Ducerf F (1979) Neonatal pharmacokinetics of valproic acid. In: Schaaf D, van der Kleijn E (eds) Progress in clinical pharmacy. Elsevier/North-Holland Biomedical Press, Amsterdam, pp 247–252

Pollack GM, Shen DD (1985) A timed intravenous pentylenetetrazol infusion seizure model for quantitating the anticonvulsant effect of valproic acid in the rat. J Pharmacol Methods 13:135–146

Rettenmeier AW, Prickett KS, Gordon WP, Bjorge SM, Chang SL, Levy RH, Baillie TA (1985) Studies on the biotransformation in the perfused rat liver of 2-n-propyl-4-pentenoic acid, a metabolite of the antiepileptic drug valproic acid. Evidence for the formation of chemically reactive intermediates. Drug Metab Dispos 13:81–96

Robbins DK, Wedlund PJ, Kuhn R, Baumann RJ, Levy RH, Chang S-L (1990) Inhibition of epoxide hydrolase by valproic acid in epileptic patients receiving carbamazepine. Br J Clin Pharmacol 29:759–762

Roberts D, Easter D, O'Bryan-Tear G (1996) Epilim^{R} chrono: a multidose, crossover comparison of two formulations of valproate in healthy volunteers. Biopharm Drug Dispos 17:175–182

Rohlfs A, Rundfeldt C, Koch R, Löscher W (1996) A comparison of the effects of valproate and its major active metabolite E-2-en-valproate on single unit activity of sustantia nigra pars reticulata neurons in rats. J Pharmacol Exp Ther 277:1305–1314

Samara E, Granneman R, Achari R, Locke C, Cavanaugh J, Boellner S (1997a) Bioavailability of a controlled-release formulation of depakote. Epilepsia 38:S102

Samara EE, Granneman RG, Witt GF, Cavanaugh JH (1997b) Effect of valproate on the pharmacokinetics and pharmacodynamics of lorazepam. J Clin Pharmacol 37:442–450

Scism JL, Powers KM, Artru AA, Shen DD (1996) The effect of probenecid on extracellular and intracellular compartmentation of valproic acid in the rabbit brain as determined by microdialysis. Pharm Res 13:S456

Semmes RLO, Shen DD (1991) Comparative pharmacodynamics and brain distribution of E-Δ^2-valproate and valproate in rats. Epilepsia 32:232–241

Shen DD, Pollack GM, Cohen ME, Duffner P, Lacey D, Ryan-Dudek P (1984) Effect of age on the serum metabolite pattern of valproic acid. Epilespsia 25:674

Shen DD, Ojemann GA, Rapport RL, Dills RL, Friel PN, Levy RH (1992) Low and variable presence of valproic acid in human brain. Neurology 42:582–585

Snead OC III, Miles MV (1985) Treatment of status epilepticus in children with rectal sodium valproate. J Pediatr 106:323–325

Sugimoto T, Muro H, Woo M, Nishida N, Murakami K (1996) Metabolite profiles in patients on high-dose valproate monotherapy. Epilepsy Res 25:107–112

Swinyard EA (1964) The pharmacology of dipropylacetic acid sodium with special emphasis on its effects on the central nervous system. Thesis, University of Utah, College of Pharmacy, Salt Lake City, pp 1–25

Ticku MK, Davis WC (1981) Effect of valproic acid on H-diazepam and H-dihydropicrotoxin in binding sites at the benzodiazepine-GABA receptor-ionophore complex. Brain Res 223:218–222

Vajda FJE, Mihaly GW, Miles JL, Donnan GA, Bladin PF (1978) Rectal administration of sodium valproate in status epilepticus. Neurology 28:897–899

Wagner ML, Graves NM, Leppik IE, Remmel RP, Shumaker RC, Ward DL, Perhach JL (1994) The effect of felbamate on valproic acid disposition. Clin Pharmacol Ther 56:494–502

Wikinski SI, Acosta GB, Rubio MC (1996) Valproic acid differs in its in vitro effect on glutamic acid decarboxylase activity in neonatal and adult rat brain. Gen Pharmacol 27:635–638

Willmore JL, Shu V, Wallin B, and the M88–194 Study Group (1996) Efficacy and safety of add-on divalproex sodium in the treatment of complex partial seizures. Neurology 46:49–53

Yoshiyama Y, Nakano S, Ogawa N (1989) Chronopharmacokinetics study of valproic acid in man: comparison of oral and rectal administration. J Clin Pharmacol 29:1048–1052

Yuen AWC, Land G, Weatherley BC, Peck AW (1992) Sodium valproate acutely inhibits lamotrigene metabolism. Br J Clin Pharmacol 33:511–513

Zeise ML, Kasparow S, Zieglgänsberger W (1991) Valproate suppresses N-methyl-D-aspartate-evoked, transient depolarizations in the rat neocortex in vitro. Brain Res 544:345–348

Zhang Y-F, Gibbs JW, Coulter DA (1996) Anticonvulsant drug effects on spontaneous thalamocortical rhythms in vitro: valproic acid, clonazepam, and α-methyl-α-phenylsuccinimide. Epilepsy Res 23:37–53

CHAPTER 14

Vigabatrin

E. BEN-MENACHEM

A. Chemistry and Use

I. Chemical Characteristics

Vigabatrin (4-amino-5-hexenoic acid; gamma-vinyl GABA; GVG) is a rationally designed, specific enzyme-activated irreversible inhibitor of GABA transaminase (LIPPERT et al. 1977; SCHECHTER et al. 1979). It is a molecular structural analogue of GABA with a vinyl appendage (Fig. 1) and is highly soluble in water but only slightly soluble in ethanol and methanol and is insoluble in hexane and toluene. It is a white to off-white crystalline solid with a melting point of 171°–177°C. Its molecular weight is 129.16 and the conversion factor (CF) is 7.75 (mg/l × CF = μmol/l).

1. Enantiomers

Vigabatrin is a racemic mixture of R(–) and S(+) isomers in equal proportions and with no optical activity. The pharmacological activity and the toxic effects of vigabatrin are associated with the S(+) enantiomer only, while the R(–) enantiomer is entirely inactive (HAEGELE and SCHECHTER 1986; REY et al. 1990). No chiral inversion exists in man. Importantly, because GABA transaminase, which is the target enzyme, has a much longer half-life than vigabatrin itself, the major pharmacological effects of the drug are determined by the half-life of the enzyme rather than by that of the drug (JUNG et al. 1977; BEN-MENACHEM et al. 1988).

II. Use

At the present time, vigabatrin is used clinically only as an anticonvulsant.

B. Pharmacodynamics

I. Biochemical Pharmacology

1. Effects on GABA and Other Amino Acids

Vigabatrin is a very specific GABA transaminase inhibitor and causes highly specific effects in the brain which are probably related to its anticonvulsant

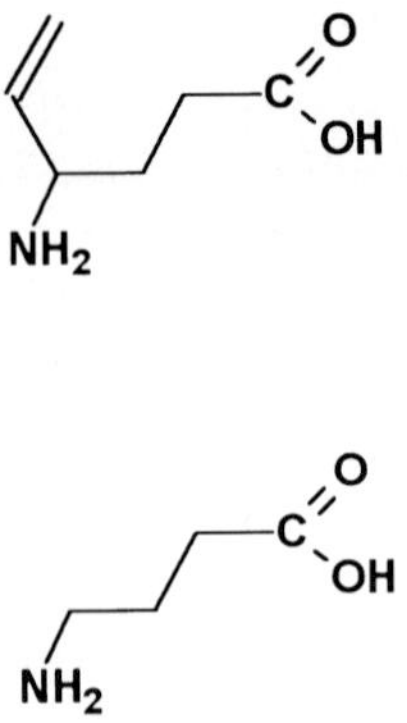

Vigabatrin

GABA

Fig. 1. Formulae of vigabatrin and GABA

activity. No other explanation has been proposed in spite of intensive research efforts in this area. The first experiments were by JUNG et al. (1977), who injected 1500 mg/kg of the compound intraperitoneally into mice and measured the brain content of GABA, GABA transaminase and glutamic acid decarboxylase over time. By 4 h a fivefold increase of whole brain GABA with a corresponding decline in GABA transaminase activity was observed. GABA transaminase concentrations recovered to 60% of their baseline levels after 5 days. A 30% decrease in glutamic acid decarboxylase was observed, but only at a very high dose of vigabatrin (1500 mg/kg). This was probably the result of a feedback mechanism following the sudden sharp increase in GABA concentration. Other studies (PALFREYMAN et al. 1980) have shown that free and total GABA and homocarnosine levels in both the brain and the CSF are increased in parallel with increasing doses of vigabatrin.

II. Animal Models

1. Anticonvulsive Effects

Vigabatrin is effective in some, but not all, experimental animal seizure models. It is inactive in such fundamental models as maximal electroshock, bicuculline (GABA antagonist) and pentylenetetrazol-induced seizures, unless injected directly into the midbrain of rats (GALE et al. 1986). After an intravenous injection of vigabatrin, seizure protection was observed after bicuculline-induced myoclonic activity (KENDALL et al. 1981), strychnine-induced tonic seizures (SCHECHTER et al. 1979), isoniazid-induced generalized seizures (SCHECHTER et al. 1979), audiogenic seizures in mice (SCHECHTER et al. 1977), photic-induced seizures in the baboon (MELDRUM and HORTON 1978) and amygdala-kindled seizures in the rat (PIREDDA et al. 1985; STEVENS et al. 1988).

Stereotaxic injections of small amounts of vigabatrin into certain specific areas of the rat brain gave seizure protection that was related to the locally increased GABA levels (GALE 1986). Protection against maximal electroshock seizures was most prominent when local GABA concentration increases were produced in the midbrain tegmentum, including the substantia nigra and the midbrain reticular formation. Injections of vigabatrin into the thalamus, hippocampus and cortex did not protect against seizures in this model. The duration of seizure protection was as long as 72h after a single injection into the substantia nigra. Only by the 5th day did the rats again respond normally to maximal electroshock. This finding supports the observations that the rate of recovery of GABA transaminase is 5 days (JUNG et al. 1977) and suggests that the anticonvulsant effect of vigabatrin is due to the local increase in GABA levels instead of being a direct effect of vigabatrin itself.

2. Prevention of Epileptogenesis

There is some indication that vigabatrin may prevent epileptogenesis. Support for this comes from the study by SHIN et al. (1986), who treated rats with either saline or vigabatrin and then proceeded to give repeated subconvulsive stimulation to the amygdala to try to produce epileptogenesis. During 16 stimulations, the saline-treated rats developed mild to fully developed generalized seizures, while the vigabatrin-treated rats remained seizure free. After a 10 day rest period, the rats which were previously treated with vigabatrin had to go through the entire kindling procedure to develop fully kindled seizures while the saline-treated rats exhibited fully developed seizures immediately.

3. Neuroprotective Effects

Stimulation of the perforant pathway is a model of status epilepticus. In a study from Finland (YLINEN et al. 1991), rats were pretreated with vigabatrin and compared with rats pretreated with saline. Stimulation of the perforant pathway caused status epilepticus in all animals. Postmortem examination of the hippocampi from the animals revealed that the saline-treated rats had evidence of cell damage and loss of somatostatin-containing interneurons in the dentate gyrus. The vigabatrin-treated rats had histologically normal hippocampi. The authors suggested that this is evidence that vigabatrin has a neuroprotective effect on the hippocampal structures during status epilepticus. In another study using the same methodology, the efficacies of carbamazepine and vigabatrin alone and in combination were assessed to determine if there was a difference between the two drugs in their capacities to prevent cell loss in the hippocampi. It was found that vigabatrin, both alone and in combination with carbamazepine, was more effective in preventing neuronal cell loss than carbamazepine monotherapy was (PITKÄNEN and HALONEN 1995).

III. Humans

1. CSF and Brain Concentrations of GABA and Other Amino Acids

The effects of vigabatrin on the human brain have been studied indirectly by measuring CSF concentrations of GABA and other neurotransmitters and amino acids. Early studies investigated the short-term relationship between vigabatrin and GABA in the CSF (Grove et al. 1981). Patients with various neurological conditions were given 0.5, 1, 2, or 6g vigabatrin daily for 3 days. Free and total GABA, beta-alanine, homocarnosine and vigabatrin increased in a dose-responsive manner. In another study (Schechter et al. 1984), ten patients were given 0.5g vigabatrin twice daily followed by 1g twice daily for 2 weeks and then spent 2 weeks receiving placebo. No changes from baseline values were found in the concentrations of homovanillic acid (the metabolite of dopamine) and 5-hydroxyindoleacetic acid (the metabolite of serotonin), but dose-related increases were seen in free and total GABA concentrations. By the end of the placebo period the levels of GABA had declined to baseline values.

No consistent changes in the concentrations of acetylcholine, somatostatin, beta-endorphins, prolactin, c-AMP, or c-GMP, amino acids, homovanillic acid or 5-hydroxyindoleacetic acid were observed in both brain tissue and CSF during chronic treatment with doses of vigabatrin up to 50mg/kg/day for 3 years (Pitkänen et al. 1987; Sivenius et al. 1987; Ben-Menachem et al. 1991). In a single dose study, however, homovanillic acid and 5-hydroxyindoleacetic acid concentrations initially increased up to 100%, but returned to the baseline level or slightly below the baseline level after 1 month of treatment (Ben-Menachem et al. 1988).

At a dose of 50mg/kg/day, vigabatrin caused a 200%–300% increase in GABA in the CSF and brain tissue (Ben-Menachem et al. 1993). A reduction of vigabatrin dose from 3g/day to 1.5g/day resulted in a proportional decrease of GABA levels in the CSF (Sivenius et al. 1987). The vigabatrin dose and the percentage increase in CSF GABA concentrations show a linear relationship, but the relationship between the dose and the efficacy appears more complex and may depend on the nature of the epilepsy that is present. Kälviäinen et al. (1993) have suggested that responders to vigabatrin monotherapy have higher glutamate levels (increased 14%) in the CSF before receiving the drug than the patients who do not respond.

2. Magnetic Resonance Spectroscopy

Recently ^{1}H-magnetic resonance spectroscopy in patients treated with vigabatrin in addition to conventional antiepileptic drugs has confirmed the observations of the CSF studies. Petroff et al. (1996) found that after a single 50mg/kg dose of vigabatrin, GABA levels, as determined by magnetic resonance spectroscopy, were increased by 40% after 2h and by 65% after 24h. By 5 days the GABA levels had declined, but were slightly above their initial values at 8 days. In another magnetic resonance spectroscopy study, GABA levels increased in a dose-dependent way during chronic intake of vigabatrin at 2g and 3g/day, but there was no further increase when the dose was increased to 6g/day (Petroff et al. 1996). These authors also found increased levels of glutamine and corresponding decreased levels of glutamate (by 9%)

in vigabatrin-treated patients compared with other patients who received conventional antiepileptic drug therapy alone (Petroff et al. 1995). The significance of this is unclear.

3. Effects on Platelets

Administration of therapeutic doses of vigabatrin causes a marked reduction in platelet GABA transaminase. Doses of 2 g/day will inhibit platelet GABA transaminase maximally, with a mean enzyme inhibition of approximately 70% (Richens 1991). The concentration of plasma vigabatrin is almost 10 times that seen in the CSF; since platelets cannot regenerate GABA transaminase, the effect of vigabatrin on this test system will also be influenced by platelet replacement rates.

4. Human Epilepsy

a) Adults with Partial Seizures

Many studies have been conducted during the 16 years of clinical investigation of vigabatrin confirming the efficacy of the drug, especially for partial seizures and infantile spasms. Consistently, patients in these studies have experienced a 50% or greater reduction in their seizure rates.

α) Major Single-Blind Studies

Meta-analysis of the first 10 single-blind studies testing the clinical efficacy of vigabatrin in 352 patients with intractable partial seizures demonstrated that 55.8% had experienced a greater than 50% seizure reduction (Gram et al. 1983; Schechter et al. 1984; Browne et al. 1987; Besser and Kramer 1989; Cocito et al. 1989; Faedda et al. 1989; Mumford and Dam, 1989; Zaccara et al. 1990; Michelucci et al. 1991; Otto and Egli 1991; Ried et al. 1991). All the patients in these studies had epilepsy that was highly intractable to standard antiepileptic drugs. One study has been carried out in patients with less severely intractable epilepsy (de Bittencourt et al. 1994). Here vigabatrin was given in a single-blind design to 19 patients with 4 partial seizures monthly. All participants had to be socially integrated and active outpatients. In this group, 14 of 19 patients had a greater than 50% seizure reduction and 10 patients (52%) had a greater than 70% seizure reduction. Two patients developed myoclonic jerks, whereas none has been reported previously. No deleterious effects on cognitive function were noted.

β) Major Double-Blind Studies

Six double-blind placebo-controlled cross-over studies, all of which were conducted in Europe, were published in the late 1980s. Two of the studies included some patients with generalized tonic-clonic seizures (Remy et al. 1986; Tassinari et al. 1987). The initial efficacy analysis, which included these particular patients, showed that the vigabatrin treatment groups did not differ significantly from the placebo groups. However, when the patients with generalized tonic-clonic seizures without partial seizures were omitted, both studies showed highly significant effects of vigabatrin, as did the other four studies which included only patients with partial seizures. In all six studies, the vigabatrin dose range was 2–3 g/day, given as add-on therapy to other standard antiepileptic drugs. Between 0% and 7% of patients became seizure-free, and the percent of patients with a greater than 50% seizure reduction varied between 33% and 64% (Rimmer and Richens 1984; Gram et al. 1985; Loiseau et al. 1986; Remy et al. 1986; Tartara et al. 1986; Tassinari et al. 1987).

In the United States, two large double-blind placebo-controlled studies with parallel rather than cross-over design were completed recently. These two trials were multicentre ones (Penry et al. 1993; French et al. 1996). All patients ($n = 356$) had complex partial seizures with or without secondary generalization. The dosing arms were 1, 3, and 6 g/day. Both trials demonstrated a statistically significant reduction in seizures when vigabatrin was compared with placebo. In the French et al. study evaluating 3 g/day, 43% of patients achieved a >50% reduction in seizures ($p < 0.001$ vs. placebo), with 5% of patients becoming seizure-free. In the Penry study, which compared 1, 3, and 6 g/day with placebo, a greater than 50% reduction in seizures was seen in 24%, 51% and 54% of patients respectively ($p < 0.0001$ for the 3 and 6 g doses versus placebo). Freedom from seizures occurred in 9.3% of the 3 g/day and 7.3% of the 6 g/day patients.

Very similar results were obtained in another placebo-controlled, double-blind, cross-over study from Australia which evaluated vigabatrin doses of 2 g/day and 3 g/day compared with placebo as add-on therapy in 97 patients with uncontrolled partial seizures (Beran et al. 1996; Table 1).

Recently a study in France (Arzimanoglou et al. 1997) has been completed in which vigabatrin was given to a group of patients with partial seizures who were usually seen in a broad routine clinical practice. Although this was not a double-blind study, it is of interest because it is a large study which reflects the type of results obtained with patients in ordinary clinical practice. These patients had less frequent seizures (<8 seizures/month) than patients who participated in the previous controlled clinical trials. A total of 397 patients between 12 and 74 years of age participated. After a 3 month baseline period, the patients were given 2 g vigabatrin/day as add-on therapy. The dose could be increased as required up to 4 g/day; the mean dose proved to be 2.2 g/day. Patients were followed for 4 months with regards to the efficacy and the tolerability of the treatment. There were 13.5% of patients who remained seizure-free for the entire 4 months and 39.8% who were seizure-free during the last month of the study. A further 17.4% experienced a 50% or greater seizure reduction. In the 77 patients with secondarily generalized seizures, 56.7% were seizure-free. Drowsiness and sleep disturbances were the most commonly reported adverse events. The drug was stopped in 8%, and the dose reduced in 6%, due to adverse events.

Table 1. Efficacy in single-blind and double-blind studies with vigabatrin (French and Ben-Menachem 1996)

Author	Year of publication	Number of patients	Percent of patients with 50% seizure reduction	Type of study	Type of epilepsy
Gram et al.	1983	15	Not available	Single-blind	Partial
Schechter et al.	1984	10	70	Single-blind	Partial
Browne et al.	1987	89	51	Single-blind	Complex partial
Cocito et al.	1989	19	63	Single-blind	Partial
Bittencourt et al.	1994	19	73	Single-blind	Partial
Rimmer and Richens	1984	22	64	Double-blind	Partial
Gram et al.	1985	18	44	Double-blind	Partial
Loiseau et al.	1986	17	53	Double-blind	Partial, but some generalized
Tartara et al.	1986	23	59	Double-blind	Partial but some with absence/atonic
Remy et al.	1986	23	7	Double-blind	Partial but some generalized
Tassinari et al.	1987	30	33	Double-blind	Partial, myoclonus, unspecified
Ring et al.	1990	33	60	Double-blind	Partial
French et al.	1996	182	44	Double-blind	Complex partial
Penry et al.	1993	172	54	Double-blind	Complex partial
Beran et al.	1997	97	Not available	Double-blind	Complex partial
Kälviänen et al.	1995	100: 50-CBZ, 50-VGB	Percent seizure-free: 50% CBZ, 42% VGB	Monotherapy, double-blind	All seizure types
Tanganelli et al.	1996	51	Percent seizure-free: 51.3% CBZ, 45.9% VGB	Monotherapy, double-blind	Complex partial

VGB, vigabatrin; CBZ, carbamazepine.

γ) Monotherapy Studies

Two single-centre trials are now completed and another large double-blind multicentre trial is currently being analysed. The single-centre open label randomized studies from Finland and Italy (Kälviänen et al. 1995; Tanganelli and Regestra 1996) compared carbamazepine and vigabatrin when used as the first drug for new onset seizures. Patients were included independent of the seizure type in the Finnish study, but only patients with partial seizures were included in the Italian study. The efficacies of the drugs during 1 year follow-up were the same in both groups for patients who had partial seizures. Twenty-one of 50 patients in the vigabatrin group and 25 of 50 in the carbamazepine group remained seizure-free in the Finnish study while 45.9% of the vigabatrin group and 51.3% of the carbamazepine group in the Italian study were seizure-free. There were more drop-outs in the carbamazepine group, due to adverse events (12 for the carbamazepine group and none in the vigabatrin group) and more drop-outs in the vigabatrin group because of lack of efficacy (14 in the vigabatrin group and 4 in the carbamazepine group) in the Finnish study. In the Italian study 41% of the carbamazepine group reported adverse events, while 21.6% did so in the vigabatrin group.

δ) Long-term Studies

There have been numerous long-term follow-up studies published. Some studies have reported follow-up for periods of more than 7 years. It is unusual for any antiepileptic drug to have such long-term results reported. For patients who were initially responders, the efficacy was maintained in about 60%. Breakthrough seizures did occur, but it is not clear if any other concomitant antiepileptic drug had had its dose reduced or had been withdrawn (Remy and Beaumont 1989; Browne et al. 1991; Sivenius et al. 1991; Tartara et al. 1992; Cocito et al. 1993; Michelucci et al. 1994). Tolerance is not thought to be a problem when vigabatrin is used, especially when its efficacy has been demonstrated to be maintained over so many years of follow-up.

b) Children with Partial Seizures

In an open trial in 135 children with various types of seizures (Livingston et al. 1989), vigabatrin was administered at doses of between 40 and 80 mg/kg/day. Eleven patients became seizure-free and another 37% had a greater than 50% reduction in seizures, a result very similar to those seen in the adult studies. Patients with partial seizures showed the best responses. In another study, 16 children with refractory epilepsy were given vigabatrin; again the patients with partial seizures responded most favourably. Myoclonic epilepsy tended to be aggravated (Luna et al. 1989). One long term follow-up study reported that after 5 years 7 of 12 children continued to have a greater than 50% reduction in seizures. The drug lost efficacy in four children (33%). One child went on to surgery, though vigabatrin was still effective at the time of surgery (Uldall et the al. 1995).

c) Children with Infantile Spasms

Infantile spasms are extremely difficult to treat. Most therapies either are not very effective or cause unacceptable side effects. Infantile spasms are included in the category of catastrophic seizure syndromes. The first report that vigabatrin could be effective in this seizure type was by CHIRON et al. (1991). These investigators found in this single uncontrolled study of 70 children that 37 had a significant reduction in spasms. The response was most impressive in the group of patients with symptomatic infantile spasms, especially those with tuberous sclerosis, of whom 71% achieved short term freedom from seizures. In the long-term follow-up, 55% continued to be seizure-free, including all those with tuberous sclerosis. APPLETON et al. (1995) reported the results from a 2 year follow-up of infantile spasms in the United Kingdom. At the time of the report 20 patients aged 3–11 months (14 with symptomatic infantile spasms) had been treated with vigabatrin as their initial drug. The drug was given at a starting dose of 50–80 mg/kg/day and increased to a maximum dose of 150 mg/kg/day. In these children, 13 of 20 patients were seizure-free for 30 months. Four children showed no response at all to vigabatrin: the other 3 had a greater than 75% seizure reduction, but were not seizure-free. The response to vigabatrin occurred within 72 h of starting the drug. No adverse side effects were seen in the 20 patients. Since then a retrospective analysis of 25 infants with infantile spasms treated with vigabatrin has been reported (AICARDI et al. 1995) and a double-blind comparison of vigabatrin with placebo for infantile spasms has just been completed and will soon be published. In the retrospective study, infants with tuberous sclerosis and those younger than 3 months at the onset of seizures did best (96% and 90% initially seizure-free, respectively). By the end of the study 96 of 192 infants who could be evaluated long term remained seizure-free. The most recent published report is a randomized comparative trial of vigabatrin or hydrocortisone in infantile spasms due to tuberous sclerosis (CHIRON et al. 1997). All patients initially treated with vigabatrin (n = 11) became seizure-free, compared with 5 of 11 patients treated with hydrocortisone. All the patients given hydrocortisone who were not seizure-free or who had adverse events (n = 7) became symptom free when treated with vigabatrin. The mean time to disappearance of infantile spasms in the vigabatrin group was 3.5 days, but 13 days in the responders to hydrocortisone.

d) Children with the Lennox-Gastaut Syndrome

There have only been a few published reports on the use of vigabatrin in treating the Lennox-Gastaut syndrome. Some have reported an increase in seizure frequency after vigabatrin therapy in patients with the syndrome and with myoclonic epilepsy (MICHELUCCI et al. 1989; LORTIE et al. 1993), whereas others have reported significant improvement (HERRANZ et al. 1991; FEUCHT et al. 1994). One factor in this discrepancy could be the dose of vigabatrin given. Patients with the Lennox-Gastaut syndrome often require lower doses than patients with other seizure types. Rarely, myoclonic jerks may develop during the course of vigabatrin treatment, necessitating withdrawal of the drug (DE BITTENCOURT et al. 1994).

C. Pharmacokinetics

I. Absorption and Bioavailability

Oral vigabatrin absorption is rapid with the peak plasma concentrations of the drug being reached within the first 2h after dosing (HAEGELE et al. 1986, 1988; SALETU et al. 1986). The absorption half-life ranges from 0.18 to 0.59h. The oral bioavailability is at least 60%–80%. There are no vigabatrin metabolites found in human urine; probably the amount of a vigabatrin dose that is not recovered in the urine simply disappears as the drug is tightly bound to GABA transaminase, which undergoes degradation within the body.

Food does not affect the extent of vigabatrin absorption. The plasma AUC for fasted and for fed volunteers did not differ significantly. Therefore the time of administration, and what and when a person eats, does not influence the clinical response to vigabatrin (FRISK-HOLMBERG et al. 1989; HOKE et al. 1991).

II. Distribution

1. Body Tissues and Fluids

The distribution of vigabatrin in the body is very wide. This is due to its water solubility and because vigabatrin does not bind to plasma proteins. The apparent volume of distribution is 0.8l/kg (total body water is 0.6l/kg) in volunteers and its half-life of distribution is 1–2h. It is estimated that between 50% and 75% of the drug in the body is outside the central blood compartment at steady state (SCHECHTER 1986).

The concentration of vigabatrin in the CSF in patients with epilepsy treated with other concomitant antiepileptic drugs was approximately 10% of the blood vigabatrin level (BEN-MENACHEM et al. 1988). The highest concentrations of vigabatrin were found in the CSF after a sampling point at 6h. By 24h only a trace was detectable in the CSF, while no vigabatrin was found at 72h or thereafter. The peak vigabatrin concentration in the blood was reached by 1h and thereafter decreased, with only small amounts being detectable by 72h. After chronic treatment with vigabatrin at 50mg/kg/day for 3 years, the levels of CSF vigabatrin were not significantly increased when compared with the concentration of vigabatrin found at 6 months (BEN-MENACHEM et al. 1991).

2. Placental Transfer

The transfer of vigabatrin from maternal to foetal blood across the placenta is low and comparable to that of other α-amino acids. The clearance for both the S(+) and R(–) enantiomers is about 27% of that of phenazone (CHALLIER et al. 1992).

III. Elimination

1. Metabolism

As mentioned above, vigabatrin is not metabolized in humans. The amount absorbed is excreted unchanged in the urine. Vigabatrin does not induce hepatic cytochrome P-450 dependent enzymes (MUMFORD 1988; RICHENS 1991).

2. Elimination Parameters

The elimination half-life of vigabatrin is 5–8h, and the total clearance about 1.7–1.9ml/min/kg, with renal clearance accounting for 70% of the total clearance. The drug's elimination is not influenced by its dose or by the duration of treatment (GRANT et al. 1991). It should be stressed that the biological half-life of the drug is of the order of days, not hours.

IV. Clinical Pharmacokinetics

The elimination of vigabatrin is slower in elderly volunteers because of their lower creatinine clearances and smaller distribution volumes. There is a direct correlation between the renal clearance of vigabatrin and the creatinine clearance. A reduced renal clearance causes an increase of the AUC/body weight ratio. Renally impaired patients therefore have higher plasma concentrations of vigabatrin and it has a longer terminal half-life. The half-life in the elderly with reduced creatinine clearances is approximately twice that in normal healthy volunteers and the AUC is 7 times higher than in the young. Analysis of AUC/body weight versus clearance shows a non-linear increase in AUC/body weight ratio as creatinine clearance falls below 60mg/min. In patients with lower renal clearances, the extrarenal clearance may compensate to some extent (HAEGELE et al. 1988).

In children the renal clearance is the same as in adults, but the plasma concentration AUC is smaller. In other words, the bioavailability is somewhat lower in children. This explains why proportionately higher doses of vigabatrin are needed to achieve the same effect in children as in adults.

D. Interactions

Because vigabatrin is not metabolized, almost the whole ingested dose being excreted unchanged in the urine, the drug does not interact significantly with other drugs except for phenytoin. Plasma phenytoin concentrations have been reported as being lower by up to 20% in two placebo controlled clinical trials

(RIMMER and RICHENS 1984; BROWNE et al. 1987). This lowering has not been a consistent observation. There is still no clear explanation of the observed reductions since no changes have been found in phenytoin protein binding, absorption, metabolism or clearance (RIMMER and RICHENS 1989; RICHENS 1991). There is no evidence that there is any loss of anticonvulsant efficacy due to these lowered concentrations. The phenytoin dosage therefore does not need to be adjusted.

E. Adverse Effects

I. General Effects

The first trials of vigabatrin were reported in 1981. Therefore reports of adverse events of the drug are based on 16 years of clinical trials as well as on vigabatrin's availability to the population with epilepsy over 8 years as a marketed drug. In clinical trials (data on file at Hoechst Marion Roussel), sedation and fatigue have been the most commonly reported side effects. In clinical trials about 2% of subjects withdrew due to drug intolerability alone.

Studies have been published on the cognitive effects of treatment with vigabatrin. While all confirm that vigabatrin does not cause deterioration of cognitive performances, some even demonstrate that an improvement performance in certain test performances can occur (DIJKSTRA et al. 1992; DODRILL et al. 1993; DE BITTENCOURT et al. 1994; GRUENEWALD et al. 1994; KÄLVIÄINEN et al. 1995; PROVINCIALI et al. 1995).

Although more than 140,000 patients are estimated to have been treated with vigabatrin with an exposure of more than 200,000 patient years, no idiosyncratic adverse events have yet been associated with the use of the drug (Table 2).

II. Psychosis

The possibility that vigabatrin may elicit a psychosis has been discussed extensively. This issue became pertinent when the first reports were published, describing 14 of 210 patients who experienced severe psychiatric reactions while taking vigabatrin (SANDER et al. 1990, 1991). Subsequently others have published case reports and issued warnings that vigabatrin can cause psychosis. The two United States multicentre, placebo-controlled double-blind studies discussed above (PENRY et al. 1993; FRENCH et al. 1996) included a careful analysis of psychiatric side effects to try to address the questions raised by the various anecdotal reports in the literature. The two studies did not, however, include patients with severe brain damage or severe psychiatric disorders, which the case reports did. The results of the two studies revealed that 2.2% in the 1 g/day treatment group ($n = 45$), 6.6% in the 3 g/day group ($n = 135$), and 7.3% in the 6 g/day group ($n = 41$) dropped out because of psychiatric

Table 2. Most frequently reported treatment-related adverse events for vigabatrin (>3% reporting) (derived from data on file MMD)

Adverse event	Multicentre placebo-controlled parallel designed studies. Placebo ($N = 135$); N (%)	Multicentre placebo-controlled parallel designed studies. Vigabatrin ($N = 222$); N (%)	All studies when treatment causality is assessed. $N = 1175$; N (%)
Whole body			
Weight increase	5 (3.7)	16 (7.2)	76 (6.5)
Asthenia	3 (2.2)	11 (5.0)	30 (2.6)
Pain	3 (3.0)	7 (3.2)	16 (1.4)
Dermatological			
Rash	6 (4.4)	7 (3.2)	16 (1.4)
Gastrointestinal			
Abdominal pain	5 (3.7)	7 (3.2)	26 (2.2)
Constipation	4 (3.0)	8 (3.6)	34 (2.9)
Diarrhoea	5 (3.7)	16 (7.2)	23 (2.0)
Dyspepsia	5 (3.7)	11 (5.0)	25 (2.1)
Nausea	8 (5.9)	15 (6.8)	31 (2.6)
CNS related			
Ataxia	9 (6.7)	20 (9.0)	51 (4.3)
Concentration impaired	2 (1.5)	11 (5.0)	29 (2.5)
Confusion	2 (1.5)	12 (6.4)	27 (2.3)
Coordination abnormal	4 (3.0)	14 (6.3)	22 (1.9)
Dizziness	18 (13.3)	46 (20.1)	95 (8.1)
Drowsiness	24 (17.8)	61 (27.5)	180 (15.3)
Fatigue	21 (15.6)	61 (27.5)	167 (14.2)
Headache	21 (15.6)	39 (17.6)	89 (7.6)
Hypoasthesia	2 (1.5)	8 (3.6)	16 (1.4)
Hyporeflexia	1 (0.7)	9 (4.1)	9 (0.8)
Nystagmus	11 (8.1)	33 (14.9)	47 (4.0)
Paresthesia	3 (2.2)	19 (8.6)	28 (2.4)
Speech disorder	1 (0.7)	7 (3.2)	22 (1.9)
Vertigo	2 (1.6)	8 (3.6)	33 (2.8)
Psychiatric			
Agitation	10 (7.4)	25 (11.3)	60 (5.1)
Depression	4 (3.0)	22 (9.9)	41 (3.5)
Thinking abnormal	1 (0.7)	11 (5.0)	16 (1.4)
Visual			
Diplopia	0 (0.0)	12 (5.4)	40 (3.4)
Vision abnormal	8 (5.9)	25 (11.3)	55 (4.7)

adverse events. This supports the contention that significant psychiatric adverse events will appear in about 5% of patients treated with vigabatrin who have not previously had psychiatric disease. In the study of Arzimanoglou et al. (1997) in which 397 patients participated, 7.1% reported irritability as an adverse event, but only 1.5% reported mood disorders and 0.7% psychic disorders.

A large postmarketing surveillance study of vigabatrin from the Drug Safety Research Unit at the University of Southampton, involving over 6000 patients, was done to try to clarify whether vigabatrin causes psychosis more often than other antiepileptic drugs. In this database, psychosis-like reactions such as manifest psychosis, hallucinations, paranoia or delusions were reported in only 88 cases, i.e. 0.64% (Data on file at Hoescht Marion Roussel), which is not greater than the rate of reported severe psychiatric adverse events seen in treatment with other antiepileptic drugs (Matsuo et al. 1993; Wolf et al. 1993; Cockerell et al. 1996). Therefore the data do not suggest that vigabatrin causes psychosis more often than any other antiepileptic drug. However, as a precaution, patients who have a history of severe psychiatric disturbances or very severe brain damage should be given low doses of vigabatrin initially, and the dose should be titrated upwards with caution. This recommendation in fact also applies to any other antiepileptic drug, especially the newer ones. Sudden withdrawal of vigabatrin can lead to postictal psychosis, so that it is important to taper vigabatrin dosage slowly, by about 500 mg every 5 days.

III. Visual Field Defects

Recently there have been reports that vigabatrin may cause visual field defects in patients who have used the drug for several years. So far only anecdotal reports have been published. Eke et al. (1997) reported visual abnormalities in 3 patients who received vigabatrin as add-on therapy but none of the cases had ever had baseline perimetry done. It is most unclear if the patients had these visual field deficits before treatment, or if other antiepileptic drugs can cause the same changes. Vigabatrin is often given as add-on therapy to severely resistant patients and is seldom given as monotherapy. This issue needs to be addressed promptly. Hoescht Marion Roussel is currently conducting further studies to attempt to determine if visual field defects are caused by vigabatrin and if other patients with partial epilepsy who have not been treated with vigabatrin have defects in their visual fields. A draft report of a pilot study (on file at Hoescht Marion Roussel) investigating the prevalence of visual field defects in patients treated with antiepileptic drugs other than vigabatrin found that 3 of 15 patients (20%) showed visual field defects of unknown origin which were mild to moderate in severity. A larger study is currently in progress.

IV. Teratogenicity

No severe teratogenic effects in animals have been reported except for an increased incidence of cleft palate in the group of rabbits receiving a very high dose of vigabatrin. Like all antiepileptic drugs, vigabatrin has a class warning against use in pregnancy, because of inadequate evidence for or against teratogenic effects. Information exists on over 100 pregnancies treated with vigabatrin, with almost all patients having taken at least one other antiepileptic drug. There do not appear to be data which suggest that vigabatrin has any specific teratogenetic effect. The results are, however, clearly inconclusive.

F. Use in Clinical Practice

I. Dosage

In clinical trials most researchers have used vigabatrin doses varying between 2 and 3g daily or up to 50mg/kg/day in adults and 150mg/kg/day in children (BEN-MENACHEM et al. 1989; CHIRON et al. 1997). In the United States double-blind placebo-controlled study (PENRY et al. 1993) where a 6g/day dose was used, the results showed that there was a somewhat higher rate of seizure-free patients, but at the cost of more side effects. The consensus today is that 3g is an average effective daily dose in adults. At this dose the CSF GABA level will increase by 200%–300%. If this dose is not effective, the drug dosage should be tapered down at a rate of about 500mg every 5days. This enables the GABA concentrations to stabilize at a new level before reducing the vigabatrin further. Hopefully this slow taper will prevent status epilepticus or the psychosis which can be elicited by rapid cessation of vigabatrin.

Vigabatrin may be given once or twice daily. The tablet is tasteless and dissolves completely in fluids and therefore can be given to infants or children in water or juice or milk. Sachets are available, which simplifies dosing in children.

II. Dose Titration

In the initial studies with vigabatrin, the full dose was given immediately. Today the practice is to increase it gradually to minimize side effects, since it has been suggested that a gradual dosage increase might reduce the frequency of reported psychiatric or behavioural side effects such as confusion or depression. In addition, some patients with milder epilepsy might respond to lower doses of vigabatrin, thereby decreasing the need to titrate the dose up to its full value.

For patients with severe brain damage, as in those with the Lennox-Gastaut syndrome, it is wise to start treatment with only one 500mg vigabatrin tablet/day and to increase the dose no faster than by 500mg weekly.

III. Laboratory Monitoring

The concentration of vigabatrin in the blood and CSF can be measured using several different methodologies. One of the easiest is a single-step protein precipitation with subsequent precolumn derivatization with *o*-phthaldialdehyde and direct injection into a Microsorb C18 column, as described by TSANCLIS et al. (1991). Other antiepileptic drugs were found not to interfere with the assay. Compared with previous methodologies for vigabatrin determination, this HPLC method requires only a small volume (50 μl) of sample for analysis and is faster and easier to use. Enantiospecific assays for the drug are mentioned in Chap. 7.

There is, however, no necessity to monitor blood vigabatrin levels in patients. Since the drug is effective only by virtue of its irreversible inhibition of GABA transaminase, the concentration of vigabatrin in the blood is not closely related to its biological effect and hence the measurement is not relevant clinically. Even when assessing compliance, measuring the blood levels of the drug is not appropriate. If the patient takes just one full dose of vigabatrin in the morning before the blood sample is collected, the blood level is likely to appear clinically acceptable.

References

Aicardi J, Sabril IS Investigator and Peer Review Groups, Mumford JP, Dumas C, Wood S (1996) Vigabatrin as initial therapy for infantile spasms: a European retrospective survey. Epilepsia 37:638–642

Appleton R (1995) Vigabatrin in the management of generalized seizures in children. Seizures 4:45–48

Arzimanoglou AA, Dumas C, Ghirardi L, and the French Neurologists Sabril Study Group (1997) Multicentre clinical evaluation of vigabatrin (Sabril) in mild to moderate partial epilepsies. Seizure 6:225–231

Ben-Menachem E, Persson L, Schechter PJ et al. (1988) Effects of single doses of vigabatrin on CSF concentrations of GABA, homocarnosine, homovanillic acid and 5-hydroxyindoleacetic acid in patients with complex partial seizures. Epilepsy Res 2:96–101

Ben-Menachem E, Persson LI, Schechter PJ et al. (1989) The effect of different vigabatrin treatment regimens on CSF biochemistry and seizure control in epileptic patients. Br J Clin Pharmac 27:79S–85 S

Ben-Menachem E, Persson LI, Mumford JP (1991) Effect of long term vigabatrin therapy on selected CSF neurotransmitter concentrations. J Child Neurology 6 [Suppl 2]:11–16

Ben-Menachem E, Mumford J, Hamberger A (1993) Effect of long-term vigabatrin therapy on GABA and other amino acid concentrations in the central nervous system – a case study. Epilepsy Res 16:241–243

Beran RG, Berkovic SF, Buchanan N et al. (1996) A double-blind, placebo-controlled cross-over study of vigabatrin 2 g/day and 3 g/day in uncontrolled partial seizures. Seizure 5:259–265

Besser R, Kramer G (1989) Long-term efficacy and safety of vigabatrin in epileptic patients. 18th International Epilepsy Congress, New Dehli Book of Abstracts, p. 155

Browne TR, Mattson RH. Penry JK et al. (1987) Vigabatrin for refractory complex partial seizures. Multicenter single-blind study and long-term follow-up. Neurology 37:184–189

Browne TR, Mattson RH, Penry JK et al. (1991) Multicenter long-term safety and efficacy study of vigabatrin for refractory complex partial seizures; an update. Neurology 41:363–364

Challier JC, Rey E, Binten T, Olive G (1992) Passage of S (+) and R (–) gamma-vinyl-GABA across the human isolated perfused placenta. Br J Clin Pharmac 34:139–143

Chiron C, Dulac O, Beaumont D et al. (1991) Therapeutic trial of vigabatrin in refractory infantile spasms. J Child Neurol 6 [Suppl 2]:S52–S59

Chiron C, Dumas C, Jambaque I, Mumford J, Dulac O (1997) Randomized trial comparing vigabatrin and hydrocortisone in infantile spasms due to tuberous sclerosis. Epilepsy Res 26:389–395

Cocito L, Maffini M, Perfumo P et al. (1989) Vigabatrin in complex partial seizures: a long-term study. Epilepsy Res 3:160–166

Cockerell C, Moriaty J, Trimble MR, Shorvon SD, Sander JWAS (1996) Epidemiological survey of acute psychological disorders in epilepsy. Epilepsy Res 25:119–131

de Bittencourt PRM, Mazer S, Marcourakis T, Bigarella MM, Ferreira ZS, Mumford JP (1994) Vigabatrin: clinical evidence supporting rational polytherapy in management of uncontrolled seizures. Epilepsia 35:373–380

Dijkstra JB, McGuire AM, Trimble MR (1992) The effect of vigabatrin on cognitive function and mood. Hum Psychopharmacol 7:329–323

Dodrill CB, Arnett JL, Sommerville KW, Sussman NM (1993) Evaluation of the effects of vigabatrin on cognitive abilities and quality of life. Neurology 43:2501–2507

Eke T, Talbot JF, Lawden MC (1997) Severe persistent visual field constriction associated with vigabatrin. Brit Med J 314:180–181

Faedda MT, Lani C, Paris L et al. (1989) Clinical results of vigabatrin treatment in patients with refractory epilepsy. In: Manelis J, Bental E, Loeber JN et al. (eds) Advances in epileptology. Raven Press, New York, pp. 170–171

Feucht M, Brantner-Inthaler S.(1994) Gamma-vinyl GABA (vigabatrin) in the therapy of Lennox-Gastaut Syndrome: an open study. Epilepsia 35:993–998

French JA, Mosier M, Walker K, Sommerville K, Sussman N and the Vigabatrin Protocol 024 Investigative Cohort (1996) A double-blind placebo-controlled study of vigabatrin three g/day in patients with uncontrolled complex partial seizures. Neurology 46:54–61

Frisk-Holmberg M, Kerth P, Meyer P (1989) Effect of food on the absorption of vigabatrin. Br J Clin Pharmac 27:23S–25 S

Gale K (1986) Role of the substantia nigra in GABA-mediated anticonvulsant actions. In: Delgado-Escueta AV, Ward AA, Woodbury DM, Porter RJ (eds) Basic mechanisms of the epilepsies. Molecular and cellular approaches. Adv Neurol 44:343–364

Gram L, Lyon BB, Dam M (1983) Gamma-vinyl GABA: a single-blind trial in patients with epilepsy. Acta Neurol Scand 68:34–39

Gram L, Klosterskov P, Dam M (1985) Gamma-vinyl GABA: a double-blind, placebo-controlled trial in partial epilepsy. Ann Neurol 17:262–266

Grant SM, Heel RC (1991) Vigabatrin: a review of its pharmacodynamic and pharmacokinetic properties and therapeutic potential in epilepsy and disorders of motor control. Drugs 4:889–926

Gruenewald RA, Thompson PJ, Corcoran R et al. (1994) Effects of vigabatrin on partial seizures and cognitive function. J Neurol Neurosurg Psych 57:1057–1063

Haegele KD, Schechter PJ (1986) Kinetics of the enantiomers of vigabatrin after an oral dose of the racemate or the active S-enantiomer. Clin Pharmac Ther 40:581–586

Haegele KD, Huebert ND, Ebel M et al. (1988) Pharmacokinetics of vigabatrin: implications of creatinine clearance. Clin Pharm and Therap 44:558–565

Herranz JL, Arteaga R, Farr IN et al. (1991) Dose-response study of vigabatrin in children with refractory epilepsy. J Child Neurol 6 [Suppl 2]:S45–S51

Hoke JF, Chi EM, Antony K et al. (1991) Effect of food on the bioavailability of vigabatrin tablets. Epilepsia 32 [Suppl 3):7

Jung MJ, Lippert B, Metcalf BW et al. (1977) Gamma-vinyl GABA (4-amino-hex-5-enoic acid), a new selective irreversible inhibitor of GABA-T: effects on brain GABA metabolism in mice. Neurochem 29:797–802

Kälviäinen R, Halonen T, Pitkänen A, Riekkinen PJ (1993) Amino acid levels in the cerebrospinal fluid of newly diagnosed epileptic patients: effect of vigabatrin and carbamazepine monotherapy. J Neurochem 60:1244–1250

Kälviäinen R, Aikia M, Saukkonen AM et al. (1995) Vigabatrin versus carbamazepine monotherapy in patients with newly diagnosed epilepsy. A randomized controlled study. Arch Neurol 52:989–996
Kendall DA, Fox DA, Enna SJ (1981) Effects of gamma-vinyl GABA on bicuculline-induced seizures. Neuropharmacol 20:351–355
Lippert B, Metcalf B, Jung MJ, Casara P (1977) 4-amino-hex-5-enoic acid, a selective catalytic inhibitor of 4-aminobutyric acid aminotransferase in mammalian brain. Eur J Biochem 74:441–445
Livingston JH, Beaumont D, Arzimanoglou A, Aicardi J (1989) Vigabatrin in the treatment of epilepsy in children. Br J Clin Pharm 27 [Suppl 1]:109S–112S
Loiseau P, Hardenberg JP, Pestre M et al. (1986) Double-blind, placebo-controlled study of vigabatrin (gamma-vinyl GABA) in drug resistant epilepsy. Epilepsia 27:115–120
Lortie A, Chiron C, Mumford J, Dulac O (1993) The potential for increasing seizure frequency, relapse, and appearance of new seizure types with vigabatrin. Neurology 43:S24–S27
Luna D, Dulac O, Pajot N, Beaumont D (1989) Vigabatrin in the treatment of childhood epilepsies. A single-blind placebo controlled study. Epilepsia 30:430–437
Matsuo F, Bergen D, Faught E, Messenheimer JA et al. (1993) Placebo-controlled study of efficacy and safety of lamotrigine in patients with partial seizures. Neurology 43:2284–2291
Meldrum BS, Horton R (1978) Blockade of epileptic responses in the photosensitive baboon, Papio papio, by two irreversible inhibitors of GABA-transaminase, gamma-acetylenic GABA (4-amino-hex-5-ynoic acid) and gamma-vinyl GABA (4-amino-hex-5-enoic acid). Psychopharacol 59:47–50
Michelucci R, Tassinari CA (1989) Response to vigabatrin in relation to seizure type. Br J Clin Pharmacol 27 [Suppl 1]:119S–124S
Michelucci R, Plasmati RM Larmeggiani L et al. (1991) Single-blind placebo-controlled dose modification study of vigabatrin in patients with refractory epilepsy. Epilepsia 32 [Suppl 1]:S102
Michelucci R, Veri L, Passarelli D et al.(1994) Long-term follow-up study of vigabatrin in the treatment of refractory epilepsy. J Epilepsy 7:88–93
Mumford JP.(1994) Epilepsy, pregnancy and vigabatrin. Intern Med Newslet 2:2–4
Mumford JP.(1988) A profile of vigabatrin. Br J Clin Pract 42 [Suppl 61]:7–9
Mumford JP, Dam M (1989) Meta-analysis of placebo controlled studies of vigabatrin in drug resistant epilepsy. Br J Clin Pharmacol 27:101S–107S
Otto FG, Egli M (1991) Effect of vigabatrin (gamma-vinyl GABA) on partial attacks of various localizations. In: Scheffner D (ed) Epilepsy 90. Einhoen-Presse Verlag, Reinbek, pp. 230–232
Palfreyman MG, Böhlen P, Huot S, Mellet M (1980) The effect of gamma-vinyl GABA and gamma-acetylenic GABA on the concentration of homocarnosine in brain and CSF of the rat. Brain Res 190:288–292
Penry JK, Wilder BJ, Sachdeo RC et al. (1993) Multicenter dose-response study of vigabatrin in adults with focal (partial) epilepsy. Epilepsia 34 [Suppl 6]:67
Petroff OAC, Rothman DL, Behar KL, Mattson RH (1995) Initial observations of effect of vigabatrin on in vivo ^{1}H spectroscopic measurements of γ-aminobutyric acid, glutamate, and glutamine in human brain. Epilepsia 36:457–464
Petroff OAC, Rothman DL, Behar KL, Collins BA, Mattson RH (1996a) Human brain GABA levels rise rapidly after initiation of vigabatrin therapy. Neurology 47:1567–1571
Petroff OAC, Rothman DL, Behar KL, Mattson RH (1996b) Human brain GABA levels rise after initiation of vigabatrin therapy but fail to rise further with increasing dose. Neurology 46:1459–1463
Piredda S, Lim CR, Gale K (1985) Intracerebral site of convulsant action of bicuculline. Life Sci 56:1295–1298

Pitkänen A, Halonen T (1995) Prevention of neuronal cell death by anticonvulsants in experimental epilepsy (extended abstract) Acta Neurol Scand [Suppl] 162:22–23

Pitkänen A, Halonen T, Ylinen A, Riekkinen P (1987) Somatostatin, β-endorphin, and prolactin levels in human cerebrospinal fluid during the gamma-vinyl GABA treatment of patients with complex partial seizures. Neuropeptides 9:185–195

Provinviali L, Bartolini M, Mari F et al. (1996) Influence of vigabatrin on cognitive performance and behaviour in patients with drug resistant epilepsy. Acta Neurol Scand 94:12–18

Remy C, Beaumont D (1989) Efficacy and safety of vigabatrin in the long-term treatment of refractory epilepsy. Br J Clin Pharmacol 27 [Suppl 1]:125S–129S

Remy C, Favel P, Tell G (1986) Double-blind, placebo-controlled, crossover study of vigabatrin in drug resistant epilepsy of the adult. Boll Lega Ital Epil 54/55:241–243

Rey E, Pons G, Richard MO, et al. (1990) Pharmacokinetics of the individual enantiomers of vigabatrin (gamma-vinyl GABA) in epileptic children. Br J Clin Pharmac 30:253–257

Reynolds EH, Ring HA, Farr IN, Heller AJ, Elwes RDC (1991) Open, double-blind and long-term study of vigabatrin in chronic epilepsy. Epilepsia 32:530–538

Richens A (1991) Pharmacology and clinical pharmacology of vigabatrin. J Child Neurology 6:2S7–2S10

Ried S, Schmidt D, Stodieck SRG et al. (1991) Vigabatrin in pharmaco-resistant epilepsies: a single-blind placebo-controlled study. In: Scheffner E (ed) Epilepsy 90. Einhorn-Presse Verlag, Reinbek, pp. 233–237

Rimmer EM, Richens A (1984) Double-blind study of gamma-vinyl GABA in patients with refractory epilepsy. Lancet 189–190

Rimmer EM, Richens A (1989) Interaction between vigabatrin and phenytoin. Br J Clin Pharmac 27:27S–33S

Saletu B, Grunberger J, Linzmayer L et al. (1986) Psychophysiological and psychometric studies after manipulating the GABA system by vigabatrin, a GABA transaminase inhibitor. Intern J Psychophysiol 4:63–80

Sander JWAS, Hart YM (1990) Vigabatrin and behavior disturbances. Lancet 335:57

Sander JWAS, Hart YM, Trimble MR, Shorvon SD (1991) Behavioral disturbances associated with vigabatrin therapy. Epilepsia 32 [Suppl 1]:12

Schechter PJ (1986) Vigabatrin. In: Meldrum B, Porter RJ (eds) New anticonvulsant drugs. Libby, London, pp. 265–275

Schechter PJ, Tranier Y (1977) Effect of elevated brain GABA concentrations of the actions of bicuculline and picrotoxin in mice. Psychopharmacol 54:145–148

Schechter PJ, Tranier Y, Grove J (1979) Attempts to correlate alterations in brain GABA metabolism by GABA-T inhibitors with their anticonvulsant effects. In: Mandel P, DeFeudes FV (eds) GABA-biochemistry and CNS Functions. Plenum Press, New York, pp. 43–57

Schechter PJ, Hanke NFJ, Grove J et al. (1984) Biochemical and clinical effects of gamma-vinyl GABA in patients with epilepsy. Neurology 34: 34–39

Shin C, Rigsbee LC, McNamara JO (1986) Anti-seizure and anti-epileptogenic effect of gamma-vinyl gamma-aminobutyric acid in amygdaloid kindling. Brain Res 398:370–374

Sivenius MRJ, Ylinen A, Murros K, Matilainen R, Riekkinen P (1987) Double-blind dose-reduction study of vigabatrin in complex partial epilepsy. Epilepsia 28:688–692

Sivenius J, Ylinen A, Murros K, Mumford JP, Riekkinen PJ (1991) Efficacy of vigabatrin in drug-resistant partial epilepsy during a 6-year follow-up period. Epilepsia 32 [Suppl 1]:11

Stevens JR, Phillips I, de Beaurepaire R (1988) Gamma-vinyl GABA in endopiriform area suppresses kindled amygdala seizures. Epilepsia 29:404–411

Tanganelii P, Regesta, G (1996) Vigabatrin versus carbamazepine monotherapy in newly diagnosed epilepsy: a randomized response conditional cross-over study. Epilepsy Res 25:257–262

Tartara A, Manni A, Galimberti CA et al. (1986) Vigabatrin in the treatment of epilepsy: a double-blind placebo controlled study. Epilepsia 27:717–723
Tartara A, Manni A, Galimberti CA et al.(1989) Vigabatrin in the treatment of epilepsy: a long-term follow-up study. J Neurol Neurosurg Psychiatry 52:467–471
Tassinari CA, Michelucci R, Ambroseetto G et al. (1987) Double-blind study of vigabatrin in the treatment of drug resistant epilepsy. Arch Neurol 44:907–910
Tsanacilis LM, Wicks J, Williams J, Richens A (1991) Determination of vigabatrin in plasma by reversed-phase high performance liquid chromatography. Ther Drug Monitor 13:251–253
Uldall P, Alving J, Gram L, Hogenhaven H (1995) Vigabatrin in childhood epilepsy: a 5-year follow-up study. Neuropediatrics 26:253–256
Wolf P (1993) The use of antiepileptic drugs in epileptology with respect to psychiatry. Neuropsychobiol 27:127–131
Ylinen A, Miettinen R, Pitkänen A, Gulyas A, Freund TF, Riekkinen PJ (1991) Enhanced GABAergic inhibition preserves hippocampal structure and function in a model of epilepsy. Proc Natl Acad Sci USA 88:7650–7653
Zaccara G, Ludice AA, Mumford J (1990) Vigabatrin as add on treatment in refractory epilepsy. A multicenter placebo-controlled study. Second International Cleveland Clinic Epilepsy Symposium. Cleveland Ohio. Abstract book:18

CHAPTER 15
Benzodiazepines

C. KILPATRICK

A. Introduction

Chlordiazepoxide, the first benzodiazepine to be used in clinical practice, was synthesized in 1955, tested in animal models and found to have hypnotic, sedative and antiepileptic activity and received marketing approval in 1960 (RANDALL et al. 1960). Although effective, the drug was noted to have significant toxicity and chemists then turned to synthesizing structural analogues in the hope of finding compounds with enhanced pharmacological activity and reduced toxicity.

Diazepam was synthesized in 1959 and its pharmacology described in 1961 (RANDALL et al. 1961). Lorazepam was synthesized by BELL et al. in 1963 and nitrazepam in the same year by STERNBACH et al. (1963). Subsequently clonazepam, a derivative of nitrazepam, was approved for use as an antiepileptic drug in 1975, and has become established as an important agent in the treatment of convulsive status epilepticus.

Clobazam was synthesized in 1972 by modification of the 1,4-benzodiazepine structure. The resultant 1,5-benzodiazepine, although introduced as an anxiolytic agent, was later found to have major antiepileptic effect in animal studies and in man (GASTAUT and LOW 1979). Midazolam, although initially used as an anaesthesia inducing agent, has more recently been used in the treatment of status epilepticus.

Over the years many benzodiazepines have been synthesized and introduced into clinical practice, most as anxiolytic and sedative drugs. Although most have antiepileptic properties, the benzodiazepines used primarily in the management of seizure disorders are diazepam, clonazepam and clobazam, and to a lesser extent nitrazepam, lorazepam and midazolam. These particular benzodiazepines will therefore be discussed individually in this chapter, following a consideration of some general properties of this group of drugs. Particular attention will be paid to aspects of their pharmacology relevant to their use in epilepsy.

B. Pharmacodynamics of Benzodiazepines in General

I. Animal Models of Epilepsy

Various benzodiazepines have been shown to have antiepileptic activity in a wide range of animal seizure models. Clonazepam, nitrazepam and diazepam are particularly sensitive in elevating the threshold for pentylenetetrazol-induced seizures (Zbinden and Randall 1967; Straw et al. 1968), often regarded as a laboratory model for absence seizures (Swinyard 1969).

Diazepam is effective in suppressing epileptiform activity in the animal model of the EEG pattern of 3 Hz spike-wave activity induced by thalamic stimulation of the cat (Guerrero-Figueroa et al. 1969b). Its antiepileptic effects have also been demonstrated against spike-wave activity in seizures secondary to picrotoxin and parenterally administered local anaesthetics (Barrada and Oftedal 1970; Feinstein et al. 1970). The benzodiazepines also inhibit photosensitivity, either occurring spontaneously as in the baboon (Stark et al. 1970), or induced by pentylenetetrazol. Nitrazepam and diazepam raise the threshold for producing spike-wave discharges by electrical stimulation of the mesencephalic reticular activating formation in the cat (Gogolak and Pillat 1965).

The benzodiazepines have been shown to have various degrees of effectiveness against maximal electroshock seizures in mice (Swinyard 1969), an animal model of tonic-clonic seizures. They are also effective against minimal electroshock seizures in mice (Randall and Schallek 1968; Randall et al. 1970). In animal models of focal or partial epilepsy involving cortical lesions induced by various irritants such as strychnine and penicillin, the benzodiazepines are effective in suppressing the spread of electrical discharges but are less effective in abolishing the focal activity at the lesion site (Browne and Penry 1973). The benzodiazepines prevent the spread of epileptogenic activity from the hippocampus and amygdala, as well as from cortical epileptogenic lesions, but they are less effective in suppressing the seizure focus itself (Guerrero-Figueroa et al. 1969a).

In summary, there is considerable experimental evidence for the antiepileptic effect of the benzodiazepines, with their ability to suppress generalized EEG discharges and epileptiform activity in several animal models of generalized seizures and, with less efficacy, in animal models of focal seizure activity.

II. Biochemical Pharmacology

Benzodiazepine actions are closely associated with the effects of the inhibitory neurotransmitter γ-aminobutyric acid (GABA) (Squires and Braestrup 1977). The pharmacological effects of the benzodiazepines are the result of these drugs acting to facilitate the synaptic action of GABA, thus enhancing inhibitory neurotransmission. Benzodiazepines have no effect on synapses where GABA does not act.

The molecular basis for the functional connection between benzodiazepines and GABA neurotransmission has been identified in recent years (De Lorey and Olsen 1992). The $GABA_A$ receptor, the main type of GABA receptor in the central nervous system, is a macromolecular complex. The complex consists of five major binding domains, including sites for: benzodiazepines, barbiturates, picrotoxin and the anaesthetic steroids. These domains modulate the $GABA_A$ receptor's response to activation by GABA. A Cl^- ion channel is an integral part of the complex. The GABA receptor is composed of protein subunits with multiple subtypes. There are five families of subunits (α, β, δ, γ and ρ). It has been shown that the $\gamma 2$ subunit is essential for the receptor to carry a benzodiazepine binding site (PRITCHETT et al. 1989). The physiology and pharmacology of the $GABA_A$ receptor depends on the particular subunits that constitute the receptor, with numerous possible combinations being assembled to form the receptors. Although the exact details are not known, it is thought that the molecular structure of the $GABA_A$ receptor-ion channel complex is that of a heteropentameric glycoprotein of about 275 kDa, composed of a combination of five polypeptide subunits which form a ring structure around an ion channel, each subunit contributing to the wall of the channel (DE LOREY and OLSEN 1992).

Benzodiazepines bind to the $GABA_A$ receptor at the so-called benzodiazepine receptor, which is in fact a modulatory site on the $GABA_A$ receptor. This binding results in an increase in the frequency of opening of the Cl^- channel and a consequent increase in GABA-mediated inhibitory neurotransmission.

Although the primary action of the benzodiazepines is to enhance GABA transmission, other actions of these drugs have been described. The benzodiazepines have been demonstrated to modify Na^+ channel function in a manner similar to phenytoin, carbamazepine and sodium valproate (MACDONALD and KELLY 1994). The benzodiazepines have also been demonstrated to reduce voltage-dependent Ca^{2+} currents. This effect, however, was produced at supratherapeutic concentrations of diazepam and is therefore unlikely to be clinically relevant (MACDONALD 1995). In support for the existence of other mechanisms of action of the benzodiazepines, in vivo studies in rats, which assessed the relationship between benzodiazepine concentration and antiepileptic effect, suggested that the efficacy of the benzodiazepines against seizure-induced cortical stimulation could not be fully explained by an interaction at the $GABA_A$-benzodiazepine receptor complex (HOOGERKAMP et al. 1996).

C. Benzodiazepine Adverse Effects and Their Mechanisms

It is now well recognized that use of the benzodiazepines is frequently associated with central nervous system and psychiatric adverse effects, as well as with tolerance and withdrawal effects. The common adverse reactions include daytime sedation, memory impairment, tolerance, hyperexcitability manifested as early morning insomnia and daytime anxiety, withdrawal effects, drug-taking behaviour and drug dependence.

The adverse effect profiles of the various benzodiazepines differ somewhat. It is postulated that this is in part due to differences in the pharmacokinetic parameters of the drugs, such as their elimination half-lives, in their routes of administration and in certain of their pharmacodynamic properties such as their receptor binding affinities and potencies, as well as in their benzodiazepine drug structures and in their effects on the locus coeruleus-noradrenaline and hypothalamic-pituitary-adrenal axes.

Central nervous system depressant effects such as daytime drowsiness are more common with drugs with long elimination half-lives (HINDMARCH 1979; JOHNSON and CHERNIK 1982). Memory-impairing effects relate to the route of administration and the drug's potency. For example, diazepam given intravenously is associated with memory impairment, but this rarely occurs when the drug is used orally, whereas highly potent benzodiazepines are associated with amnesia after oral administration. Receptor binding affinity is also relevant. Drugs with low affinities are infrequently associated with memory impairment, as compared with drugs with high affinities (BIXLER et al. 1979; VGONTZAS et al. 1995). Although it has been hypothesized that increased sedation associated with increased benzodiazepine potency accounts for memory loss following use of these drugs, studies suggest that the effect of benzodiazepines on memory is specific (LISTER et al. 1988). It is also suggested that the memory-impairing effects of the benzodiazepines relate both to suppression and to activation of the locus coeruleus-noradrenaline system (VGONTZAS et al. 1995).

The development of tolerance appears to be quicker for rapidly eliminated benzodiazepines such as temazepam (BIXLER et al. 1978) and triazolam (KALES et al. 1986b) than for more slowly eliminated congeners such as diazepam and clonazepam (KALES et al. 1986a). Tolerance is also thought to be related to the receptor affinities of the drugs and to their effects on the noradrenaline- and hypothalamic-pituitary-adrenal systems. Studies have shown that downregulation of benzodiazepine receptor binding and decreased $GABA_A$ receptor function are closely associated with tolerance to benzodiazepines (MILLER et al. 1988), and withdrawal effects are associated with upregulation of $GABA_A$ receptor function (GALPERN et al. 1991).

Similarly, development of hyperexcitability is more common with rapidly eliminated benzodiazepines such as triazolam and midazolam (KALES et al. 1983a) and with drugs with high receptor affinities. There is evidence to suggest that it is in part related to alternating activation and suppression of the noradrenaline- and hypothalamic-pituitary-adrenal systems. Hyperexcitability following regular nocturnal use of benzodiazepines as hypnotics can lead to drug-taking behaviour and drug dependence (MARTINEZ-CANO and VELA-BUENO 1993).

It has been postulated that rebound insomnia resulting from the abrupt withdrawal of benzodiazepine drugs may be due to a lag in the production and replacement of endogenous benzodiazepine-like compounds (KALES et al. 1983b). Withdrawal effects are more common with benzodiazepines which have short elimination half-lives and high receptor binding affinities (VGONTZAS et al. 1995).

The triazolo benzodiazepines are associated with more severe and frequent central nervous system and psychiatric reactions than the other benzodiazepines, probably due to a direct effect on the locus coeruleus-noradrenaline system and the hypothalamic-pituitary-adrenal axis (KALOGERAS et al. 1990).

Thus rapid eliminations, high receptor binding affinities and effects on the locus coeruleus-noradrenaline and hypothalamic-pituitary-adrenal axes together with the possession of a triazolo structure influence the severity and frequency of central nervous system and psychiatric adverse reactions associated with use of the benzodiazepines.

D. Diazepam

I. Chemistry

Diazepam (7-chloro-1-methyl-5-phenyl-1,3-dihydro-2*H*-1,4-benzodiazepine-2-one) is insoluble in water. Because of this insolubility, the drug is dissolved in a mixture of 40% propylene glycol, 10% ethyl alcohol and an aqueous sodium benzoate/benzoic acid buffer to provide a parenteral preparation (SCHMIDT 1995). The chemical structure of diazepam is shown below.

II. Pharmacodynamics

1. Humans

Diazepam was the first benzodiazepine to be used in the treatment of epilepsy, NAQUET et al. (1965) and GASTAUT et al. (1965) reporting its effects in status epilepticus. Diazepam's role in the acute treatment of seizures is based on the

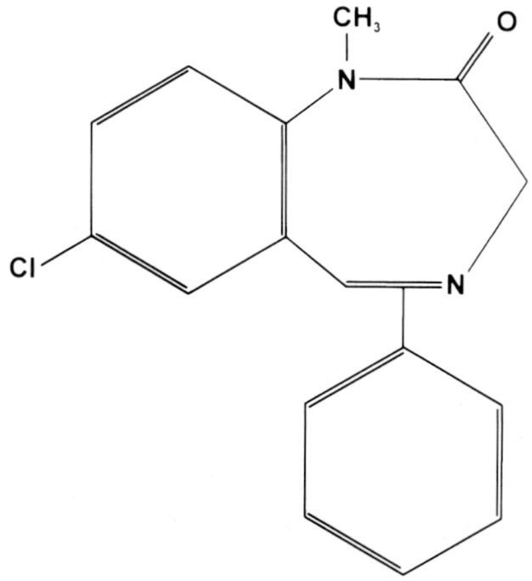

drug's rapidity of absorption and brain penetration and brain receptor binding (BOREA and BONORA 1983). Due to diazepam's sedative effects, the difficulty in maintaining its plasma concentrations at effective values, and the development of tolerance to it, the drug has no role in the chronic management of seizure disorders.

III. Pharmacokinetics

1. Absorption

Diazepam is rapidly and almost completely absorbed following oral administration, with mean peak plasma levels being achieved within 30–90 min of intake (SCHWARTZ et al. 1965; GARATTINI et al. 1973a; KAPLAN et al. 1973; HILLSTAD et al. 1974; GAMBLE et al. 1975; FRIEDMAN et al. 1992). The patient's age influences the drug's absorption, an earlier peak being seen in children and a delayed and lower peak in the elderly (GARATTINI et al. 1973a). Peak plasma diazepam concentrations increase in proportion to the drug dose, but the time to the peak is dose-independent (FRIEDMAN et al. 1992). Peak plasma levels following oral diazepam are significantly lower than those achieved following intravenous use of the drug (BOOKER and CELESIA 1973).

Lower, delayed and more erratic absorption of diazepam is to be expected with rectal suppository use as compared with oral administration of the drug. Therefore diazepam suppositories should not be used in the acute treatment of seizures (AGURELL et al. 1975; KNUDSEN 1977; MILLIGAN et al. 1982). Similarly, poor and irregular diazepam absorption is seen after intramuscular administration, the drug's plasma levels being approximately 60% of those attained when it is given orally (HILLSTAD et al. 1974; GAMBLE et al. 1975). The drug is rapidly and well absorbed rectally when given in solution, with peak plasma concentrations in adults being reached within 60 min of the administration of 10 mg diazepam and with a significant reduction in spike frequency in the EEG appearing within 15 min, associated with a mean plasma diazepam level of 210 (range 80–410) ng/ml (MILLIGAN et al. 1982).

2. Distribution

Studies in the dog, mouse and rat have shown diazepam to be rapidly and widely distributed in all tissues following both oral and parenteral administration (COUTINHO et al. 1970; GARATTINI et al. 1970; MARCUCCI et al. 1970). The drug enters adipose tissue quickly and crosses the blood-brain barrier rapidly.

The apparent volume of distribution of diazepam in humans ranges from 1 to 2 l/kg (KLOTZ et al. 1975; HVIDBERG and DAM 1976; GREENBLATT et al. 1989; SCHMIDT 1995) and has been shown to be influenced by age and sex, being larger in females and in the elderly (GREENBLATT et al. 1980).

a) Cerebrospinal Fluid

The concentration of diazepam in cerebrospinal fluid has been shown to correspond to that of the drug's free (unbound) fraction in plasma (KANTO et al. 1975).

b) Brain

Following parenteral administration, diazepam enters the brain rapidly, with its maximum concentration being reached within minutes (GARATTINI et al. 1973b). Studies in cats have shown that maximum drug concentrations occur initially in the grey matter, and that there is a longer accumulation phase for diazepam and its metabolites in the white matter (MORSELLI et al. 1973). The rapid attaining of peak diazepam brain levels correlates with the rapid antiepileptic effect of the drug noted in humans (GASTAUT et al. 1965). This correlates with the rapid response of the EEG following intravenous injection of diazepam, with suppression of spike-wave activity and the onset of benzodiazepine-induced fast rhythms (LOMBROSO 1966; GREENBLATT et al. 1989) and by the timing of the EEG changes following oral diazepam administration (FRIEDMAN et al. 1992).

c) Plasma Protein Binding

Diazepam is highly bound to plasma proteins (range 96%–99%, according to KLOTZ et al. 1975, 1976a,b; GREENBLATT et al. 1980). The binding is independent of the drug's total concentration (THIESSEN et al. 1976). A lower percentage for the drug's plasma protein binding has been reported in the newborn (KANTO et al. 1974), in chronic liver disease (KLOTZ et al. 1975; KOBER et al 1978) and in uraemia (KOBER et al. 1979). The apparent association constant (K_{app}) is $1.3\,M^{-1}\,10^{-4}$ for normal serum and $0.9\,M^{-1}\,10^{-4}$ for liver disease and uraemic serum (KOBER 1978, 1979). A similar extent of binding has been reported for the diazepam metabolite desmethyldiazepam (KLOTZ et al. 1976a).

3. Elimination

Diazepam is eliminated predominantly by biotransformation.

a) Metabolism

Diazepam undergoes biotransformation in the liver. The major steps in the metabolism of the drug are demethylation at N1 to form *N*-desmethyldiazepam, and oxidation at C3 to yield *N*-methyloxazepam. In man, the main intermediate product of biotransformation is the *N*-demethylated derivative *N*-desmethyldiazepam (SCHWARTZ et al. 1965). Both metabolites are eventually degraded to the *N*-demethylated C3-hydroxylated product, oxazepam, which is conjugated with glucuronic acid before being excreted (SCHWARTZ et al. 1965; SCHWARTZ and POSTMA 1968).

There are significant species differences in the metabolism of diazepam (MARCUCCI et al. 1970). Oxidations of diazepam and *N*-desmethyldiazepam, *N*-methyloxazepam and oxazepam at C4 have been described in different animal species (SCHWARTZ et al. 1965). Whereas the N-demethylation is relatively rapid, the oxidation steps are slower. The rapid antiepileptic effect achieved after intravenous administration of diazepam, before appreciable concentrations of *N*-desmethyldiazepam are achieved, indicates that diazepam per se possesses antiepileptic activity. *N*-desmethyldiazepam is, however, a pharmacologically significant metabolite with sedative, anxiolytic and antiepileptic properties (RANDALL et al. 1965). In mice, *N*-desmethyldiazepam, oxazepam and *N*-methyloxazepam have anti-pentylenetetrazol activities comparable to that of diazepam (MARCUCCI et al. 1971). Because of the low plasma concentrations of oxazepam and *N*-methyloxazepam that occur, these metabolites do not contribute significantly to the antiepileptic effect of diazepam in humans.

b) Elimination Parameters

A two compartment model is often used to describe the elimination kinetics of the benzodiazepines, including diazepam. Diazepam administered intravenously enters the central compartment of the model (blood and extracellular fluid) directly. The drug then distributes rapidly to the peripheral compartment (in particular fat and muscle) with a distribution half-life ($t_{1/2\alpha}$) of approximately 1 h. The value of this parameter increases with chronic treatment due to changes in the distribution rate constant ratio k_{12}/k_{21}, reflecting a change in the rate of transfer of the drug from the central compartment to the peripheral compartment as the peripheral compartment becomes relatively saturated by the drug (KLOTZ et al. 1976b; Fig. 1). Diazepam is eliminated from the central compartment by hepatic metabolism and renal excretion at a rate quantified by the elimination half-life ($t_{1/2\beta}$). For diazepam the value of this elimination half-life is 20–50 h (KLOTZ et al. 1975, 1976a,b). It is independent of the drug's mode of administration (KAPLAN et al. 1973), and is shorter in patients treated with microsomal enzyme-inducing drugs (HEPNER et al. 1977). It increases with increasing age (KLOTZ et al. 1975), and is increased in chronic liver disease (KLOTZ et al. 1975) and following long term treatment with the drug, probably due to an

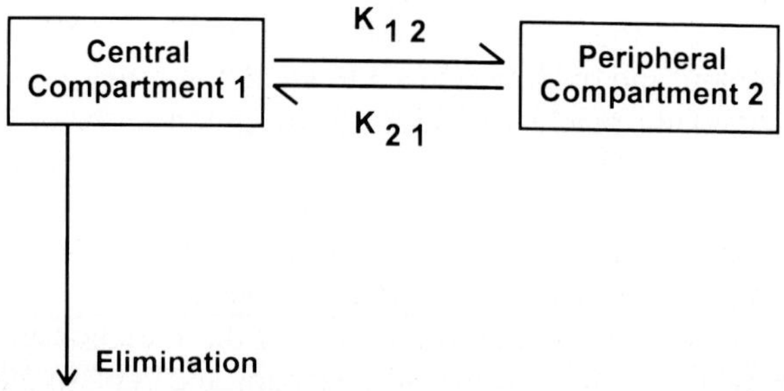

Fig. 1. Diagram of the two compartment model, showing the intercompartmental rate constants referred to in the text

inhibitory effect of the metabolite desmethyldiazepam on diazepam metabolism (KLOTZ et al. 1976b). The increase in the elimination half-life of diazepam in chronic liver disease is due to a reduction in the total plasma clearance of the drug, resulting from the algebraic sum of the effects of an increase in the drug's free fraction in plasma, a reduction in its intrinsic clearance, and an increase in its volume of distribution (KLOTZ et al. 1975). Because of the length of its half-life, diazepam is classed as a long acting benzodiazepine.

The total plasma clearance of diazepam in volunteers is approximately 26 ml/min and is proportional to the drug's plasma protein binding, suggesting that diazepam is cleared restrictively, i.e. that its clearance is altered by changes in the percentage of the unbound drug in plasma (KLOTZ et al. 1976a). Hypoalbuminaemic states are associated with reduced protein binding of the drug and hence with an increase in its free fraction. This results in an increased total plasma clearance of the drug and a reduced elimination half-life (KLOTZ et al. 1976a; THIESSEN et al. 1976).

The elimination half-life of desmethyldiazepam is longer than that of diazepam, being 50–120 h (KAPLAN et al. 1973; MAHON et al. 1976; KLOTZ et al. 1977), but its volume of distribution (TOGNONI et al. 1975; MANDELLI et al. 1978) and plasma protein binding (KLOTZ et al. 1976b) are similar in value to those of its parent substance.

The pharmacokinetic properties of diazepam are summarized in Table 1.

c) Excretion

The excretion of diazepam in humans takes place primarily in the kidneys, and to a lesser extent in the faeces (SCHWARTZ et al. 1965). In humans, dogs and mice, little unchanged diazepam is found in the urine, because the majority of a dose of the drug is metabolized to N-desmethyldiazepam and oxazepam and these are then excreted after conjugation with glucuronic acid (SCHWARTZ et al. 1965; KAPLAN et al. 1973). In humans diazepam is not excreted in bile (KLOTZ et al. 1976b).

4. Clinical Pharmacokinetics

Plasma diazepam concentrations differ widely following a single oral dose of the drug (GAMBLE et al. 1975; MANDELLI et al. 1978; REIDENBERG et al. 1978). A similar variation in plasma levels is seen following intramuscular (GAMBLE et al. 1975), intravenous and rectal administrations (AGURELL et al. 1975; MILLIGAN et al. 1982). Intravenous injection of 10 mg and 20 mg diazepam results in plasma concentrations of 700–800 ng/ml and 1100–1607 ng/ml respectively, occurring within 3–15 min (HILLESTAD et al. 1974). A plasma diazepam concentration of greater than 500 ng/ml, the level which has been suggested as needed to suppress seizure activity (BOOKER and CELESIA 1973), can be achieved within 1 min with an intravenous 30 mg dose of the drug (HARAM et al. 1978).

Table 1. Pharmacokinetic parameters for diazepam

Plasma protein binding (%)		
Volunteers	96–98	KLOTZ et al. (1975, 1976a, 1976b)
Newborns	84	KANTO et al. (1974)
Chronic liver disease	95	KLOTZ et al. (1975)
Uraemia	92	KOBER et al. (1979)
Volunteers	99.1–96.3	GREENBLATT et al. (1980)
Clearance (ml/min)		
Enzyme inducing drugs	18.7 ± 2.3	HEPNER et al. (1977)
Volunteers (single i.v. dose)	26.6 ± 4.1	KLOTZ et al. (1975)
Volunteers (single i.v. dose)	15.1 ± 1.8	HEPNER et al. (1977)
Chronic liver disease	13.8 ± 2.4	KLOTZ et al. (1975)
Chronic liver disease	9.8 ± 1.8	HEPNER et al. (1977)
Volume of distribution (l/kg)		
Volunteers	1.13 ± 0.28	KLOTZ et al. (1975)
Volunteers	0.7–4.66	GREENBLATT et al. (1980)
Chronic liver disease	1.74 ± 0.21	HEPNER et al. (1977)
Distribution half-life ($t_{1/2\alpha}$) (h)		
Volunteers (single i.v. dose)	0.82 ± 0.23	KLOTZ et al. (1975)
Volunteers (single i.v. dose)	1.1 ± 0.3	KLOTZ et al. (1976b)
Single i.v. dose	0.95–3.1	KAPLAN et al. (1973)
Volunteers (single i.v. dose)	0.96 ± 0.34	KLOTZ et al. (1976a)
Volunteers (subchronic treatment)	4.2 ± 2.3	KLOTZ et al. (1976b)
Elimination half-life ($t_{1/2\beta}$) (h)		
Volunteers (single i.v. dose)	53.1 ± 5.6	HEPNER et al. (1977)
Single i.v. dose	26.7–36.5	KAPLAN et al. (1973)
Volunteers (single i.v. dose)	36.0 ± 11.8	KLOTZ et al. (1976b)
Volunteers (single i.v. dose)	32.9 ± 8.8	KLOTZ et al. (1976a)
Volunteers (single i.v. dose)	46.6 ± 14.2	KLOTZ et al. (1975)
Single oral dose	21.0–46.2	KAPLAN et al. (1973)
Volunteers (subchronic treatment)	53.0 ± 17.4	KLOTZ et al. (1976b)
Subchronic treatment and chronic liver disease	107.6 ± 25.1	KLOTZ et al. (1977)
Young age (20 years) (single i.v. dose)	20	KLOTZ et al. (1975)
Old age (80 years) (single i.v. dose)	90	KLOTZ et al. (1975)
Chronic liver disease (single i.v. dose)	99.2 ± 23.3	KLOTZ et al. (1977)
Chronic liver disease (single i.v. dose)	105.6 ± 15.2	KLOTZ et al. (1975)
Chronic liver disease (single i.v. dose)	116 ± 9.8	HEPNER et al. (1977)
Enzyme inducing drugs (single i.v. dose)	36.4 ± 4.9	HEPNER et al. (1977)
Single i.v. dose	20.4–198	GREENBLATT et al. (1980)
Young males	36 (mean)	GREENBLATT et al. (1980)
Elderly males	98.5 (mean)	GREENBLATT et al. (1980)

a) Plasma Concentration: Clinical Effect Relationships

A correlation between plasma levels of diazepam and desmethyldiazepam and the drug's clinical effects has not been found, although it has been shown that diazepam has antiepileptic effects at a peak plasma level of 400–500 ng/ml (HVIDBERG and DAM 1976), while plasma diazepam levels from 600–2000 ng/ml suppress interictal generalized paroxysmal discharges (BOOKER and CELESIA 1973). As mentioned above, these authors suggested that plasma diazepam levels of 500 ng/ml or greater were needed to achieve a therapeutic effect in epilepsy. However, MILLIGAN et al. (1982) found no correlation between serum diazepam concentrations and the percentage reduction in the spike count in the interictal EEG. A relationship between plasma diazepam concentration and benzodiazepine type EEG changes has been reported (GREENBLATT et al. 1989). A recent study reviewing the literature on the plasma concentration-effect relationships for the benzodiazepines in humans and experimental animals reported a relationship for a wide range of benzodiazepine effects, but a model allowing prediction of the effects has not yet been established (LAURIJSSENS and GREENBLATT 1996).

b) Treatment of Status Epilepticus

The management of status epilepticus requires rapid attainment of a therapeutically adequate brain concentration of the antiepileptic drug used. This necessitates the administration of a drug which is highly lipid soluble and which therefore crosses the blood-brain barrier readily. Benzodiazepines are highly lipophilic and do enter the brain rapidly. It has been estimated that plasma diazepam levels of at least 500 ng/ml are needed to achieve initial seizure control, and levels of at least 200 ng/ml to maintain the control (BOOKER and CELESIA 1973). Intravenous administration of diazepam results in the drug entering the central pharmacokinetic compartment (blood and extracellular fluid) directly and then being distributed into the brain rapidly. Due to the drug's lipophilic nature it will also be distributed rapidly to the peripheral compartment, in particular fat and muscle. This pattern of distribution leads to a fall in the plasma drug concentration, following the peak plasma level. Thus following a single intravenous injection of 10–20 mg of diazepam in adults, and of 0.2–0.3 mg/kg in children, given at a rate of 2–5 mg/min, a brain concentration of the drug may be achieved which is responsible for an acute antiepileptic effect, but this effect may then be lost rapidly following redistribution of the drug to the peripheral compartment. Repeated bolus doses or infusions of diazepam may therefore be needed to maintain the drug's plasma levels and brain concentrations, and thus to allow its antiepileptic effects to persist.

However, with repeated administration of diazepam there will be an accumulation of the drug within the peripheral compartment, which increasingly becomes saturated with it. When this happens, the drug no longer redistributes from the central compartment to the peripheral compartment and its clearance from the central compartment becomes dependent solely on the drug's elimination half-life. In this situation the administration of further boluses, or of an infusion of diazepam, may result in a significant increase in its plasma and brain levels. Adverse effects, with hypotension and respiratory depression, may then occur. This pharmacokinetic prediction of events is consistent with the finding of significantly higher plasma levels of diazepam following chronic administration of the drug as compared with those found after a single dose of the drug. This is consistent with saturation of tissue stores having occurred (DE SILVA et al. 1966). Once the diazepam infusion is stopped, the drug will redistribute back from the peripheral compartment (which will then act as a reservior) to the central compartment. This may lead to a late increase in plasma diazepam concentration. Hence, because of these redistribution effects, after stopping a diazepam infusion a patient may remain drowsy for a much longer period than expected from the value of the elimination half-life of the drug.

Several studies have documented the effectiveness of diazepam in the treatment of status epilepticus and the drug has become the agent of choice in this clinical situation (LEPPIK et al. 1983). Given the potential danger in using multiple boluses or an infusion of diazepam, an intravenous load of phenytoin following the initial use of diazepam has been suggested: only if seizures persist is a diazepam infusion recommended (DELGADO-ESCUETO and ENRILE-BACSAL 1983).

Although intravenous therapy for the treatment of status epilepticus is preferred, this is not always possible. Rectal administration of diazepam can achieve therapeutic plasma levels of the drug within minutes. HOPPER and SANTAVOURI (1981) reported the use of rectal diazepam solutions in ten children, 80% of whose convulsions were stopped within 15 min. A more recent study reported success in 85% of patients treated at home with rectal diazepam, and with a low rate of adverse effects (KRIEL et al. 1991). The recommended dose of rectal diazepam is 30 mg in adults and 0.5 mg/kg in children.

IV. Interactions

There are no significant interactions between diazepam and other drugs.

V. Adverse Effects

There is a reasonable correlation between plasma diazepam concentrations and the sedative effects of the drug (HILLSTAD et al. 1974; KANTO 1975), with most patients becoming drowsy with levels of 200 ng/ml or greater. The major risks of intravenous administration of diazepam in the management of status epilepticus are apnoea, hypotension and obtundation. Similar concern relates to the use of rectal diazepam.

E. Clobazam

I. Chemistry

Clobazam is a 1,5-benzodiazepine derivative and differs from the 1,4-benzodiazepines in that the nitrogen atoms in its 7-membered heterocyclic ring are located at positions 1 and 5, rather than at positions 1 and 4, and an oxo- substituent is present on the carbon atom at position 4. Chemically clobazam is 7-chloro-1-methyl-5-phenyl-1,5-benzodiazepine-2,4-dione. It is relatively insoluble in water and no preparation for its intravenous or intramuscular injection is available. The chemical structure of clobazam is shown below.

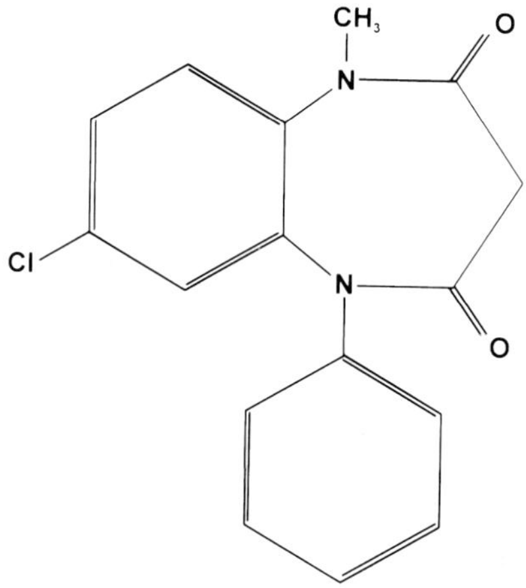

II. Pharmacodynamics

1. Mechanism of Action

Caccia et al. (1980) studied brain concentrations of clobazam and *N*-desmethylclobazam and antileptazol (anti-pentylenetetrazole) activity in the mouse and rat. Their findings suggested that the antileptazol effect of the drug in mice is mediated by both clobazam and its metabolite *N*-desmethylclobazam. Meldrum and Croucher (1982) demonstrated that *N*-desmethylclobazam had antiepileptic activity in DBA/2 mice with audiogenic seizures and in the photosensitive epilepsy of the *Papio papio* baboon. More recently, Nakamura et al. (1996) showed that both clobazam and desmethylclobazam enhance $GABA_A$ activated currents in a dose-dependent manner in rat cerebral neurons in culture. Flumazenil, a selective antagonist at the benzodiazepine receptor, inhibited both clobazam and desmethylclobazam enhancement of GABA currents. It was therefore assumed that, like the 1,4-

benzodiazepines, clobazam and *N*-desmethylclobazam bind to the benzodiazepine receptor to increase the frequency of Cl^- currents. In this study *N*-desmethylclobazam exhibited the identical dose-dependent enhancement that clobazam did. Because the metabolite *N*-desmethylclobazam is pharmacologically active and maintains a serum concentration 10–20 times higher than that of clobazam during chronic therapy (Koeppen et al. 1987), it is generally believed that the antiepileptic effect of clobazam in long-term therapy is predominantly due to its metabolite *N*-desmethylclobazam (Shorvon 1995).

2. Animal Models

Clobazam has been studied in several animal models and has been demonstrated to have a potent broad-spectrum antiepileptic effect. Fielding and Hoffman (1979) showed that in mice clobazam was active against seizures induced by pentylenetetrazol and maximal electroshock. It has also been shown to have a similar potency to diazepam in suppressing sound-induced seizures in mice and photically induced seizures in the baboon (Chapman et al. 1978; Meldrum et al. 1979). In animal models of chemically induced seizures, clobazam is a more potent antiepileptic drug than phenytoin, carbamazepine, phenobarbitone, diazepam and valproate (Shenoy et al. 1982; Kruse 1985).

3. Human Studies

Clobazam has been shown to be an effective antiepileptic drug in both double-blind placebo-controlled trials and open studies (Gastaut and Low 1979; Critchley et al. 1981; Feely et al. 1982, 1984; Allen et al. 1983; Dellaportas et al. 1984; Aucamp 1985; Wilson et al. 1985; Robertson 1986; Schmidt et al. 1986; Kilpatrick et al. 1987; Koeppen et al. 1987; Bardy et al. 1991). Most of the studies assessing the effectiveness of clobazam as adjunctive therapy have used doses ranging from 10 to 80 mg/day. In a recent large Canadian study, 40% of patients with a single seizure type achieved a 50% or greater reduction in seizure frequency (Canadian 1991). Although some authors have reported a better response of certain seizure types than others to the drug (Allen et al. 1983; Aucamp 1985; Bardy et al. 1991), this has not been a consistent finding.

Although epilepsy in a high proportion of patients responds to clobazam, at least initially, the frequent development of tolerance limits the drug's long term use (Schmidt et al. 1986; Kilpatrick et al. 1987; Bardy et al. 1991). The time of onset of tolerance varies, but in many patients it develops within weeks of the initial exposure to the drug (Kilpatrick et al. 1987). Intermittent or occasional treatment, as in the use of clobazam in catamenial epilepsy, may limit the development of tolerance (Feely et al. 1982, 1984). In one study the use of a moderate to low dose of clobazam did not reduce the development of tolerance (Kilpatrick et al. 1987).

III. Pharmacokinetics

1. Absorption

At least 87% of an oral dose of clobazam is absorbed, as indicated by urinary recovery of labelled material (RUPP et al. 1979). Following oral administration, peak plasma clobazam levels are reached within 0.5–4h (VALLNER et al. 1978, 1980; RUPP et al. 1979; TEDESCHI et al. 1981; GREENBLATT et al. 1981; JAWAD et al. 1984). Absorption of the drug is not influenced by the patient's age but its peak plasma levels are lower in males than in females (GREENBLATT et al. 1981). Rectal administration of the drug in solution results in rapid absorption with peak plasma levels equivalent to those after oral administration. Absorption of the drug from a suppository is slow (SHORVON 1995).

2. Distribution

The apparent volume of distribution of clobazam (0.87–1.83 l/kg) increases with age and is greater in women than in men (GREENBLATT et al. 1981). Clobazam and *N*-desmethylclobazam concentrations in saliva correlate reasonably well with the serum concentrations of these substances (BARDY et al. 1991).

a) Protein Binding

In humans, 85%–91% of the clobazam in plasma is bound to plasma proteins (VOLZ et al. 1979; GREENBLATT et al. 1981). The extent of the protein binding is independent of the plasma concentration of clobazam, but decreases with increasing age of the patient (GREENBLATT et al. 1981).

3. Elimination

Clobazam is eliminated mainly by virtue of metabolism.

a) Metabolism

The metabolism of clobazam has been studied in humans and in other species (VOLZ et al. 1979). In humans, clobazam's main metabolic pathways involve demethylation to *N*-desmethylclobazam, and hydroxylation at the 4′-position to 4′-hydroxy-*N*-desmethylclobazam. Clobazam, unlike the 1,4-benzodiazepines, does not undergo hydroxylation at the 3-position of the heterocyclic ring (VOLZ et al. 1979). In dogs, hydroxylation occurs at the 9-position, resulting in the formation of the metabolite 9-hydroxy-*N*-desmethylclobazam, a pattern of biotransformation by which this species is distinguished from humans, rats and monkeys. Other clobazam metabolites found in human urine are the dihydriols of clobazam (clobazam-3′,4′-dihydriol) and *N*-desmethylclobazam (*N*-desmethylclobazam-3′,4′-dihydriol) and phenolic derivatives of clobazam and *N*-desmethylclobazam.

b) Elimination Parameters

The distribution half-life of clobazam is 0.45–1.17 h (TEDESCHI et al. 1981), and its elimination half-life is 10–37 h (mean 18 h) (RUPP et al. 1979; VALLNER et al. 1980; TEDESCHI et al. 1981). The half-life is longer in the elderly (GREENBLATT et al. 1981), and in young patients is longer (30.7 h vs. 16.6 h) in women than in men (GREENBLATT et al. 1981).

In men, GREENBLATT et al. (1981) showed that the total plasma clearance of the drug was lower in the elderly (0.36 ml/min/kg) than in the young (0.63 ml/min/kg).

AUCAMP (1982) found that the elimination half-life of clobazam's principal metabolite *N*-desmethylclobazam (mean 42 h) was longer than that of the parent drug substance (mean 18 h). *N*-desmethylclobazam reaches higher serum levels (approximately tenfold higher) than those of clobazam itself, especially in long term use (RUPP et al. 1979).

The pharmacokinetic properties of clobazam are summarized in Table 2.

4. Clinical Pharmacokinetics

RUPP et al. (1979) and TEDESCHI et al. (1981) have demonstrated in adults that there is a correlation between plasma concentrations of clobazam and the clobazam dose. Others, however, could not confirm this finding, but did report a linear relationship between the clobazam dose and the plasma concentra-

Table 2. Pharmacokinetics of clobazam

Protein binding (% bound)		
Volunteers	85 ± 3	VOLZ et al. (1979)
Volunteers	85–91.4	GREENBLATT et al. (1981)
Clearance (ml/min per kg)		
Volunteers (single oral dose)		
Elderly males	0.22–0.64 (mean 0.36)	GREENBLATT et al. (1981)
Young males	0.40–0.76 (mean 0.63)	
Volume of distribution (l/kg)		
Volunteers (single oral dose)	0.7–2.2	GREENBLATT et al. (1981)
Distribution half-life ($t_{1/2\alpha}$) (h)		
Volunteers (single oral dose)	0.45–1.17	TEDESCHI et al. (1981)
Elimination half-life ($t_{1/2\beta}$) (h)		
Volunteers (single oral dose)	10.2–37.9	TEDESCHI et al. (1981)
Epilepsy patients (chronic treatment)	10.2–57.9	TEDESCHI et al. (1981)
Volunteers (single oral dose)	9.7–20.3	RUPP et al. (1979)
Volunteers (single oral dose)	7.7–30.9 (mean 18.0)	VALLNER et al. (1980)
Volunteers (single oral dose)	11–72	GREENBLATT et al. (1981)
Young males	11–23 (mean 16.6)	GREENBLATT et al. (1981)
Elderly males	29–77 (mean 47.7)	GREENBLATT et al. (1981)

tion of the main metabolite, *N*-desmethylclobazam (KILPATRICK et al. 1987). GOGGIN and CALLAGHAN (1985) reported a good correlation between clobazam plasma concentration and the dose of the drug in individual patients. However, due to large interindividual variations, it has been suggested that the plasma levels cannot be used to predict the daily dosage of the drug (VALLNER et al. 1980).

Studies have found no clear correlation between the efficacy of the drug and plasma clobazam concentrations (HAIGH et al. 1984; KILPATRICK et al. 1987; BARDY et al. 1991). This is not surprising given that both clobazam and its metabolite *N*-desmethylclobazam have antiepileptic effects and their pharmacokinetic interrelationship is complex. A correlation between plasma desmethylclobazam concentration and toxic effects of the drug has been reported (HAIGH et al. 1984; GOGGIN and CALLAGHAN 1985; KILPATRICK et al. 1987; BARDY et al. 1991).

IV. Interactions

Clobazam intake may increase the plasma concentrations of phenytoin, valproate and phenobarbitone (GOGGIN and CALLAGHAN 1985). The plasma *N*-desmethylclobazam/clobazam ratio increased when patients were co-medicated with the liver enzyme-inducing drugs carbamazepine, phenytoin or phenobarbitone (BARDY et al. 1991; SENNOUNE et al. 1991).

V. Adverse Effects

Adverse effects of treatment with clobazam are common, but overall are relatively mild. The most frequent are neurotoxic ones such as drowsiness, dizziness and fatigue. KOEPPEN et al. (1985) reviewed 23 open studies of clobazam in the treatment of epilepsy and noted an incidence of adverse effects of 33%. The drug has no effect on haematological and biochemical parameters (KOEPPEN et al. 1981, 1985). Withdrawal of clobazam, like other benzodiazepines, may precipitate seizures. Therefore withdrawal of the drug should always be done slowly (CRITCHLEY et al. 1981).

Tolerance to the drug is common, as mentioned above, and limits the drug's use in the treatment of chronic seizure disorders.

F. Clonazepam

I. Chemistry and Use

1. Chemistry

Clonazepam is a 1,4-benzodiazepine with a nitro substituent at the 7-position of ring A and a chlorine atom at the ortho position of ring C. Chemically, it is 5-(2-chlorophenol)-1,3-dihydro-7-nitro-2*H*-1,4-benzodiazepin-2-one. The chemical structure of clonazepam is shown below.

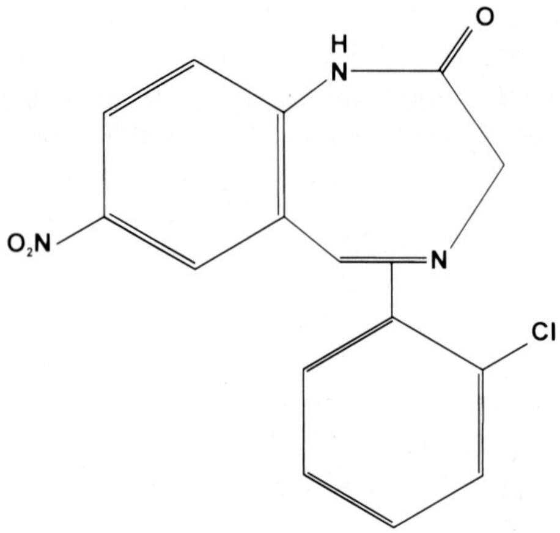

2. Use

Clonazepam is used as adjunctive therapy in the management of chronic seizure disorders, or as acute treatment of serial seizures or status epilepticus, but rarely as a primary antiepileptic drug. The drug's major role is in the treatment of status epilepticus, both convulsive and non-convulsive, and either partial or generalized. Clonazepam has been shown to be useful as adjunctive therapy in intractable absence seizures and tonic-clonic seizures (Mireles and Leppik 1985). It has also been shown to provide useful alternative therapy in the treatment of the Lennox-Gastaut syndrome (Roussounis and Rudolf 1977) and in the therapy of myoclonic seizures (Mikkelson et al. 1976). The drug is less effective for treating partial seizures.

II. Pharmacodynamics

1. Tolerance

As is the case for other benzodiazepines, tolerance to the effects of clonazepam limits its use in the chronic treatment of seizure disorders. In a study of the ability of benzodiazepines to raise the threshold for pentylenetetrazol-induced seizures in mice (Gent et al. 1985), tolerance was slower to develop than with clobazam, which is consistent with clinical observations. Similar differences in tolerance to benzodiazepines have been reported in the amygdala-kindled rat (Rosenberg et al. 1989) and in the genetically epilepsy prone rat (De Sarro et al. 1992). Whether or not the drug's high-affinity binding to benzodiazepine receptors, relative to that of other benzodiazepines, is relevant to the development to tolerance is uncertain (Greenblatt et al. 1987). Development of tolerance to the effects of clonazepam has also been studied clinically (Specht et al. 1989). A reduced tolerance when using an alternate day clonazepam dosage regimen has been reported in both an animal model (Suzuki et al. 1993) and in clinical use (Sher 1985).

III. Pharmacokinetics

1. Absorption

Clonazepam is well absorbed (at least 80% of the dose) following oral administration, with its peak plasma concentration usually being achieved within 1–4h of intake (BERLIN and DAHLSTROM 1975), though the peak may occur as late as 8h from dosage (SATO 1989).

2. Distribution

Because of clonazepam's high lipid solubility, its distribution within the body is rapid. Its apparent volume of distribution ranges from 1.5 to 4.4 l/kg (BERLIN and DAHLSTROM 1975). Clonazepam in plasma is 86% protein bound (BENET and SHEINER 1985).

3. Elimination

Clonazepam is extensively metabolized with less than 0.5% of the dose being recovered unchanged in the urine (KAPLAN et al. 1974; SJO et al. 1975).

a) Metabolism

Metabolism of the nitrobenzodiazepines, such as clonazepam, does not result in important pharmacologically active metabolites (GREENBLATT et al. 1987). Clonazepam is extensively biotransformed, principally by reduction of its nitro group to form 7-aminoclonazepam, followed by acetylation of this derivative to 7-acetaminoclonazepam, but trace amounts of a 3-hydroxy derivative, a 3-hydroxy-7-amino derivative and a 3-hydroxy-7-acetamino derivative occur (PINDER et al. 1976). The nitro compounds are pharmacologically active but their amino derivatives are not. However, the plasma level of the 3-hydroxy-7-nitro metabolite suggests that it is not likely to contribute significantly to the pharmacological effect after the parent drug is administered.

b) Elimination Parameters

DREIFUSS et al. (1975) determined the elimination half-life of clonazepam as 22–33h, with a mean of 28.7h, whereas GREENBLATT et al. (1987) reported that its elimination half-life ranged from 20 to 80h. BERLIN and DAHLSTROM (1975) reported that the elimination half-life was similar following oral and intravenous administration of the drug, with there being no significant change following long term use of the drug, which suggested that clonazepam has no enzyme-inducing effects. A clonazepam elimination half-life of 20–43h has been reported in the newborn (ANDRE et al. 1986). The drug is classed as an intermediate acting benzodiazepine.

Clonazepam has a total plasma clearance of 0.091/kg/h. The value is increased by co-medication with carbamazepine (GREENBLATT et al. 1987).

Table 3. Pharmacokinetics of clonazepam

Protein binding (% bound)		
In vitro studies	86 ± 0.5	Benet and Sheiner (1985)
Volume of distribution (l/kg)		
Volunteers	1.5–4.4	Berlin and Dahlstrom (1975)
Elimination half-life ($t_{1/2\beta}$) (h)		
Patients with epilepsy	22–33 (mean 28.7)	Dreifuss et al. (1975)
Volunteers (single i.v. dose)	24–60	Berlin and Dahlstrom (1975)
Volunteers (single oral dose)	18.7–99	Kaplan et al. (1979)
Volunteers (single oral dose)	19–42	Berlin and Dahlstrom (1975)
Volunteer (chronic treatment)	31–42	Berlin and Dahlstrom (1975)
Newborn	20–43	Andre et al. (1986)

Plasma clonazepam concentrations vary widely between individuals (Berlin and Dahlstrom 1975; Dreifuss et al. 1975). There is no good correlation between the plasma levels and the therapeutic efficacy of the drug (Dreifuss et al. 1975; Sato 1989).

The pharmacokinetic properties of clonazepam are summarized in Table 3.

IV. Interactions

There are no significant interactions between clonazepam and other drugs.

V. Adverse Effects

The adverse effects of clonazepam occur frequently and limit the long term use of the drug orally. The unwanted effects include drowsiness, ataxia and incoordination, and behavioural and personality change. Hypersecretion and hypersalivation may be a problem in children (Sato and Malow 1995).

Exacerbation of seizures and psychiatric reactions such as rebound insomnia, and anxiety are well documented following clonazepam withdrawal (Sironi et al. 1984).

G. Lorazepam

Lorazepam is a 1,4-benzodiazepine, chemically 7-chloro-5(*o*-chlorophenyl)-1,3-dihydro-3-dihydroxy-2*H*-1,4-benzodiazepine-2-one. The drug is rapidly absorbed following oral administration, with peak plasma levels occurring within 90–120 min of intake. The distribution half-life of the drug is 2–3 h and its elimination half-life 15 h (Homan and Treiman 1995). Approximately 90% of the drug in plasma is protein bound.

Lorazepam has been shown to be an anticonvulsant agent with a potency equivalent to that of clonazepam, and with a high benzodiazepine receptor binding affinity (SQUIRES and BAESTRUP 1977). The antiepileptic effect of lorazepam has been studied in a variety of animal models. It is effective against audiogenic seizures in DBA/3 mice (JENSEN et al. 1983), maximal electroshock seizures in mice (STERU et al. 1986), pentylenetetrazol-induced convulsions in mice (MARCUCCI et al. 1972), myoclonic seizures in the photosensitive baboon *Papio papio* (VALIN et al. 1981), convulsive status epilepticus in rats (WALTON and TREIMAN 1990) and pentylenetetrazol-induced seizures in pigs (PRATT and SPIVEY 1989).

The major clinical use of lorazepam has been in status epilepticus, where several open studies have reported its effectiveness (HOMAN and TREIMAN 1995). A potential advantage of lorazepam over diazepam in the treatment of status epilepticus is that lorazepam plasma levels remain at a therapeutic level for longer (COMER and GIESECKE 1982), although the onset of its antiepileptic effect probably is slower (AALTONEN et al. 1980). There appear to be no significant differences between the efficacies of diazepam, clonazepam and lorazepam in treating status epilepticus (TREIMAN 1989).

H. Nitrazepam

Nitrazepam, chemically 1,3-dihydro-7-nitro-5-phenyl-2*H*-1,4-benzodiazepine-2-one, is well absorbed, with peak plasma levels being achieved within 1 h after oral administration. The distribution half-life of the drug is about 17 min and its elimination half-life 20–36 h. Its apparent volume of distribution is approximately 2 l/kg and in plasma it is approximately 87% protein bound (JOCHEMSEN et al. 1982). Nitrazepam is metabolized predominantly by reduction of its nitro group to the corresponding amine, which is then acetylated to a 7-acetamido derivative (REIDER and WENDT 1973).

Nitrazepam's major use is as an hypnotic and it is now less commonly used in the treatment of epilepsy. Its main role as an antiepileptic has been in the management of intractable seizures associated with the Lennox-Gastaut syndrome. The adverse effects of sedation and tolerance limit its use.

I. Midazolam

Midazolam is a 1,4-benzodiazepine, chemically 8-chloro-6-(2-fluorophenyl)-1-methyl-4*H*-imidazo-[1,5-a][1,4]-benzodiazepine. In recent years midazolam been used in the treatment of status epilepticus. The drug is water soluble and at physiological pH is lipid soluble, so that it can be given intramuscularly, rapidly achieving therapeutic plasma levels. The distribution half-life (0.06 ± 0.03 h) following intravenous administration is brief, and its elimination half-life, whether given intramuscularly or intravenously, is also brief (1.5 ± 0.3 h and 2.6 ± 1.7 h, respectively). These pharmacokinetic properties provide the advantage of a shorter duration of sedation following termination of intake of the drug, compared with the other benzodiazepines (BELL et al. 1991). JAWAD et al. (1986) reported the rate of onset and duration of effect of intravenous diazepam and intramuscular midazolam on interictal epileptiform spikes and concluded that intramuscular midazolam is a useful alternative to diazepam in the treatment of status epilepticus.

References

Aaltonen L, Kanto J, Salo M (1980) Cerebrospinal fluid concentrations and serum protein binding of lorazepam and its conjugate. Acta Pharmacol Toxicol 46:156–158

Agurell S, Berlin A, Ferngren H, Hellstrom B (1975) Plasma levels of diazepam after parenteral and rectal administration in children. Epilepsia 16:277–283

Allen J, Oxley J, Robertson M, Richens A, Jawad S (1983) Clobazam as adjunctive treatment in refractory epilepsy. Br Med J 286:1246–1247

Andre M, Boutroy MJ, Dubruc C et al. (1986) Clonazepam pharmacokinetics and therapeutic efficacy in neonatal seizures. Eur J Clin Pharmacol 30:585–589

Aucamp AK (1982) Aspects of the pharmacokinetics and pharmacodynamics of benzodiazepines with particular reference to clobazam. Drug Devel Res [Suppl 1]: 117–126

Aucamp AK (1985) Clobazam as adjunctive therapy in uncontrolled epileptic patients. Curr Ther Res 37:1098–1103

Bardy AH, Seppala T, Salokorpi T, Granstrom M-L, Santavuori P (1991) Monitoring of concentrations of clobazam and norclobazam in serum and saliva of children with epilepsy. Brain Dev 13:174–179

Barrada O, Oftedal SI (1970) The effect of diazepam (Valium) and nitrazepam (Mogadon) on picrotoxin induced seizures in rabbits. Electroenceph Clin Neurophysiol 29:220–221

Bell SC, McCarlly RJ, Gochman C, Childress SJ, Gluckman MI (1963) 3-Substituted 1,4-benzodiazepin-2-ones. J Med Chem 11:457–461

Bell DM, Richards G, Dhillon S et al. (1991) A comparative pharmacokinetic study of intravenous and intramuscular midazolam in patients with epilepsy. Epilepsy Res 10:183–190.

Benet LZ, Sheiner LB (1985) Appendix II. Design and optimization of dosage regimens: pharmacokintic data. In: Gilman AG, Goodman LS, Rall, TW, Murad F (eds) The pharmacological basis of therapeutics. 7th edn, Macmillan, New York, pp. 1663–1733

Berlin A, Dahlstrom H (1975) Pharmacokinetics of the anticonvulsant drug clonazepam evaluated from single oral and intravenous doses and by repeated oral administration. Eur J Clin Pharmacol 9:115–159

Bixler EO, Kales A, Soldatos CR, Scharf MB, Kales JD (1978) Effectiveness of temazepam with short-, intermediate-and long-term use: sleep laboratory evaluation. J Clin Pharmacol 18:110–118

Bixler EO, Scharf MB, Soldatos CR, Mitsky DJ, Kales A (1979) Effects of hypnotic drugs on memory. Life Sci 25:1388

Booker HE, Celesia GG (1973) Serum concentrations of diazepam in subjects with epilepsy. Arch Neurol 29:191–194

Borea PA, Bonora (1983) Brain receptor binding and lipophilic character of benzodiazepines. Biochem Pharmacol 32:603–607

Browne TR, Penry JK (1973) Benzodiazepines in the treatment of epilepsy, a review. Epilepsia 14:277–310

Caccia S, Guiso G, Garattini S (1980) Brain concentrations of clobazam and N-desmethylclobazam and antileptazol activity. J Pharm Pharmacol 32:295–296

Canadian Clobazam Cooperative Group (1991) Clobazam in treatment of refractory epilepsy: the Canadian experience. A retrospective study. Epilepsia 32:407–416

Chapman AG, Horton RW, Meldrum BS (1978) Anticonvulsant action of a 1,5-benzodiazepine, clobazam, in reflex epilepsy. Epilepsia 19:293–299
Comer WH, Giesecke AH Jr (1982) Injectable lorazepam (Ativan). Semin Anesth 1:33–39
Coutinho CB, Cheripko JA, Carbone JJ (1970) Correlation between the duration of the anticonvulsant activity of diazepam and its physiological disposition in mice. Biochem Pharmacol 19:363–379
Critchley EMR, Valil SD, Hayward HW, Owen MVH, Cocks A, Freemantle NP (1981) Double-blind clinical trial of clobazam in refractory epilepsy. In Hindmarch, I, Stonier, PD (eds) Clobazam. Royal Society of Medicine, London, pp. 159–163
Delgado-Escueta AV, Enrile-Bacsal F (1983) Combination therapy for status epilepticus; intravenous diazepam and phenytoin. Adv Neurol 34:477–485
Dellaportas CI, Wilson A, Clifford Rose F (1984) Clobazam as adjunctive treatment in chronic epilepsy. In Porter RJ, Mattson RH, Ward Jr AA, Dam M (eds) Advances in epileptology: XVth Epilepsy International Symposium, Raven Press, New York:363–367
De Lorey TM, Olsen RW (1992) GABA receptor structure and function. J Biol Chem 267:16747–16750
De Sarro GB, Rotiroti D, Gratteri S, Sinopoli S, Juliano M, De Sarro A (1992) Tolerance to anticonvulsant effects of clobazam, diazepam and clonazepam in genetically epilepsy prone rats. In: Biggio G, Concas A, Costa E (eds) GABAergic synaptic transmission. Raven Press, New York, pp. 249–254
de Silva AJ, Koechlin DA, Bader G (1966) Blood level distribution patterns of diazepam and first major metabolite in man. J Pharm Sci 55:692–702
Dreifuss FE, Penry JK, Rose SW, Kupferberg HJ, Dyken P, Sato S (1975) Serum clonazepam concentrations in children with absence seizures. Neurology 23:255–258
Feely M, Gibson J (1984) Intermittent clobazam for catamenial epilepsy: avoid tolerance. J Neurol Neurosurg Psychiatry 47:1279–1282
Feely M, Calvert R, Gibson J (1982) Clobazam in catamenial epilepsy. A model for evaluating anticonvulsants. Lancet 2:71–73
Feinstein MB, Lenard W, Mathias J (1970) The antagonism of local anaesthetic induced convulsions by the benzodiazepine derivative diazepam. Arch Int Pharmacodyn 187:144–153
Fielding S, Hoffmann I (1979) Pharmacology of antianxiety drugs with special reference to clobazam. Br J Clin Pharmacol 7:7S–15S
Friedman H, Greenblatt DJ, Peters GR et al. (1992) Pharmacokinetics and pharmacodynamics of oral diazepam: effect of dose, plasma concentration and time. Clin Pharmacol Ther 52:139–150
Galpern WR, Lumpkin M, Greenblatt DJ, Shader RJ, Miller LG (1991) Chronic benzodiazepine administration. Psychopharmacology 104:225–230
Gamble JAS, Dundee JW, Assaf RAE (1975) Plasma diazepam levels after single dose oral and intramuscular administration. Anaesthesia 30:164–169
Garattini S, Marcucci F, Mussini E (1970) Studies on the anticonvulsant action of diazepam. Br J Pharmacol 38:455–457
Garattini S, Marcucci F, Morselli PL, Mussini E (1973a) The significance of measuring blood levels of benzodiazepines. In: Davies and Prichard (eds) Biological effects of drugs in relation to their plasma concentrations. MacMillan, London, pp. 211–225
Garrattini S, Mussini E, Marcucci F, Guaitani A (1973b) Metabolic studies on benzodiazepines in various animal species. In: Garattini S, Mussini E, Randall LO (eds) The benzodiazepines. Raven Press, New York, pp. 75–97
Gastaut H, Low MD (1979) Antiepileptic properties of clobazam, 1,5-benzodiazepine in man. Epilepsia 20:437–446
Gastaut H, Naquet R, Poire R, Tassinari CA (1965) Treatment of status epilepticus with diazepam. Epilepsia 6:167–182

Gent JP, Feely MP, Haigh JRM (1985) Differences between the tolerance characteristics of two anticonvulsant benzodiazepines. Life Sci 37:849–856
Goggin T, Callaghan N (1985) Blood levels of clobazam and its metabolites and therapeutic effect. In Hindmarch I, Stonier PD, Trimble MR (eds) Clobazam: human psychopharmacology and clinical applications. Royal Society of Medicine, London, pp. 149–153.
Gogolak G, Pillat B (1965) Effect of Mogadon on arousal reaction in rabbits. In: Akert K, Bally C, Schade JP (eds) Sleep mechanisms (Progress in Brain Research, Vol. 18) Elsevier, Amsterdam, pp. 229–230
Greenblatt DJ, Allen MD, Harmatz JS, Shader RI (1980) Diazepam disposition determinants. Clin Pharmac Ther 27:301–312
Greenblatt DJ, Divoll M, Puri SK, Ho I, Zinny MA, Shader RI (1981) Clobazam kinetics in the elderly. Br J Pharmacol 12:631–636
Greenblatt DJ, Miller LG, Shader RI (1987) Clonazepam pharmacokinetics, brain uptake, and receptor interactions. J Clin Psychiatry 48 [Suppl]:4–11
Greenblatt DJ, Ehrenberg BL, Gunderman J, Locniskar A, Scavone JM, Harmatz JS, Shader RI (1989) Pharmacokinetic and electroencephalographic study of intravenous diazepam, midazolam and placebo. Clin Pharmacol Ther 45:356–365
Guerrero-Figueroa R, Rye MM, Heath RG (1969a) Effects of two benzodiazepine derivates on cortical and subcortical epileptogenic tissues in the cat and monkey, Part 2 (cortical and centrencephalic structures). Curr Ther Res 11:40–50
Guerrero-Figueroa R, Rye MM, Heath RG (1969b) Effects of two benzodiazepine derivatives on cortical and subcortical epileptogenic tissues in the cat and monkey, Part 1 (cortical and centrencephalic structures). Curr Ther Res 11:27–39
Haigh JRM, Gent JP, Calvert R (1984) Plasma levels of clobazam and its N-desmethyl metabolite: protection against pentylene-tetrazone-induced convulsions in mice. J Pharm Pharmacol 36:636–638
Haram K, Bakke OM, Johannessen KH, Lund T (1978) Transplacental passage of diazepam during labor: influence of uterine concentrations. Clin Pharmacol Ther 24:590–599
Hepner GW, Vesell ES, Lipton A, Harvey HA, Wilkinson GR, Schenker S (1977) Disposition of aminopyrine, antipyrine, diazepam and indocyanine green in patients with liver disease or on anticonvulsant drug therapy. Diazepam breath test and correlations in drug elimination. J Lab Clin Med 90:440–456
Hillestad L, Hansen T, Melsom H, Drivenes A (1974) Diazepam metabolism in normal man. 1. Serum concentrations and clinical effects after intravenous, intramuscular, and oral administration. Clin Pharmacol Ther 16:479–484
Hindmarch I (1979) Effects of hypnotic and sleep-inducing drugs on objective assessment of human psychomotor performance and subjective appraisals of sleep and early morning behaviour. Br J Pharmacol 8:435–465
Homan RW, Treiman DM (1995) Benzodiazepines lorazepam. In: Levy RH, Mattson RH, Meldrum BS (eds) Antiepileptic drugs. 4th edn, Raven Press, New York, pp. 779–790
Hoogerkamp A, Arends RH, Bomers AM, Mandema JW, Vaskuyl RA, Danhof M (1996) Pharmacokinetics/pharmacodynamic relationship of benzodiazepines in the direct cortical stimulation model of anticonvulsant effect. J Pharmacol Exp Ther 279:803–812
Hopper K, Santavuori P (1981) Diazepam rectal solution for home treatment of acute seizures in children. Acta Paediatr Scand 70:369–372
Hvidberg EF, Dam M (1976) Clinical pharmacokinetics of anticonvulsants. Clin Pharmacokinet 1:161–188
Jawad S, Oxley J, Wilson J, Richens A (1986) A pharmacodynamic evaluation of midazolam as an antiepileptic compoud. J Neurol Neurosurg Psychiat 49: 1050–1054.
Jawad S, Richens A, Oxley J (1984) Single dose pharamcokinetic study of clobazam in normal volunteers and epileptic patients. Br.J Clin Pharmacol 18:873–877

Jensen LH, Petersen EN, Braestrup C (1983) Audiogenic seizures in DBA/2 mice discriminate sensitively between low efficacy benzodiazepine receptor agonists and inverse agonits. Life Sci 33:393–399

Jochemsen R, Hogendoorn JJH, Dingemanse J, Hermans J, Boeijinga JK, Breimer DD (1982) Pharmacokinetics and bioavailability of intravenous, oral and rectal nitrazepam in humans. J Pharmacokinet Biopharm 10:231–245

Johnson LC, Chernik DA (1982) Sedative-hypnotics and human performance. Psychopharmacology 72:101–113

Kales A, Soldatos CR, Bixler EO, Kales JD (1983a) Early morning insomnia with rapidly eliminated benzodiazepines. Science 220:95–97

Kales A, Soldatos CR, Bixler EO, Kales JD (1983b) Rebound insomnia and rebound anxiety: a review. Pharmacology 26:121–137

Kales A, Bixler EO, Soldatos CR, Vela-Bueno A, Jacoby JA, Kales JD (1986a) Quazepam and temazepam: effects of short and intermediate-term use and withdrawal. Clin Pharmacol Ther 39:345–353

Kales A, Bixler EO, Vela-Bueno A, Soldatos CR, Niklaus DE, Manfredi RL (1986b) Comparison of short and long half-life benzodiazepine hypnotics: triazolam and quazepam. Clin Pharmacol Ther 40:378–386

Kalogeras KT, Calogero AE, Kuribayiashi T, Khan I, Galluci WT, Kling MA, Chrousos GP, Gold PW (1990) In vitro and in vivo effects of the triazolobenzodiazepine alprazolam on hypothalamic-pituitary-adrenal function: Pharmacological and clinical implications. J Clin Endocrinol Metab 70:1462–1471

Kanto J (1975) Plasma concentrations of diazepam and its metabolites after peroral, intramuscular, and rectal administration. Int J Clin Pharmaol 12:427–432

Kanto J, Erkkola R, Sellman R (1974) Distribution and metabolism of diazepam in early and late human pregnancy. Postnatal metabolism of diazepam. Acta Pharmacol et Toxicol 35 [Suppl 1]:36

Kanto J, Kangas L, Siirtola T (1975) Cerebrospinal fluid concentrations of diazepam and its metabolites in man. Acta Pharmacologica 36:328–334

Kaplan SA, Alexander K, Jack ML, Puglisi DV, de Silva JAF, Lee TL, Weinfeld RE (1974) Pharmacokinetic profiles of clonazepam in dog and humans and of flunitrazepam in dog. J Pharm Sci 63:527–532

Kaplan SA, Jack ML, Alexander K, Weinfeld RE (1973) Pharmacokinetic profile of diazepam in man following single intravenous and oral and chronic oral administrations. J Pharm Sci 63:1789–1796

Kilpatrick C, Bury R, Fullinfaw R, Moulds R (1987) Clobazam in the treatment of epilepsy. Clin Exp Neurol 23:139–144

Klotz U, Avant GR, Hoyumpa A, Schenker S, Wilkinson GR (1975) The effects of age and liver disease on the disposition and elimination of diazepam in adult man. J Clin Inv 55:347–359

Klotz U, Antonin K-H, Bieck PR (1976a) Pharmacokinetics and plasma binding of diazepam in man, dog, rabbit, guinea pig and rat. J Pharmacol Exp Ther 199:67–73

Klotz U, Antonin K-H, Bieck PR (1976b) Comparison of the pharmacokinetics of diazepam after single and subchronic doses. Eur J Clin Pharmacol 10:121–126

Klotz U, Antonin KH, Brugel H, Bieck PR (1977) Disposition of diazepam and its major metabolite desmethyldiazepam in patients with liver disease. Clin Pharm Ther 21:430–436

Knudsen FU (1977) Plasma-diazepam in infants after rectal administration in solution and by suppository. Acta Paed Scandinav 66:563–567

Kober A, Jenner A, Sjoholm I, Borga O, Odar-Cederlof I (1978) Differentiated effects of liver cirrhosis n the albumin binding sites for diazepam, salicylic acid and warfarin. Biochem Pharmacol 27:2729–2735

Kober A, Sjoholm I, Borga O, Odar-Cederlof I (1979) Protein binding of diazepam and digitoxin in uremic and normal serum. Biochem Pharmacol 28:1037–1042

Koeppen D (1981) Clinical experience with clobazam (1968–1981). In: Hindmarch I, Stonier PD (eds) Clobazam. Royal Society of Medicine, London, pp. 193–198

Koeppen D (1985) A review of clobazam studies in epilepsy. In: Hindmarch I, Stonier PD, Trimble MR (eds) Clobazam:human psychopharmacology and clinical applications. Royal Society of Medicine, London, pp. 207–215

Koeppen D, Baruzzi A, Capozza M, Chauvel P, Courgon J, Favel P, Harmant J et al. (1987) Clobazam in therapy resistant patients with partial epilepsy: a double blind placebo controlled crossover study. Epilepsia 28:495–506

Kriel RL, Cloyd JC, Hadsall RS, Carlson AM, Floren KL, Jones-Saete CM (1991) Home use of rectal diazepam for cluster and prolonged seizures: efficacy, adverse reactions, quality of life, and cost analysis. Ped Neurol 7:13–17

Kruse HJ (1985) Psychopharmacology of clobazam with special reference to its anticonvulsant activity. In: Hindmarch I, Stonier PD, Trimble MR (eds) Clobazam. Royal Society of Medicine, London, pp. 113–120

Laurijssens BE, Greenblatt DJ (1996) Pharmacokinetic pharmacodynamic relationships for benzodiazepines. Clin Pharmacokinet 30:52–76

Leppik IE, Derivan AT, Homan RW, Walker J, Ramsay RE, Patrick B (1983) Double blind study of lorazepam and diazepam in status epilepticus. J Amer Med Assoc 249:1452–1454

Lister RG, Weingartner H, Eckhardt MJ, Linnoila M (1988) Clinical relevance of effects of benzodiazepines on learning and memory. Psychopharmacology 6:117–127

Lombroso CT (1966) Treatment of status epilepticus with diazepam. Neurology 16:629–634

Macdonald RL (1995) Benzodiazepines, mechanisms of action. In: Levy RH, Matson TT, Meldrum BS (eds) Antiepileptic drugs. 4th edn, Raven Press, New York, pp. 695–703

Macdonald RL, Kelly RM (1994) Drug mechanisms of action of currently prescribed and newly developed antiepileptic drugs. Epilepsia 35:S41–S50

Mahon WA, Inaba T, Umeda T, Tsutsumi E, Stone R (1976) Biliary elimination of diazepam in man. Clin Pharmacol Ther 19:443–450

Mandelli M, Tognoni G, Garattini S (1978) Clinical pharmacokinetics of diazepam. Clin Pharmacokinet 3:72–91

Marcucci F, Fanelli R, Mussini E, Garattini S (1970) Further studies on species differences in diazepam metabolism. Eur J Pharmacol 9:253–256

Marcucci F, Mussini E, Guaitaini A, Fanelli R, Garattini S (1971) Anticonvulsant activity and brain levels of diazepam and its metabolites in mice. Eur J Pharmacol 16:311–314

Marcucci F, Mussini E, Airoldi, L, Guaitani A, Garattini S (1972) Brain concentrations of lorazepam and oxazepam at equal degree of anticonvulsant activity. J Pharm Pharmacol 24:63–64

Martinez-Cano H, Vela-Bueno A (1993) Daytime consumption of triazolam. Acta Psychiatr Scand 88:286–288

Meldrum BS, Croucher MJ (1982) Anticonvulsant action of clobazam and desmethylclobazam in reflex epilepsy in rodents and baboons. Drug Devl Res [Suppl 1]: 33–38

Meldrum BS, Chapman AG, Horton RW (1979) Clobazam: anticonvulsant action in animal models of epilepsy. Br J Clin Pharmacol 7:595–605

Mikkelsen B, Birket-Smith E, Brandt S et al. (1976) Clonazepam in the treatment of epilepsy. A controlled clinical trial in simple absences, bilateral massive epileptic myoclonus, and atonic seizures. Arch Neurol 33:322–325

Miller LG, Greenblatt DJ, Barnhill JG, Shader RI (1988) Chronic benzodiazepine administration. I. Tolerance is associated with benzodiazepine down regulation and decreased $GABA_A$ receptor function. J Pharmacol Exp Ther 246:170–176

Milligan N, Dhillon S, Oxley J, Richens A (1982) Absorption of diazepam from the rectum and its effects oninterictal spikes in the EEG. Epilepsia 23:323–331

Mireles R, Leppik IL (1985) Valproate and clonazepam comedication in patients with intractable epilepsy. Epilepsia 26:122–126

Morselli PL, Cassano GB, Placidi GF, Muscettola GB, Rizzo M (1973) Kinetics of the distribution of C^{14}-diazepam an its metabolites in various areas of cat brain. In: Garattini S, Mussini E, Randall L (eds) The benzodiazepines. Raven Press, New York, pp. 129–143
Nakamura F, Suzuki S, Nishimura S, Yagi K, Seino M (1996) Effects of clobazam and its active metabolite on GABA-activated currents in rat cerebral neurons in culture. Epilepsia 37:728–735
Naquet R, Soulayrol R, Dolce G, Tassinari CA, Broughton R, Loeb H (1965) First attempt at treatment of experimental status epilepticus in animals and spontaneous status epilepticus in man with diazepam (Valium®). Electroencephalogr Clin Neurophysiol 18:427
Pinder RM, Brogden RM, Speight TM, Aver GS (1976) Clonazepam: a review of its pharmacological properties and therapeutic efficacy in epilepsy. Drugs 12:321–361
Pratt LF, Spivey WH (1989) Suppression of pentylenetetrazol-elecited seizure activity by intraosseous lorazepam in pigs. Epilepsia 30:480–486
Pritchett DB, Sontheimer H, Shivers BD, Ymer S, Kettenmann H, Schofield PR, Seeburg PH (1989) Importance of a novel $GABA_A$ receptor sumunit for benzodiazepine pharmacology. Nature 338:582–588
Randall LO, Schallek W (1968) Pharmacological activity of certain benzodiazepines. In: Efron DH (ed) Psychopharmacology. A review of progress 1957–1967. Public Health Service Publication No 1836, US Government Printing Office, Washington DC
Randall LO, Schallek W, Heise GA, Keith EF, Bagdon RE (1960) The psychosedative properties of methaminodiazepoxide. J Pharmacol Exp Ther 129:163–171
Randell LO, Heise GA, Shallek W et al. (1961) Pharmacology and clinical studies on Valium. A new psychtherapeutic agent of the benzodiazepine class. Curr Ther Res 3:405–425
Randell LO, Scheckel CL, Banzinger RF (1965) Pharmocolgy of the metabolites of chlordiazepoxide and diazepam. Curr Ther Res 7:590–606
Randall LO, Scheckel CL, Pool W (1970) Pharmacology of medazepam and metabolites. Arch Int Pharmacodyn 185:135–148
Reidenberg MM, Levy M, Warner H, Coutinho CB, Schwartz MA, Yu G, Cheripko J (1978) Relationship between diazepam dose, plasma level, age, and central nervous system depression. Clin Pharmacol Ther 23:371–374
Reider J, Wendt G (1973) Pharmacokinetics and metabolism of the hypnotic nitrazepam. In: Garattini S, Mussini E, Randall L (eds) The benzodiazpines. Raven Press, New York, pp. 99–127
Robertson MM (1986) Current status of the 1,4 and 1,5 benzodiazepines in the treatment of epilepsy: the place of clobazam. Epilepsia 27 [Suppl 1]:S27–S41
Rosenberg HC, Tietz EI, Chiu TH (1989) Tolerance to anticonvulsant effects of diazepam, clonazepam, and clobazam in amygdala-kindled rats. Epilepsia 30:276–285
Roussounis SH, Rudolf NM (1977) A long term electroclinical study of clonazepam in children with intractable seizures. Electroencephalogr Clin Neurophysiol 43:528–529
Rupp W, Badian M, Christ O et al. (1979) Pharmacokinetics of single and multiple doses of clobazam in humans. Br J Clin Pharmacol 7 [Supp 1]:51S-57S
Sato S (1989) Benzodiazepines: Clonazepam. In: Levy R, Mattson R, Meldrum B, Penry JK, Dreifuss FE (eds) Antiepileptic drugs. 3rd edn. Raven Press, New York, pp. 765–784
Sato S, Malow BA (1995) Benzodiazepines: Clonazepam. In: Levy R, Mattson RH, Meldrum BS (eds) Antiepileptic drugs. 4th edn, Raven Press, New York, pp. 725–734
Schmidt D (1995) Benzodiazepines: Diazepam. In: Levy RH, Mattson RH, Meldrum BS (eds) Antiepileptic drugs. 4th edn, Raven Press, New York, pp. 705–724

Schmidt D, Rhode M, Wolf P, Roeder-Warner U (1986) Tolerance to the antiepileptic effect of clobazam. In: Frey H-H, Froscher W, Koella WP, Meinardi H (eds) Tolerance to beneficial and adverse effects of antiepileptic drugs. Raven Press, New York, pp. 109–118
Schwartz MA, Postma E (1968) Metabolism of diazepam in vitro. Biochem Pharmacol 17:2443–2449
Schwartz MA, Koechlin BA, Postma E, Palmer S, Krol G (1965) Metabolism of dizepam in rat, dog and man. J Pharmacol Exp Ther 149:423–435
Sennoune S, Mesdjian E, Bonneton J, Genton P, Dravet C, Roger J (1992) Interactions between clobazam and standard antiepileptic drugs in patients with epilepsy. Ther Drug Monit 14:269–274
Shenoy AK, Miyahara JT, Swinyard EA, Kupferberg, HJ (1982) Comparative anticonvulsant activity and neurotoxicity of clobazam, diazepam, phenobarbital and valproate in mice and rats. Epilepsia 23:399–408
Sher PK (1985) Alternate day clonazepam treatment of intractable seizures. Arch Neurol 42:787–788
Shorvon SD (1995) Benzodiazepines: clobazam. In: Levy RH, Mattson RH, Meldrum BS (eds) Antiepileptic drugs. 4th edn, Raven Press, New York, pp. 763–777
Sironi VA, Miserocchi G, DeRiu PL (1984) Clonazepam withdrawal syndrome. Acta Neurol 6:134–139
Sjo O, Hvidberg EF, Naestoft J, Lund M (1975) Pharmacokinetics and side effects of clonazepam and its 7-amino-metabolite in man. Eur J Clin Pharmacol 8:249–254
Specht U, Boenigk HE, Wolf P (1989) Discontinuation of clonazepam after long-term treatment. Epilepsia 20:458–463
Squires RF, Braestrup C (1977) Benzodiazepine receptors in rat brain. Nature 266:732–734
Stark LG, Killam KF, Killam EK (1970) The anticonvulsant effects of phenobarbital, diphenylhydantoin and two benzodiazepines in the baboon, Papio papio. J Pharmacol Exp Ther 173:125–132
Sternbach LH, Fryer RI, Keller O, Metlesics W. Sach G, Sterger N (1963) Quinazolines and 1–4 bezodiazepines X. Nitro-substituted 5-phenyl-1,4-benzodiazepine derivatives. J Med Pharm Chem 6:261–265.
Steru L, Chermat R, Millet B, Mico JA, Simon P (1986) Comparative study in mice of ten 1.4-benzodiazepines and of clobazam:anticonvulsant, anxiolytic, sedative, and myorelaxant effects. Epilepsia 27 [Suppl 1]:S14-S17
Straw RN (1968) The effect of certain benzodiazepines on the threshold for pentylenetchazol-induced seizures in the cat. Arch Int Pharmacodyn Ther 171:464–469
Suzuki Y, Edge J, Mimaki T, Walson PD (1993) Intermittent clonazepam treatment prevents anticonvulsant tolerance in mice. Epilepsy Res 15:15–20
Swinyard EA (1969) Laboratory evaluation of antiepileptic drugs. Review of laboratory methods. Epilepsia 10:107–119
Tedeschi G, Riva R, Baruzzi A (1981) Clobazam plasma concentrations: pharmacokinetic study in healthy volunteers and data in epileptic patients. Br J Clin Pharmacol 11:619–621
Thiessen JJ, Sellers EM, Denbeigh P, Dolman L (1976) Plasma protein binding of diazepam and tolbutamide in chronic alcoholics. J Clin. Pharmacol 16:345–351
Tognoni G, Gomeni R, De Maio D, Alberti GG, F anciosi P, Scieghi G (1975) Pharmacokinetics of N-desmethyldiazepam in pateints suffering from insomnia and treated with notriptyline Br J Clin Pharmacol 2:227–232.
Treiman DM (1989) Pharmacokinetics and lcinical use of benzodiazepines in the management of status epilepticus. Epilepsia 30 [Suppl 2]:S4-S10
Valin A, Cepeda C, Rey E, Naquet R (1981) Opposite effects of lorazepam on two kinds of myoclonus in the photosensitive Papio papio. Electroenceph Clin Neurophysiol 52:647–651

Vallner JJ, Needham TE, Jun HW, Brown WJ, Stewart JT, Kotzan JA, Honigberg IL (1978) Plasma levels of clobazam after three oral dosage forms in healthy subjects. J Clin Pharmacol 18:319–324

Vallner JJ, Kotzan JA, Stewart JT, Honigberg IL, Needham TE, Brown J (1980) Plasma levels of Clobazam after 10, 20 and 40 mg tablet doses in health subjects. J Clin Pharmcol 20:445–451

Vgontzas AN, Kales A, Bixler EO (1995) Benzodiazepine side effects; role of pharmacokinetics and pharmacodynamics. Pharmacology 51:205–223

Volz M, Christ O, Kellner H-M et al. (1979) Kinetics and metabolism of clobazam in animal and man. Br J Clin Pharmacol 7 [Suppl 1]:41S-50S

Walton NY, Treiman DM (1990) Lorazepam treatment of experimental status epilepticus in the rat: relevance to clinical practice. Neurology 40:990–994

Wilson A, Dellaportas CI, Clifford Rose F (1985) Low-dose clobazam as adjunctive therapy in chronic epilapsy. In Hindmarch I, Stonier PD, Trimble MR (eds) Clobazam: human psychopharmacology and clinical applications. Royal Society of Medicine, London 172–178

Zbinden G, Randall LO (1967) Pharmacology of benzodiazepines: laboratory and clinical correlations. Adv Pharmacol 5:213–291

CHAPTER 16

Gabapentin

F.J.E. Vajda

A. Introduction

Gabapentin ("Neurontin") has been shown in extensive preclinical and clinical studies to be an effective anticonvulsant drug, which appears to have novel mechanisms of action. Although designed as a GABA analogue it is clearly not GABAmimetic, although GABAergic mechanisms may be involved in its mechanisms of action. In clinical trials, gabapentin has shown efficacy in patients with refractory partial epilepsy. Because of its simple pharmacokinetic profile, minimal propensity for drug interactions, and lack of demonstrable or reported idiosyncratic reactions to date, the drug may have advantages in the treatment of epilepsy, when used as add-on therapy.

B. Chemistry and Use

I. Chemical Structure and Properties

Gabapentin (1-(aminoethyl)-cyclohexaneacetic acid) is a conformationally restricted analogue of γ-aminobutyric acid (GABA) which has a higher lipid solubility than the naturally occurring inhibitory transmitter (Rogawski and Porter 1990). Structurally, gabapentin incorporates a GABA moiety into a cyclohexane ring. It is a bitter tasting crystalline substance with a molecular weight of 171.34. Gabapentin is highly water soluble (octanol/aqueous pH 7.4, buffer partition coefficient log P = –1.10). It has 2 pK_a values at 25°C (3.68 and 10.70) and is a zwitterion at physiological pH (Bartoszyk et al. 1986). It resembles the bulky hydrophobic amino acids L-leucine and L-phenylalanine, despite not having a chiral carbon atom (therefore there are no enantiomers) or an amino group in an α-position in relation to the carboxyl group. Gabapentin was designed as a structural analogue of GABA which, unlike GABA, would cross the blood-brain barrier (McLean 1994). Gabapentin possesses this capacity (Ojemann et al. 1988; Ben Menachem et al. 1990). However, it does not interact with GABA receptors, and the mechanism of its anticonvulsant activity is still not fully elucidated (Rogawski and Porter 1990; Taylor 1994).

Gabapentin has a melting point of 165°–167°C. As confirmed by X-ray structure analysis, the pseudo ring configuration of the GABA molecule is integrated into a lipophilic cyclohexane moiety (Schmidt 1989). A character-

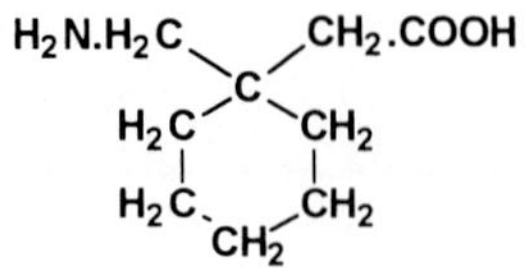

istic of the GABA molecule is its considerable degree of structural flexibility in that it can adopt a variety of almost equi-energetic configurations (PULLMAN et al. 1975). Investigation of the structurally more rigid analogues of GABA, like gabapentin, contributes to attempts to understand better the molecular process involved in the interaction of GABA with specific binding sites (BARTOSZYK et al. 1986).

II. Analytical Methods for Measuring Gabapentin

Gabapentin concentrations in plasma can be measured by high performance liquid chromatographic methods (HENGY and KOLLE 1995) or by gas liquid chromatography (HOOPER et al. 1990). The former method is based on derivatization of gabapentin followed by ultraviolet photometric detection and has a detection limit of 10 ng/ml. The latter method also involves derivatization and has a detection limit of 0.2 μg/ml in plasma and 5 μg/ml in urine. The results obtained by these methods correlate closely. The conversion factor for gabapentin is 5.84, i.e. 1 μg/ml = 5.84 μmol/l (MCLEAN 1994).

III. Use

At present, gabapentin is used in human medicine mainly as add-on therapy for partial epilepsy, but other possible uses are being explored.

C. Pharmacodynamics

I. Biochemical Pharmacology

1. Effects on GABAergic Mechanisms

In order to test whether gabapentin was GABAmimetic, a series of ligand binding and GABA turnover experiments was carried out, using mainly valproate or tritiated ligands as positive controls (SCHMIDT 1989). The conclusion drawn was that although gabapentin is a GABA analog it shows no direct GABAmimetic action. Prominent effects on monoamine neurotransmitter release were observed with gabapentin concentrations even lower than those which apply after moderate in vivo dosage (SCHLICKER et al. 1985; REIMANN 1988). Gabapentin significantly reduced stimulation-evoked neurotransmitter release from brain slices preincubated with monoamines. The release of acetylcholine was not altered by gabapentin, and the effects of gabapentin were not antagonized by bicuculline. Interactions with $GABA_A$ agonists showed that the effects of gabapentin were additive to the effects of the GABA agonists through a different, as yet unidentified, mode of action. This was explored further, utilizing numerous approaches.

a) Effects on GABA Accumulation

Gabapentin increases aminooxyacetic acid-induced GABA accumulation (Löscher et al. 1991). In the 12 brain areas examined, the time course of GABA accumulation differed from region to region. The areas where the GABA accumulation time course paralleled the time course of the anticonvulsant effect of gabapentin were the substantia nigra, amygdala and thalamus. Although Löscher et al. (1991) suggested that increased GABA synthesis may be involved in the mechanism of action of gabapentin, this has not been confirmed by later studies. In a study of rat hippocampal slices maintained in vitro and treated with microappliactions of nipecotic acid, which promotes the release and blocks the uptake of GABA, synaptically evoked excitatory population postsynaptic potentials were assessed before and after the application of gabapentin. Gabapentin treatment did not alter the population excitatory postsynaptic potential amplitude to multiple stimuli, but nearly doubled the shunting effects of nipecotic acid on the potentials. This shunting effect was bicuculline sensitive, indicating that there was $GABA_A$ receptor activation. It is suggested that gabapentin may increase free GABA levels in hippocampal cells, under conditions of promoted GABA release (Honmou et al. 1995b). Kocsis and Honmou (1994) noted that gabapentin appears to enhance the releasable pool of GABA in rat neonatal optic nerves, studied in a sucrose-gap chamber. Nipecotic acid resulted in bicuculline-sensitive depolarization and gabapentin pretreatment resulted in a near doubling of this effect, but gabapentin by itself did not alter the membrane potential. Similar results were obtained from whole cell patch clamp recordings from CA_1 pyramidal neurons in vitro (Honmou et al. 1995a).

b) Effects on GABA and Glutamate Metabolic Pathways

Gabapentin was tested for its effects on seven enzymes in the metabolic pathways of glutamate and GABA (Goldlust et al. 1993). The results suggest that gabapentin may significantly reduce the synthesis of glutamate from the branched chain amino acids L-leucine, L-isoleucine and L-valine in the brain, by acting on branched chain amino acid-transferase.

c) Effects on Receptors and Ion Channels

The effects of gabapentin on inhibitory (GABA and glycine) and excitatory (NMDA and non-NMDA) amino acid receptors and on repetitive firing of Na^+ action potentials and on voltage-dependent Ca^{2+} currents were tested in cultured rodent neurons using intracellular, whole cell or single channel recording techniques. Gabapentin in therapeutic concentrations had no significant effect (ROCK et al. 1993). In contrast, in another study it was noted that gabapentin limited the repetitive firing of Na^+ dependent action potentials in the mouse spinal cord and in neocortical neurons in monolayer dissociated cell culture, but the mechanism involved was unproven and may be an indirect one (WAMIL and MCLEAN 1993).

GEE et al. (1996) recently reported the isolation and characterization of a ^3H-gabapentin binding protein from membranes of pig cerebral cortex. The protein was purified and found to have a terminal amino acid sequence identical to that reported for the α-2-δ subunit of the L-type calcium channel prepared from rabbit skeletal muscle. High levels of tritiated gabapentin binding sites were found in membranes prepared from rat brain, heart and skeletal muscle. Further characterization was consistent with expression of an α-2-δ protein. Purified L-type Ca^{2+} channel complexes were fractionated under dissociating conditions on an ion exchange column. Tritiated gabapentin activity closely followed the elution of the α-2-δ subunit. These studies suggest that gabapentin may exert at least part of its pharmacological effect by its interaction with a subunit of a voltage-dependent Ca^{2+} channel.

2. Effects on Membrane Amino Acid Transport

Specialized membrane-bound proteins have evolved to facilitate the passage of various amino acids across cell membranes. Since gabapentin is an artificial amino acid, existing as a zwitterion at physiological pH, TAYLOR (1994) postulated that its passage across cell membranes would be severely limited without facilitated transport by one of the specialized membrane transport systems. Several studies indicate that the system utilized by the molecule may have a significant effect on the distribution of gabapentin into specific sites and tissues (STEWART et al. 1993). A lack of proportionality between tissue and plasma gabapentin levels after oral dosage was thought due to the existence of a saturable transport system, similar to the one which transports the drug across the gut membrane into the blood stream, the large, non-sodium-dependent neutral amino acid transport system (system L), which is ordinarily concerned with L-leucine and L-phenylalanine transport. In gut rings in vivo, STEWART and KUGLER (1993) have shown that gabapentin and the amino acids have mutually inhibitory and concentration-dependent effects on their trans-membrane transport, and have similar affinities for the transport mechanism. There are three neutral amino acid transport systems in Chinese hamster ovary cells. In this system also, gabapentin and L-leucine uptakes were mutually and competitively inhibited by each other (SU et al. 1995). It has been postulated that gabapentin entry through the blood-brain barrier may involve the L-amino acid transport system, as in other tissues where gabapentin is a substrate. THURLOW et al. (1993) examined the ability of large amino acids to interact with a site in mouse and pig brain labelled by ^3H-gabapentin. Gabapentin was bound with a high affinity to synaptic plasma membranes from the cerebral cortex. The presence of a submaximal concentration of leucine reduced ^{3}H-gabapentin binding, but did not affect the maximum number of binding sites, suggesting that there was competition between leucine and gabapentin for the binding proteins. These results suggest that gabapentin may label a site in the brain that resembles a large amino acid transporter system. A study of the anticonvulsant action of gabapentin in rats indicated that there was a discrepancy between the peak gabapentin concentrations in plasma and in brain microdialysate. WELTY et al. (1993) reported that the concentration-time profiles of ^{14}C-gabapentin in plasma and in interstitial fluid showed a progressive decline in plasma gabapentin concentrations whilst brain interstitial fluid concentrations peaked at 1 h, before declining linearly in parallel with the plasma concentration. Throughout the brain, the interstitial fluid concentration of the drug was approximately 3%–6% of that of the ^{14}C-gabapentin concentration in plasma, but the two concentrations became equal 4 h postdose. The anticonvulsant effect lagged behind both the plasma and the brain interstitial fluid concentrations of gabapentin and appeared to be delayed by time-dependent events other than the distribution of the drug from blood to brain. WELTY et al. (1993) also speculated whether gabapentin competes for the branched chain amino acid transport mechanism and thereby reduces the influx of isoleucine, leucine and valine into brain capillary, astrocyte or neuronal membranes. It is thought possible that increased cystosolic gabapentin concentrations and reduced branched chain amino acid concentrations would result in a net decrease in the rate of glutamate synthesis and a possible decline in neuronal neurotransmitter glutamate levels. The means by which an interaction with a neuronal transport system might reduce the paroxysmal neuronal discharges associated with epilepsy remains to be determined.

3. Studies on the Gabapentin Binding Site in Animal Brains

TAYLOR et al. (1993) studied the potent and stereospecific anticonvulsant activity of 3-isobutyl GABA in relation to its in vitro binding at a novel site labelled by tritiated gabapentin. They showed that the S(+)-enantiomer of 3-isobutyl GABA blocked maximal electroshock seizures in mice and also displaced tritiated gabapentin from the high affinity binding site in a brain membrane fraction. The R(–)-enantiomer of 3-isobutyl GABA was much less active both as an anticonvulsant and as a ligand, suggesting that the gabapentin binding site is involved in the anticonvulsant activity of L-isobutyl GABA. Further characterization of ^{3}H-gabapentin binding to a novel site in rat brain was performed by SUMAN-CHAUHAN et al. (1993). ^{3}H-Gabapentin bound with high affinity to a single population of sites on purified plasma membranes prepared from rat cerebral cortex ($K_d = 38 \pm 2.8$ nM). The binding was potently inhibited by a range of gabapentin analogues, and by 3-alkyl substituted GABA derivatives, whilst GABA itself, and the selective $GABA_B$ ligand baclofen, were only weakly active. Gabapentin binding studies in brain tissue reveal a specific binding site not present in other organs or tissues (TAYLOR 1994).

Scatchard analysis of specific binding affinities suggests that there is a single site, probably a protein, whose specific activity is abolished by heating to denaturing temperatures. High levels of binding were seen in synaptosomal brain fractions, suggesting that the protein is probably membrane-bound. The binding site is located mainly on neurons (HILL et al. 1993) and shows a discrete localization in eight regions associated with an excitatory amino acid input. These findings do not support previous indications of an association between the gabapentin binding site and the NMDA-glycine receptor complex. HILL et al. (1993) confirmed that gabapentin binding was potently inhibited by the neutral amino acids and that the gabapentin binding site closely resembled the L-system amino acid transporter.

a) Distribution of Gabapentin Specific Binding Sites

Gabapentin has been shown to bind most specifically in those areas of the brain where glutamatergic synapses are predominant, such as the superficial layers of the neocortex (layers 1 and 2), the dendritic layers of the hippocampus (CA_1, CA_2 and CA_3 subfields) and the dentate gyrus and the molecular layer of the cerebellum (TAYLOR 1994). However, the distribution of gabapentin binding sites differs from the distribution of NMDA-sensitive glutamate receptors. The binding of gabapentin at its binding sites is not altered by carbamazepine, phenytoin, valproate, ethosuximide, phenobarbitone or diazepam, but gabapentin is consistently and stereospecifically displaced from the sites by L-leucine and various other L-amino acids.

4. Overview of Biochemical Pharmacology

According to TAYLOR (1994), gabapentin has a pharmacological profile distinct from that of other antiepileptic drugs. In clinically relevant concentrations it does not interact with GABA, benzodiazepine, glutamate or NMDA receptors, or with Na^+ or Ca^{2+} channels. It appears to have a high affinity for a specific site on brain neuronal cell bodies, which is apparently associated with the system L neutral amino acid transporter. Gabapentin interacts with at least three cytosolic enzymes involved in branched chain amino acid metabolism, which convert leucine, isoleucine and valine into glutamate. The drug also enhances the activity of glutamate dehydrogenase and is a weak inhibitor of GABA transaminase. Gabapentin has a considerable structural similarity to L-leucine, and its anticonvulsant action may result from producing an alteration in brain amino acid concentrations.

II. Studies at a Cell or Tissue Level

Although early research suggested that gabapentin may act on GABAergic neurotransmitter systems (BARTOSZYK et al. 1983), subsequent preclinical studies have failed to demonstrate a specific effect of the drug on these systems

(Reimann 1983; Schlicker et al. 1985; Kondo et al. 1991; Rock et al. 1993; Taylor 1994).

1. Hippocampal Slices

GABAergic mechanisms have been studied by paired pulse orthodromic stimulation of rat hippocampal cells. Gabapentin decreased GABAergic inhibition at intraperitoneal doses of 3 mg/kg and above. Phenytoin had a similar effect at its anticonvulsant doses. It was concluded that gabapentin and phenytoin affect GABAergic inhibition in the rat hippocampus in a manner opposite to those of diazepam and pentobarbitone (Dooley et al. 1985). Haas and Wieser (1986) found gabapentin did not interfere with inhibition due to Cl^- or K^+ channel activation in rat hippocampal slices. These results suggest that a direct interaction of gabapentin with $GABA_A$ or $GABA_B$ receptors is unlikely.

2. Cultured Neurons

Taylor (1994) studied the effects of gabapentin on cultured spinal neurons in vitro. At concentrations up to 30 μg/ml, gabapentin did not change postsynaptic GABA or glutamate responses, did not depress spontaneous neuronal activity and did not block high frequency sustained repetitive action potentials. This contrasts with the effects of phenytoin, carbamazepine and valproate, all of which at low concentrations may interact with voltage-sensitive Na^+ channels to block sustained firing.

III. Animal Models of Epilepsy

1. Spectrum of Activity

Gabapentin has a broad spectrum of anticonvulsant activity similar to that of valproate (Rogawski and Porter 1990). Like valproate, it is effective in preventing tonic seizures induced by various chemical convulsants in mice. It is also effective in the maximal electroshock test in rats. In addition to its effect on tonic seizures, gabapentin is weakly effective against clonic seizures induced by pentylenetetrazole in mice, and it blocks the occurrence of reflex seizures in several species of animals (Bartoszyk and Hamer 1987), and seizures in genetically epilepsy-prone rats (Naritakou et al. 1988). The drug does not prevent photosensitive myoclonic epilepsy in baboons. Administered intraperitoneally, it was active against hippocampal kindled seizures in rats (a model of partial seizures) and reduced the duration of afterdischarging (Taylor 1993). The spectrum of antiepileptic activity of the drug, as predicted from these studies, would be expected to include both partial seizures and generalized seizures (Goa and Sorkin 1993). Kondo et al. (1991) considered that the antiepileptic profile of gabapentin, based on the feline trigeminal complex model, corresponded most closely to those of carbamazepine and phenytoin.

2. Standard Seizure Models in Mice and Rats

Bartoszyk et al. (1983) administered gabapentin orally in saline or in 0.8% hydroxypropyl methyl cellulose to male mice of the NMRI strain to investigate various models of seizures. Gabapentin protected mice from tonic extension provoked by bicuculline, picrotoxin, 3-mercaptopropionic acid, isonicotinic acid and semicarbazide. Bicuculline, an antagonist at postsynaptic $GABA_A$ receptors, was given subcutaneously in a convulsive dose of 3 mg/kg: picrotoxin, a blocker of GABA-regulated Cl^- channels, was given subcutaneously in a dose of 15 mg/kg; 3-mercaptopropionic acid, an inhibitor of GABA synthesis, was given intraperitoneally in a dose of 55 mg/kg; the other drugs, which inhibit pyridoxal phosphate, a co-factor for glutamate decarboxylase, were given in doses of 200 and 1000 mg/kg respectively (Bartoszyk et al. 1986). Gabapentin also protected mice from seizures induced by the glycine antagonist strychnine (11 mg/kg subcutaneously) and was effective in the pentylenetetrazole maximum test, related to the maximum electroshock test (Desmedt et al. 1976).

a) *Maximal Electroshock Testing*

The maximal electroshock procedure in mice showed that gabapentin had no pronounced efficacy, but in rats an oral ED_{50} value of 9.4 mg /kg was obtained, after 2 h premedication with the drug. Taylor (1993) found that gabapentin was about as effective as phenytoin in preventing the hind limb extension phase of induced seizures in rats (ED_{50} 9.1 mg/kg orally and 2.1 mg/kg intravenously compared with an ED_{50} for phenytoin of 9.5 mg/kg orally or intravenously – Foot and Wallace 1991; Taylor 1993).

b) *Seizures Induced by Glutamate, Aspartate and Kainic Acid*

The excitatory amino acids glutamate and aspartate may provoke seizures in animals leading to clonic convulsions, tonic extension and death (Watkins and Evans 1981; Zaczek and Coyle 1982). Gabapentin given intraperitoneally in doses of 30–240 mg/kg before seizure provocation prolonged the latency of the onset of seizures induced by 1 mmol/kg *N*-methyl-D-aspartic acid (NMDA). Gabapentin did not affect either the time of onset or the severity of convulsions in the kainic acid or quisqualate models (Foot and Wallace 1991).

c) *Hippocampal Kindled Seizures*

The method of Albright and Burnham (1980) and Zorumski et al. (1982) was used to test the effect of gabapentin on the threshold of hippocampal afterdischarging in a rodent model of partial seizures. Gabapentin had no significant effect (Bartoszyk et al. 1986). McLean (1995) reported that the lowest effective dose of gabapentin for blocking kindled hippocampal seizures in rats was 30 mg/kg. Doses of up to 100 mg/kg intraperitoneally did not completely block partial seizures in this kindling model.

d) Audiogenic Seizures in Mice

All commonly used antiepileptic drugs are effective in modifying audiogenic seizures in susceptible strains of mice, so that this test is not specific for particular agents (CHAPMAN et al. 1984). Gabapentin given orally in the 30–60 min prior to seizure provocation had ED_{50} values of over 80–16 mg/kg for protection against clonic activity and of 16–3 mg/kg for protection against tonic extension, respectively.

e) Seizures in the Photosensitive Baboon

In the photosensitive baboon, gabapentin did not display anticonvulsant effects in doses up to 240 mg/kg intravenously, in contrast to drugs which act on GABAergic systems (MELDRUM and HORTON 1978; MELDRUM 1986).

f) Reflex Epilepsy

The action of gabapentin in this form of epilepsy, in selectively inbred male epileptic gerbils, was evaluated by BARTOSZYK et al. (1986). The animals were shaken for 30 s or until the onset of seizures, and the seizures were evaluated by the method of LOSKOTA et al. (1974). The mongolian gerbils were protected by oral gabapentin at doses of 10–40 mg/kg given 30–240 min before the testing. This effect is regarded as a indication of a drug's capacity to protect against major seizures (LÖSCHER et al. 1983, 1984).

g) Classical Absences

Gabapentin was ineffective against classic absence epilepsy, but did not make it worse (TRUDEAU et al. 1993).

IV. Antinociceptive Effects

The GABAergic system appears to mediate antinociceptive effects. Several GABAergic drugs have analgesic properties, but gabapentin showed no analgesic effect following oral doses of 250 mg/kg in the phenyl-*p*-quinone writhing test in mice, and no antinociceptive effect occurred in the tail flick test in rats (BARTOSZYK 1986).

V. Antispasticity Effects

In animal models gabapentin showed a strong antispasticity potency comparable to, or superior to, that of the antispasticity $GABA_B$ agonist baclofen. Sedation in mice occurred following high doses of gabapentin. An oral gabapentin dose of 400 mg/kg resulted in a 40%–80% decrease in motility.

VI. Human Studies

There have been numerous controlled clinical trials of gabapentin as add-on therapy for partial seizures (CRAWFORD et al. 1987; BAUER et al. 1989; SIVENIUS 1991; UK GABAPENTIN STUDY GROUP 1990; ABOU-KHALIL et al. 1990; WIENER et al. 1990; CHADWICK 1991; SCHEAR et al. 1991; OJEMANN et al. 1992; BROWNE 1993; US GABAPENTIN STUDY GROUP No. 5 1993; ANHUT et al. 1994). The consensus of the results of these studies indicates that gabapentin is an effective treatment in patients with partial epilepsy refractory to standard antiepileptic therapy, and it is fairly well tolerated and appears to have a favourable ratio of efficacy to toxicity.

In the UK GABAPENTIN STUDY (1990), 50% of patients showed a 25% or greater reduction in seizures, compared to a 9.8% reduction in those receiving placebo. In the study of SIVENIUS (1991) there was a mean 57% decrease in seizure frequency at a gabapentin dose of 1200mg daily. In the US GABAPENTIN STUDY GROUP (1993) trial, 306 patients with refractory partial seizures were studied and 18 patients were excluded. Of the remaining patients, 18%–26% experienced a 50% or greater reduction in seizure frequency, compared with an 8% reduction in those receiving placebo. However, an increase in seizure frequency was experienced by 19%–26% of patients. Studies are continuing in children and in patients with other seizure types. Myoclonus seems to worsen in those taking gabapentin, and the drug appears to have little effect in symptomatic generalized epilepsies (West's syndrome, the Lennox-Gastaut syndrome). Higher gabapentin doses than those initially employed in the clinical trials (i.e. doses above 1800mg/day in adults) appear to be safe and studies are continuing to evaluate the optimal tolerated dose of the drug (SHORVON 1996).

D. Pharmacokinetics

I. Pharmacokinetics in Animals

BARTOSZYK (1986) investigated the absorption, metabolism and excretion of gabapentin following administration of the ^{14}C-labelled drug. Its distribution in rats was studied by VON HODENBERG and VOLLMER (1983) and by VOLLMER (1986). Gabapentin is well absorbed in rats and dogs, with 70% of the dose being excreted renally in 24h. The elimination half-life of gabapentin ranged from 2 to 3h in rats, and from 3 to 4h in dogs. Following intravenous administration to rats, similar gabapentin concentrations were present in the blood and the brain after time for a short distribution phase. In rats more than 93% of gabapentin radioactivity was eliminated renally, as the unchanged substance, and biotransformation to *N*-methyl gabapentin was found to occur only in dogs. The drug's pharmacokinetics were linear over the dosage range of 4–500mg/kg, when given intravenously to rats. The pharmacokinetics in animals were not sex dependent and were not altered after multiple doses had been taken (VOLLMER et al. 1986). Gabapentin is distributed to virtually all body tissues in rats, with highest concentrations occurring in the pancreas and kidneys.

II. Pharmacokinetics in Humans

1. Absorption and Bioavailability

There is evidence suggesting that the extent of the absorption of orally administered gabapentin diminishes as the dose increases (see below). This needs to be kept in mind in interpreting the findings described below. VOLLMER et al. (1989) investigated the absolute bioavailability of gabapentin. The area under the plasma concentration-time curve after oral administration of the drug in capsules or solution was about 60% of that after intravenous administration. After intravenous administration of 150 mg of the drug and oral administration of 300 mg (in capsules or in solution), the linear terminal phase contributed 90% to the total area under the plasma concentration-time curve, which may be of significance to the matter of the drug's penetration through the blood-brain barrier. The capsule formulation and a solution of the drug were found to be bioequivalent.

2. Distribution

The apparent volume of distribution of gabapentin at steady state was calculated to be approximately 50–58 l (MCLEAN 1994). No binding of gabapentin to plasma proteins has been observed.

a) Brain, CSF and Plasma Gabapentin Concentration Relationships

Maximum brain gabapentin levels are expected 1 h after intravenous administration of the drug. Gabapentin levels in the human brain were shown to be 80% of those in serum, in keeping with the findings of animal distribution studies (OJEMANN et al. 1988; FOOT and WALLACE 1991). Gabapentin concentrations in human CSF were 5%–35% of its plasma levels, and the drug's tissue concentrations were approximately 80% of its plasma levels (OJEMANN et al. 1988; BEN-MENACHEM et al. 1990; MCLEAN 1995). BEN-MENACHEM et al. (1992) evaluated the penetration of gabapentin into human CSF and the drug's effects on free and total GABA, homovanillic acid and 5-hydroxyindoleacetic acid concentrations by studying five patients taking a placebo, who were given a single oral dose of gabapentin, 600 mg in four patients and 1200 mg in one patient. Their plasma and CSF were collected for 72 h. The CSF to plasma gabapentin concentration ratio was 0.1 after 6 h. After 24 h, gabapentin could be recovered only from the patient who was given 1200 mg of the drug. The free and total GABA concentrations were unchanged, but the CSF 5-

hydroxyindoleacetic acid and homovanillic acid concentrations were increased at 24 and 72h.

3. Elimination

a) Metabolism

Gabapentin is not metabolized in humans and does not induce microsomal oxidative enzymes (SCHMIDT 1989; RICHENS 1993). A double-blind, phenytoin controlled parallel group trial of gabapentin in healthy volunteers was carried out, using antipyrine clearance as a measure of enzyme induction, to investigate the possible influence of prolonged gabapentin administration on liver enzyme activity. None of the antipyrine parameters was affected by gabapentin administration (SCHMIDT 1989).

b) Elimination Parameters

After intravenous administration, the elimination kinetics of gabapentin are tri-exponential with half-life values of 0.1, 0.6 and 5.3h for the three phases, respectively (SCHMIDT 1989). In the dosage range of 25–300mg, the pharmacokinetics of gabapentin are not dose-dependent. The elimination half-life of gabapentin, given orally as monotherapy, is approximately 6–9h (ANHUT et al. 1988; GRAVES et al. 1989; HOOPER et al. 1990; BEN MENACHEM et al. 1992; RICHENS 1993). These half-life values suggest that steady-state plasma concentrations of gabapentin can be reached within 1–2days of starting therapy in patients with normal renal function (MCLEAN 1995). After multiple oral doses, dose linearity of the kinetics has been demonstrated (TURCK et al. 1989).

Since the absorbed dose of gabapentin is excreted completely unchanged in urine, the plasma clearance of the drug should equal its renal clearance, which in the normal subject is of the order of 120–130ml/min, i.e. the glomerular filtration rate.

4. Clinical Pharmacokinetics

a) Plasma Concentration-Dose Relationships

Following a single gabapentin dose of 300mg in a capsule preparation, plasma gabapentin concentrations of 2.7 μg/ml were obtained after 2–3h, whilst following oral administration of 300mg every 8h, peak plasma levels of the drug averaged 4 μg/ml.

Plasma concentrations of gabapentin, when the drug is given in doses above 1800mg/day, continue to increase, but deviate increasingly from simple linear proportionality, and begin to plateau at doses of approximately 3600mg/day. At dosages of 4800mg/day, the oral bioavailabilty of the drug was estimated to be 35% (RICHENS 1993).

At dosages of 300–600mg t.i.d., trough plasma gabapentin concentrations are generally in the range of 1–10 μg/ml (MCLEAN 1994).

b) Effects of Food, Multiple Dosing, Age and Disease

Gabapentin's absorption pharmacokinetics are not altered by food or by multiple doses of the drug. Its accumulation following multiple dose administration is predictable from single dose data (VOLLMER 1992; RICHENS 1993). Abrupt discontinuation of gabapentin has been accomplished without significant increases in seizure frequency (MCLEAN 1994).

c) Gabapentin and Renal Function

Because gabapentin's elimination is affected by disease-related and age-related decreases in renal function, the drug's dosage guidelines are related to the patient's renal function. In patients with impaired renal function, peak plasma gabapentin levels are increased compared with those in persons with normal renal function (COMSTOCK et al. 1990). Following a single oral dose of gabapentin, the drug's elimination half-life was increased to a mean of 16h in patients with a mean creatinine clearance of 41 ml/min, and to 43h in those with a mean creatinine clearance of 13 ml/min. The effect of age on the single dose pharmacokinetics of gabapentin was studied in 38 patients ranging in age from 20 to 78 years. The decline in renal clearance with age paralleled the decline in creatinine clearance, which is age-related.

Gabapentin is removed from the body by haemodialysis and the maintenance dose after each dialysis should provide steady state plasma concentrations comparable to those attained in the setting of normal renal function (BOYD 1990; HALTENSON et al. 1992).

d) Plasma Gabapentin Concentrations and Therapeutic Effects

SIVENIUS et al. (1991) reported that a therapeutic effect was evident with gabapentin only when its plasma levels exceeded 2 μg/ml. In one major study, the mean gabapentin level in plasma was higher in responders than in non-responders, while higher drug levels were related to an increased efficacy of the drug (UK GABAPENTIN STUDY GROUP 1990). In the US GABAPENTIN GROUP STUDY (1993), improved seizure control tended to correlate with the drug dose. Further studies are indicated to define the relationships between plasma gabapentin concentrations and the therapeutic effects of the drug (MCLEAN 1994).

E. Interactions

I. Effect of Gabapentin on Other Drugs

Gabapentin appears to have minimal potential for drug interactions, as it is not metabolized, does not induce or inhibit hepatic microsomal oxidative enzymes, and is not bound to plasma proteins. It may conceivably interact with certain drugs which are eliminated unchanged, predominantly by renal mechanisms, but clinically significant interactions of this type have not yet been noted (McLEAN 1994).

1. Other Antiepileptic Drugs

As most of the absorbed gabapentin, approximately 10% of the absorbed lamotrigine and 50% of the absorbed felbamate are excreted unchanged in the urine, the potential exists for gabapentin to interact with the latter two drugs at a renal site. Concomitant administration of gabapentin has not affected the plasma concentrations of carbamazepine or of its epoxide metabolite, phenobarbitone, phenytoin or valproate (COMSTOCK et al. 1990; GRAVES et al. 1989, 1990; UTHMANN et al. 1990; HOOPER et al. 1991). Phenytoin monotherapy patients who had gabapentin added to their treatment in a controlled study showed no significant changes in phenytoin concentrations (GRAVES et al. 1989). CHADWICK (1994) reported that gabapentin has not produced any clinically significant drug interactions with other antiepileptic drugs. These findings are consistent with the effects of gabapentin observed in clinical studies using the drug (CRAWFORD et al. 1987; UK GABAPENTIN STUDY GROUP 1990; US GABAPENTIN STUDY GROUP 1993), and in other interaction studies related to the new antiepileptic drugs (ANHUT et al. 1988; YUEN et al. 1991).

a) Multiple Drug Interactions

TYNDEL (1994), in a case report, indicated that when gabapentin was added to three antiepileptic drugs being taken concurrently (phenytoin, carbamazepine and clobazam), there was a rise in phenytoin plasma levels that was clinically significant, causing signs of phenytoin toxicity. After cessation of gabapentin, the concentrations of phenytoin returned to their previous values, but rechallenge with gabapentin caused evidence of renewed toxicity and a rise in the plasma phenytoin level.

2. Oral Contraceptives

The effects of gabapentin on oral contraceptive steroids were studied by ELDON et al. (1993). Administration of gabapentin on days 16–22 of the last of three consecutive menstrual cycles in healthy women taking oral contraceptives did not alter the pharmacokinetics of the contraceptive components.

II. Effects of Other Drugs on Gabapentin

Gabapentin has been reported to interact with an aluminium hydroxide- and magnesium hydroxide-containing antacid (BUSCH et al. 1992). The concentration of gabapentin was decreased by 15%, which was not thought to be of clinical significance (McLEAN 1994). Cimetidine also caused a similar effect, via a renal mechanism (RICHENS 1993).

F. Adverse Effects

I. Animal Studies

1. Acute Exposure

The acute toxicology of gabapentin was investigated in 2-week-old and adult mice and rats of both sexes. Even at the highest gabapentin doses tested (8000 mg/kg orally, 4000 mg/kg subcutaneously, and 2000 mg/kg intravenously) no deaths occurred within the 2 week observation period. Autopsies showed no substance-related damage to any internal organ (Bartoszyk 1986).

2. Subacute Exposure

In a 6 months study in rats, a slight impairment of liver function was noted, with recovery 3 weeks after gabapentin dosing was ceased.

3. Chronic Exposure

Toxicology data from 2 year bioassay studies conducted in rats and mice showed an increase in the incidence in acinar cell carcinomas of the pancreas in male rats. The tumours were not seen in mice or in female rats. The doses of gabapentin used were up to 2000 mg/day for 2 years, resulting in plasma gabapentin concentrations of up to 85 mg/l, approximately 6 times those produced by therapeutic doses of the drug in humans (Foot and Wallace 1991). These findings caused clinical trials on the drug to be suspended for over 2 years, pending investigation.

4. Mutagenicity

No mutagenic activity was observed in standard tests, and daily gabapentin doses of 1500 mg/kg given to pregnant rats did not cause malformations. In human safety studies involving 14 volunteers and 70 spastic patients, no dose-related adverse reactions were noted (Schmidt 1989).

5. Carcinogenicity

Reports of the development of acinar carcinoma of the pancreas in aged male rats of a specific strain, following prolonged intake of gabapentin, were not confirmed in other species. The rats in question are generally prone to this particular malignancy, which is atypical and slow growing. The survival of the rats was not affected significantly by gabapentin intake, the gabapentin treated animals actually living longer. There were no metastases and no local invasion. The tumours were similar to those seen in concurrent control animals, although they were more frequent in the treated animals. Human pancreatic cancers tend to be ductal rather than acinar, so that the relevance of the animal tumours to any human carcinogenic risk is unclear (McLean 1995).

6. Teratogenicity

Gabapentin was found to be foetotoxic in rodents. Delayed ossification of the long bones, skull and vertebrae was observed in some foetuses exposed to dosages the equivalent (on a mg/m^2 basis) of up to 14,400 mg/day, given to patients. Hydroureters and hydronephrosis were also seen in the rats. Other significant malformations were not increased in frequency in mice, rats and rabbits at gabapentin doses of between 4 and 8 times the daily human dose on an mg/m^2 basis.

II. Human Studies

1. Add-on Pivotal Placebo-Controlled Studies in Refractory Patients

Of the three main trials, the UK GABAPENTIN STUDY GROUP (1990) compared the efficacy of 1200 mg gabapentin daily with that of placebo in 113 evaluable patients, the US GABAPENTIN STUDY GROUP (1993) compared the efficacies in 288 evaluable patients and the INTERNATIONAL GABAPENTIN STUDY GROUP (ANHUT et al. 1994) enrolled 245 evaluable patients with refractory partial seizures, in an add-on comparison against placebo. The most common side effects of gabapentin were CNS related, mild to moderate in severity, and were characterized as somnolence, dizziness and fatigue.

2. Monotherapy Trials in Previously Untreated Patients

a) Early Clinical Trials

Clinical safety data from 14 healthy volunteers and 70 spastic patients receiving gabapentin monotherapy revealed no dose-related adverse effects associated with gabapentin monotherapy in dosages up to 3600 mg/day (BARTOSZYK et al. 1986).

3. Particular Adverse Effects in Humans

In general, all studies have reported no evidence of alarming, idiosyncratic or major adverse effects of gabapentin, apart from mild to moderate fatigue and drowsiness when the drug was taken in higher dosages. As gabapentin has a relatively short half-life (5–9 h), it has been recommended for 3 times a day dosing. The dosages can be increased to a target of 1200–3600 mg/day (ABOU-KHALIL 1992) and a dose of 4800 mg/day is under evaluation (MCLEAN 1995). No withdrawal seizures have been reported after abrupt cessation of intake of the drug, but tapering the dose over a week is recommended if intake of the drug is to be discontinued.

a) Quality of Life

The neuropsychological, mood and psychosocial effects of gabapentin were studied in 15 patients whose treatment had been stabilized using phenytoin. Later they were given gabapentin alone, carbamazepine alone, and gabapentin plus carbamazepine. Neuropsychological testing at the end of the study periods showed that gabapentin monotherapy was associated with the best performance on 16 out of the 18 variables tested (DODRILL et al. 1992). The effect of gabapentin on cognitive functioning and mood was studied by ARNETT and DODRILL (1995). The quality-of-life-related side effects, obtained from data obtained in placebo-controlled clinical trials involving 921 patients, were examined by LEIDERMANN et al. (1993). Confusion, insomnia, psychoses, anxiety, apathy, emotional lability and hostility occurred less frequently in the patients who received gabapentin whilst agitation, depression and nervousness occurred more frequently. The differences between the treatment groups were small. WOLF et al. (1994) reported the occurrence of behavioural change, in the absence of other signs of toxicity, as a manifestation of gabapentin toxicity in children who were taking other antiepileptic drugs. These authors' claim that this manifestation may have been idiosyncratic is not supported by other evidence.

4. Overdosage

FISHER et al. (1994) reported a lack of serious toxicity following a massive gabapentin overdose in a 16 year old girl (48,900 mg of the drug taken as 163 capsules, each containing 300 mg of the drug). After 8 h the patient was lethargic, but rousable. Her vital signs were stable throughout, and her plasma gabapentin levels reached 62 μg/ml, 8 h after ingestion of the drug. Eighteen hours after the overdose there were no abnormal signs or symptoms. The only complicating factors were the existence of cocaine abuse, and the development of abstinence symptoms.

5. Laboratory Abnormalities

Results from the three main large scale controlled clinical trials of gabapentin and reports subsequent to the registration of the drug for clinical use have revealed no significant or clinically relevant changes in laboratory parameters, including haematological, renal, hepatic, electrolyte or endocrine laboratory values (MCLEAN 1995).

6. Pregnancy

There are few reports of human exposure to gabapentin in pregnancy, as pregnant women were deliberately excluded from the pre-marketing studies of the drug for ethical reasons (MCLEAN 1995). The total number of successful outcomes of pregnancies in women taking gabapentin is documented in a register established in the United States for this purpose.

References

Abou Khalil B, McLean M, Casiro O, Courville K (1990) Gabapentin in the treatment of refractory partial seizures. Epilepsia 31:644

Abou Khalil B, Shellenberger MK, Anhut H (1992) Two open label multicentre studies of the safety and efficacy of gabapentin in patients with refractory partial epilepsy. Epilepsia 33 [Suppl 3]:77
Albright PS, Burnham WM (1980) Development of a new pharmacological seizure model: effects of anticonvulsants on cortical and amygdala-kindled seizures in the rat. Epilepsia 21:681–6
Anhut H, Leppik I, Schmidt B, Thomann P (1988) Drug interaction study on the new anticonvulsant gabapentin with phenytoin in epileptic patients. Naunyn-Schmiedeberg's Arch Pharmacol 337 [Suppl]:29
Anhut H, Ashman P, Feuerstein TJ, Sauerrnann W, Saunders M, Schmidt B (1994) Gabapentin (Neurontin) as add-on therapy in patients with partial seizures: a double-blind, placebo controlled study. The International Gabapentin Study Group. Epilepsia 35:795–801
Arnett JL, Dodrill CB (1995) Effects of gabapentin (GBP, Neurontin) on cognitive functioning and mood. Epilepsia 38 [Suppl 3]:S32
Bartoszyk GD, Hamer M (1987) The genetic animal model of reflex epilepsy in the mongolian gerbil: differential efficacy of new anticonvulsive drugs and prototype antiepileptics. Pharmacol Res Commun 19:429–440
Bartoszyk GD, Fritschi E, Herrmann M, Satzinger G (1983) Indications for an involvement of the GABA-system in the mechanism of action of gabapentin. Naunyn-Schmiedeberg's Arch Pharmacol 322:94
Bartoszyk GD, Meyerson N, Reimann W, Satzinger G, von Hodenberg A (1986) Gabapentin. In: Meldrum BS, Porter RJ (eds) New anticonvulsant drugs. Libbey, London, pp. 147–164
Bauer G, Bechinger D, Castell X et al. (1989) Gabapentin in the treatment of drug-resistant epileptic patients. In: Manelis J, Bental E, Loeber JN, Dreifuss FE (eds) XVIIth Epilepsy International Symposium. Raven Press, New York, Advances in Epileptology 17:219–221
Ben-Menachem E, Hedner T, Persson LI, Soderfeldt H (1990) Seizure frequency and CSF gabapentin, GABA, and monoamine metabolite concentrations after 3 months' treatment with 900 mg or 1,200 mg gabapentin daily in patients with intractable complex partial seizures. Neurology 40 [Suppl 1]:158
Ben-Menachem E, Persson LI, Hedner T (1992) Selected CSF biochemistry and gabapentin concentrations in the CSF and plasma in patients with partial seizures after a single oral dose of gabapentin. Epilepsy Res 11:45–49
Boyd RA, Bockbrader HN, Türck D, Sedman AJ, Posvar EL, Chang T (1990) Effect of subject age on the single dose pharmacokinetics of orally administered gabapentin (CI-945). Pharm Res 7 [Suppl 9]:S215
Browne T, and the Gabapentin Study Groups (1993) Long-term efficacy and toxicity of gabapentin. Neurology 43:A307
Busch JA, Radulovic LI, Bockbrader HN, Underwood BA, Sedman AJ, Chang T (1992) Effect of Maalox TC® on single-dose pharmacokinetics of gabapentin capsules in healthy subjects. Pharm Res 9 [Suppl 10]:S315
Chadwick D (1991) Gabapentin. In: Pisani F, Perucca E, Avanzini G, Richens A (eds) New antiepileptic drugs. Elsevier, Amsterdam, pp. 183–186
Chadwick D (1994) Gabapentin. Lancet 343:89–91
Chapman AG, Croucher MJ, Meldrum BS (1984) Evaluation of anticonvulsant drugs in DBA/2 mice with sound-induced seizures. Arzneimittel-Forsch 34: 1261–1264
Comstock TI, Sica DA, Bockbrader HN, Underwood BA, Sedman AJ (1990) Gabapentin pharmacokinetics in subjects with various degrees of renal function. J Clin Pharmacol 30:862
Crawford P, Ghadiali E, Lane R, Blumbardt I, Chadwick D (1987) Gabapentin as an antiepileptic drug in man. J Neurol Neurosurg Psychiatry 50:682–686
Desmedt LKC, Niemegeers CJE, Lewi PJ, Janssen PAJ (1976) Antagonism of maximal metrazol seizures in rats and its relevance to an experimental classification of antiepileptic drugs. Arzneimittel-Forsch 26:1592–1603

Dodrill CB, Wilensky AJ, Ojemann LM, Temkin NR, Shellenberger K (1992) Neuropsychological, mood, and psychosocial effects of gabapentin. Epilepsia 33 [Suppl 3]:117

Dooley DJ, Bartoszyk GD, Hartensein J, Reimann W, Rock DM, Satzinger G (1986) Preclinical pharmacology of gabapentin. In: Golden Jubilee Conference and Northern European Epilepsy Meeting (University of York) Abstract 8

Eldon MA, Underwood BA, Randinitis EJ, Posvar EL, Sedman AJ (1993) Lack of effect of gabapentin on the pharmacokinetics of a norethidrone acetate/ethinyl oestradiol containing oral contraceptive. Neurology 43 [Suppl 4]:A307–A308

Fischer JH, Barr AN, Rogers SL, Fischer PA, Trudeau VL (1994) Lack of serious toxicity following gabapentin overdose. Neurology 44:982–983

Foot M, Wallace J (1991) Gabapentin. In: Pisani F, Perucca E, Avanzani G, Richens A (eds) New antiepileptic drugs. Elsevier, Amsterdam, pp. 109–114

Gee NS, Brown JP, Dissanayake VUK, Offord J, Thurlow R, Woodruff GN (1996) The novel anticonvulsant drug gabapentin (Neurontin) binds to the 2delta subunit of a Ca^{++} channel. J Biol Chem 271:5768–5776

Goa KL, Sorkin EM (1993) Gabapentin: a review of its pharmacological properties and clinical potential in epilepsy. Drugs 46:409–427

Goldlust A, Su T-Z, Welty DF, Taylor CP, Oxender DL (1995) Effects of anticonvulsant drug gabapentin on the enzymes in metabolic pathways of glutamate and GABA. Epilepsy Res 22:1–11

Graves NM, Holmes GB, Leppik E, Rask C, Slavin M, Anhut H (1989) Pharmacokinetics of gabapentin in patients treated with phenytoin. Pharmacotherapy 9: 196

Graves NM, Leppik IE, Wagner ML, Spencer MM, Erdman GR (1990) Effect of gabapentin on carbamazepine levels. Epilepsia 31:644–645

Haas HI, Wieser HG (1986) Gabapentin: action on hippocampal slices of the rat and effects in human epileptics. Proceedings of the Golden Jubilee Conference and Northern Europe Epilepsy Meeting. York, Abstract 9

Haltenson CE, Keane WF, Turck D, Bockbrader HN, Eldon MA et al. (1992) Disposition of gabapentin (GAB) in hemodialysis (HD) patients. J Clin Pharmacol 32: 751

Hengy H, Kölle EU (1985) Determination of gabapentin in plasma and urine by high-performance liquid chromatography and pre-column labelling for ultraviolet detection. J Chromatogr 341:473–478

Hill DR, Suman-Chahaun N, Woodruff GN (1993) Localization of $[^3H]$gabapentin to a novel site in rat brain: autoradiographic studies. Europ J Pharmacol – Molec Pharmacol Section 244:303–309

Honmou O, Kocsis JD, Richerson GB (1995a) Gabapentin potentiates the conductance increase induced by nipecotic acid in CA_1 pyramidal neurons in vitro. Epilepsy Res 20:193–202

Honmou O, Oyelese AA, Kocsis JD (1995b) The anticonvulsant gabapentin enhances promoted release of GABA in hippocampus: a field potential analysis. Brain Res 692:273–277

Hooper WD, Kavanagh MC, Dickinson RB (1990) Determination of gabapentin in plasma and urine by capillary column gas chromatography. J Chromatog 529: 167–174

Hooper WD, Kavanagh MC, Herkes GK, Eadie MJ (1991) Lack of a pharmacokinetic interaction between phenobarbitone and gabapentin. Brit J Clin Pharmacol 31: 171–174

Kocsis JD, Honmou O (1994) Gabapentin increases GABA-induced depolarization in rat neonatal optic nerve. Neurosci Lett 169:181–184

Kondo T, Fromm GH, Schmidt B (1991) Comparison of gabapentin with other antiepileptic and GABAergic drugs. Epilepsy Res 8:226–231

Leiderman D, Koto E, Lamoreaux L (1993) Gabapentin therapy and quality of life: side effects in placebo-controlled studies. Epilepsia 34 [Suppl 6]:45

Löscher W, Frey HH (1984) Evaluation of anticonvulsant drugs in gerbils with reflex epilepsy. Arzneimittel-Forsch 34:1484–1488

Löscher W, Frey HH, Reiche R, Schultz D (1983) High anticonvulsant potency of γ-aminobutyric acid (GABA) mimetic drugs in gerbils with genetically determined epilepsy. J Pharmacol Exp Ther 226:839–844

Löscher W, Honack D, Taylor CP (1991) Gabapentin increases aminooxyacetic acid-induced GABA accumulation in several regions of rat brain. Neurosci Lett 128: 150–154

Loskota WJ, Lomax P, Rich ST (1974) The gerbil as a model for the study of epilepsies. Epilepsia 15:109–119

McLean MJ (1994) Clinical pharmacokinetics of gabapentin. Neurology 44 [Suppl 5]:S17–S22

McLean MJ (1995) Gabapentin. Epilepsia 36 [Suppl 2]:S73–S85

Meldrum B, Horton R (1978) Blockade of epileptic responses in the photosensitive baboon, Papio papio, by two irreversible inhibitors of GABA-transaminase, γ-acetylenic GABA (4amino-hex-5-ynoic acid) and γ-vinyl GABA (4-amino-5-enoic acid). Psychopharmacol 59:47–50

Meldrum BS (1986) Preclinical test systems for evaluation of novel compounds. In: Meldrum BS, Porter RJ (eds) New anticonvulsant drugs. Libbey, London, pp. 31–48

Naritaku DK, Stryker MT, Mecozzi LB, Copley CA, Faingold CL (1988) Gabapentin reduces the severity of audiogenic seizures in the genetically epilepsy-prone rat. Epilepsia 29:693

Ojemann LM, Friel PH, Ojemann GA (1988) Gabapentin concentration in human brain. Epilepsia 29:694

Ojemann LM, Wilensky AJ, Temkin NR, Chmelir T, Ricker RA, Wallace J (1992) Long-term treatment with gabapentin for partial epilepsy. Epilepsy Res 13: 159–165

Pullman B, Berthod J (1975) Molecular orbital studies in the confirmation of GABA. Theoret Chim Acta 36:317–328

Reimann W (1983) Inhibition by GABA, baclofen and gabapentin of dopamine release from rabbit caudate nucleus: are there common or different sites of action? Eur J Pharmacol 94:341–344

Richens A (1993) Clinical pharmacokinetics of gabapentin. In: Chadwick D (ed) New trends in epilepsy management: the role of gabapentin. Royal Society of Medicine Services, London, pp. 41–46

Rock DM, Kelly KM, Macdonald RL (1993) Gabapentin actions on ligand and voltage-gated responses in cultured rodent neurons. Epilepsy Res 16:89–98

Rogawski MA, Porter RJ (1990) Antiepileptic drugs: pharmacological mechanisms and clinical efficacy with consideration of promising developmental stage compounds. Pharmacol Rev 42:223–286

Schear MJ, Wiener JA, Rowan AJ (1991) Long-term efficacy of gabapentin in the treatment of partial seizures. Epilepsia 32 [Suppl 3]:6

Schlicker E, Reimann W, Gother M (1985) Gabapentin decreases monoamine release without affecting acetylcholine release in the brain. Arzneimittel Forsch 35: 1347–1349

Schmidt B (1989) Potential antiepileptic drugs: gabapentin. In: Levy RH, Dreifuss FE, Mattson RH, Meldrum BS, Penry JK (eds) Antiepileptic drugs. 3rd edn. Raven Press, New York, pp. 925–935

Shorvon SD (1996) Gabapentin in treatment of epilepsy. In: Shorvon S, Dreifuss F, Fish D, Thomas D (eds) Blackwell Science, Oxford, pp. 429–443

Sivenius J, Kïlviïnen R, Ylinen A et al. (1991) Double blind study of gabapentin the treatment of partial seizures. Epilepsia 32:539–542

Stewart BH, Kugler AR, Thompson PR, Bockbrader HN (1993) A saturable transport mechanism in the intestinal absorption of gabapentin is the underlying cause of the lack of proportionality between increasing dose and drug levels in plasma. Pharmac Res 10:276–281

Su T-Z, Lunney B, Campbell G, Oxender DL (1995) Transport of gabapentin, a g-amino acid drug, by system L α-amino acid transporters: A comparative study in astrocytes, synaptosomes and CHO cells. J Neurochem 64:2125–2131

Suman-Chauhan N, Webdale L, Hill DR, Woodruff GN (1993) Characterisation of [^{3}H]gabapentin binding to a novel site in rat brain, homogenate binding studies. Eur J Pharmacol 244:293–301

Taylor CP (1993) Mechanism of action of new anti-epileptic drugs. In: Chadwick D (ed) New trends in epilepsy management: the role of gabapentin. Royal Society of Medicine Services Ltd, London, pp. 13–40

Taylor CP (1994) Emerging perspectives on the mechanism of action of gabapentin. Neurology 44 [Suppl 5]:S10–S16

Taylor CP, Vartanian MG, Yuen PW, Bigge C, Suman-Chauhan N, Hill DR (1993) Potent and stereospecific anticonvulsant activity of 3-isobutyl GABA relates to in vitro binding at a novel site labelled by tritiated gabapentin. Epilepsy 14:11–15

Thurlow RJ, Brown JP, Gee NS, Hill DR, Woodruff GN (1993) [^{3}H]Gabapentin may label a system-L-like neutral amino acid carrier in brain. Eur J Pharm 247: 341–345

Trudeau V, Leiderman D, Garafalo E, La Moreaux L (1993) Gabapentin (Neurontin) in patients with absence seizures: two double blind placebo controlled studies. Epilepsia 34 [Suppl 6]:45

Turck D, Vollmer KO, Bockbrader HN, Sedman A (1989) Dose-linearity of the new anticonvulsant gabapentin after multiple oral doses. Eur J Clin Pharmacol 36:A310

Tyndel (1994) Interaction of gabapentin with other antiepileptics. Lancet 343:1363–1364

UK Gabapentin Study Group (1990) Gabapentin in partial epilepsy. Lancet 335: 1114–1117

US Gabapentin Study Group No. 5 (1993) Gabapentin as add-on therapy in refractory partial epilepsy: a double-blind, placebo controlled, parallel-group study. Neurology 43:2292–2298

Uthmann BM, Hammond EJ, Wilder BJ (1990) Absence of gabapentin and valproate interaction: an evoked potential and pharmacokinetic study. Epilepsia 31:645

Vollmer KO, von Hodenberg A, Kölle EU (1986) Pharmacokinetics and metabolism of gabapentin in rat, dog and man. Arzneimittel Forsch 36:830–839

Vollmer KO, Anhut H, Thomann P, Wagner F, Jïhnchen D (1989) Pharmacokinetic model and absolute bioavailability of the new anticonvulsant gabapentin. In: Manelis J et al. (eds) Advances in epileptology, Raven Press, New York, 17: 209–211

Vollmer KO, Turek D, Bockbrader HN et al. (1992) Summary of Neurontin (gabapentin) clinical pharmacokinetics. Epilepsia 33 [Suppl 3]:77

Von Hodenberg A, Vollmer KO (1983) Metabolism of ^{14}C-gabapentin in rat, dog and man. Naunyn-Schmiedeberg's Arch Pharmacol 324:R74

Wamil AW, McLean MJ (1994) Limitation by gabapentin of high frequency action potential firing by mouse central neurons in cell culture. Epilepsy Res 17:1–11

Watkins JC, Evans RH (1981) Excitatory amino acid transmitters. Ann Rev Pharmacol Toxicol 21:165–204

Welty DF, Schielke GP, Vartanian MG, Taylor CP (1993) Gabapentin anticonvulsant action in rats: dizequilibrium with peak drug concentrations in plasma and brain microdialysate. Epilepsy Res 16:175–181

Wiener JA, Schear MJ, Rowan AJ, Wallace JD (1990) Safety and effectiveness of gabapentin in the treatment of partial seizures. Epilepsia 31:3

Wolf SA, Shinnar S, Kang H, Ballaban-Gil K, Moshe S (1994) Abstract. Epilepsia 35 [Suppl 8]:38

Yuen AWC (1991) Lamotrigine. In: Pisani F, Perucca E, Avanzini G et al (eds) New antiepileptic drugs. Elsevier, New York, pp. 115–123

Zaczek R, Coyle IT (1982) Excitatory amino acid analogues: neurotoxicity and seizures. Neuropharmacol 21:15–26
Zorumski CF, Lothman EW, Hatlelid JM (1982) Rapid kindling in the hippocampus. Soc Neurosci Abstr 8:287.26

CHAPTER 17

Tiagabine

S.C. SCHACHTER

A. Introduction

Tiagabine (TGB) was synthesized by Novo Nordisk A/S and has been co-developed with Abbott Laboratories. France and other European countries recently approved tiagabine for use as adjunctive therapy in patients with partial seizures. Other countries in Europe are currently reviewing the application. Abbott Laboratories filed a new drug application for tiagabine with the Food and Drug Administration in the United States for its use as add-on therapy for partial seizures and the drug was approved September, 1997.

This chapter will review the mechanism of action of tiagabine, and its metabolism and pharmacokinetics, the clinical development program of tiagabine, and the safety profile of tiagabine. Unless otherwise referenced, all study-related data are on file at Abbott Laboratories, Abbott Park, Illinois, USA, or Novo Nordisk, Bagsvaerd, Denmark.

B. Chemistry and Use

Nipecotic acid has an anticonvulsant effect when injected into the cerebral ventricles of mice and has been shown to inhibit the reuptake of gamma-aminobutyric acid (GABA) in cultured astrocytes and neurons (KROGSGAARD-LARSEN et al. 1987). However, nipecotic acid does not cross the blood-brain barrier. Tiagabine hydrochloride [(R)-n-(4,4-di(3-methyl-thien-2-yl)-but-3-enyl-nipecotic acid hydrochloride] is formed by linking nipecotic acid to a lipophilic anchor via an aliphatic chain, which allows tiagabine to cross the blood-brain barrier easily (Fig. 1).

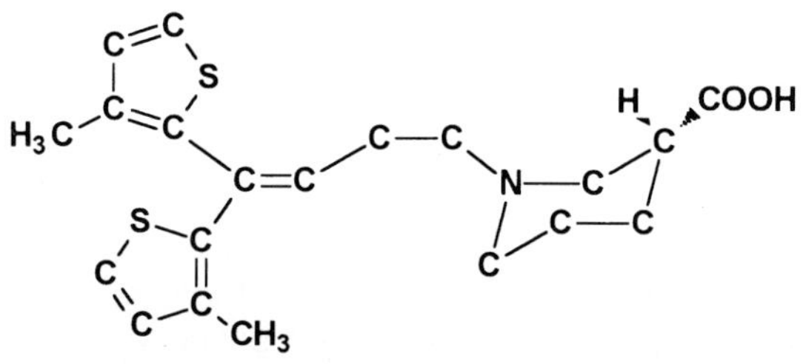

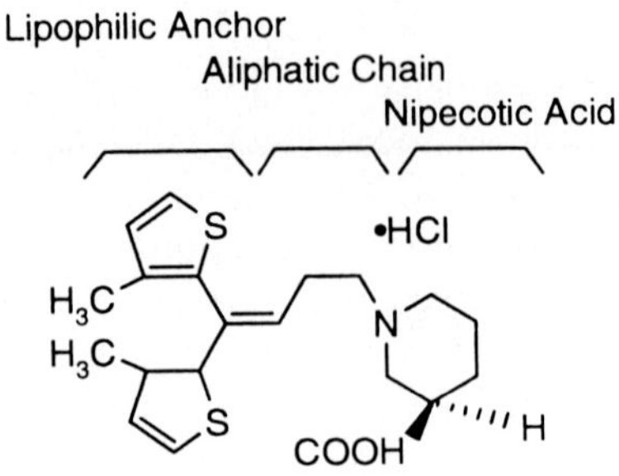

Fig. 1. Chemical structure of tiagabine (SCHACHTER 1996)

C. Pharmocodynamics

I. Biochemical Pharmacology

Tiagabine selectively binds to a single class of high-affinity binding sites associated with, but not identical to, the GABA uptake carrier GAT-1 (BORDEN et al. 1994; SUZDAK and JANSEN 1995). The mechanism of action of tiagabine is novel in that it enhances GABA-mediated inhibition by blocking the neuronal and glial reuptake of GABA (BRAESTRUP et al. 1990; GIARDINA 1994). The drug is a potent inhibitor of [^{3}H]GABA uptake into synaptosomal membranes (IC_{50} = 67 nM) or neurons (IC_{50} = 446 nM) and glial cells (IC_{50} = 182 nM) in primary cell culture. It is 2.5 times more potent in inhibiting glial than neuronal GABA uptake. Unlike nipecotic acid, tiagabine is not transported by means of the GABA uptake carrier in a synaptosomal preparation, nor does it stimulate [^{3}H]GABA release from cerebral cortical neurons in culture. Tiagabine has greater physiological specificity than GABA receptor agonists and benzodiazepine agonists because it affects only endogenously produced GABA.

Tiagabine has no significant affinity for other uptake sites, such as those for dopamine, noradrenaline, acetylcholine, adenosine, serotonin, histamine (H_2 and H_3), opiate, glycine, glutamate, or GABA (i.e. at the GABA receptor). It has only weak affinity for benzodiazepine receptors and does not affect Na^+ or Ca^{2+} channel function (BRODIE 1995; SUZDAK and JANSEN 1995).

II. Electrophysiology

Evoked inhibitory postsynaptic potentials (IPSPs) in the hippocampus result from an early $GABA_A$ receptor-mediated increase in Cl^- conductance. IPSPs play a major role in epileptic discharges, as impairment of IPSPs can result in epileptic discharges, whereas enhancement of IPSPs results in a reduction of epileptic discharges (ANDERSON et al. 1980; COLLINGRIDGE et al. 1984; STREIT et al. 1989). REKLING et al. (1990) studied the effects of tiagabine on the responses to exogenous GABA and on GABA-mediated IPSPs in pyramidal neurons of the CA1 region of hippocampal slices in culture. GABA application to the hippocampal pyramidal cell dendritic region resulted in a depolarization that was prolonged by the co-application of tiagabine (0.1 mM). In addition, GABA application to the region of the somas resulted in a hyperpolarization that was also prolonged by tiagabine (0.1 mM). Perfusion of the hippocampal slice culture with the drug also increased the amplitude of antidromic IPSPs produced by electrical stimulation of the pyramidal cell axons.

FINK-JENSEN et al. (1992), using in vivo microdialysis, examined the effect of tiagabine on changes in extracellular GABA overflow in the globus pallidus, ventral pallidum and substantia nigra in awake Sprague-Dawley rats. Tiagabine administered at either 11.5 or 21 mg/kg intraperitoneally (doses respectively corresponding to the ED_{50} and ED_{85} for inhibiting pentylenetetrazole-induced seizures in Sprague-Dawley rats) dose dependently increased extracellular GABA overflow, with peak values 200%–350% over basal ones. The maximal increase in extracellular GABA occurred at 40 min (both doses), and the increase returned to baseline at time points between 120 min (11.5 mg/kg) and 160 min (21 mg/kg).

III. Animal Seizure Models

1. Electrically and Chemically Induced Epilepsy Models

Tiagabine shows efficacy against maximal electroshock-induced seizures, bicuculline-induced seizures in rats (SUZDAK and JANSEN 1995), and picrotoxin-induced convulsions in mice (NIELSEN et al. 1991). In amygdala-kindled rats, tiagabine decreases both the severity and duration of convulsions (SUZDAK and JANSEN 1995). Tiagabine inhibits pentylenetetrazole (PTZ)-induced tonic and clonic convulsions in rats and mice, although it is slightly less potent in rats than in mice. Vigabatrin, which irreversibly inhibits GABA transaminase and thus also raises synaptic GABA concentrations, does not inhibit PTZ-induced seizures. Tiagabine also exerts potent anticonvulsant activity against DMCM-induced clonic seizures. DMCM and pentylenetetrazole produce convulsions by impairing GABAergic neurotransmission at different receptor sites associated with the postsynaptic $GABA_A$ receptor complex (ENNA 1981; ENNA and MOHLER 1987; SCHWARTZ 1988). The ability to inhibit pentylenetetrazole-induced clonic and tonic convulsions has been suggested to predict efficacy against absence seizures and/or myoclonic seizures (LÖSCHER and SCHMIDT 1988).

Tolerance to the anticonvulsant effects of tiagabine does not appear to develop during chronic administration; further, the pentylenetetrazole seizure threshold returns to the pretreatment level after tiagabine discontinuation (JUDGE et al. 1990; SUZDAK 1993).

2. Genetic Epilepsy Models

Intravenous doses of 0.25–1 mg/kg tiagabine produce partial protection against photically induced myoclonus in the photosensitive baboon for up to 3 h (SUZDAK and JANSEN 1995). Intraperitoneal doses up to 60 mg/kg tiagabine dose dependently block audiogenic convulsions in genetically epilepsy-prone rats (FAINGOLD et al. 1994). Convulsions are completely eliminated in most animals with no overt signs of sedation.

After chronic (21 day) tiagabine administration at either 15 or 30 mg/kg orally (already described), the therapeutic ratio (defined as the ratio of the ED_{50} for inhibiting exploratory locomotor activity and the ED_{50} value for inhibiting DMCM-induced clonic convulsions) significantly increased in NMRI mice from 14 (chronic vehicle-treated mice) to 28 [chronic tiagabine-treated (30 mg/kg orally) group (SUZDAK 1993)]. These data suggest that tiagabine may induce a lower incidence of side effects during long-term treatment of epilepsy.

3. Anxiolytic Effects

NIELSEN (1988) demonstrated that tiagabine was active in the modified Vogel water-lick suppression test for anxiolytic activity, with an ED_{50} = 10 mg/kg intraperitoneally.

4. Analgesic Effects

The analgesic effect of tiagabine has been investigated in various mouse and rat analgesic tests (SHEARDOWN et al. 1989). The drug has potent analgesic effects in the mouse acetic acid writhing test (ED_{50} = 0.18 mg/kg subcutaneously), mouse hot-plate test (ED_{50} = 3.7 mg/kg intraperitoneally), mouse grid shock test (ED_{50} = 1.75 mg/kg intraperitoneally), and the rat Randall Selitto test (ED_{50} = 12 mg/kg intraperitoneally).

5. Effect on Cerebral Ischaemia

JOHANSEN and DIEMER (1991) examined the effect of tiagabine on the loss of hippocampal CA_1 pyramidal cells produced in the rat four-vessel occlusion model of transient global ischaemia. Tiagabine administered at a dose of 50 mg/kg intraperitoneally, immediately before and 1, 24 and 48 h after ischaemia, significantly reduced the ischaemic CA_1 pyramidal cell loss. This protection against ischaemic CA_1 cell death may have been due to the increased GABA levels resulting from inhibition of GABA uptake, leading to a decrease in excitation in the hippocampus.

IV. Human Studies

Five multicentre, double-blind, randomized, placebo-controlled trials have been performed in 951 patients with refractory partial-onset seizures, including 675 patients aged 12–72 years who were randomized to tiagabine (LASSEN et al. 1995). Two studies had crossover designs (ØSTERGAARD et al. 1995; RICHENS et al. 1995); the other three had parallel-group, add-on designs, viz. the dose response, the dose frequency, and the three times daily (TID study) dosing studies (BEN-MENACHEM 1995).

1. Adult Add-on, Parallel-Design Trials

a) Study Designs

The objective of the dose-response study was to confirm the efficacy of add-on tiagabine in complex partial seizures and to demonstrate a dose-response relationship. During the first 4 weeks of the 16-week treatment phase, treatment doses were increased weekly to one of the target daily dosages: placebo, 16 mg tiagabine, 32 mg tiagabine, and 56 mg tiagabine, all taken in four divided doses (UTHMAN et al. 1997).

The dose-frequency study compared tiagabine 32 mg/day, given as 16 mg twice a day (BID group) or 8 mg four times a day (QID group), with placebo. During the 1st month of the 12-week treatment phase, doses were increased weekly to the target dosage (SACHDEO et al. 1997).

The TID dosing study compared 10 mg/day tiagabine t.i.d. with placebo. During the 1st month of the 18-week treatment phase, tiagabine and placebo doses were increased weekly till tiagabine 10 mg t.i.d. or a similar number of placebo tablets were taken (BEN-MENACHEM 1995).

b) Enrolment Information

Overall, the placebo and treatment groups were well-matched. The median duration of epilepsy for both groups was 23 years, and patients in both groups had taken a median of nearly six antiepileptic drugs in the past. Patients with primary generalized seizures were excluded.

c) Results

The primary efficacy parameters for these three studies were (1) the median reduction in 4-week complex partial seizure rates from their baseline number, and (2) the proportion of patients who achieved at least a 50% reduction in 4-week complex partial seizure rates during the treatment period, as compared with the baseline rate. Figure 2 shows the reduction in 4-week rates of complex partial seizure for each of the three studies. The seizure rate reduction in each treatment group is compared with that in the placebo group. Figure 3 shows the proportion of patients with a 50% reduction in 4-week complex partial seizure rates.

In the dose-response study, the median reduction in complex partial seizure and simple partial seizures from their baseline rates in the 32 mg and 56 mg groups combined (as specified in the protocol) was statistically significant compared to placebo. The minimum effective dose was 32 mg/day.

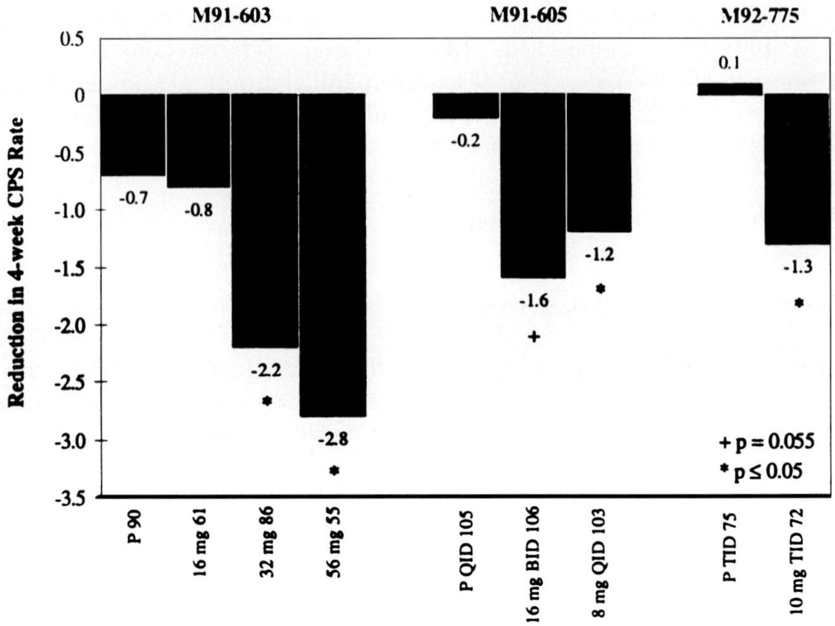

Fig. 2. Tiagabine efficacy in parallel, add-on studies: reduction in 4-week complex partial seizures (SCHACHTER 1996). M91-603, dose-response study; M91-605, dose-frequency study; M92-775, TID dosing study

In the dose-frequency study, the seizure reduction in the 8 mg QID group was statistically significant and the reduction in the 16 mg BID group was significant at the $p = 0.055$ level. The median changes in 4-week complex partial seizure rates were –1.6 ($p = 0.06$) for the 16 mg BID group and –1.2 ($p = 0.02$) for the 8 mg QID group.

In the TID dosing study, 30 mg/day tiagabine was significantly more effective than placebo in reducing the median 4 week complex partial seizure rate (–1.3 vs. +0.1; $p = 0.05$), the simple partial seizure rate (–1.0 vs. +0.6; $p = 0.05$), and the rate for all seizure types combined.

2. Open-label, Long-term Treatment

There are six ongoing, long-term trials; three are extensions of the placebo-controlled, add-on studies, whilst the other three phase III studies enrolled patients with any type of uncontrolled seizure. As of May 1997, over 1200 patients had received tiagabine for at least 1 year. The maximum daily dose of tiagabine allowed was 120 mg in two of the studies, 80 mg in two of the studies, and 64 mg in two studies. The mean and median daily dosages appeared to stabilize around 45 mg/day after 6 months of treatment. Some patients benefitted from doses up to 80 mg/day. Some 30%–40% of the

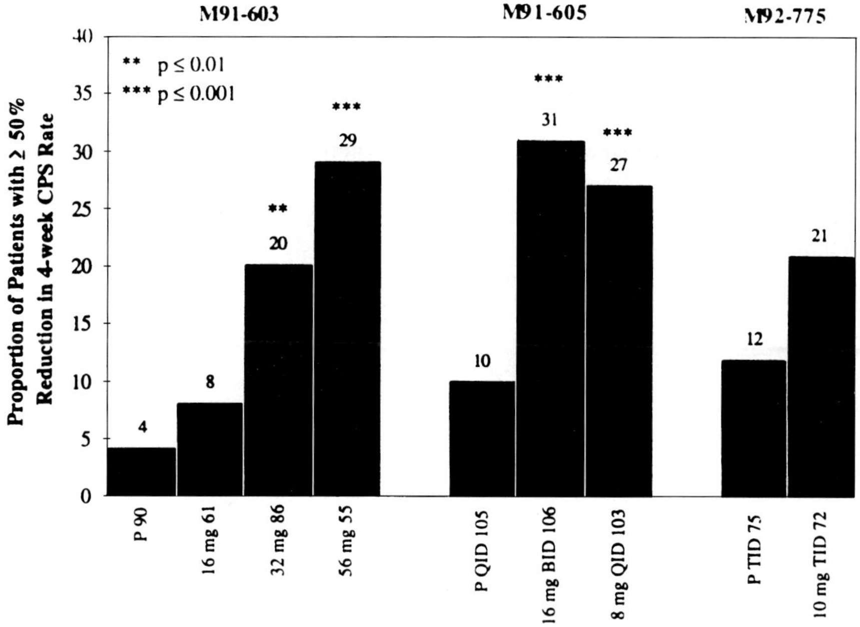

Fig. 3. Tiagabine efficacy in parallel, add-on studies: proportion of patients with a 50% reduction in 4-week complex partial seizures (SCHACHTER 1996). M91-603, dose-response study; M91-605, dose-frequency study; M92-775, TID dosing study

patients in the extension studies had a favourable response to treatment; the median reduction in complex partial seizure rate was 28.4% after 3–6 months of treatment and increased to 44% after 12 months.

3. Monotherapy Studies

a) Dose-Ranging, Tiagabine-Substitution Study

The objective of the dose-ranging, tiagabine-substitution study was to determine the maximum tolerated dose of tiagabine monotherapy (SCHACHTER 1995). Patients were tapered off their baseline antiepileptic drugs over 3 weeks as tiagabine was added. Daily tiagabine doses could be increased up to 80 mg or 0.6 mg/kg, as tolerated (SCHACHTER et al. 1995). Thirty-one patients with epilepsy for a median time of over 20 years and who were refractory to at least two previous antiepileptic drugs entered the study. The treatment of 19 patients (61%) was converted successfully to tiagabine monotherapy, of whom 12 completed the study. Nineteen patients withdrew prematurely from the study, including seven whose treatment had been converted to tiagabine monotherapy. The mean daily tiagabine dose for those who completed the study was 38.4 mg (range 24–54 mg).

b) Multicentre High- Versus Low-Dose Study

The high- versus low-dose study was a multicentre, double-blind, randomized, parallel-group study that compared the safety and efficacy of 6 mg and 36 mg tiagabine daily when administered as monotherapy to patients with complex partial seizures, with or without secondarily generalized tonic-clonic seizures (SCHACHTER 1995). Dosages were titrated over 2 weeks and, over the following 4 weeks, concomitant antiepileptic drugs were withdrawn. Of the 198 patients randomized in the study, 34 patients in the low-dose group and 23 patients in the high-dose group completed treatment. For both dosage groups, the median complex partial seizure rates decreased significantly during tiagabine monotherapy when compared with their baseline values in patients who completed 12 weeks of the treatment phase ($p = <0.05$). In addition, nearly twice as many patients in the 36-mg-daily group experienced a reduction in their complex partial seizure rate of at least 50% when compared with patients in the 6-mg-daily group (30% vs. 18%; $p = 0.038$).

4. Paediatric Trials

In a single-blind study in children with either partial or generalized seizures that were unsatisfactorily controlled with other antiepileptic drugs, approximately 20% of those with partial seizures achieved a reduction in their seizure rates of 50% or more; generalized seizures responded less well (ULDALL et al. 1995).

Twenty-five children aged 3–11 who had epilepsy were enrolled in a polytherapy, single-dose pharmacokinetic study (BOELLNER et al. 1996). In most of these children, one or two trials of antiepileptic drugs had failed in the past. During a subsequent long-term safety study, the treatment of 16 was converted to tiagabine monotherapy successfully. After approximately 1 year of tiagabine therapy, these 16 children were seizure-free for at least 2 months at a dose of 4–14 mg/day.

D. Pharmacokinetics

I. Animal Pharmacokinetics

This topic was admirably reviewed by SUZDAK and JANSEN (1995). The absorption of tiagabine, when administered orally in aqueous solution, was rapid, giving a T_{max} of 10 min in mice, 30 min in rats, and 1 h in dogs. After the administration of tiagabine capsules to dogs, the T_{max} was 0.75–2.2 h. The bioavailability of the drug was 25% in rats and 54% in dogs. In rats administered 27 mg/kg tiagabine intraperitoneally twice daily for 7 or 14 days, the bioavailability increased to 54% and 74%, suggesting a saturation of first-pass metabolism. In mice, the bioavailability was 92%. The volume of distribution was 1.41 and 1.28 l/kg in rats and dogs, respectively. The plasma protein binding was 92%–93% in dogs (SUZDAK and JANSEN 1995). After the administration of [^{14}C]-labelled tiagabine, the levels of radioactivity in most tissues were similar to that in plasma. Only eliminating organs had considerably higher levels, with tissue/plasma ratios of 9 (rats) and 15 (dogs) in the liver, and 3.2 (rats) and 4.0 (dogs) in the kidney, and 1.2 (rats) in the lung 30 min after the administration of the isotopic drug. The decrease in tissue levels of labelled tiagabine followed the decrease in plasma levels. The brain to plasma ratio in rats remained constant at 0.24.

Tiagabine is extensively metabolized in rats and dogs. The major metabolic pathway is thiophene oxidation, leading to geometric 5-oxo-thiolene isomers. In rats, a dioxidized metabolite conjugated with glutathione was found in bile, whereas in dogs the oxo-thiolene isomers were further metabolized either by hydroxylation of the methyl group or by conjugation with glucuronic acid. An acyl glucuronic acid conjugate was noted in both dogs and rats. The metabolic pathway of the drug in rats and dogs has not been elucidated completely.

II. Human Pharmacokinetics

1. Absorption and Bioavailability

Tiagabine is quickly and nearly completely absorbed after oral administration (Mengel 1994); its bioavailability is 89%. When tiagabine is taken without food, the maximum serum concentration (C_{max}) is reached in 60–90 min. When taken with food, the time to the C_{max} is increased to 2.6 h and the C_{max} is halved, although the area under the curve (AUC) is unchanged (Brodie 1995). Therefore, food appears to reduce the rate, but not the extent, of tiagabine absorption. After oral administration of tiagabine (2, 4, 6, 8, or 10 mg) once daily for 5 days, the time of occurrence of the peak serum concentration appears to be independent of both the size and the number of doses administered. Although C_{max} values vary both within and among subjects, the overall dose-adjusted C_{max} is independent of the dose, its value being approximately 16.0–26.5 ng/ml/mg tiagabine.

2. Distribution

Tiagabine is widely distributed throughout the body; its apparent volume of distribution is approximately 1 l/kg, and it is approximately 96% protein bound in plasma.

3. Elimination

a) Metabolism

Tiagabine is oxidized in the liver by the cytochrome isoenzyme CYP3 A (Bopp et al. 1995a). The E- and Z-5-oxo-tiagabine isomers are the only prominent metabolites found in plasma (Østergaard et al. 1995). Some 25% of the administered dose of tiagabine is excreted in the urine, mainly as the 5-oxo isomer metabolites. Tiagabine is subject to extensive hepatic metabolism and only 2% of the administered dose is excreted in urine as the unchanged parent drug (BOPP et al. 1995b; ØSTERGAARD et al. 1995). Within 3–5 days after a tiagabine dose, the remainder of the administered drug is eliminated in the faeces as two unidentified metabolites (ØSTERGAARD et al. 1995).

b) Elimination Parameters

The plasma elimination half-life of tiagabine in patients whose hepatic function is not induced is 5–8h (GUSTAVSON and MENGEL 1995). The half-life is reduced to 2–3h by the co-administration of hepatic enzyme-inducing antiepileptic drugs (BRODIE 1995).

4. Applied Pharmacokinetics

There is a linear relationship between daily dosages of tiagabine and serum concentrations in subjects, whether or not hepatic function is induced (GUSTAVSON and MENGEL 1995; SO et al. 1995). For the same daily dose, un-induced patients achieve higher tiagabine serum concentrations than induced patients. Consequently, tiagabine concentrations may rise in patients who are tapered off concomitant therapy with enzyme-inducing antiepileptic drugs (SCHACHTER 1995).

5. Special Patient Groups

a) Hepatic and Renal Impairment

Plasma concentrations of both total and unbound tiagabine are increased in association with hepatic dysfunction (LAU et al. 1997), and the elimination half-life is slowed to approximately 12–16h. The pharmacokinetic profile of tiagabine is unaffected in patients with renal failure (CATO et al. 1995). Consequently, dosage adjustments appear to be unnecessary in patients with reduced renal function.

b) The Elderly and Children

The pharmacokinetics of tiagabine have been studied in a limited number of subjects up to 81 years of age and appear to be similar to those of younger patients (SNEL et al. 1993). Hence, there is no apparent need for dosage modification in the elderly (ØSTERGAARD et al. 1995). Children eliminate tiagabine slightly faster than adults, but this appears to be clinically insignificant (GUSTAVSON et al. 1997).

E. Interactions

I. Pharmacodynamic Interactions

No potentiation of cognitive impairment has been noted when tiagabine is taken together with triazolam or alcohol, both of which are GABA agonists.

II. Pharmacokinetic Interactions

1. Effect of Tiagabine on the Pharmacokinetics of Other Drugs

Tiagabine does not displace other tightly plasma protein-bound drugs, including phenytoin, valproate, amitriptyline, tolbutamide and warfarin (Brodie 1995; Gustavson et al. 1995).

The clearance of antipyrine is unaffected by tiagabine, suggesting that this drug neither induces nor inhibits hepatic enzymatic function (Gustavson and Mengel 1995). The steady-state pharmacokinetics of carbamazepine and phenytoin are unchanged by the addition of tiagabine, whereas the mean steady-state AUC and C_{max} for valproate are reduced by 10%–12%, decreases that are probably of limited clinical importance (Gustavson et al. 1995). Tiagabine does not significantly affect the pharmacokinetics of other hepatically metabolized drugs, including theophylline, warfarin, and digoxin (Mengel et al. 1995). At a dosage of 8mg/day, tiagabine has no effect on the metabolism of oral ethinyloestradiol (30 μg) plus 150 μg levonorgestrel or desogestrel (Mengel et al. 1994). The potential effects of higher tiagabine doses on contraceptive metabolism and efficacy remain to be determined.

2. Effects of Other Drugs on the Pharmacokinetics of Tiagabine

When 800mg/day cimetidine is added to 8mg/day tiagabine, there is an approximate 5% increase in trough plasma tiagabine concentrations and AUC at steady state, increases that are unlikely to be clinically important (Mengel et al. 1995). The tiagabine clearance is increased by antiepileptic drugs that induce cytochrome P450, and tiagabine is displaced from serum proteins by naproxen, salicylates, and valproate.

F. Adverse Effects

I. Animal Animal Toxicology

1. Acute Toxicity

Single-dose tiagabine studies in rats and mice showed no adverse effects with clinically relevant doses, though sedation occurred at dosages higher than those needed for anticonvulsant activity (Pierce et al. 1991; Mengel 1994). There were no clinically significant cardiovascular effects in rats or dogs, even at doses that produce plasma concentrations many times higher than those produced by the maximum recommended human dosage.

2. Chronic Toxicity

Three-month treatment in rats with tiagabine doses considerably higher than therapeutic ones (100mg/kg/day) produced no systemic organ toxicity other than abdominal swelling. However, in this species doses above 25mg/kg/day may cause hepatic cellular hypertrophy, consistent with the occurrence of enzyme induction. In dogs, doses up to 15 times the therapeutic doses are not associated with systemic organ toxicity. After the twice-daily injection of tiagabine (30 mg/kg intraperitoneally) for 4 days, acute treatment at 10 mg/kg intraperitoneally produced a memory deficit (a 59% reduction in the latency to drink). There were no effects at a 3 mg/kg intraperitoneal dose. In the chronic vehicle-treated group, acute tiagabine treatment at both 3 and 10 mg/kg significantly reduced the latency to drink. A parallel set of experiments, using the same dosing regimen, showed no tolerance to the anticonvulsant effects of the drug (JUDGE et al. 1990).

Tolerance developed to the motor-impairing side effects of tiagabine in mice treated for 21 days with 15 or 30 mg/kg of the drug (JUDGE et al. 1990).

3. Teratogenicity, Carcinogenicity, Mutagenicity

Tiagabine does not impair fertility in male or female rats or show teratogenicity in rats or rabbits. In rats, the no-adverse-effect dosage for both parental and fetal toxicity is at least 6 times the therapeutic dosage. In mice and rats that have received tiagabine for 2 years (10–250 mg/kg per day and 10–200 mg/kg per day, respectively), the only drug-related increases in tumor incidence observed were at the high-dose levels (>200 mg/kg/day), and consisted of Leydig cell testicular tumours and liver adenomas in the rats.

In vitro mutagenicity tests have shown no consistent increases in mutation frequency in the presence of tiagabine.

II. Human Studies

1. Add-on, Parallel-Group Studies

Overall, 91% of tiagabine-treated patients and 79% of placebo-treated patients reported one or more treatment-emergent adverse event in the add-on, parallel-group studies; most unwanted effects were mild or moderate, occurred during dose titration, and resolved spontaneously. Three or four doses a day were better tolerated than two doses a day. The adverse events that occurred significantly more often with tiagabine than with placebo were dizziness, asthenia (fatigue or generalized muscle weakness), nervousness, tremor, abnormal thinking (trouble concentrating, mental lethargy, or slowness of thought), depression, and aphasia (dysarthria, difficulty speaking, or speech arrest). Nine percent of tiagabine-treated patients and 5% of placebo-treated patients reported severe adverse events, mostly somnolence, asthenia, and headache (SCHACHTER 1997).

In double-blind, placebo-controlled, parallel-group studies, 13% of tiagabine-treated patients prematurely discontinued the therapy because of adverse events, compared with 5% of placebo-treated patients. The most common reasons for ceasing treatment were confusion (1.4%), somnolence (1.2%), ataxia (<1%), asthenia (<1%), and dizziness (<1%) (SCHACHTER 1997).

2. Monotherapy Trials

The adverse events seen in the high- versus low-dose monotherapy study were similar to those described above. In addition, speech disorder, somnolence, and blurred vision (amblyopia) occurred statistically more often with the 36-mg-daily than the 6-mg-daily treatment (BRODIE 1997).

In the dose-ranging, open-label, tiagabine-substitution monotherapy study, the most common adverse events were asthenia, dizziness, difficulty concentrating, insomnia, nervousness, somnolence, and impaired memory. The adverse events leading to premature discontinuation resolved when tiagabine was stopped. Every patient experienced at least one treatment-emergent adverse event because patients were dosed to their limit of tolerance (SCHACHTER 1995).

3. Long-term Studies

In the long-term studies, 1236 patients received tiagabine for at least 1 year. Excluding accidental injury and infection, the five most frequently reported adverse events were dizziness, somnolence, asthenia, headache, and tremor. The incidence of these events appeared to peak within the first 30–45 days of treatment. There were no indications that new or more severe types of adverse events developed during long-term therapy compared with short-term therapy (LEPPIK 1995).

4. Special Safety Issues in Humans

a) Death

There were 35 deaths in patients treated in the various tiagabine studies (total patient exposure approximately 3831 patient-years). The most commonly identified cause of mortality was sudden unexpected death in epilepsy (10), accounting for 0.0026 deaths per patient-year. Two of the deaths were thought to be possibly related to tiagabine; one patient, who had been taking tiagabine for more than 1000 days, was a smoker with hypertension and a previous stroke, and was found dead in bed. No autopsy was performed, and hypertensive atherosclerotic cardiovascular disease was cited as an alternative explanation. The other patient died from a cerebral neoplasm; neurofibromatosis was cited as a possible alternative aetiology.

b) Rash, Psychosis, Status Epilepticus

The occurrence of rash and psychosis was similar in tiagabine-treated patients and patients treated with placebo. Status epilepticus occurred in approximately 0.8% of patients receiving tiagabine and in 0.7% receiving placebo in the double-blind, parallel studies. All episodes of status were either complex partial or simple partial status epilepticus. No instances of convulsive status occurred in these controlled trials.

c) Overdosage

As of August 1996, there had been 11 reported instances of overdosage with tiagabine during clinical trials of the drug. In all 11 instances, the patients recovered completely, generally within 24h, even at tiagabine doses up to 800mg (PARKS et al. 1997). In all these cases, supportive care with gastric lavage and the use of activated charcoal was helpful in the treatment of tiagabine overdose. Since tiagabine is highly protein bound and largely metabolized by the liver, dialysis would not be expected to be beneficial.

The most common reported symptoms of overdosage were confusion, somnolence, agitation, hostility, speech difficulty, weakness, impaired consciousness and myoclonus. There was one case of convulsive status epilepticus after a patient ingested 400mg tiagabine. The patient responded to intravenous phenobarbitone and made a full recovery (PARKS et al. 1997).

d) Laboratory Values

In the parallel-group, add-on, double-blind studies, no clinically important changes in haematological and biochemical test results, vital signs, or electrocardiograms were attributable to tiagabine (LEPPIK 1995).

e) Neuropsychological Function and Cognitive Effects

In the double-blind, add-on, crossover study, there were no significant differences in neuropsychological test scores, mood, or behavioural rating scales between patients receiving tiagabine and those receiving placebo. Similarly, in the add-on, dose-response study, neuropsychological testing showed no evidence of worsening in mood or cognitive abilities (DODRILL et al. 1997). In the high-dose, low-dose monotherapy study, patients improved modestly on tests of mental abilities and on four measures of adjustment when their treatment was converted to tiagabine monotherapy ($p = <0.05$ – DODRILL et al. 1996).

f) Pregnancy

The safety of tiagabine in pregnancy is unknown. As of 15 October, 1996, 22 pregnancies had occurred in patients exposed to tiagabine or blinded drug in the clinical trials (COLLINS et al. 1997). Nine patients carried their babies to term, and eight of these patients delivered healthy offspring. The ninth patient had a Caesarean section delivery for a breech presentation; the baby had hip displacement, which was attributed to the breech presentation. Five patients underwent elective abortion, four patients had miscarriages, one patient underwent dilation and curettage with suction for a blighted ovum, and another patient underwent right salpingectomy for an ectopic pregnancy. One patient, who had discontinued tiagabine 3 months previously, drowned in a bathtub from a seizure during her 5th month of pregnancy. She had a pre-existing cerebral neoplasm when she entered the trial. The outcome was not then available for one patient.

References

Andersen P, Dingledine R, Gjerstad L, Langinden LA, Mosfeldt Laursen A (1980) Two different responses of hippocampal pyramidal cells to application of gamma-amino butyric acid. J Physiol 305:270–296

Ben-Menachem E (1995) International experience with tiagabine add-on therapy. Epilepsia 36 [Suppl 6]:S14–S21

Boellner S, McCarty J et al. (1996) Pilot study of tiagabine in children with partial seizures. Epilepsia 37 [Suppl 4]:S92

Bopp BA, Nequist GE et al. (1995a) Role of the cytochrome P450 3 A subfamily in the metabolism of [14 C] tiagabine by human hepatic microsomes. Epilepsia 36 [Suppl 2]:S159

Bopp B, Gustavson L et al. (1995b) Pharmacokinetics and metabolism of [14 C tiagabine] after oral administration to human subjects. Epilepsia 36 [Suppl 2]:S158

Borden LA, Dhar TGM et al. (1994) Tiagabine, SK&F 89976-A, CI-966, and NNC-711 are selective for the cloned GABA transporter GAT-1. Eur J Pharmacol 269: 219–224

Braestrup C, Nielsen EB et al. (1990) (R)-N-(4,4-bis(3-methyl-2-thienyl)but-3-en-1-yl)nipecotic acid binds with high affinity to the brain GABA uptake carrier. J Neurochem 54:639–664

Brodie MJ (1995) Tiagabine pharmacology in profile. Epilepsia 36 [Suppl 6]:S7–S9

Brodie MJ (1997) A monotherapy approach with tiagabine. Presented at the 22nd International Epilepsy Congress Satellite Symposium, Dublin, June 30, 1997

Cato A, Qian JX et al. (1995) Pharmacokinetics and safety of tiagabine in subjects with various degrees of renal function. Epilepsia 36 [Suppl 3]:S159

Collingridge GL, Gage PW, Robertson B (1984) Inhibitory postsynaptic currents in rat hippocampal CA1 neurons. J Physiol 356:551–564

Collins SD, Donnelly J et al. (1997) Pregnancy and tiagabine exposure. Neurology 48 [Suppl 2]:A38

Dodrill CB, Arnett JL et al. (1996) Changes in mental abilities and adjustment with conversion to tiagabine monotherapy. Neurology 46 [Suppl]:A277

Dodrill CB, Arnett JL et al. (1997) Cognitive and quality of life effects of differing dosages of tiagabine in epilepsy. Neurology 48:1025–1031

Enna SJ (1981) Neuropharmacological and clinical aspects of GABA. In: Palmer G (ed) Neuropharmacology of central nervous system GABA and behavioral disorders. New York, Academic Press, pp. 507–516

Enna SJ, Mohler H (1987) GABA receptors and their association with benzodiazepine recognition sites. In: Meltzer HY, ed. Psychopharmacology: the third generation of progress. New York: Raven Press, pp. 265–274

Faingold CL, Randall ME et al. (1994) Blockade of GABA uptake with tiagabine inhibits audiogenic seizures and reduces neuronal firing in the inferior colliculus of the genetically epilepsy-prone rat. Exp Neurol 126:225–232

Fink-Jensen A, Suzdac RD, Sweberg MD, Judge ME, Hansen L, Nielsen PG (1992) The GABA uptake inhibitor, tiagabine, increases extracellular brain levels of GABA in awake rats. Eur J Pharmacol 20:197–201

Giardina WJ (1994) Anticonvulsant action of tiagabine, a new GABA-uptake inhibitor. J Epilepsy 7:161–166

Gustavson LE, Mengel HB (1995) Pharmacokinetics of tiagabine, a gamma-aminobutyric acid-uptake inhibitor, in healthy subjects after single and multiple doses. Epilepsia 36:605–611

Gustavson LE, Cato A et al. (1995) Lack of clinically important drug interactions between tiagabine and carbamazepine, phenytoin, or valproate. Epilepsia 36:S159

Gustavson LE, Boellner SW et al. (1997) A single-dose study to define tiagabine pharmacokinetics in pediatric patients with complex partial seizures. Neurology 48: 1032–1037

Johansen FF, Diemer NH (1991) Enhancement of GABA neurotransmission after cerebral ischemia in the rat reduces loss of hippocampal CA1 pyramidal cells. Acta Neurol Scandinav 84:1–5

Judge ME, Swedberg MDB et al. (1990) Tolerance to the cognitive impairing effects, but not to the anticonvulsant effects, of NO-328: a selective GABA uptake inhibitor. Eur J Pharmacol 183:467

Krogsgaard-Larsen P, Falch E et al. (1987) GABA uptake inhibitors: relevance to antiepileptic drug research. Epilepsy Res 1:77–93

Lassen LC, Sommerville K et al. (1995) Summary of five controlled trials with tiagabine as adjunctive treatment of patients with partial seizures. Epilepsia 36 [Suppl 3]: S148

Lau AH, Gustavson LE et al. (1997) Pharmacokinetics and safety of tiagabine in subjects with various degrees of hepatic function. Epilepsia 38:445–451

Leppik IE (1995) Tiagabine: the safety landscape. Epilepsia 36 [Suppl 6]:S10–S13

Löscher W, Schmidt D (1988) Which animal models should be used in the search for new antiepileptic drugs? A proposal based on experimental and clinical considerations. Epilepsy Res 2:145–181

Mengel H (1994) Tiagabine. Epilepsia 35 [Suppl 5]:S81–S84

Mengel HB, Houston A et al. (1994) An evaluation of the interaction between tiagabine and oral contraceptives in female volunteers. J Pharm Med 4: 141–150

Mengel H, Jansen JA et al. (1995) Tiagabine: evaluation of the risk of interaction with theophylline, warfarin, digoxin, cimetidine, oral contraceptives, triazolam, or ethanol. Epilepsia 36 [Suppl 3]:S160

Nielsen EB (1988) Anxiolytic effect of NO-328, a GABA-uptake inhibitor. Psychopharmocology 96, N:42

Nielsen EB, Suzdak PD et al. (1991) Characterization of tiagabine (NO-328), a new potent and selective GABA uptake inhibitor. Eur J Pharmacol 196:257–266

Østergaard LH, Gram L et al. (1995) Potential antiepileptic drugs. Tiagabine. In: Levy RH, Mattson RH, Meldrum BS (eds) Antiepileptic drugs. Raven Press, New York, pp. 1057–1061

Parks BR, Flowers WC et al. (1997). Experience with clinical overdoses of tiagabine. 8th International Bethel-Cleveland Clinic Epilepsy Symposium, Bielefeld, Germany

Pierce MW, Suzdak PD et al. (1991) Tiagabine. In: Pisani F, Perucca E, Avansini G, and Richens A (eds) New antiepileptic drugs. Elsevier, Amsterdam, pp. 157–160

Rekling JC, Jahnsen H, Laursen AM (1990) The effect of two lipophilic GABA uptake blockers in CA1 of the rat hippocampual slice. Br J Pharmacol 99:103–107

Richens A, Chadwick DW et al. (1995) Adjunctive treatment of partial seizures with tiagabine: a placebo-controlled trial. Epilepsy Res 21:37–42

Sachdeo RC, Leroy RF et al. (1997) Tiagabine therapy for complex partial seizures. Arch Neurol 54:595–601

Schachter SC (1995) Tiagabine monotherapy in the treatment of partial epilepsy, Epilepsia 36 [Suppl 6]:S2–S6

Schachter SC (1996) Tiagabine: current status and potential clinical applications. Exp Opin Invest Drugs 5:1377–1387

Schachter SC (1997) Therapeutic choices and decisions. Presented at the 22nd International Epilepsy Congress Satellite Symposium, Dublin, June 30, 1997

Schachter SC, Cahill WT, Wannamaker BB, Shu VS, Sommerville KW. Open-label dosage and tolerability study of tiagabine monotherapy in patients with refractory partial seizures. J Epilepsy 1998;11:248–255

Schwartz RD (1988) The GABA-A receptor-gated ion channel: biochemical and pharmacological studies of structure and function. Biochem Pharmacol 27: 3369–3378

Sheardown MJ, Weis JU, Knutsen LIS et al. (1989) Analgesic effect of the GABA uptake inhibitor NO-328. Soc Neurosci Abst 15:602

Snel S, Mukherjee S et al. (1993) Pharmacokinetics of tiagabine in the elderly. Epilepsia 34 [Suppl 2]:S157

So EL, Wolff D et al. (1995) Pharmacokinetics of tiagabine as add-on therapy in patients taking enzyme-inducing antiepilepsy drugs. Epilepsy Res 22:221–226
Streit P, Thompson SM, Gahwiler AM (1989) Anatomical and physiological properties of GABAergic neurotransmission in organotypic slice cultures in rat hippocampus. Eur J Neurosci 1:603–615
Suzdak PD (1993) Lipophilic GABA uptake inhibitors: biochemistry, pharmacology and therapeutic potential. Drugs of the Future 18:1129–1136
Suzdak PD, Jansen JA (1995) A review of the preclinical pharmacology of tiagabine: a potent and selective anticonvulsant GABA uptake inhibitor. Epilepsia 36:612–626
Uldall P, Bulteau C et al. (1995) Single-blind study of safety, tolerability, and preliminary efficacy of tiagabine as adjunctive treatment of children with epilepsy. Epilepsia 36 [Suppl 3]:S147–S148
Uthman BM, Rowan AJ et al. (1997) Tiagabine for complex partial seizures: a randomized, add-on, dose-response trial. Arch Neurol 1998;55:56–62

CHAPTER 18

Topiramate

D. HEANEY and S. SHORVON

A. Introduction

Topiramate is a new antiepileptic drug that has been approved for use in epilepsy by the regulatory authorities of many countries as adjunctive treatment for partial seizures whether or not they become secondarily generalized, for seizures associated with the Lennox-Gastaut syndrome and for primary generalized tonic-clonic seizures. Recent studies have described topiramate's pharmacodynamic profile and have demonstrated that its antiepileptic action may be a result of several mechanisms including effects on sodium and potassium channels, a novel interaction with the $GABA_A$ receptor and inhibition of the action of kainate on the kainate/AMPA subtype of glutamate receptor.

Six large randomized, placebo-controlled, double-blind clinical trials have evaluated topiramate as add-on therapy in partial epilepsy and there have been over 500,000 patient months of exposure to the drug as of December 1997. Topiramate is rapidly and well absorbed and is excreted largely unchanged in the urine. It is not prone to enzyme inhibition or induction and has no significant interactions with other antiepileptic drugs. Topiramate continues to be investigated for use in other forms of epilepsy, such as the primary generalized variety, the Lennox-Gastaut syndrome and various childhood epilepsies.

B. Chemistry

Topiramate (2,3:4,5-bis-*0*-(1-methylethylidene)-*β*-D-fructopyranose sulphamate) is a sulphamate-substituted monosaccharide derived from D-fructose (SHANK 1994). It is structurally unrelated to the other antiepileptic drugs. It has a molecular weight of 339.37 daltons, a pK_a of 8.61 at 25°C and a solubility of 9.8mg/ml at pH6.7 (data from Janssen-Cilag Ltd.).

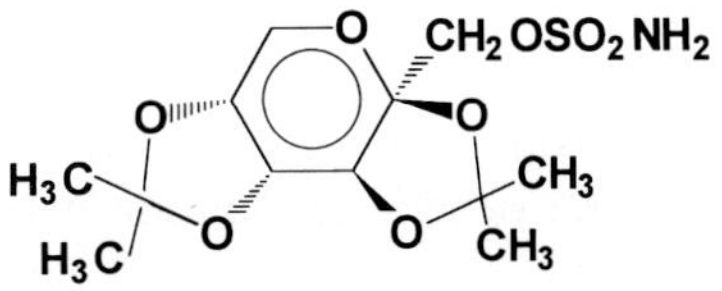

C. Pharmacodynamics

I. Animal Models of Epilepsy

Topiramate is active in several animal models of epilepsy. The effects of antiepileptic drugs in these models are to some extent predictive of their efficacies in human epilepsy (WHITE et al. 1997). Several types of animal model of epilepsy exist which are thought to correlate with particular forms of human epilepsy. However, while aspects of the aetiology and pathophysiological mechanisms responsible for human epilepsy remain poorly understood these models are inevitably of limited utility.

Topiramate has been shown to be active in the maximal electroshock test in rats and mice (SHANK et al. 1994), a model which is thought to correlate well with partial and secondarily generalized seizures in humans. In contrast, topiramate is inactive in chemically induced seizures such as those evoked by pentylenetetrazol, picrotoxin and bicuculline (SHANK et al. 1994), although it may elevate the seizure threshold for subcutaneous pentylenetetrazol-induced seizures (SHANK 1994). Topiramate's activity in maximum electroshock testing and its inactivity in chemically induced seizure models raise the possibility that the drug may act primarily by blocking the spread of seizures rather than by altering the seizure threshold.

Topiramate is active in other animal models including the rat and mouse hereditary epilepsy model (NAKAMURA et al. 1994), stroke-induced epilepsy in rats (EDMONDS et al. 1991) and kindled epilepsy models which are thought to be comparable with human complex partial seizures (NAKAMURA et al. 1993; WAUQUIER et al. 1996). These findings suggest that topiramate might be effective against a broad range of seizure types, including partial, generalized tonic-clonic and absence varieties.

II. Biochemical Pharmacology

In vitro evidence suggests that topiramate affects neuronal activity and produces its antiepileptic effect by several mechanisms, including modification of Na^+ and/or Ca^{2+} dependent action potentials, enhancement of γ-aminobutyric acid (GABA) activity and inhibition of kainate mediated conductance at glutamate receptors of the kianate type. It also appears that topiramate acts indirectly on α- or β-adrenergic neurotransmission. Topiramate has a weak inhibitory effect on some carbonic anhydrase isoenzymes, although this action is thought not to be related to its antiepileptic effect.

1. Na^+ Channels

Electrophysiological studies have demonstrated topiramate's activity on cultured rat hippocampal neurons. Topiramate (10 mmol/l) reduced both the burst duration and the number of action potentials within each burst (COULTER et al. 1993). In common with both phenytoin and carbamazepine, topiramate (20 mmol/l) reduced the frequency of action potentials elicited by a depolarizing electrical current. These effects are consistent with the hypothesis that topiramate blocks state-dependent voltage-sensitive Na^+ and/or Ca^{2+} channels (Coulter et al. 1993; Sombati et al. 1995), a mechanism of action shared with other antiepileptic drugs such as phenytoin and carbamazepine.

2. GABA-Mediated Cl^- Influx

GABA is one of the major inhibitory neurotransmitters in the central nervous system. Topiramate, in common with other antiepileptic drugs, has been shown to enhance GABA-mediated Cl^- flux into neurons. In cultured cerebellar granule cells, topiramate (10 mmol/l) significantly enhanced the rate of Cl^- influx into Cl^- depleted neurons (Brown et al. 1993). Topiramate also increased the frequency of GABA-mediated activation of $GABA_A$ receptors in cultures of cerebellar and cortical neurons (Brown et al. 1993; White et al. 1995).

Ligand binding studies have demonstrated that topiramate does not interact with the GABA or benzodiazepine binding sites on the $GABA_A$ receptor (Sedor and Oldham 1985). However, topiramate enhances $GABA_A$ mediated Cl^- currents in a benzodiazepine-like manner and enhances $GABA_A$ evoked currents in human embryonic kidney (HEK293) cells transfected with $GABA_A$ receptors (White et al. 1995). These effects are not blocked by the benzodiazepine antagonist, flumazenil. Topiramate therefore must exert its effect on $GABA_A$ mediated currents through a novel interaction with the $GABA_A$ receptor, but the detailed mechanism is not clear. It has been hypothesized that only certain $GABA_A$ receptor subtypes mediate topiramate's antiepileptic effects and that these effects may result in a relatively slow desensitization of the receptor (Gordey et al. 1995).

3. Glutamate Receptors

Topiramate (10–100 mmol/l) has little effect on NMDA-type excitatory amino acid receptors but inhibits the activity of kainate on the kainate/AMPA receptor subtype in a concentration-dependent manner (Coulter et al. 1995; Severt et al. 1995). The blocking of kainate-evoked potentials reduces neuronal excitability. This effect of topiramate could contribute to the drug's antiepileptic action. This selective blockade at glutamate receptors seems to represent a novel mechanism of action for an antiepileptic drug.

Further studies have shown intraperitoneal administration of topiramate reduces the abnormally high basal levels (approximately twice normal) of glutamate and aspartate in the hippocampi of spontaneously epileptic rats by approximately 45% (Kanda et al. 1992) but has no effects on glycine, GABA or taurine levels (Kanda et al. 1992; Shank et al. 1994). In normal Wistar rats, topiramate has no effect on hippocampal levels of these amino acids (Kanda et al. 1992).

4. Carbonic Anhydrase

Topiramate weakly inhibits the type II and IV isoenzymes of carbonic anhydrase, though less potently than acetazolamide. K_i values in lysed human erythrocytes are 119 mmol/l for topiramate and 4.6 nmol/l for acetazolamide (SHANK et al. 1994). It is assumed that the antiepileptic actions of topiramate are independent of this effect (BROWN et al. 1993), as acetazolamide-tolerant mice are not tolerant to the antiepileptic effects of topiramate (SHANK 1994).

5. Other Actions

In vitro receptor binding studies have indicated that topiramate has no direct effect at $GABA_A$, NMDA, α- or β- adrenergic, dopamine D_1 and D_2, serotonin, muscarinic or benzodiazepine receptors in rat brains. Furthermore, topiramate does not inhibit synaptosomal uptake of GABA, adenosine, noradrenaline, dopamine, serotonin or α-ketoglutarate (SHANK 1991, 1994). However, topiramate's anticonvulsant activity in mice is markedly reduced following pretreatment with the monoamine depleters, reserpine and tetrabenzine, suggesting that topiramate acts at least in part indirectly by altering adrenergic neurotransmission (SHANK et al. 1994).

III. Toxicology

1. Systemic Toxicity

The preclinical studies of the acute toxicology of topiramate have been reviewed by RIEFE (1997). Data from the RW Johnson Research Institute were analysed. These studies demonstrated that topiramate was well tolerated when administered orally to mice, rats and dogs and its intraperitoneal administration was well tolerated in rats and mice. The LD_{50} in mice and rats was between 2338 and 3745 mg/kg. Dogs are more sensitive than rodents. The acute toxicity was primarily related to the central nervous system.

Multiple dose preclinical toxicity studies have also been performed to evaluate topiramate over 3 and 12 month periods. Weight change, increases in kidney and liver weights, hepatocyte hypertrophy, urothelial hyperplasia, fluid and electrolyte shifts and central nervous system signs were observed. The increases in liver weight and hepatocyte hypertrophy were thought due to induction of drug metabolizing enzymes (RIEFE 1997). Topiramate's weak effect on carbonic anhydrase activity is thought to be responsible for the gastric changes (viz. gastric hyperplasia, reduced gastric acid secretion, increased blood gastrin levels) and the renal changes (viz. urothelial hyperplasia and urinary microcalculi) that have been noted. In a study of eight humans receiving long term treatment with topiramate (200–500 mg/day), endoscopic gastric examination including histological review, and measurement of serum gastrin levels, were performed after 15 months and seven of the patients were reviewed after 3 years. No changes in upper gastrointestinal tract were detected that could be attributed to topiramate (BEN-MENACHEN and ABRAHAMSSON 1994).

2. Carcinogenicity

There was no evidence of carcinogenicity in 12 and 24 month studies of topiramate in rats and mice (ZIMMER 1992). An increase in a species specific bladder tumour was observed in a rat study (JOHNSON et al. 1993). No genotoxic potential was demonstrated in in vitro or in vivo mutagenic assays which included the Ames *Salmonella*/microsomal activation assay, the *E. coli* bacterial/microsomal activation assay, the primary rat hepatocyte/DNA repair assay, the mouse lymphoma mutagenic assay and an in vitro cytogenetics assay (NEWMAN and OLDHAM 1985; OLDHAM 1984a,b; OLDHAM et al. 1985; SEDOR and OLDHAM 1985; PRESTON and OLDHAM 1989).

3. Reproductive and Teratology Studies

Animal studies showed that topiramate has little effect on reproductive potential but is teratogenic. No effect on fertility or on pup survival was demonstrated at daily doses of 10–100 mmol/l (DAVIS and OLDHAM 1988). In teratology studies topiramate was associated with right sided ectrodactyly in rats, rib and vertebral malformations in rabbits, and decreased foetal weight and delayed skeletal ossification in mice (RIEFE 1997). These teratogenic effects are similar to those seen with acetazolamide and other carbonic anhydrase inhibitors in susceptible animal species (HIRSCH et al. 1978; SCOTT et al. 1981; NAKATSUKA et al. 1992; SCHARDEIN 1993). It should be noted that carbonic anhydrase inhibitors have not been associated with congenital malformations in monkeys (SCHARDEN 1976) or humans (WYETH PHARMACEUTICALS 1998).

Clinical data regarding the safety of topiramate in pregnancy are very limited. Evidence from animal studies suggests that there is likely to be an increased incidence of congenital malformations in babies born to mothers taking topiramate.

IV. Human Studies

1. Placebo-Controlled Double-blind Add-on Trials

Six placebo-controlled, double-blind multicentre parallel-group trials have been performed to assess the efficacy of topiramate as an add-on therapy for patients with refractory partial epilepsy whether or not their seizures became secondarily generalized. These trials were performed in Europe (TASSINARI 1995; BEN-MENACHEM 1996; SHARIEF et al. 1996) and North America (FAUGHT 1996; PRIVITERA 1996; ROSENFELD 1996) and involved similar protocols which allowed their data to be pooled for meta-analysis. All trials recorded seizure frequency during a baseline phase and then observed the effects of adding

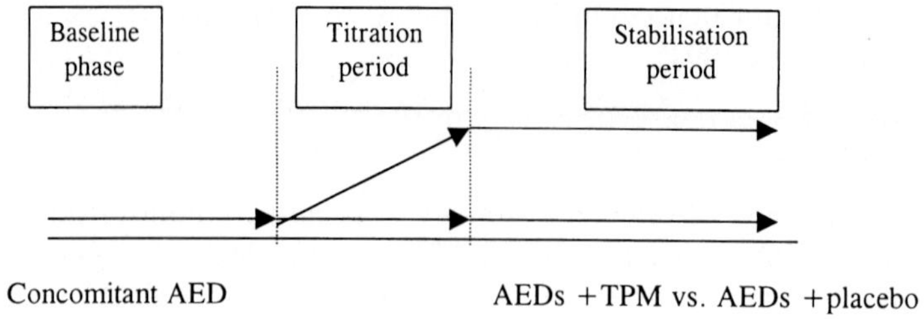

Fig. 1. Clinical trials of topiramate

topiramate during an active treatment phase lasting between 11 and 19 weeks (Table 1).

The European and North American trials differed in terms of the duration of the baseline and stabilization periods (8 weeks vs. 12 weeks respectively) and the numbers of patients recruited (Fig. 1) and in that the European trials included patients established on clobazam therapy.

In all six of the trials, patients were included if they had one or more seizures per week during the baseline stabilization period. The primary outcome measure was "treatment response", defined as a greater than 50% reduction in seizure frequency. Other measures of outcome included the median seizure frequency reduction, the frequency of generalized seizures and the investigator and patient global treatment evaluations. Overall, 743 patients were randomized in these studies, of whom 527 were assigned to topiramate and 216 to placebo.

Statistically significant ($p < 0.05$) "treatment responses" were observed in the patient groups receiving topiramate 400-1000 mg/day (35%–52%) as compared with patient groups receiving placebo (0%–19%). Other measures of seizure reduction also demonstrated a significant effect of topiramate ($p < 0.05$). Median reductions in seizure frequency ranged from 30% to 51% over a topiramate dose range of 200–1000 mg/day, compared with a –18% to 13% reduction in the placebo group. The patient and investigator "global evaluation" measure also demonstrated a statistically significant benefit of topiramate over placebo.

The trials indicated that a topiramate dosage of 200 mg/day did not produce a statistically significant benefit when compared with placebo. Higher doses (>400 mg/day) produced benefit but there were no further significant improvements using topiramate dosages greater than 400 mg/day. In clinical practice, however, patients who do not respond to lower doses of topiramate may respond to doses in excess of 800 mg/day. In some of the open extension trials, doses of up to 1600 mg/day of the drug have been used, with benefit.

The effect of topiramate on the subgroup with generalized epilepsy (either primary or secondarily generalized) was examined in four of the trials (BEN-MENACHEM 1996; FAUGHT 1996; PRIVITERA 1996; SHARIEF et al. 1996).

Table 1. Summary of the clinical efficacy of topiramate (TPM) in controlled trials (all randomized patients)

Authors	Drug and target daily dose (mg)	Daily dose achieved (mg)	*n*	Reduction in seizure rate from baseline (%)	Treatment responders[a] (%)	Reduction in generalized seizure rate (%)	Investigator global evaluation[b]	Patient assessment[c]
Ben-Menachem et al. (1996)	TPM 800	568	28	36***	43***	90*	3.7***	2.4**
	Placebo		28	18 increase	0	19	2.3	1.8
Sharief et al. (1996)	TPM 400	387	23	41	35*	84**	3.5***	2.3*
	Placebo		24	1	8	9	2.2	1.4
Tassinari et al. (1996)	TPM 600	519	30	46**	47***	NS	3.3**	2.3**
	Placebo		30	12 increase	10	NS	2.5	1.6
Rosenfeld et al. (1996b)	TPM 1000	832	167	51***	52***	NS	NS	NS
	Placebo		42	1		NS	NS	NS
Faught et al. (1996)	TPM 200	200	45	30	19	62	3.3**	2.6*
	TPM 400	387	45	48**	27	100	3.8***	2.8**
	TPM 600	556	45	45***	47*	89	3.6***	2.6
	Placebo		45	13.1	18	1	2.7	2.2
Privitera et al. (1996)	TPM 600	544	48	41***	44***	86	3.5***	2.6***
	TPM 800	739	48	41***	40***	44	3.5***	2.6***
	TPM 1000	799	47	38***	38***	78	3.5***	2.4*
	Placebo		47	1	9	40	2.4	1.9

* $p < 0.05$; ** $p < 0.01$; *** $p < 0.001$.
[a] Treatment responder, i.e. patient with >50% reduction in seizure rate.
[b] Investigator improvement rating (1, worse; 2, none; 3, minimal; 4, moderate; 5, marked).
[c] Subject's rating of medication (1, poor; 2, fair; 3, good; 4, excellent).

Treatment responses occurred in 47%–87% in the topiramate 200-1000 mg/day group, compared with 21%–38% in the placebo group. Complete seizure freedom occurred in 21%–53% of the topiramate 200-mg/day group, compared with 0%–25% in the placebo recipients.

The similar trial protocols used allowed meaningful meta-analysis to be performed (CHADWICK 1997). The studies demonstrated that topiramate is of significant benefit in simple partial, complex partial and secondarily generalized seizures. The results were not confounded by the effects of age, gender, race, background antiepileptic drug use or the baseline seizure frequency.

2. Non-Controlled Add-on Trials

In addition to the six double blind randomized controlled trials, several uncontrolled, open trials have been carried out. These trials have varied in terms of their inclusion criteria, durations, rates of dosage titration and topiramate dosages used. Although less definitive than double-blind trials, such studies offer the opportunity of observing the effect of topiramate in a variety of different clinical situations. At present most of these trials have been published only in the form of abstracts, but overall they have demonstrated that topiramate is an effective add-on treatment. The results are consistent with those observed in the large blinded, randomized controlled trials. Several trials demonstrated a continuing clinical benefit when prescribing topiramate for periods greater than 12 months, suggesting that in at least certain patients topiramate is well tolerated over long periods (ROSENFELD et al. 1997).

3. Monotherapy Studies

There is some evidence that topiramate monotherapy can be achieved and maintained. In a double-blind study of 48 patients, topiramate monotherapy (1000 mg/day) was shown to be more effective than 100 mg/day (SACHDEO et al. 1997). Patients were observed during an 8 week "baseline" period and then topiramate, either 100 mg or 1000 mg/day, was introduced whilst other antiepileptic drugs were withdrawn. Topiramate monotherapy was maintained over an 11 week "active" period. Patients "exited" the trial if their seizures increased in frequency or severity. Thirteen of 24 patients taking 1000 mg/day reached the end of the trial, compared with 4 of 24 taking 100 mg/day; 11 of 24 achieved a greater then 50% reduction in seizure frequency and 3 of 24 were seizure free at the end of the 11 week period in the topiramate 1000 mg/day group, compared with 3 of 24 and 0 of 24 respectively in the topiramate 100 mg/day group.

Two other open studies have followed up patients receiving topiramate monotherapy for longer periods. In one study 32 patients received topiramate monotherapy for a mean period of 20.5 months. Of these, 19 became seizure free (SACHDEO and ROSENFELD 1997). In a further study of 45 patients with partial epilepsy whose treatment had been converted successfully to topiramate monotherapy, this treatment was tolerated for a mean period of 22 months. In seven patients with complex partial seizures, topiramate monotherapy was associated with a reduction in severity of the epilepsy so that the seizures the patients continued to experience were classified as simple partial ones only; 28 patients became seizure free for 3 months and 13 could legally drive a car, under United States regulations (ROSENFELD et al. 1997).

4. Add-on Therapy for Generalized Seizures

Several small trials which have examined topiramate as add-on therapy for generalized tonic-clonic seizures have been reported in the form of abstracts.

In an open-label follow-up study to a multicentre double-blind, placebo-controlled study, eight patients with primary generalized seizures were treated with topiramate as add-on therapy for up to 12 months. Two patients were seizure free for at least 3 months and three patients had a greater than 50% reduction in their seizure frequency (CRAWFORD 1997). The preliminary findings from a similar study of 33 patients maintained on open-label topiramate for at least 12 weeks following completion of double-blind studies have been reported. The mean duration of treatment was 10.5 months and 67% of patients had a reduction in seizure frequency of 50% or more, as compared with their baseline seizure frequency. Three patients were seizure free for at least 3 months (BEN-MENACHEM 1996).

Two other smaller studies have reported the use of topiramate in generalized seizures and have concluded that the drug is a useful add-on therapy in secondary generalized tonic-clonic, complex-partial and absence seizures (DURISOTTI 1996; LEUF et al. 1996).

A pooled analysis of these trials has also been published (ANONYMOUS 1997). In this pooled analysis, 160 patients with 3 or more generalized tonic-clonic seizures observed during an 8 week baseline period were identified. All these patients were receiving one or more standard antiepileptic drugs. The patients were randomized to topiramate or placebo for an 8 week titration period and a 12 week stabilization period. In terms of a reduction in median seizure frequency, a reduction in seizure frequency by 50% or more and a reduction in seizure frequency by 75% or more, topiramate was superior to placebo in patients with generalized tonic-clonic seizures ($p < 0.005$).

5. The Lennox-Gastaut Syndrome

Topiramate may benefit patients with the Lennox-Gastaut syndrome. In a double-blinded study of 98 patients with the Lennox-Gastaut syndrome aged between 2 and 42 years, topiramate was statistically significantly superior to placebo as add-on therapy (GLAUSER at al 1997). Patients were enrolled and observed over an 8 week baseline phase. Patients with drop attacks, atypical seizures and greater than 60 seizures/month were recruited. The topiramate dose was titrated over 3 weeks and then maintained for an 8 week active treatment period. The maximum dose of topiramate used was 600 mg. The authors concluded that topiramate 6 mg/kg/day appeared to be effective adjunctive therapy in the management of seizures associated with the Lennox-Gastaut syndrome. It significantly reduced the frequency of drop-attacks compared with placebo, and the parent or guardian global evaluation scores of seizure severity were significantly reduced by the drug.

An open-labelled extension study was conducted in 97 patients with the Lennox-Gastaut syndrome, following their participation in a double-blind, placebo-controlled trial. Topiramate therapy was initiated in patients who had been treated with placebo during the double-blind phase. The results in patients maintained on open-label topiramate for at least 3 months at an average dose of 8.4 mg/kg/day were that seizures were reduced by 50% from base-line in 53% of patients, with a reduction of at least 75% in 37%, whilst 14% had been seizure free during the previous 3 months. Overall, 30% of the patients discontinued participation in the trial. The authors concluded that topiramate appeared to be well tolerated during long-term therapy in patients with the Lennox-Gastaut syndrome and the majority of the patients were successfully maintained on topiramate for periods of up to 3 years (RITTER et al. 1997).

D. Pharmacokinetics

There have been several studies of the pharmacokinetics of topiramate in animals, healthy volunteers and people with epilepsy receiving concomitant medication. Here, the focus is on human studies.

I. Absorption

Topiramate absorption has been studied using single and multiple dose protocols. The peak plasma concentration is usually attained within 2–3 h of intake (EASTERLING et al. 1988; DOOSE 1995; TAKAHASHI et al. 1995). Although no studies with intravenously administered topiramate have been performed to measure the absolute oral bioavailablity of the drug, it appears that it is well absorbed from the gastrointestinal tract. In studies where ^{14}C-labelled topiramate was administered to healthy volunteers, renal and non-renal clearance data have given an estimate of the bioavailablity of topiramate as being 80%–95% (NAYAK et al. 1994; PERUCCA and BAILER 1996). The extent of the absorption of topiramate is not significantly reduced by food, although high fat meals may slow its absorption (DOOSE et al. 1996).

II. Distribution

Topiramate appears to be distributed throughout body water, the drug's volume of distribution being between 0.6 and 0.8 l/kg (EASTERLING et al. 1988). Approximately 15% of the circulating topiramate is bound to plasma proteins (DOOSE et al. 1995). Significant binding to high affinity, low capacity binding sites on erythrocytes has been noted (Doose et al. 1995), relating to the drug's carbonic anhydrase inhibiting action. This is of clinical importance in monitoring topiramate plasma levels. The proportion of topiramate bound to erythrocytes is higher at low plasma concentration (<4 mg/l) than at high concentrations, resulting in a higher blood to plasma concentration ratio of the drug at low doses (Doose et al. 1995).

III. Elimination

1. No Interacting Drug Present

In the absence of P450 enzyme inducing co-medication, topiramate is not metabolized in vivo to a significant extent. A single 100 mg dose of ^{14}C-labelled topiramate was administered to six fasting healthy volunteers. Less than 5% of the total excreted radioactivity was accounted for by metabolites and 78% of the radioactivity in the plasma was unchanged drug (Wu et al. 1994). More than 60% of the topiramate was eliminated unchanged, by the renal route. After 48 h, approximately 40% of the radioactivity in the excreta was unchanged drug whilst after 10 days, 80.6% of the total drug had been recovered in the urine and 0.7% in the faeces. Two hydoxy metabolites, two diol metabolites and glucuronides of 10-hydroxy and 2,3-diol topiramate were formed. The metabolites are not thought to have significant clinical activity (Johannesson 1997). In the presence of enzyme-inducing drugs there is increased metabolism of topiramate and the proportion of the dose eliminated unchanged may fall to as little as 30% (Sachdeo et al. 1996).

The half-life of topiramate has generally been found to be between 20 and 30 h (Doose et al. 1988, 1996; Easterling et al. 1988), although a Japanese study observed a slightly longer half-life (Takahashi A et al. 1995). The oral clearance of the drug is estimated to be 1.2–2.4 l/h. The renal clearance of topiramate is 0.78–0.88 l/h.

The elimination of topiramate at steady state is similar to that after single doses of the drug. In healthy volunteers at steady state the Cl/F, CL_{renal} and $T_{1/2(\beta)}$ were similar over three dosage regimens (50 mg or 100 mg once a day for 14 days, then twice daily for 14 days, or 200 mg once daily for 20 days) with the mean values of 1.27 l/h and 0.79 l/h and 25.4 l/h respectively (Doose et al. 1988).

2. Interacting Drugs Present

Concomitant antiepileptic drug therapy may affect the pharmacokinetics of topiramate. When the treatment of patients receiving topiramate and phenytoin was converted to topiramate monotherapy, the mean oral clearance of topiramate was reduced by 59% and significantly higher mean steady-state concentrations, maximal plasma concentrations, times to reach peak plasma concentrations and plasma AUCs of the drug were seen (Gisclon et al. 1994a,b).

During concomitant administration of carbamazepine 900–2400 mg/day and topiramate in doses below 800 mg/day, the mean topiramate AUC_{0-12}, C_{max} and minimum plasma concentrations were all approximately 40% lower than during topiramate monotherapy. Topiramate oral and non-renal clearance rates were two- to threefold higher, whereas the topiramate renal clearance was unchanged during concomitant carbamazepine intake (SACHDEO et al. 1996).

IV. Special Situations

It has been demonstrated that children eliminate topiramate at a faster rate than adults. The drug's plasma concentration for the same mg/kg dose is approximately 30% lower in children than in adults. Coadministration of an enzyme inducing antiepileptic drug can alter the clearance of topiramate by as much as twofold (ROSENFLED 1997).No formal pharmacokinetic studies of topiramate in the elderly have been performed. The clearance of topiramate is partially dependent on renal function and the reduction of the glomerular filtration rate with normal age is likely to be associated with a reduced topiramate clearance rate in the elderly.

E. Interactions

I. Pharmacodynamic Interactions

To the time of writing, topiramate has been used mainly as add-on therapy in the presence of other antiepileptic drugs. In these circumstances, additive pharmacodynamic effects are likely which may enhance seizure control, but which may also lead to an increased severity of adverse effects, particularly those of a sedative type.

II. Pharmacokinetic Interactions

1. Effects of Other Drugs on Topiramate

As was mentioned in the section on the elimination of the drug, concurrent treatment with phenytoin or carbamazepine enhances the clearance of topiramate. The addition or withdrawal of valproate has not been shown to have a clinically significant effect on the blood concentration of topiramate.

2. Effects of Topiramate on Various Drugs

a) Antiepileptic Drugs

The mechanisms involved in the pharmacokinetic effects of topiramate on other drugs are not yet fully understood. Both its capacity for protein binding and its ability to inhibit the CYP2C19 isoform of cytochrome P450 may be involved (DOOSE et al. 1995; LEVY et al. 1995). Substrates for this isoform include mephenytoin, omeprazole and diazepam. There is no evidence that topiramate affects other P450 isoforms.

Topiramate affects the pharmacokinetics of phenytoin. In a study of 12 patients prescribed topiramate in addition to phenytoin, phenytoin AUC values at steady state in 6 patients were increased by an average of 125% compared with those seen with monotherapy. Some authors believe that this increase warrants monitoring of plasma phenytoin concentrations before and after topiramate dosage changes.

No significant effect of topiramate on the pharmacokinetic profile of concurrently administered carbamazepine or carbamazepine-10,11-epoxide has been demonstrated (Bourgeois 1996; Sachdeo et al. 1996).

Topiramate has been demonstrated to interact pharmacokinetically with valproic acid. Mean valproic acid plasma concentrations and $AUC_{0-12\ hour}$ values decreased by 11% and the CL/F increased by 13% during concomitant steady-state topiramate 200–800 mg/day administration, as compared with the corresponding values during valproic acid monotherapy (Bourgeois 1996; Rosenfeld et al. 1997). The authors commented that these changes were unlikely to be of clinical significance. This prediction has been borne out in clinical practice. Topiramate has also been demonstrated to produce a decrease in urinary glucuronide conjugates and an increase in the oxidative metabolites of valproic acid (Bourgeois 1995).

b) Other Drugs

The effects of coadministering topiramate and two important drugs, digoxin and oral contraceptives, have been investigated although no studies have been performed to establish the effects of these drugs on the pharmacokinetics of topiramate. In a study of 12 healthy male volunteers pretreated with topiramate 200 mg/day for 6 days, the plasma digoxin C_{max} and AUC after a single oral 0.6 mg dose of the drug were reduced by 16% and 12% respectively and the CL/F was increased by 13% when compared with the corresponding values after administration of digoxin alone. Topiramate did not significantly alter the CL_{renal} or the $T_{1/2}$ of digoxin (Liao et al. 1993). In view of these findings it is recommended that plasma digoxin levels be monitored carefully if topiramate is added to or withdrawn from the therapy of a person being treated with digoxin.

Topiramate intake also leads to an increased clearance of the oestrogenic component of the oral contraceptive pill. In a study of 12 women with epilepsy taking an ethinyloestradiol 35 μg plus norethindrone 1 mg oral contraceptive combination, topiramate (200–800 mg/day) reduced the serum ethinyloestradiol concentrations by 15%–30% and increased its CL/F values by 15%–33% (Rosenfeld et al. 1997). It is generally recommended that women taking topiramate should be given an oral contraceptive pill with a oestradiol content of greater than, or equal to, 50 μg and that they should also report any intermenstrual bleeding.

F. Adverse Effects

The data on adverse effects associated with topiramate come from clinical trials and from long term monitoring after the drug's use was licensed. Clinical trials use strict protocols to observe and record treatment-emergent adverse experiences, but as these trials are designed primarily to satisfy regulatory authorities, the strict adherence to titration rates and dosage schedules which they involve may produce side effect profiles that may not reflect those which will be observed in everyday clinical practice. Furthermore, in clinical trials of an add-on therapy, treatment-emergent adverse experiences may be due to potentiation of toxicity between drugs that share a similar side-effect profile. In the random-blinded controlled trials on topiramate used as add-on therapy for partial epilepsy, the WHO-ART dictionary of side effects was used. Using this dictionary the side effects with an incidence of 10% or more were ataxia (18%), impairment of concentration (13%), confusion (17%), dizziness (31%), fatigue (24%), paraesthesia (15%), somnolence (27%) and abnormal thinking (25%).

In these trials the number of patients who withdrew prematurely from treatment because of adverse effects was 3% in the placebo group and 14% in the topiramate group. The most frequent causes of discontinuation in these trials were central nervous system side effects. Approximately 75% of those who withdrew, did so within the first 2 months of treatment. This may have related to the rapid titration dosage schedules used in these trials and the target doses, which may have been too high for individual patients.

There is no evidence to date of clinically significant haematotoxicity, hepatotoxicity, cardiotoxicity or gastrointestinal toxicity from the drug.

The risk of renal calculi in those treated with topiramate has been estimated to be approximately 1%–2% (Wasserstein et al. 1995; Shorvon 1996). The stones were passed spontaneously in those affected, and most patients elected to continue topiramate despite this adverse effect (Wasserstein et al. 1995). Stone formation is believed to be related to an increase in urinary pH and a reduced excretion of citrate associated with topiramate's carbonic anhydrase inhibiting activity (Wasserstein et al. 1995). The risk is likely to be higher in those patients predisposed to renal stone formation, e.g. those who have previously had renal stones or a family history of renal stones or hypercalcuria. Those at risk are advised to maintain adequate hydration, although there are no guidelines for the monitoring of patients by ultrasound examination or intravenous pyelonephrogram. The concomitant use of carbonic anhydrase inhibitors such as acetazolamide should be avoided.

Weight loss has been observed during topiramate therapy. This has usually been mild and appears to be dose related. The mean decreases have ranged from 1.1kg in patients receiving 200mg/day topiramate to 5.9kg in those receiving greater than 800mg/day (Shorvon 1996). In some cases the weight loss appears to be partially reversible after prolonged intake of the drug (Sander 1997).

G. Clinical Use

Topiramate is a relatively new antiepileptic drug and as a result its place in the treatment of patients with epilepsy has not yet been clearly defined, although it shows great promise in view of its impressive efficacy profile and its apparent broad spectrum of activity.

I. Indications

There is evidence to suggest that topiramate is an effective adjunctive agent for treating patients with partial and secondarily generalized epilepsy. Comparison with other new antiepileptic drugs is difficult in view of the differences in methodology between the trials assessing these drugs, but it would appear that topiramate is at least as effective as vigabatrin, zonisamide, lamotrigine, felbamate, tiagabine and gabapentin. Indeed, in most reviews topiramate is regarded as marginally more effective than these other drugs (MARSON et al. 1996; CHADWICK 1997). Anecdotal evidence suggests that topiramate may be effective in a wide variety of epilepsy types including absence seizures and primary generalized tonic-clonic seizures. More information is required before recommendations can be made regarding these potential additional indications. The decision to use topiramate in patients with epilepsy who have difficulty communicating (for instance people with learning difficulties or other severe disabilities) should be made in the realization that such patients may not be able to report the symptoms of potentially serious side-effects such as renal calculi.

II. Dosage and Administration

Topiramate is administered orally, usually in two divided doses each day. In adults and the elderly the minimal effective dose is at least 100 mg/day, but the maintenance dose in most patients is between 200 and 600 mg/day, taken in divided doses. The maximum recommended dose is 800 mg/day, but with careful monitoring patients may be treated with higher doses with an associated reduction in seizure frequency. In the elderly, the reduced glomerular filtration rate may mean that higher doses of topiramate may not be tolerated.

Topiramate therapy should not be started in pregnancy or during lactation. However, if a patient taking topiramate becomes pregnant the risks of withdrawing the therapy should be carefully weighed against the unknown risks to the foetus.

1. Dosage Titration

Topiramate dosages should be titrated slowly. Our practice is to begin with 25 mg/day for 2 weeks and then increase the daily dose by 25–50 mg/day at 2 weekly intervals until the patient is taking 200 mg/day, and after that prescribe fortnightly increments of 100 mg/day. Higher doses are prescribed if tolerated, and if adequate seizure control has not been achieved. More rapid dosage titration is possible, but may be associated with an increased incidence of adverse effects. Where side-effects occur, the usual practice is to delay further dosage increases for 1–2 weeks or until the symptoms that have troubled the patient are no longer present. Other options include reducing the dosage of topiramate to the previous dose level or reducing the dosage of another antiepileptic drug which is being taken concomitantly. Titration of topiramate dosage can be resumed when the side effect resolves.

2. Patient Monitoring

Patients maintained on topiramate therapy do not need to have blood levels of topiramate measured routinely, as there is very little correlation between the blood concentrations and the clinical effects of the drug. Patients should be monitored for the development of adverse effects, in particular the formation of renal stones, which may present with haematuria or abdominal pain. No specific recommendations have been made regarding the monitoring of patients who may be at an increased risk of developing renal stones.

3. Overdosage

In acute topiramate overdosage, the stomach should be emptied by lavage or by induced emesis. Charcoal has been shown not to absorb topiramate and therefore its use is not recommended. Haemodialysis is an effective method of clearing topiramate from the blood. Supportive treatment should be used as appropriate.

4. Discontinuation of Topiramate

Discontinuation of topiramate intake should be considered if adverse effects continue after dose reduction or if at any point become unacceptable to the patient, or if no antiepileptic response is obtained at the maximal tolerated dosage of the drug. Topiramate should be withdrawn in 100 mg/day decrements at fortnightly intervals.

H. Conclusions

Topiramate is a new antiepileptic drug with several mechanisms of action and a favourable pharmacokinetic profile. It has been tested in preclinical and clinical trials and has proved comparable to other antiepileptic drugs. Recent trials have demonstrated its effectiveness in primary generalized epilepsy and the Lennox-Gastaut syndromes, although the numbers of subjects involved in the relevant trials have been small. Topiramate has predominantly the central nervous system side effects that are common to most antiepileptic drugs, and these side effects often occur during rapid dosage titration. Long term side effects may include the development of renal stones (ca. 1%/year incidence).

Topiramate is indicated as adjunctive therapy for adults and children over 2 years of age with partial seizures whether or not they become secondarily generalized, with the Lennox-Gastaut syndrome and with primary generalized tonic-clonic seizures, which are inadequately controlled by conventional first line antiepileptic drugs.

Experience of the side effects, safety, tolerability and use of topiramate in specific epilepsy syndromes and patient populations is accumulating. Only after many years of clinical experience will the eventual role of topiramate (as, indeed, of any other newly introduced antiepileptic drug) in the management of epilepsy be established. Nevertheless, all the evidence at present available suggests that topiramate is a welcome addition to the drugs available for treating refractory epilepsy.

References

Anonymous (1997) Topiramate as adjunctive therapy in partial onset seizures: the spectrum in adults to children. AED News June 29:1

Ben-Menachem E, Abrahamsson H (1994) Gastroscopic evaluation of patients with complex partial seizures treated with topiramate (abstract). Epilepsia 35 [Suppl 8]:116

Ben-Menachem E, Henriksen O, Dam M et al. (1996) Double-blind, placebo-controlled trial of topiramate as add-on therapy in patients with refractory partial seizures. Epilepsia 37:539–43

Bourgoeois BFD (1996) Drug interaction profile of topiramate. Epilepsia 37 [Suppl 2]:S14–17

Brown SD, Wolf HH, Swyniard EA et al. (1993) The novel anticonvulsant topiramate enhances GABA-medicated chloride flux (abstract). Epilepsia 34 [Suppl 2]:122–123

Chadwick DW (1997) An overview of the efficacy and tolerability of new antiepileptic drugs. Epilepsia 38 [Suppl 1]:S59–S62

Coulter DA, Sombati S, DeLorenzo RJ (1993) Selective effects of topiramate on sustained repetitive firing and spontaneous bursting in cultured hippocampal neurones (abstract). Epilepsia 34 [Suppl 2]:123

Coulter DA, Sombati S, DeLorenzo RJ (1995) Topiramate effects on excitatory aminoacid mediated responses in cultured hippocampal neurones: selective blockade of kianate currents (abstract). Epilepsia 36 [Suppl 3]:S40

Crawford PM (1997) Use of topiramate in primary generalised seizures (abstract). Epilepsia 38 [Suppl 3]:80

Doose DR, Scott VV, Margul BL et al. (1988) Multiple-dose pharmacokinetics of topiramate in healthy male subjects (abstract). Epilepsia 29:662

Doose DR, Gisclon LG, Liao S et al. (1995a) Pharmacokinetics of topiramate. Advances in Antiepileptic Drug Therapy 1:7–16

Doose DR, Walker SA, Pledger G et al. (1995b) Evaluation of phenobarbital and primidone/phenobarbital (primidone's active metabolite) plasma concentrations during administration of add-on topiramate therapy in five multi-centre, double-blind, placebo controlled trials in out-patients with partial seizures (abstract). Epilepsia 36 [Suppl 3]:S158

Doose DR, Walker SA, Gisclon LG et al. (1996) Single-dose pharmacokinetics and effect of food on the bioavailability of topiramate, a novel antiepileptic drug. J Clin Pharmacol 36:884–891

Durisotti C, Garofalo P, DiFazo M (1996) Topiramate as add-on, open therapy in drug resistant epilepsies: one year of follow-up (abstract). Epilepsia 37 [Suppl 4]:89
Easterling DE, Zakszewski T. Moyer MD et al. (1988) Plasma pharmacokinetics of topiramate, a new anticonvulsant, in humans. Epilepsia 29: 662
Edmonds H, Jiang D, Zhang P et al. (1991) Topiramate in a rat model of posttraumatic epilepsy (abstract). Epilepsia 32 [Suppl 3]:15
Faught E, Wilder BJ, Ramsay RE et al. (1996) The topiramate YD Study Group. Topiramate placebo-controlled dose-ranging trial in refractory epilepsy using 200, 400 and 600 mg daily dosages. Neurology 46:1684–1690
Gisclon LG, Curtin CR, Kramer LD (1994) The steady-state (SS) pharmacokinetics (PK) of phenytoin (Dilantin [RM]) and topiramate (Topamax[RM]) in epileptic patients on monotherapy, and during combination therapy (abstract). Epilepsia 35 [Suppl 8]:54
Glauser TA, Sachdeo RC, Ritter FJ et al. (1997) A double-blind trial of topiramate in LennoxGastaut Syndrome (abstract). Neurology 48:1729
Gordey M, Delorey TM, Olsen RE (1995) Topiramate modulates GABA responses in Xenopus oocytes expressing recombinant receptor subunit combinations (abstract). Epilepsia 36 [Suppl 4]:34
Graves NM, Leppik IE (1991) Antiepileptic medications in development. DICP 25:978–986
Harden CL (1994) New antiepileptic drugs. Neurology 44:787–795
Hirsch KS, Scott WJ, Hurley LS (1978) Acetazolamide teratology; the presence of carbonic anhydrase during the sensitive stage of rat development. Teratology 17:38 A
Johannessen SI (1997) Pharmacokinetics and interaction profile of topiramate: review and comparison with other newer antiepileptic drugs. Epilepsia 38 [Suppl l]:S18–23
Kanda T, Nakamura J, Kurokawa M et al. (1992) Inhibition of excessive releases of excitatory amino acids in hippocampus of spontaneously epileptic rate (SER) by topiramate (KW-6485), Jap J Pharmacol 58 [Suppl 1]:92P
Kimishima K, Wang Y, Tanebe K (1992) Anti-convulsant activities and properties of topiramate (abstract). Jap J Pharmacol 58 [Suppl 1]:211P
Leuf G, Bauer G (1996) Topiramate in drug-resistant partial and generalised epilepsies (abstract). Epilepsia 37 [Suppl 4]:69
Levy RH, Bishop F, Streeter AJ et al. (1995) Explanation and prediction of drug interactions with topiramate using a CYP450 inhibition spectrum (abstract). Epilepsia 36 [Suppl 4]:47
Liao S, Palmer M (1993) Digoxin and topiramate drug interaction study in male volunteers (abstract). Pharmacol Res 10 [Suppl]:S-405
Liao S, Rosenfeld WE, Palmer M et al. (1994) Steady-state pharmacokinetics of topiramate and valproic acid in patients with epilepsy on monotherapy, and during combination therapy (abstract). Epilepsia 35 [Suppl 8]:117
Marson AG, Kadir ZA, Chadwick DW (1996) New anti-epileptic drugs: a systematic review of their efficacy and tolerability. Brit Med J 313:1169–1174
Martinez-Lage J, Ben-Menachem E, Shorvon SD et al (1995) Double-blind, placebo controlled trial of 400 mg per day topiramate as add-on therapy in patients with refractory partial epilepsy. Epilepsia 36 [Suppl 3]:149–150
Montouris GD, Biton V (1997) Long-term topiramate therapy in generalised seizures of nonfocal origin (abstract). Epilepsia 38 [Suppl 3]:82
Nakamura F, Hiyoshi T, Kudo T et al. (1993) Anticonvulsant effects of topiramate (2,3:4,5 bis-O-(1-methylethylidene)-beta-D-fructopyranose sulphate) on amygdaloid kindled seizures in the cat. Jap J Psychiat Neurol 47:394–395
Nakamura J, Tamura S, Kanda T et al. (1994) Inhibition by topiramate of seizures in spontaneously epileptic rats and DBA/2 mice. Europ J Pharmacol 11:83–89
Nakatsuka T, Komatsu T, Fujii T (1992) Axial skeletal malformations induced by acetozolamide in rabbits. Teratology 45:629–636

Nayak RK, Gisclon LG, Curtin CA et al. (1994) Estimation of the absolute bioavailability of topiramate in humans without intravenous data. J Clin Pharmacol 34:1029

Perruca E, Bailer M (1996) The clinical pharmacokinetics of the newer antiepileptics: focus on topiramate, zonisamide and tiagabine. Clin Pharmacokinet 31:29–46

Pritchard JF (1985) Binding of McN-4853 to plasma and erythrocytes of rat, mouse, rabbit, dog, monkey and human to human serum. Data on file at RWJPRI

Privitera M, Fincham R, Penry J et al. (1996) The topiramate YE Study Group. Topiramate placebo-controlled dose-ranging trial in refractory partial epilepsy using 600, 800 and 100 mg daily dosages. Neurology 46:1678–1683

Rangel RJ, Penry JK, Wilder BJ et al. (1988) Topiramate: a new antiepileptic drug for complex-partial seizures – first use in epileptic patients (abstract). Neurology 38 [Suppl 1]:234

Reife RA (1997) Topiramate. In: Shorvon SD, Driefuss F, Fish D, Thomas D (eds) The treatment of epilepsy. Blackwell, Oxford, pp. 471–481

Ritter FJ, Sachdeo RC, Glauser TA and the Topiramate YL Study Group (1997) Topiramate as open-label adjunctive therapy in Lennox-Gastaut Syndrome (poster). 22nd Epilepsy Conference, Dublin, Eire

Rosenfeld WE, Doose DR, Walker SA et al. (1995) Steady state pharmacokinetics of topiramate as adjunctive therapy in paediatric subjects with epilepsy (abstract). Epilepsia 36 [Suppl 3]:S158

Rosenfeld WE, Abou-Khalil B, Morrell M et al. (1996a) Double-blind placebo controlled trial of topiramate adjunctive therapy for partial-onset therapy. Epilepsia 37 [Suppl 4]:5

Rosenfeld WE, Abou-Khalil B, Reife R et al. (1996b) The Topiramate YF/YG Study Group. Placebo controlled trial of topiramate as adjunctive therapy to carbamazepine phenytoin for partial onset epilepsy. Epilepsia 37 [Suppl 5]:153

Rosenfeld WE, Doose DR, Walker SA et al. (1997a) Effect of topiramate on the pharmacokinetics of an oral contraceptive containing norethindrone and ethinyl estradiol in patients with epilepsy, Epilepsia 38:317–323

Rosenfeld WE, Liao S, Kramer LD et al. (1997b) Comparison of steady-state pharmacokinetics of topiramate and valproate in patients with epilepsy during monotherapy and concomitant therapy. Epilepsia 38:324–333

Rosenfeld WE, Sachdeo RC, Faught RE et al. (1997c) Long-term experience with topiramate as adjunctive therapy and as monotherapy in patients with partial onset seizures: retrospective survey of open-label treatment. Epilepsia 38 [Suppl 1]:S34–S36

Sachdeo RC, Rosenfeld WE (1997) Experience with long-term topiramate monotherapy (abstract). Epilepsia 38 [Suppl 3]:59

Sachdeo RC, Sachdeo SK, Walker SA et al. (1996) Steady state pharmacokinetics of topiramate and carbamazepine in patients with epilepsy during monotherapy and concomitant therapy. Epilepsia 37:774–780

Sachdeo RC, Riefe RA, Lim P et al. (1997) Topiramate monotherapy for partial onset seizures. Epilepsia 38:294–300

Sander JWAS (1997) Practical aspects of the use of topiramate in patients with epilepsy. Epilepsia 38 [Suppl 1]:S56–S58

Schardein JL (1993) Chemically induced birth defects, 2nd edn. Marcel Dekker, New York, pp 84–85

Scott WJ, Hirsch KS, De Sesso JM et al. (1981) Comparative studies on acetozolamide teratogenesis in pregnant rats, rabbits and rhesus monkeys. Teratology 24:37–42

Severt L, Coulter DA, Sombati S et al. (1995) Topiramate selectively blocks kianate currents in cultured hippocampal neurones. Epilepsia 26 [Suppl 4]:38

Shank RP, Vaught JL, Raffa RB et al. (1991) Investigation of the mechanism of topiramate's anticonvulsant activity (abstract). Epilepsia 32[Suppl 3]:7

Shank PS, Gardocki JF, Vaught JL et al. (1994) Topiramate: preclinical evaluation of a structurally novel anticonvulsant. Epilepsia 35:450–460

Sharief M, Viteri C, Ben-Menachem E et al. (1996) Double-blind placebo controlled trial of topiramate adjunctive therapy for partial-onset epilepsy (abstract) Epilepsy Research 25:217–224

Shorvon SD (1996) Safety of topiramate: adverse events and relationship to dosing. Epilepsia 37 [Suppl 2]:S18–22

Takahashi A, Kasahara T, Sugiyama T et al. (1995) Phase 1 study of topiramate in Japanese subjects (abstract). Epilepsia 36 [Suppl 3]:149

Tassinari CA, Michelucci R, Chauvel P et al. (1996) Double-blind, placebo-controlled trial of topiramate (600 mg daily) for the treatment of refractory partial epilepsy. Epilepsia 37:763

Wasserstein A, Reife R, Rak I (1995) Topiramate and nephrolithiasis. Epilepsia 36 [Suppl 3]:S153

Wauquier A, Zhou S (1996) Topiramate: a potent antiepileptic in the amygdala kindled rat. Epilepsy Res 24:73–77

White HS (1997) Clinical significance of animal seizure models and mechanism of action studies of potential antiepileptic drugs. Epilepsia 38 [Suppl 1]:S9–S17

White HS, Brown D, Skeen GA et al. (1995) The anticonvulsant topiramate displays a unique ability to potentiate GABA-evoked chloride currents (abstract). Epilepsia 36 [Suppl 3]:39–40

Wu WN, Heebner JB, Streeter AJ et al. (1994) Evaluation of the absorption, excretion, pharmacokinetics and metabolism of the anticonvulsant, topiramate in healthy men (abstract). Pharmacol Res 11 [Suppl]:S336

CHAPTER 19

Zonisamide

I.E. LEPPIK

A. Chemistry and Use

Zonisamide is a synthetic 1,2-benzisoxazole derivative (1,2-benzisoxazole-3-methanesulphonamide). The anticonvulsant properties of zonisamide were not predicted from its chemistry; rather they were discovered by routine screening of various 1,2-benzisoxazole derivatives. Its formula is $C_8H_8N_2O_3S$, and its molecular weight is 212. It has a pK_a of 9.66, so that its water solubility is dependent on the pH. Below a pH of 8, it has a solubility of only 0.8 mg/ml, but it has a marked increase in solubility as the pH increases into the alkaline range. Although zonisamide is quite soluble in acetone it is much less soluble in methanol, ethanol, ether and chloroform. Its synthesis was first accomplished in 1972 by UNO et al. (1976).

B. Pharmacodynamics

I. Studies in Animals

In animal models, zonisamide appears to be a broad spectrum antiepileptic drug, as it shows activity in epilepsy models in which phenytoin, carbamazepine and valproate are effective. Like carbamazepine and phenytoin, zonisamide prevents the tonic extensor component of maximal electroshock seizures in mice, rats, rabbits and dogs (MASUDA et al. 1980), restricts the spread of focal seizures created by electrical stimulation of the visual cortex in cats (ITO et al. 1980; WADA et al. 1990) and prevents propagation of seizures to subcortical structures in visual cortex-kindled cats (WADA et al. 1990). In addition, zonisamide suppresses spikes induced by the cortical application of tungstic acid gel in rats, an effect shared with valproate but not carbamazepine or phenytoin (HORI et al. 1979; ITO et al. 1979). Both zonisamide and valproate also abolish spike-wave discharges produced by the application of conjugated oestrogens to the cortex of cats (ITO et al. 1986). Zonisamide is also effective in the single neuron feline spiral trigeminal nucleus model developed by FROMM et al. (1987). Because zonisamide has a sulphamoyl group, it was suspected that it may exert its anticonvulsant activity by inhibiting carbonic anhydrase and thus have an effect similar to that of acetazolamide. However, zonisamide is much less potent an inhibitor than acetazolamide and does not

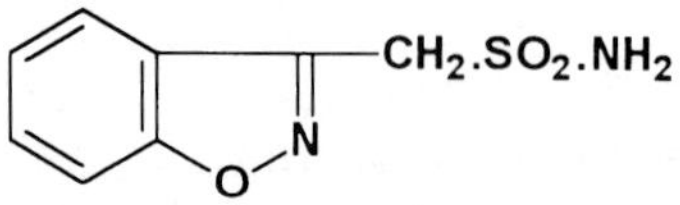

exert its anticonvulsant effect by this mechanism (Seino et al. 1995). At the cellular level, zonisamide blocks the sustained repetitive firing of voltage sensitive Na^+ channels in cultured spinal cord neurons from mouse embryos. Furthermore, it reduces voltage-dependent T-type Ca^{2+} currents without affecting L-type Ca^{2+} currents in rat embryo cerebral cortex neurons (Suzuki et al. 1992).

Based on the experimental evidence from cellular and animal models of epilepsy, zonisamide, like carbamazepine and phenytoin, would be predicted to be effective against partial and secondarily generalized tonic-clonic seizures in humans. However, like valproate, it also is active in models predictive of effectiveness against absence and myoclonic seizures. Therefore, zonisamide might be expected to prove to be a broad-spectrum antiepileptic drug in clinical use.

II. Studies in Humans

Early pilot studies of zonisamide showed it to be a promising antiepileptic drug. In one investigation, zonisamide was given to ten adult patients during a phase I study of its pharmacokinetics. In most patients, the seizure frequency was reduced after zonisamide was substituted for a standard antiepileptic drug (Sackellares et al. 1985). In an open crossover study, zonisamide was compared with carbamazepine in eight adult patients initially treated with phenytoin as monotherapy; in five zonisamide was found to have definite antiseizure activity (Wilensky et al. 1985).

Although zonisamide is presently marketed only in Japan and Korea, many studies on the drug have been done in the United States and Europe. Some of the United States studies were done in the mid-1980s as Parke-Davis was preparing for a New Drug Application to the Food and Drug Administration. The appearance of renal calculi in the late phases of the study, however, led to the termination of this work. Subsequently, Dainippon resumed testing in the United States and filed a New Drug Application based on these studies during 1997.

1. Efficacy in Localization-Related Epilepsies

There have been 4 randomized controlled and 3 open-label trials in adults and children, involving more than 1500 subjects.

A double-blind, multicentre placebo-controlled study of zonisamide when added to treatment with one or two marketed antiepileptic drugs was performed in the United States during the early and mid-1980s (Wilder et al. 1986). Adult patients ($n = 152$) with four or more complex partial seizures with or without secondary generalization were randomized to zonisamide ($n = 78$) or placebo ($n = 74$). The final median daily dose in responders in the zonisamide group was 7.2 mg/kg (given in divided doses twice a day) with a mean blood zonisamide level of 14.7 μg/ml, whilst the corresponding figures for the non-responders were 6.7 mg/kg and 16.8 μg/ml, respectively. These differences were not statistically significant. The observation period was 12 weeks and the median percent change in seizure frequency was a 30.1% decrease in the zonisamide group compared with a 0.3% increase in the placebo group ($p < 0.01$). The percentages of patients with a 50% or greater decrease in seizures was 28.6% in the zonisamide group and 13.2% in the placebo group ($p = 0.03$) (Wilder et al. 1986).

In the European multicentre double-blind placebo-controlled study, 139 adult patients with 4 or more complex partial seizures per month were randomized to zonisamide ($n = 71$) or placebo ($n = 68$) (Schmidt et al. 1993). The median daily dose was 7.8 mg/kg, with a mean blood level of 17.0 μg/ml, in zonisamide responders, and 6.8 mg/kg with a mean blood level of 15.2 μg/ml, in non-responders. In the 12 week observation period, the final median seizure change was a 27.7% reduction in the zonisamide group and an increase of 3.9% in the placebo group ($p = 0.01$). In the zonisamide group, 30.3% had a 50% or larger decrease in seizures compared with a 12.7% decrease in the placebo group ($p < 0.02$) (Schmidt et al. 1993).

A double-blind study of zonisamide compared with carbamazepine was performed by Seino et al. (1995). Of the 123 adult subjects, 59 received zonisamide and 64 received carbamazepine in addition to one to three standard antiepileptic drugs. Subjects needed to have two or more simple or complex partial and/or secondarily generalized seizures per month for inclusion in the study. The final mean drug dose was 330 mg/day in the zonisamide group and 600 mg/day in the carbamazepine group. In the zonisamide treatment group, the final mean percent decrease in simple/complex partial seizures was 68.4% and in secondarily generalized tonic-clonic seizures the decrease was 69.7%. For carbamazepine, the reductions were 46.6% and 70.2% respectively. Overall, 66.1% of the patients in the zonisamide group "improved" compared with 65.1% in the carbamazepine group (Seino et al. 1995).

In a large, open-label multicentre study of the safety of zonisamide in adults, 169 subjects with refractory partial seizures (4 or more a month) received zonisamide as add-on therapy for 16 weeks. Subjects completing the 16 weeks were permitted to continue the therapy, and alterations in other antiepileptic drugs were permitted after the initial study period. A total of 113 subjects entered the longer study period and 76 patients continued zonisamide intake for more than 1 year (Leppik et al. 1993). The median daily dose of zonisamide was 500 mg (range 50–1100 mg). The median seizure frequency of 11.5 seizures/month during the baseline period decreased to 5.5/month during the last month (weeks 13–16) of the study. Overall, there was a 41.4% decrease in all seizures, but the decrease was more impressive for secondarily generalized tonic-clonic seizures (75.3%) than for complex partial seizures

(40.6%). The percentage of subjects with a decrease of 50% or more for all seizures was 41.0%, the figure being 67.5% for those with generalized tonic-clonic seizures, and 43.2% for those with complex partial seizures (LEPPIK et al. 1993).

Evaluation of zonisamide in long-term use indicates that its efficacy is maintained, and there is no evidence of tachyphylaxis (BROWN et al. 1997). At months 5–7, 120 patients had a median reduction of seizures from baseline of 42.1%. To the present, 95 patients have been followed for 8–10 months with a 45.2% seizure reduction, 74 for 11–13 months with a 50.7% reduction, 63 for 14–16 months with a 43.9% reduction, and 40 for 16 or more months with a 45.9% reduction (BROWN et al. 1997).

ONO and collaborators (SEINO et al. 1995) performed a study of zonisamide added to other antiepileptic drugs in 538 adult Japanese subjects with partial and generalized seizures which were intractable to standard antiepileptic drugs (an average of 2.9 such drugs per patient). The average final dose of zonisamide was 6.1 mg/kg and the average plasma drug concentration was 19.90 μg/ml. Overall, 59.0% of patients with partial seizures were "improved".

In a study of children, 17 of 24 cases of symptomatic partial epilepsy had complete remission of seizures (KUMAGAI et al. 1991).

Thus zonisamide appears to be effective in localization-related epilepsies, both for partial seizures and secondarily generalized tonic-clonic seizures, in both adults and children.

2. Efficacy in Generalized Epilepsies

OGUNI and colleagues (SEINO et al. 1995) investigated zonisamide in comparison with valproate in a randomized study involving paediatric subjects (15 years of age or younger). Entry criteria included four or more convulsive and/or non-convulsive generalized seizures per month. The seizures were either untreated or were uncontrolled by treatment with one to three standard antiepileptic drugs. Of the 34 subjects, 18 were randomly assigned to zonisamide and 16 to valproate, and were then monitored for 8 weeks. The final mean daily doses were 7.3 mg/kg for zonisamide and 27.6 mg/kg for valproate. The final mean reduction in the frequency of generalized tonic-clonic seizures was 81.2% in the zonisamide group and 43.8% in the valproate group. Overall, 50.0% of the subjects in the zonisamide group and 43.8% in the valproate group were "improved" (SEINO et al. 1995). This study confirmed zonisamide to be as useful as valproate in treating tonic-clonic seizures, generalized tonic-clonic seizures and atypical absence seizures (SEINO et al. 1995).

One open study included 44 paediatric subjects aged from 8 months to 15 years. Zonisamide was started at a dose of 2–4 mg/kg per day and the dose was increased until toxicity or a satisfactory response occurred, the maximum dose being 12 mg/kg/day. Control was attained in all five cases of idiopathic generalized epilepsy, and in seven of eight cases of symptomatic generalized epilepsy (KUMAGAI et al. 1991).

Zonisamide monotherapy was reported effective in two cases of "absence seizures", one with a 3 Hz generalized spike-wave pattern and 3 Hz high voltage bursts in the right occipital area, and the other with 3.5–4 Hz generalized spike-wave patterns and focal spike-wave complexes in the left frontal to central areas (KOTANI 1994).

Zonisamide, given alone or with valproate, resulted in marked reduction of spasms and improvement in the EEG in four patients with infantile spasms (SEINO et al. 1997). In these subjects, the onset of the seizures was between 3 and 6 months of age, the EEG showed hypsarrhythmia, and computed tomography indicated the presence of some lesions.

Myoclonic epilepsies also appear to benefit from zonisamide. Two patients with progressive myoclonic epilepsy of the Unuerricht-Lundborg type had a dramatic improvement following the initiation of zonisamide intake. The doses used were 8.8 and 10.5 mg/kg/day, yielding mean serum zonisamide concentrations of 43 and 27 μg/ml respectively (HENRY et al. 1988). A report of seven cases of progressive myoclonic epilepsy from Sweden indicated that a dramatic decrease in seizures was observed, but in three patients the decrease appeared less dramatic 2–4 years later (KYLLERMAN and BEN-MENACHEM 1996). In one patient with the progressive myoclonic epilepsy with ragged-red fibres syndrome (MERRF), the addition of zonisamide resulted in disappearance of the seizures (YAGI and SEINO 1992).

In one study, 10 of 20 patients with the Lennox-Gastaut syndrome treated with zonisamide had a greater than 50% reduction in seizures (YAMATOGI and OHTAHARA 1991).

III. Measurement in Biological Fluids

A number of methods for measuring zonisamide in various biological fluids and tissues have been developed. The earlier methods used high-performance liquid chromatography (ITO et al. 1982; MATSUMOTO et al. 1983) and gas chromatography. High performance liquid chromatography is now the most commonly used method and has the advantage of being able to detect other antiepileptic drugs in the same sample (JUERGENS 1987; FURUNO et al. 1994). Recently, enzyme immunoassay methods for the drug have been developed (KAIBE et al. 1990). These methods are more rapid than high performance liquid chromatography, but can measure only one antiepileptic drug per assay.

C. Pharmacokinetics

Zonisamide has a pharmacokinetic profile which is favourable for its clinical use. It has a rapid and full absorption, long half-life, and relatively low plasma protein binding. It is partially metabolized by the liver and some is excreted in the urine as the unchanged drug.

Table 1. Pharmacokinetic parameters of zonisamide in human volunteers (modified from SEINO et al. 1995)

Dose (mg)	*N*	t_{max} (h)	C_{max} (μg/ml)	$t_{1/2}$ (h)
200	12	2.4	2.27	62.5
400	12	2.8	5.16	52.1
800	12	3.6	12.5	49.7

Values of the pharmacokinetic parameters of zonisamide in human volunteers following oral administration of the drug are shown in Table 1.

I. Absorption

The absorption of zonisamide from the gastrointestinal tract in experimental animals is rapid and almost complete, as determined after the oral administration of [^{14}C]-zonisamide. Zonisamide is rapidly absorbed in humans, with a mean t_{max} of 2.8–3.3 h in normal volunteers and with an overall range of 2–5 h (TAYLOR et al. 1986; BUCHANAN et al. 1996).

II. Distribution

Zonisamide has an interesting distribution profile. Studies of [^{14}C]-zonisamide administered either as a single dose or over 14 consecutive days to rats showed an unusual pattern. The radioactivity in most tissues was similar to that in plasma, but concentrations in erythrocytes, liver, kidneys, and adrenals was twice that of plasma and other tissues (SEINO et al. 1995). A study of the drug's distribution in the rat brain demonstrated a high concentration in the cerebral cortex and midbrain (MIMAKI et al. 1994). Zonisamide is transferred across the placenta, and levels in the foetus are similar to those in the plasma of the maternal rat. In lactating rats, it has been shown the drug's concentrations in milk are similar to those in maternal plasma (SEINO et al. 1995).

III. Elimination

1. Elimination Parameters

The elimination half-life of zonisamide in human volunteer receiving no other medication is long. In 24 volunteers, the terminal $t_{1/2}$ after 28 days of use was 63–69 h (PAGE et al. 1996). After a single dose of 300 mg, the $t_{1/2}$ was 56 h, and using [^{14}C]-zonisamide, the mean $t_{1/2}$ was 78 h after 4 days of treatment (BUCHANAN et al. 1996). In using zonisamide according to the proposed United States product labelling, the serum steady state concentration (C_{ss}) of the drug fluctuated by 14% when zonisamide was given every 12 h (PAGE et al. 1996). Thus, twice a day dosing appears appropriate. Administered once a day, the fluctuation around the mean steady-state zonisamide concentration was 27%.

2. Metabolism and Excretion

Zonisamide has a number of metabolites, formed principally via reductive and conjugative mechanisms, with oxidation being of minor metabolic significance (Stiff and Zemitis 1990). In rats, 86.5% of a 100 mg/kg intraperitoneal radioactive dose was recovered in the urine as unchanged drug and eight metabolites. Overall, unmetabolized zonisamide comprised 32.8% of the urine metabolites, 2-(sulphamoylacetyl)-phenol glucuronide 12.6%, *N*-acetyl-3-(sulphamoylmethyl)-1, 2-benzisoxazole 7.7%, zonisamide glucuronide 7.6% whilst the remaining substances found in urine were unidentified or comprised less than 5% of the dose (Stiff and Zemitis 1990). The formation of 2-(sulphamoylacetyl)-phenol glucuronide occurs by reductive cleavage of the 1,2-benzisoxazole ring (Sugihara et al. 1996). Cultured aerobic and anaerobic intestinal flora are involved in the reduction of numerous nitro, azo, and *N*-oxide compounds but do not play a significant role in zonisamide metabolism (Stiff et al. 1992). A marked gender difference between male and female rats has been reported, with 2-(sulphamoylacetyl)-phenol glucuronide production being 4 times lower in female rats than in male rats (Nakasa et al. 1993a).

Studies using microsomes from human liver samples indicated that a cytochrome P450 is involved in the metabolism of zonisamide to 2-(sulphamoylacetyl)-phenol glucuronide (Nakasa et al. 1993b). Further characterization of this process indicated that 2-(sulphamoylacetyl)-phenol glucuronide formation correlated closely with the concentration of the P450 3 A isoenzyme, moderately well with P450 2D6, but not with P450 2 C. The metabolism of zonisamide to 2-(sulphamoylacetyl)-phenol glucuronide was almost completely inhibited by anti-P450 3A4 antibody, demonstrating the importance of the 3 A family in this pathway (Nakasa et al. 1993b). The conversion of zonisamide to 2-(sulphamoylacetyl)-phenol glucuronide is markedly inhibited by cimetidine (Nakasa et al. 1992, 1996).

Zonisamide and its metabolites are excreted mainly in the urine, with little being found in the faeces. In rats, after oral administration, approximately 85% of a dose of radioactive zonisamide is found in the urine, and only 15% in faeces (Matsumoto et al. 1983). In humans, the major substance found in urine is unmetabolized zonisamide, and 48%–60% of a dose is present in urine either as zonisamide or its major metabolite 2-(sulphamoylacetyl)-phenol glucuronide (Ito et al. 1982).

D. Interactions

I. Pharmacokinetic Interactions

Because zonisamide is not highly bound to plasma proteins, one would not expect it to be affected by, or to affect, the plasma protein binding of other antiepileptic drugs. This has been confirmed by in vitro studies which demonstrated that zonisamide binding to human serum protein was not affected by phenytoin and valproate (the two most highly bound antiepileptic drugs), by phenobarbitone and by carbamazepine (MATSUMOTO 1983).

Zonisamide elimination may be affected by other antiepileptic drugs. In rats, pretreatment with carbamazepine or phenobarbitone significantly decreased the $t_{1/2}$ of zonisamide (KIMURA et al. 1992). A long term study evaluating the concentration to dose ratio of zonisamide in patients found that phenobarbitone, phenytoin and carbamazepine significantly decreased the ratio, whereas clonazepam and valproate did not (SHINODA et al. 1996). In a human study, patients receiving either phenytoin or carbamazepine as monotherapy were given a single 400 mg oral dose of zonisamide. The plasma $t_{1/2}$ of zonisamide in the carbamazepine patients was 36.4 h, and in the phenytoin patients, the $t_{1/2}$ of zonisamide was 27.1 h (OJEMANN et al. 1986). In another study in which patients were receiving two to four other antiepileptic drugs (carbamazepine, phenytoin, phenobarbitone and valproate), the mean half-life of zonisamide was 28.4 h (SACKELLARES 1985). These findings suggest that phenytoin and carbamazepine double the rate of zonisamide elimination. A report regarding two patients who received lamotrigine indicated that this drug may inhibit the clearance of zonisamide. Concentrations of zonisamide had been stable for over a year in both patients (around 27 μg/ml and 33 μg/ml) but rose to 61 μg/ml and 64 μg/ml respectively when doses of lamotrigine reached 400 mg/day (MCJILTON et al. 1996). Non-linear kinetics of zonisamide have been reported in patients receiving other antiepileptic drugs, but this phenomenon needs to be studied further (WAGNER et al. 1984). In humans, 266 serum concentration-dose pairs from 68 adults were analysed using the non-linear mixed effects model (NONMEM) for estimating population pharmacokinetic parameters. This analysis showed that the V_{max} for zonisamide was increased by 13% in patients receiving carbamazepine (HASHIMOTO et al. 1994). Thus, zonisamide doses may need to be modified in the presence of concomitant antiepileptic drug therapy, with larger zonisamide doses being needed to achieve similar concentrations of the drug if zonisamide is used with antiepileptic drugs known to induce its metabolism.

A number of studies have evaluated the effect of zonisamide on the pharmacokinetics of other drugs including antiepileptic drugs. Because of the high concentration of zonisamide in erythrocytes, an interaction between it and other sulphonamide derivatives was postulated, but this does not occur (MATSUMOTO et al. 1989). A study in rats investigating the effect of zonisamide on other antiepileptic drugs indicated that the $t_{1/2}$ and area under the plasma concentration-time curve values were slightly increased by zonisamide coadministration, but overall zonisamide had little effect on other antiepileptic drugs (KIMURA et al. 1993). In patients receiving carbamazepine or phenytoin as monotherapy, the addition of zonisamide was observed to result in a small but significant increase in phenytoin serum concentrations but not in carbamazepine concentrations (KANEKO 1993). An evaluation of 21 paediatric

Table 2. Interactions between zonisamide and other antiepileptic drugs

Effect of other antiepileptic drugs on zonisamide concentrations	
Carbamazepine	Decrease
Phenytoin	Decrease
Valproate	No change
Clonazepam	No change
Lamotrigine	Increase
Effect of zonisamide on other antiepileptic drugs	
Carbamazepine	No change
Carbamazepine-epoxide	Increase
Phenytoin	No change
Valproate	No change

patients demonstrated that the addition of zonisamide did not result in a significant change of total or unbound (free) concentrations of phenytoin and valproate (TASAKI et al. 1995). However, another human study found that the ratio of the plasma concentration of carbamazepine-10,11-epoxide (the major metabolite of carbamazepine) to the plasma concentration of carbamazepine was significantly decreased by concomitant administration of zonisamide (SHINODA et al. 1996). These findings suggest that zonisamide may inhibit the metabolism of carbamazepine to carbamazepine-10,11-epoxide, but not affect plasma concentrations of carbamazepine, phenytoin or valproate to a clinically significant degree (Table 2).

E. Adverse Effects

I. Clinical Trials

In the double-blind, placebo-controlled studies, the most common adverse events reported from zonisamide were somnolence, ataxia, anorexia, confusion, abnormal thinking, nervousness, fatigue and dizziness (WILDER et al. 1986; SCHMIDT et al. 1993). The overall rate of adverse effects in the United States study was 92% in the treated and 58% in the placebo group (WILDER et al. 1986). In the European study, the rates were 59% for zonisamide- and 28% for placebo-treated subjects (SCHMIDT et al. 1993). Although the United States study reported a higher rate for both treatment and placebo, the effect attributable to zonisamide was similar, i.e. 92% – 58% = 34% for United States compared with 59% – 27% = 32% for Europe. Most of the adverse events reported were minor and did not lead to discontinuation of zonisamide intake. In the Japanese series of 1008 patients, adverse events were reported by 51.3%, and 185 (18%) discontinued zonisamide (SEINO et al. 1991). In this study the most common adverse events were: drowsiness (24%), ataxia (13%), anorexia (11%), gastrointestinal symptoms (7%), decrease in spontaneity (6%) and slowing of mental activity (5%). Some adverse events were decreased with zonisamide monotherapy; for example, drowsiness occurred in only 9%. Other adverse effects, however, were similar in frequency during zonisamide monotherapy (loss of appetite 7%; gastrointestinal symptoms 7%; loss or decrease in spontaneity 6%). In 17 patients, zonisamide was discontinued because of leucopenia or elevation of hepatic enzyme levels on plasma (SEINO et al. 1991).

A major difference between the Japanese experience and that in Europe and United States is the occurrence of renal calculi. Overall, 13 of 505 subjects (2.6%) in the United States and European series developed kidney stones. Four urinary stones have been analysed. One was mostly urate and the others were primarily calcium oxalate and calcium phosphate (SEINO et al. 1995). In the current United States studies, renal ultrasound studies are being performed before the initiation of zonisamide and then at yearly intervals. The development of renal calculi during zonisamide treatment has been observed, but almost all have been less than a few millimetres in size, and some have resolved spontaneously. Overall, 13 of 505 (2.6%) of patients have developed nephrolithiasis. Most calculi were small and did not require treatment (PADGETT et al. 1996). In Japan only 2 of 1008 subjects (0.2%) developed this complication. YAGI and colleagues measured the 24 h urine calcium, magnesium, citrate and phosphate excretion, and found a significant decrease in urine citrate excretion but no change in excretion of the other substances (SEINO et al. 1995).

One study evaluated cognitive functioning before and after zonisamide intake. Steady-state concentrations of zonisamide above 30 μg/ml were associated with decreased acquisition and consolidation of new information (BERENT et al. 1987). However, previously learned material such as vocabulary and psychomotor performance was not affected.

There is one report in the literature of zonisamide-induced mania (CHARLES et al. 1990). The affected subject participated in the United States trial. He was normally a quiet, shy individual but during the study became acutely manic, was hospitalized, and all his symptoms resolved after zonisamide was discontinued, with no subsequent recurrence. In children, a few instances of zonisamide-induced behavioural disorders have been reported (KIMURA 1994).

II. Overdosage

One case of zonisamide overdose as a suicide attempt has been reported (NAITO et al. 1988). A dose of 7400 mg zonisamide was ingested together with 120 mg clonazepam and 4000 mg carbamazepine. Initially, the patient was comatose, but after emergency treatment, she became conscious 10 h after drug ingestion. The blood concentrations of zonisamide, clonazepam and carbamazepine were 100.1 μg/ml, 376 mg/ml, and 3.6 mg/ml respectively, 31 h after drug ingestion. Zonisamide disappeared from the blood with a half-life of 56 h (NAITO et al. 1988).

III. Teratogenicity

Zonisamide has been evaluated in pregnant animals by Terada and co-workers (Seino et al. 1995). In mice, rats, and dogs, increased external and visceral abnormalities were observed. In a prospective evaluation of Japanese women receiving zonisamide, 26 offspring exposed in utero to zonisamide with or without other antiepileptic drugs were identified. Malformations were detected in two offspring exposed to zonisamide polypharmacy (one anencephaly, one an atrial septal defect). In both, plasma zonisamide levels were low (6.1 and 6.3 μg/ml). Zonisamide could not be definitely implicated because of the polypharmacy and the low plasma zonisamide levels (Kondo et al. 1996).

F. Dose and Administration

The recommended initial daily dose of zonisamide is 100–200 mg for adults and 2–4 mg/kg for children. A steady state is achieved in 7–10 days, so that it is reasonable to increase zonisamide doses at 2-week intervals. In adults, maintenance doses of the drug are generally 200–400 mg in adults (in Japan) and 400–600 mg (in the United States), but higher doses have been used by the author. The recommended schedule is twice a day administration. In children, the maintenance dose is 4–8 μg/kg and the maximum dose is considered to be 12 mg/kg. Monitoring plasma zonisamide levels is useful, levels of 20–30 μg/ml appearing to be appropriate.

Acknowledgement. This study was supported in part by NIH NINDS P50 NS16308.

References

Berent S, Sackellares JC, Giordani B, Wagner JG, Donofrio PD, Abou-Khalil B (1987) Zonisamide (CI-912) and cognition: results from preliminary study. Epilepsia 28:61–67
Browne TR, Leppik IE, Penry JK, Dean C, Buchanan RA (1998) Zonisamide efficacy in long term studies. Epilepsia (in press)
Buchanan RA, Bockbrader HN, Chang T, Sedman AJ (1996) Single-and multiple-dose pharmacokinetics of zonisamide. Epilepsia 37 [Suppl 5]:172
Charles CL, Stoesz L, Tollefson G (1990) Zonisamide-induced mania. Psychosomatics 31:214–217
Fromm GH, Shibuya T, Terrence CF (1987) Effect of zonisamide (CI-912) on a synaptic system model. Epilepsia 28:673–679
Furuno K, Oishi R, Gomita Y, Eto K (1994) Simple and sensitive assay of zonisamide in human serum by high-performance liquid chromatography using a solid-phase extraction technique. J Chromatogr B Biomed Appl 656:456–459
Hashimoto Y, Odani A, Tanigawara Y, Yasuhara M, Okuno T, Hori R (1994) Population analysis of the dose-dependent pharmacokinetics of zonisamide in epileptic patients. Biol Pharm Bull 17:323–326
Henry T, Leppik IE, Gumnit RJ, Jacobs M (1988) Progressive myoclonus epilepsy treated with zonisamide. Neurology 38:928–931

Hori M, Ito T, Yoshida K, Shimizu M (1979) Effect of anticonvulsants on spiking activity induced by cortical freezing in cats. Epilepsia 20:25–36

Ito T, Hori M, Yoshida K, Shimizu M (1979) Effect of anticonvulsants on experimental cortical epilepsy induced by tungstic acid gel in rats. Arch Int Pharmacodyn 241:287–299

Ito T, Hori M, Masuda Y, Yoshida K, Shimizu M (1980) 3-Sulfamoylmethyl-1,2-benzisoxazole, a new type of anticonvulsant drug. Electroencephalographic profile. Arzneimittelforsch 30:603–609

Ito T, Yamaguchi T, Miyazaki H et al. (1982) Pharmacokinetic studies of AD-810, a new antiepileptic compound, Phase I trials. Arzneimittelforsch 32:1581–1586

Ito T, Hori M, Kadokawa T (1986) Effects of zonisamide (AD-810) on tungstic acid gel-induced thalamic generalized seizures and conjugated estrogen-induced cortical spike-wave discharges in cats. Epilepsia 27:367–374

Juergens U (1987) Simultaneous determination of zonisamide and nine other antiepileptic drugs and metabolites in serum. A comparison of microbore and conventional high-performance liquid chromatography. J Chromatogr 385:233–240

Kaibe K, Nishimura S, Ishii H, Sunahara N, Naruto S, Kurooka S (1990) Competitive binding enzyme immunoassay for zonisamide, a new antiepileptic drug, with selected paired-enzyme labeled antigen and antibody. Clin Chem 36:24–27

Kaneko S, Hayashimoto A, Niwayama H, Fukushima Y (1993) Effects of zonisamide on serum levels of phenytoin and carbamazepine. Jpn J Epilepsy Soc 11:31–35 (in Japanese)

Kimura S (1994) Zonisamide-induced behavior disorder in two children. Epilepsia 35:403–405

Kimura M, Tanaka N, Kimura Y, Miyake K, Kitaura T, Fukuchi H (1992) Pharmacokinetic interaction of zonisamide in rats; effect of other antiepileptics on zonisamide. J Pharmacobio Dyn 15:631–639

Kimura M, Tanaka N, Kimura Y, Miyake K, Kitaura T, Fukuchi H (1993) Pharmacokinetic interaction of zonisamide in rats. Effect of zonisamide on other antiepileptics. Biol Pharm Bull 16:722–725

Kondo T, Kaneko S, Amano Y, Egawa I (1996) Preliminary report on teratogenic effects of zonisamide in the offspring of treated women with epilepsy. Epilepsia 37:1242–1244

Kumagai N, Seki T, Yamawaki H et al. (1991) Monotherapy for childhood epilepsies with zonisamide. Jpn J Psychiatr Neurol 45:357–359

Kyllerman M, Ben-Menachem E (1996) Long-term treatment of progressive myoclonic epilepsy syndromes with zonisamide and n-acetylcysteine. Epilepsia 37 [Suppl 5]:172

Leppik IE, Willmore LJ, Homan RW et al. (1993) Efficacy and safety of znoisamide: results of a multicenter study. Epilepsy Res 14:165–173

Masuda Y, Karasawa T, Shiraishi Y, Hori M, Yoshida K, Shimizu M (1980) 3-Sulfamoylmethyl-1,2-benzisoxazole, a new type of anticonvulsant drug. Pharmacological profile. Arzneimittelforsch 30:477–483

Matsumoto K, Miyazaki H, Fujii T, Kagemoto A, Maeda T, Hashimoto M (1983) Absorption, distribution and excretion of 3-(sulfamoyl[^{14}C]-methyl)-1,2-benzisoxazole (AD-810) in rats, dogs and monkeys and of AD-810 in man. Arzneimittelforsch 33:961–968

Matsumoto K, Miyazaki H, Fujii T, Miyazaki H, Hashimoto M (1989) Binding of sulfonamides to erythrocyte proteins and possible drug-drug interaction. Chem Pharm Bull 37:2807–2810

McJilton J, DeToledo J, DeCerce J, Huda S, Abubakr A, Ramsay RE (1996) Cotherapy of lamotrigine/zonisamide results in significant elevation of zonisamide levels. Epilepsia 37 [Suppl 5]:173

Mimaki T, Tanoue H, Matsunaga Y, Miyazaki H, Mino M (1994) Regional distribution of [^{14}C]zonisamide in rat brain. Epilepsy Res 17:223–236

Naito H, Itoh N, Matsui N, Eguchi T (1988) Monitoring plasma concentrations of zonisamide and clnazepam in an epileptic attempting suicide by an overdose of the drugs. Curr Ther Res 43:463–467

Nakasa H, Komiya M, Ohmori S, Kitada M, Rikihisa T, Kanakubo Y (1992) Formation of reductive metabolite, 2-sulfamoylacetylphenol, from zonisamide in rat liver microsomes. Res Commun Chem Pathol Pharmacol 77:31–41

Nakasa H, Komiya M, Ohmori S, Rikihisa T, Kitada M (1993a) Rat liver microsomal cytochrome P-450 responsible for reductive metabolism of zonisamide. Drug Metab Dispos 21:777–781

Nakasa H, Komiya M, Ohmori S, Rikihisa T, Kiuchi M, Kitada M (1993b) Characterization of human liver microsomal cytochrome P450 involved in the reductive metabolism of zonisamide. Mol Pharmacol 44:216–221

Nakasa H, Ohmori S, Kitada M (1996) Formation of 2-sulphamoylacetylphenol from zonisamide under aerobic conditions in rat liver microsomes. Xenobiotica 26:495–501

Ojemann LM, Shastri RA, Wilensky AJ, Friel PN, Levy RH, McLean JR, Buchanan RA (1986) Comparative pharmacokinetics of zonisamide (CI-912) in epileptic patents on carbamazepine or phenytoin monotherapy. Ther Drug Monit 8:293–296

Padgett CS, Bergen DC, French JA, Buchanan RA (1997) Renal calculi associated with zonisamide. Epilepsia 37 [Suppl 5]:173

Page JG, Kochak GM, Polvino WJ, Buchanan RA (1996) Multiple dose zonisamide metabolism. Epilepsia 37 [Suppl 5]:172

Rock DM, Macdonald RL, Taylor CP (1989) Blockade of sustained repetitive action potentials in cultured spinal cord neurons by zonisamide (AD 810, CI 912), a novel anticonvulsant. Epilepsy Res 3:138–143

Sackellares JC, Donofrio PD, Wagner JG, Abou-Khalil B, Berent S, AAsved-Hoyt K (1985) Pilot study of zonisamide (1,2-benzisoxazole-3-methanesulfonamide) in patients with refractory partial seizures. Epilepsia 26:206–211

Schmidt D, Jacob R, Loiseau P et al. (1993) Zonisamide for add-on treatment of refractory partial epielpsy: a European double blind trial. Epilepsy Res 15:67–73

Seino M, Miyazaki H, Ito T (1991) Zonisamide. In: Pisani F, Perucca E, Avanzini G, Richens A (eds) New antiepileptic drugs (Epilepsy Res Suppl 3). Elsevier, New York, p. 169

Seino M, Naruto S, Ito T, Miyazaki H (1995) Other antiepileptic drugs. In: Levy RH, Mattson RH, Meldrum BS (eds) Antiepileptic drugs, 4th edn, Raven Press, New York, p. 1011

Shinoda M, Akita M, Hasegawa M, Hasegawa T, Nabeshima T (1996) The necessity of adjusting the dosage of zonisamide when coadministered with other antiepileptic drugs. Biol Pharm Bull 19:1090–1092

Stiff DD, Zemaitis MA (1990) Metabolism of the anticonvulsant agent zonisamide in the rat. Drug Metab Dispos 18:888–894

Stiff DD, Robicheau JT, Zemaitis MA (1992) Reductive metabolism of the anticonvulsant agent zonisamide, a 1,2-benzisoxazole derivative. Xenobiotica 22:1–11

Sugihara K, Kitamura S, Tatsumi K (1996) Involvement of mammalian liver cytosols and aldehyde oxidase in reductive metabolism of zonisamide. Drug Metab Dispos 24:199–202

Suzuki S, Kawakami K, Nishimura S et al. (1992) Zonisamide blocks T-type calcium channel in cultured neurons of rat cerebral cortex. Epilepsy Res 12:21–27

Tasaki K, Minami T, Ieiri I, Ohtsubo K, Hirakawa Y, Ueda K, Higuchi S (1995) Drug interactions of zonisamide with phenytoin and sodum valproate: serum concentrations and protein binding. Brain Develop 17:182–185

Taylor CP, McLean JR, Bockbraer HN et al. (1986) Zonisamide (AD-810, CI-912). In: Meldrum BS, Porter RJ (eds) New anticonvulsant drugs. John Libbey, London, pp. 277–294

Uno H, Kurokawa M, Natsuka K, Yamato Y, Nishimura H (1976) Studies on 3-substituted 1,2-benzisoxazole derivatives. Chem Pharm Bull 24:632–643

Wada Y, Hasegawa H, Okuda H, Yamaguchi N (1990) Anticonvulsant effects of zonisamide and phenytoin on seizure activity of the feline visual cortex. Brain Dev 12:206–210

Wagner JG, Sackellares JC, Donofrio PD, Berent S, Sakmer E (1984) Nonlinear pharmacokinetics of CI-912 in adult epileptic patients. Ther Drug Monit 6:277–283

Wilder BJ, Ramsay RE, Guterman A et al. (1986) A double-blind multicenter placebo-controlled study of the efficacy and safety of zonisamide in the treatment of complex partial seizures in medically refractory patients. Internal report of Dainippon Pharmaceutical Co, Ltd

Wilensky AJ, Friel PN, Ojemann LM, Dodrill CB, McCormick KB, Levy RH (1985) Zonisamide in epilepsy: a pilot study. Epilepsia 26:212–220

Yagi K, Seino M (1992) Open clinical trial of new antiepileptic drug, zonisamide (ZNA) on 49 patients with refractory epileptic seizures. Clin Psychiat 29:111–119 (in Japanese)

Yamatogi Y, Ohtahara S (1991) Current topics of treatment. In: Ohtahara S, Roger J (eds). Proceedings of the international symposium, new trends in pediatric epileptology. Okayama University Medical School, pp. 136–148

CHAPTER 20
Felbamate

W.H. Theodore

A. Introduction

Felbamate is a relatively new antiepileptic drug which has pharmacological activity in animal models of both partial and generalized seizures, as well as clinical efficacy in patients with localization-related and generalized epilepsies. It is structurally dissimilar to any other antiepileptic drug in current clinical use, and has a different spectrum of dose-related side effects. Initial excitement about the drug was tempered by the appearance of idiosyncratic haematological and hepatic toxicity, and the number of patients taking the drug fell dramatically. Felbamate remains, however, a useful agent for patients with uncontrolled seizure disorders. In addition, it may have some neuroprotective activity in animal models of cerebral ischaemia, and an effect on neuropathic pain.

B. Chemistry and Use

In chemical structure, felbamate (2-phenyl-1,3-propanediol dicarbamate; FBM; MW 238.24) is related to the antianxiety drug meprobamate. Although relatively insoluble in water or ethanol, it penetrates the central nervous system readily and is distributed uniformly (Perhach et al. 1986; Cornford et al. 1992, 1996). Felbamate is available in 400 and 600 mg scored tablets, and a 600 mg/5 ml suspension. There is no difference in bioavailability between the formulations.

C. Pharmacodynamic Studies

I. Animal Models of Epilepsy

Felbamate is active in the maximal electroshock, pentylenetetrazole, bicuculline and picrotoxin seizure models in experimental animals, suggesting that it has a broad spectrum of antiepileptic activity (Palmer et al 1993). Its protective index (TD_{50}/ED_{50}) in the rat maximum electroshock seizure model is 63, compared to 100 for phenytoin, and in the pentylenetetrazole model 12, versus 1.6 for valproic acid (Perhach et al. 1986). No pharmacodynamic evidence of tolerance to felbamate was found in 15-day studies in rats and mice.

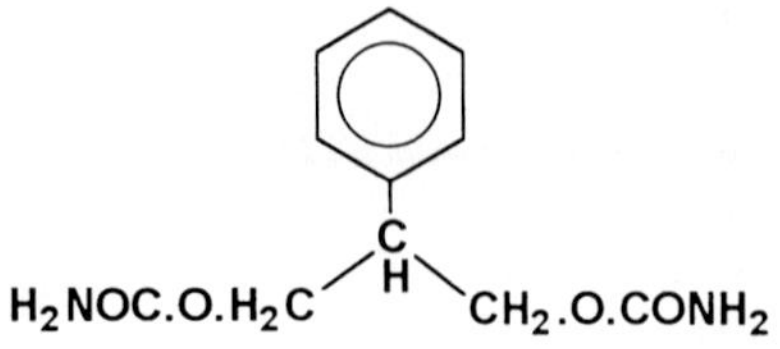

II. Biochemical Actions

In cultured hippocampal neurons, felbamate has an unusual pattern of activity, blocking currents evoked by *N*-methyl-D-aspartate (NMDA), but facilitating GABAergic responses (TICKU et al. 1991; WHITE et al. 1992; RHO et al. 1994). These features may explain both felbamate's antiepileptic drug spectrum, and its stimulant-like side effects at doses used clinically. Felbamate, unlike meprobamate, does not appear to have direct $GABA_A$ agonist activity; the evidence suggests it has a relatively weak barbiturate-like modulatory effect (RHO et al. 1994, 1997). GABAergic activity does not seem essential for its anticonvulsant effect (SERRA et al. 1997). The proposed sites for the NMDA receptor interaction of the drug include competitive antagonism at the glycine site, open channel blocking, or a non-competitive allosteric channel effect. In audiogenic seizure-susceptible mice, D-serine, a glycine agonist, blocks the anticonvulsant activity of felbamate as well as its glycine receptor binding (WHITE et al. 1995). Felbamate also binds to strychnine-insensitive glycine receptors in the human brain (WARMSLEY et al. 1995). Other investigators, however, have not found that felbamate blocks NMDA at the glycine site (SUBRAMANIAM et al. 1995). Some studies have suggested that both glycine-NMDA and AMPA-kainate receptor complexes may be important for the action of felbamate (DE SARRO et al. 1994; DOMENICI et al. 1996; PUGLIESE et al. 1996).

Felbamate has neuroprotective effects which could be mediated at NMDA receptors distinct from the strychnine-insensitive site, and related to a decrease in NMDA- and glutamate-induced neuronal Ca^{2+} influx (MCCABE et al. 1993; KANTHASAMY et al. 1995). At concentrations of 30–100 nM, felbamate produces a significant inhibition of high-voltage-activated Ca^{2+} currents (STEFANI et al. 1996). Felbamate inhibits NMDA-glycine-stimulated increases in intracellular Ca^{2+} with a minimal effective concentration of 100 μM (TAYLOR et al. 1995).

In a model of fluid percussion injury, felbamate protected CA_1 neurons at concentrations similar to those reported after monotherapy for seizures, even when the drug was given 15 min after the injury (WALLIS et al. 1995). However, in a gerbil global ischaemia model, effective neuroprotection required doses higher than those used for anticonvulsant treatment (WASTERLAIN et al. 1996). Interestingly, the protective effect against forebrain ischaemia in gerbils was greater when felbamate was given 30 min after the ischaemia (SHUAIBE et al. 1996). The drug's mechanism of neuroprotective effect may be distinct from antagonism of NMDA, or potentiation of GABA responses (LONGO et al. 1995).

Felbamate may also share some neuronal membrane effects with other antiepileptic drugs. Its inhibitory effect on veratridine-induced release of glutamate may be due to inactivation of voltage-sensitive Na^+ channels (SRINIVASIN et al. 1996). Felbamate (1 mM) caused a marked inhibition of voltage-dependent Na^+ currents expressed in *Xenopus* oocytes (TAGLIALATELA et al. 1996). Like some other antiepileptic drugs, felbamate seems to bind preferentially to, and stabilize, the inactivated state of the Na^+ channel, in this respect resembling the action of local anaesthetics. The drug has been shown to be effective in a rat model of neuropathic pain (IMAMURA et al. 1995). It has been used successfully to treat trigeminal neuralgia (CHESHIRE 1995).

III. Human Studies

1. Partial Epilepsy

Felbamate is effective against simple partial, complex partial and generalized tonic-clonic seizures in patients with localization-related epilepsy. These trials were carried out in patients with intractable seizures, which had failed to respond to a number of other antiepileptic drugs. Many patients were candidates for surgery. Two add-on studies (to carbamazepine plus phenytoin and to carbamazepine alone) showed a reduction of about 15%–30% in seizure frequency compared with placebo at felbamate doses of 2300–3600 mg/day, and plasma felbamate levels of 30–40 mg/l (LEPPIK et al. 1991; THEODORE et al. 1991). In two short-term (10 and 14 day) monotherapy trials, patients treated with felbamate had a seizure rate significantly lower than that of patients receiving placebo alone (DEVINSKY et al. 1995; THEODORE et al. 1995).

Three studies used a "survival" rather than a seizure frequency endpoint. In an add-on trial after surgical monitoring, patients receiving felbamate were less likely to develop a fourth seizure in 28 days than those receiving placebo (BOURGEOIS et al. 1993). Two studies compared felbamate 3600 mg/day with valproate 15 mg/kg/day over 112* days (SACHDEO et al. 1992; FAUGHT et al. 1993). Other antiepileptic drugs were tapered by day 28. Some 18%–40% of patients taking felbamate, compared with 78%–91% taking valproate, dropped out due to an increased seizure frequency or severity: 29% of patients receiving felbamate, compared with 11% receiving low-dose valproate, had a reduction in seizure frequency of 50% or greater, compared with their baseline value (JENSEN 1993).

2. Generalized Epilepsy

Felbamate was effective in a multicentre add-on study of patients with the Lennox-Gastaut syndrome (FELBAMATE STUDY GROUP 1993). Overall seizure counts by the parents or guardians were 19% lower in subjects taking felbamate at a dose of 45 mg/kg (3600 mg/day, with a mean blood felbamate level of 43.8 mg/l) compared with their baseline values, while the counts were only 7% lower in those taking placebo ($p = 0.01$). The atonic seizure frequency was reduced 34% by felbamate but only 9% by placebo ($p = 0.002$). Felbamate's effect may have been greater at a dose of 45 mg/kg/day than at one of 15 mg/kg/day. Subsequent data analysis (JENSEN 1994) showed that 47% of patients had a reduction of at least 50% in their total number of seizures, and of 57% in their number of atonic seizures. In this study, phenytoin and valproate levels varied by up to 22%. In a smaller, single centre study, felbamate added to valproate reduced the atonic seizure frequency by 40%. However, the mean valproate level was higher when felbamate was taken (OLETSKY et al. 1996).

Several preliminary reports in small patient groups have suggested that felbamate may be effective in other generalized seizure syndromes seizure types such as absence or juvenile myoclonic epilepsy when other drugs have failed (THEODORE et al. 1995). Although the results are consistent with the effect found in Lennox-Gastaut syndrome, they have not yet been confirmed by controlled studies. In a single case report, a patient with acquired epileptic aphasia experienced complete seizure control and almost complete return of language skills following the addition of felbamate to therapy (GLAUSER et al. 1995).

Felbamate may be more or less useful than other new antiepileptic drugs in any given patient. It is very difficult to compare efficacy data across clinical trials, or to judge the relative effectiveness of antiepileptic drugs. Even within a single trial, the effect of the design may vary with seizure type. Felbamate appeared to be more effective against complex partial seizures than generalized tonic-clonic seizures (THEODORE et al. 1991). However, the difference may have been due to the better baseline control of the latter achieved by carbamazepine in this particular add-on study.

Most clinical trials have a relatively short duration, particularly when compared to the course of seizure disorders. Over the course of long open-label, follow-up periods, there is a tendency for patients to discontinue most experimental drugs gradually (THEODORE et al. 1995). A high seizure frequency when treated with standard antiepileptic drugs is a criterion for entry to trials, and surgery is an alluring alternative. Although it has proved difficult to taper baseline antiepileptic drugs during open-label follow-up after felbamate add-on studies, the drug's efficacy does appear to be maintained during long-term treatment in patients with the Lennox-Gastaut syndrome as well as localization-related epilepsy (JENSEN 1993, 1994; WAGNER et al. 1993).

Several large, longer term, but uncontrolled open-label studies have been performed. AVANZINI et al. (1996) studied 246 patients with localization-related epilepsy. Of these, 52% (126/246) achieved a seizure reduction of 50% or more, including 10% (25/246) who became seizure-free. There was no difference in the response rate between adults and children. Of 80 patients with a diagnosis of Lennox-Gastaut syndrome, 60% (48/80) achieved a seizure reduction of 50% or more, and 6% (5/80) became seizure-free. Of 25 patients with generalized epilepsy (other than the Lennox-Gastaut syndrome), 60% (15/25) achieved a seizure reduction of 50% or more; 12% (3/24) became seizure-free (AVANZINI et al. 1996). LI et al. (1996) followed 111 adults for a mean of 4 months. Fifty-seven percent were still taking felbamate. The reasons for discontinuing felbamate were adverse events in 21%, an increase in seizures in 10%, and a lack of efficacy in 12%. Behavioural disturbance occurred in 14 patients, and was the most likely adverse event to result in discontinuation of therapy. No cases of aplastic anaemia or liver failure were observed in this group. Seven percent of the patients had a more than 95% seizure reduction (2 became seizure free), and 13% had a greater than 50% reduction in seizure frequency. An open label add-on study in children aged 2–17 years showed an overall decrease in seizure frequency of 53% (CARMANT et al. 1994). The drug was well tolerated; one of 30 children discontinued it, due to a rash.

D. Pharmacokinetics

I. Absorption

About 90% of an oral felbamate dose is absorbed (WILENSKY et al. 1985). The bioavailability is similar for the suspension, and the chewable and standard tablets, and is not affected by food (PALMER and MCTAVISH 1993). Peak plasma concentrations of the drug are reached 2–6h after dosing (WILENSKY et al. 1985). With monotherapy at a dose of 3600mg/day, plasma felbamate concentrations ranged from 60 to 90mg/l, while patients receiving hepatic enzyme-inducing drugs had felbamate levels of 30–70mg/l. Plasma felbamate concentration, AUC and C_{max} values increase linearly with dose (PALMER and MCTAVISH 1993).

II. Distribution

The apparent volume of distribution of felbamate, about 0.8l/kg, is the same after single dose or chronic administration. Felbamate is relatively lipid soluble and readily crosses the blood-brain barrier (CORNFORD et al. 1992). Some 20%–25% of the drug in plasma is reversibly bound to plasma protein, mainly albumin. It does not show preferential accumulation in any peripheral organ or specific brain region. Its pharmacokinetic parameters are stable on chronic administration (CORNFORD et al. 1992).

III. Elimination

Felbamate is metabolized by the cytochrome P450 system, and this probably accounts for its interactions with other antiepileptic drugs (PERHACH et al. 1986). Its terminal elimination half-life ranges from 13 to 23h. About 40%–50% of the absorbed dose appears unchanged in the urine. The drug's metabolites include *p*-hydroxyphenyl felbamate, 2-hydroxyfelbamate, monocarbamate derivatives, and polar compounds, including conjugates, none of which has significant antiepileptic activity, and which make up about 15% of plasma radioactivity when labelled felbamate is given (PALMER and MCTAVISH 1993). Children may metabolize the drug more quickly than adults. Felbamate had a decreased bioavailability in beagle pups, but an unchanged absorption and volume of distribution, compared with adult beagles, suggesting that there was faster elimination (ADSUMALLI et al. 1992). In humans, the apparent clearance was highest in the very young and decreased during adolescence. The mean clearance was approximately 40% higher in subjects under 12 years of age. The clearance is reduced, and the half-life increased, in the elderly (RICHENS et al. 1997). However, there do not seem to be any gender differences in the elimination parameters (BANFIELD et al. 1996; KELLEY et al. 1997). Felbamate blood levels are stable during chronic treatment, and there is no evidence of autoinduction of its metabolism (LI et al. 1996). Renal clearance accounts for about 30% of felbamate's disposition; the drug's half-life, and maximum concentration, are increased in patients with renal failure, who should therefore probably be given lower doses (GLUE et al. 1997).

E. Interactions

When felbamate is used, drug interactions may be important. Felbamate reduces blood carbamazepine levels by about 20%, while levels of the active metabolite, carbamazepine-epoxide, are increased by 25%–50% (FUERST et al. 1988; GRAVES et al. 1989; ALBANI et al. 1991). Several investigators (WILENSKY et al. 1985; GRAVES et al. 1989; LEPPIK et al. 1991; WAGNER et al. 1991; REIDENBERG et al. 1995) have reported that felbamate increases phenytoin, valproate, and phenobarbitone (due to reduced parahydroxylation) levels. WAGNER et al. (1994) showed that the coadministration of felbamate decreased steady-state valproate clearance (28% and 54%, respectively; $p < 0.01$). This effect is probably due to inhibition of valproate β-oxidation (HOOPER et al. 1996). The doses of these drugs may need to be reduced by 10%–30% to maintain their plasma levels at constant values when felbamate is given concurrently, although the effect varies from patient to patient. Felbamate does not appear to have clinically significant interactions with clonazepam, lamotrigine, oxcarbazepine, or vigabatrin (HULSMAN et al. 1995; THEODORE et al. 1995; COLUCCI et al. 1996).

Carbamazepine and phenytoin increase the clearance of felbamate by about 30% and, consequently, lower blood felbamate levels. In patients receiving hepatic enzyme inducers and felbamate at a maximum daily dose of 3000 mg, plasma felbamate levels were in the range of 30–40 mg/l compared with 70–80 mg/l in those receiving felbamate monotherapy at 3600 mg/day (LEPPIK et al. 1991; THEODORE et al. 1991; SACHDEO et al. 1992; FAUGHT et al. 1993). Valproate decreases felbamate clearance by about 15% (PALMER and MCTAVISH 1993). The protein binding of other antiepileptic drugs does not seem to be affected by felbamate (FUERST et al. 1988; PALMER and MCTAVISH 1993). Carbamazepine and phenytoin increased the clearance of felbamate by 49% and 40% respectively, whilst valproate decreased it by 21%. Barbiturate had no significant effect on felbamate clearance (KELLEY et al. 1997). Although drug interactions may complicate therapy with felbamate, they are probably no more extensive than those that occur with phenobarbitone, phenytoin and carbamazepine. Felbamate does not have a significant effect on lamotrigine plasma levels (GIDAL et al. 1997). The small effect the drug has on vigabatrin clearance (a 13% increase in the AUC and an 8% increase in urinary excretion of S(+)-vigabatrin), is not clinically significant (REIDENBERG et al. 1995). The efficacy of low-dose combination oral contraceptives may be adversely affected during felbamate treatment (SAANO et al. 1995).

F. Adverse Effects

I. Dose-Related Adverse Effects

The LD_{50} of felbamate could not be established in rats, as the animals did not succumb after ingestion of 3g felbamate, the maximum dose that could be administered (PERHACH et al. 1986). A patient who took 8 times her daily dose in an attempted suicide suffered only mild side effects (NAGEL et al. 1995). Felbamate was well tolerated in clinical trials: only about 7% of patients stopped treatment with the drug prematurely due to adverse events. In clinical trials, adverse effects that occurred significantly more often with felbamate than with placebo included nausea and vomiting, weight loss, diplopia, blurred vision, headache, ataxia, and insomnia (JENSEN et al. 1993, 1994). However, these effects were more common in add-on than in monotherapy trials and often disappeared when the other coadministered drugs, particularly phenytoin, were ceased.

In adults receiving felbamate monotherapy, insomnia and weight loss tend to be the most frequently reported side effects. Stimulant-like effects are prominent (KETTER et al. 1996). Some patients may experience an anxiety-dysphoria syndrome, in addition to insomnia. Isolated cases of tremor, involuntary movements, and psychosis have been reported, which may or may not have been due to felbamate. At least one patient taking felbamate monotherapy had a new onset psychosis (MCCONNELL et al. 1997). Children may experience sleepiness (perhaps analogous to the paradoxical effect of amphetamine-like drugs), as well as prominent weight loss. Unlike antiepileptic drugs such as carbamazepine, felbamate does not appear to have anxiolytic effects, or to attenuate the adverse psychological consequences of antiepileptic drug withdrawal (KETTER et al. 1996). As is common with antiepileptic drugs, the elderly may have more frequent adverse effects from felbamate, due to either pharmacokinetic or pharmacodynamic factors (RICHENS et al. 1997).

Patients tend either to like felbamate very much, experiencing increased energy and well-being, along with better seizure control, or to tolerate it poorly. Oesophageal burning can be a troubling and persistent symptom. Felbamate side effects such as anorexia, headache, insomnia, or anxiety usually do not remit on continued treatment, although one study reported that headache, which occurred in 33% of patients, seemed to be dose-related (ETTINGER et al. 1996). Laboratory studies suggest that felbamate can exacerbate acute intermittent porphyria (HAHN et al. 1997).

II. Idiosyncratic Adverse Effects

Initially, little systemic toxicity of the drug was reported. There was no evidence of clinically significant hepatic or haematological changes in the clinical trials, although mild elevation of liver function tests and other clinical laboratory abnormalities were noted occasionally (JENSEN 1993, 1994; PALMER and MCTAVISH 1993). Rashes and hypersensitivity reactions, sometimes including fever and lymphadenopathy, occurred in 3%–4% of patients. The number of patients studied, about 1600, would have been too small to detect the incidence of the haematological and hepatic toxicity that has begun to be reported since, with the wider clinical use of felbamate.

Aplastic anaemia has been reported in 32 patients receiving felbamate (Wallace Laboratories, data on file). The patients, 19 of whom were women, ranged in age from 13 to 70 (mean 41) years, and had been exposed to the drug for 72–354 days (mean 174 days). However, only 23 met International Agranulocytosis and Aplastic Anaemia Study criteria, while there were insufficient data in 2 others (KAUFMAN et al. in press). KAUFMAN et al. found that only 3 of the 23 definite cases had no confounding variable, such as exposure to another drug associated with aplastic anaemia, parvovirus infection, or a history of diseases such as rheumatoid arthritis. Eleven had exposure to a confounding agent, but felbamate was still thought to be the most likely cause. Seven died. The lowest estimate of the incidence was 27 cases per million felbamate users (the 3 cases without confounding), and the highest 209 per million (all confirmed cases), and the most probable 127 per million (the 14 for whom felbamate was judged the "likely" cause). Thus, the true magnitude of the risk of aplastic anaemia is uncertain. By comparison, the best estimate for the incidence of aplastic anaemia associated with carbamazepine is 39 cases per million (KAUFMAN et al. 1996).

Eighteen cases of liver failure (with 9 deaths so far) have been reported (O'NEIL et al. 1996). These patients ranged in age from 3 to 56 years; 6 were children. The exposure to the drug had ranged from 14 to 265 days; some of the patients had a rash as well as liver toxicity. All the patients were taking other antiepileptic drugs. Seven (including four who died) had been in status epilepticus when the hepatic failure occurred.

The manufacturer now advises that patients treated with felbamate should have blood counts and liver function tests every 1–2 weeks. Unfortunately, even this high degree of caution may not detect incipient toxicity. Aplastic anaemia and hepatic failure may not be reversible even if detected early.

Moreover, patients may develop symptoms after the drug has been stopped. Platelets and white blood cells have a short lifespan, but red cells live 120 days, so peripheral evidence of marrow injury may have a delayed appearance. Mild hepatic enzyme elevations are often found in patients taking antiepileptic drugs, and may not necessarily be an indication of "toxicity". Reactive aldehyde metabolites may play a role in the toxicity (Thompson et al. 1996).

Other unusual side effects of felbamate include involuntary movements, which may in part have been due to drug interactions (Kerrick et al. 1995). Skin rashes, including toxic epidermal necrolysis, have occurred sporadically (Travaglini et al. 1995). Teratology studies in rats and rabbits have been negative, and there are no human data.

G. Use of Felbamate in Practice

Although rapid escalation of felbamate dosage has been carried out in clinical trials, a slow dosage titration schedule may lead to fewer initial adverse effects, particularly gastrointestinal disturbances, insomnia, and anxiety. The drug seems to be better tolerated when taken with meals, and the individual doses spread out as much as possible. Felbamate can be started in a dose of 400 mg 3 times a day, with dosage increases of 400–600 mg/day every 1–2 weeks. Some patients, particularly the elderly, may need lower starting doses and slower increases in dose. For children, an initial felbamate dose of 15 mg/kg/day, with weekly increases to 45 mg/kg/day, seems reasonable.

Felbamate decreases phenytoin and valproate clearances. To maintain steady state plasma levels of these drugs, it may be necessary to reduce their doses when starting felbamate intake. However, this dose reduction should be done cautiously to avoid seizure exacerbation, since it may take several weeks to reach therapeutic doses of felbamate.

The highest felbamate dose used in adult clinical trials has been 3600 mg/day, but some patients have received 5000–6000 mg/day. The maximum dose tried in the Lennox-Gastaut trial was 45 mg/kg or 3600 mg/day. Clinical experience will have to determine the true upper limit of the dose. In some patients, because of gastrointestinal discomfort, the maximally tolerated dose is in the range of 2400–3000 mg/day. Children usually are more rapid metabolizers of the drug than adults, and need relatively more drug to maintain effective blood levels. The pharmacology of felbamate has not been studied in elderly patients, but its metabolism is likely to be reduced in this age group. Moreover, the elderly are usually more sensitive to the CNS side effects of antiepileptic drugs. The starting dose, and subsequent dosage increases, should probably be reduced by about one-third in the elderly.

I. Role of Felbamate Blood Levels

There are few data on the relation of plasma felbamate levels to the clinical response to the drug. Children in the Lennox-Gastaut syndrome trial tended to have fewer seizures at plasma felbamate levels of 45 mg/l than at levels of 18 mg/l (FELBAMATE STUDY GROUP 1993). In an uncontrolled study, patients with felbamate levels above 44 mg/l were more likely to have both side effects and improved seizure control (HARDEN et al. 1996). Although the data are not directly comparable, the response in adult trials may have been better with felbamate levels in the 60–80 mg/l than the 30–40 mg/l range (LEPPIK et al. 1991; THEODORE et al. 1991; SACHDEO et al. 1992; BOURGEOIS et al. 1993; FAUGHT et al. 1993). Since felbamate clearance is increased by carbamazepine and phenytoin, higher felbamate doses may be necessary to achieve comparable plasma levels when these drugs are given at the same time.

II. Managing Drug Interactions

Drug interactions may play an important role in the frequency of side effects experienced by patients treated with felbamate. Increased phenytoin and valproate levels may contribute to nausea and vomiting, diplopia, blurred vision, and ataxia. Even though carbamazepine levels fall, levels of the pharmacologically active metabolite, carbamazepine-epoxide, may increase. This compound could also contribute to side effects, since it has lower protein binding than carbamazepine itself, and may penetrate the brain more readily.

However, it is possible that some of the therapeutic effect of felbamate in add-on trials could also have been related to drug interactions, particularly those which increased phenytoin and valproate levels. One study suggested that the fall in carbamazepine levels might lead to reduced seizure control, despite increased carbamazepine-epoxide levels (THEODORE et al. 1991). It may be valuable to measure the levels of the epoxide as well as those of carbamazepine itself when patients are taking both felbamate and carbamazepine. There is considerable individual variation in felbamate's effects on other antiepileptic drugs. Rather than automatically adjusting the doses of the other drugs, it is important to measure the levels of the drugs that are present. Since felbamate does not have an appreciable effect on the protein binding of other drugs, it is not necessary to measure free antiepileptic drug levels.

III. Stopping Felbamate

Because of the risk of aplastic anaemia or liver disease, felbamate intake should be stopped when the drug appears not to be working. On the other hand, since felbamate is likely to be used when all other appropriate agents have failed, patients may be willing to tolerate side effects that are not life-threatening. Insomnia, gastrointestinal distress, and weight loss may be less discomforting to some patients than the side effects of other drugs, particularly if seizures are controlled by felbamate.

There is no evidence for any acute exacerbation of seizures during felbamate withdrawal, which has been carried out rapidly in clinical trials. Certainly the drug should be stopped abruptly if there is evidence of haematological or liver disease. When reports of such complications began to appear, many asymptomatic patients were tapered off felbamate over 1–2 weeks without a sudden increase in seizures, although many experienced a chronic rise in seizure frequency, despite higher doses, or the addition, of other drugs.

H. Conclusions

Felbamate has a broad antiepileptic spectrum. Children with the Lennox-Gastaut syndrome and related secondary generalized epileptic syndromes, for whom few therapeutic options exist, may benefit most from felbamate. It can also be tried in patients with refractory partial and secondarily ed seizures which have not responded to other drugs. There may be some patients who have attained seizure control with other drugs only at the cost of unacceptable central nervous system depressant side effects, who are not candidates for surgery, and who are willing to accept the risk of felbamate's systemic toxicity. Since felbamate appears to be less sedating than other antiepileptic drugs, it may be useful for patients who find sedation particularly debilitating. Felbamate should be used only when seizures have not been controlled by other drugs. Results of clinical laboratory tests should be monitored closely and the drug stopped if any abnormalities are detected. It may be prudent to avoid combinations of felbamate with other drugs that can cause hepatic or haematological dysfunction, such as valproate or carbamazepine. Women taking felbamate may be more likely to develop aplastic anaemia than men. Felbamate should not be given to patients with a history of blood dyscrasias or autoimmune disorders. Patients with a history of psychiatric disorders may be more likely to experience acute anxiety or even psychosis when being treated with felbamate.

References

Adusumalli VA, Gilchrist JR, Wichmann JK, Kucharcyzk N, Sofia RD (1992) Pharmacokinetics of felbamate in pediatric and adult dogs. Epilepsia 33:955–960

Albani F, Theodore WH, Washington P et al. (1991) Effect of felbamate on plasma levels of carbamazepine and its metabolites. Epilepsia 32:130–132

Avanzini G, Canger R, Dalla Bernardina B, Vigevano F (1996) Felbamate in therapy-resistant epilepsy: an Italian experience. Epilepsy Res 25:249–255

Banfield CR, Zhu GR, Jen JF et al. (1996) The effect of age on the apparent clearance of felbamate: a retrospective analysis using nonlinear mixed-effects modelling. Ther Drug Monit 18:19–29

Bergen DC, Ristanovic RK, Waicosky K, Kanner A, Hoeppner TJ (1995) Weight loss in patients taking felbamate. Clin Neuropharmacol 18:23–27

Bourgeois B, Leppik IE, Sackellares JC et al. (1993) Felbamate: a double-blind controlled trial in patients undergoing presurgical evaluation of partial seizures. Neurology 43:693–696

Carmant L, Holmes GL, Sawyer S, Rifai N, Anderson J, Mikati MA (1994) Efficacy of felbamate in therapy for partial epilepsy in children. J Pediatr 125:481–486

Cheshire WP (1995) Felbamate relieved trigeminal neuralgia. Clin J Pain 11:139–142

Colucci R, Glue P, Holt B et al. (1996) Effect of felbamate on the pharmacokinetics of lamotrigine. J Clin Pharmacol 36:634–638
Cornford EA, Young D, Paxton JA, Sofia RD (1992) Blood-brain barrier penetration of felbamate. Epilepsia 33:944–955
Cornford EM, Truong HV, Sofia RD, Kucharczyk N (1996) Distribution of felbamate in brain. Epilepsia 37:15–18
De Sarro G, Ongini E, Bertorelli R, Aguglia U, De Sarro A (1994) Excitatory amino acid neurotransmission through both NMDA and non-NMDA receptors is involved in the anticonvulsant activity of felbamate in DBA/2 mice. Eur J Pharmacol 262:11–19
Devinsky O, Faught RE, Wilder BJ, Kanner AM, Kamin M, Kramer LD, Rosenberg A (1995) Efficacy of felbamate monotherapy in patients undergoing presurgical evaluation of partial seizures. Epilepsy Res 20:241–246
Domenici MR, Marinelli S, Sagratella S (1996) Effects of felbamate, kynurenic acid derivatives and NMDA antagonists on in vitro kainate-induced epileptiform activity. Life Sci 58:PL391–396
Ettinger AB, Jandorf L, Berdia A, Andriola MR, Krupp LB, Weisbrot DM (1996) Felbamate-induced headache. Epilepsia 37:503–505
Faught E, Sachdeo RC, Remler MP et al. (1993) Felbamate monotherapy for partial-onset seizures: an active control trial. Neurology 43:688–692
Felbamate Study Group in the Lennox-Gastaut Syndrome (1993) Efficacy of felbamate in childhood epileptic encephalopathy (Lennox-Gastaut Syndrome). N Engl J Med 328:29–33
Fuerst RH, Graves NM, Leppik IE, Brundage RC, Holmes GB, Remmel RP (1988) Felbamate increases phenytoin but decreases carbamazepine concentrations. Epilepsia 29:488–491
Gidal BE, Kanner A, Maly M, Rutecki P, Lensmeyer GL (1997) Lamotrigine pharmacokinetics in patients receiving felbamate. Epilepsy Res 27:1–5
Glauser TA, Olberding LS, Titanic MK, Piccirillo DM (1995) Felbamate in the treatment of acquired epileptic aphasia. Epilepsy Res 20:85–89
Glue P, Sulowicz W, Colucci R, Banfield C, Pai S, Lin C, Affrime MB (1997) Single-dose pharmacokinetics of felbamate in patients with renal dysfunction. Br J Clin Pharmacol 44:91–93
Graves NM, Holmes GB, Fuerst RH, Leppik IE (1989) Effect of felbamate on phenytoin and carbamazepine serum concentrations. Epilepsia 30:225–229
Hahn M, Gildemeister OS, Krauss GL, Pepe JA, Lambrecht RW, Donohue S, Bonkovsky HL (1997) Effects of new anticonvulsant medications on porphyrin synthesis in cultured liver cells: potential implications for patients with acute porphyria. Neurology 49:97–106
Harden CL, Trifiletti R, Kutt H (1996) Felbamate levels in patients with epilepsy. Epilepsia 37:280–283
Hooper WD, Franklin ME, Glue P et al. (1996) Effect of felbamate on valproic acid disposition in healthy volunteers: inhibition of beta-oxidation. Epilepsia 37:91–97
Hulsman JA, Rentmeester TW, Banfield CR et al. (1995) Effects of felbamate on the pharmacokinetics of the monohydroxy and dihydroxy metabolites of oxcarbazepine. Clin Pharmacol Ther 58:383–389
Imamura Y, Bennett GJ (1995) Felbamate relieves several abnormal pain sensations in rats with an experimental peripheral neuropathy. J Pharmacol Exp Ther 275:177–182
Jensen PK (1993) Felbamate in the treatment of refractory partial onset seizures. Epilepsia 34 [Suppl 7]:S25–S29
Jensen PK (1994) Felbamate in the treatment of Lennox-Gastaut Syndrome. Epilepsia 35 [Suppl 5]:S54–S57
Kanthasamy AG, Matsumoto RR, Gunasekar PG, Trunong DD (1995) Excitoprotective effect of felbamate in cultured cortical neurons. Brain Res 705:97–104

Kaufman DW, Kelly JP, Jurgelon J et al. (1996) Drugs in the etiology of agranulocytosis and aplastic anemia. Eur J Hematol 57 [Suppl 60]:23–30

Kaufman DW, Kelly JP, Anderson T, Harmon DC, Shapiro S (1998) An evaluation of case reports of aplastic anemia among individuals using felbamate. Epilepsia (in press)

Kelley MT, Walson PD, Cox S, Dusci LJ (1997) Population pharmacokinetics of felbamate in children. Ther Drug Monit 19:29–36

Kerrick JM, Kelley BJ, Maister BH, Graves NM, Leppik IE (1995) Involuntary movement disorders associated with felbamate. Neurology 45:185–187

Ketter TA, Malow BA, Flamini R, Ko D, White SR, Post RM, Theodore WH (1996) Felbamate monotherapy has stimulant-like effects in patients with epilepsy. Epilepsy Res 23:129–137

Leppik IE, Dreifuss FE, Pledger GW et al. (1991) Felbamate for partial seizures; results of a controlled clinical trial. Neurology 41:1785–1789

Li LM, Nashef L, Moriarty J, Duncan JS, Sander JW (1996) Felbamate as add-on therapy. Eur Neurol 36:146–148

Longo R, Domenici MR, Scotti de Carolis A, Sagratella S (1995) Felbamate selectively blocks in vitro hippocampal kainate-induced irreversible electrical changes. Life Sci 56:PL409–414

McCabe RT, Wasterlain CG, Kucharcyzk N, Sofia RW, Vogel JR (1993) Evidence for anticonvulsant and neuroprotectant action of felbamate mediated by strychnine-insensitive glycine receptors. J Pharmacol Exp Ther 264:1248–1252

McConnell H, Snyder PJ, Duffy JD et al. (1996) Neuropsychiatric side effects related to treatment with felbamate J Neuropsychiatry Clin Neurosci 8:341–346

Nagel TR, Schunk JE (1995) Felbamate overdose: a case report and discussion of a new antiepileptic drug. Pediatr Emerg Care 11:369–371

O'Neil MG, Perdun CS, Wilson MB, McGown ST, Patel S (1996) Felbamate-associated fatal acute hepatic necrosis. Neurology 46:1457–1459

Oletsky H, Kelley K, Stertz B, Reeves-Tyer P, Flamini R, Malow B, Theodore WH (1996) The efficacy of felbamate as add-on therapy to valproic acid in the Lennox-Gastaut syndrome. Epilepsia 37 [Suppl 5]:155

Palmer KJ, McTavish D (1993) Felbamate: a review of its pharmacodynamic and pharmacokinetic properties, and therapeutic efficacy in epilepsy. Drugs 45: 1041–1065

Perhach JL, Weliky I, Newton JJ, Sofia RD, Romayshyn WM, Arndt WF Jr (1986) Felbamate. In: Porter RJ, Meldrum BS (eds) New anticonvulsant drugs. Libby, London, pp. 117–124

Pugliese AM, Passani MB, Pepeu G, Corradetti R (1996) Felbamate decreases synaptic transmission in the CA1 region of rat hippocampal slices. J Pharmacol Exp Ther 279:1100–1108

Reidenberg P, Glue P, Banfield C et al. (1995a) Pharmacokinetic interaction studies between felbamate and vigabatrin. Br J Clin Pharmacol 40:157–160

Reidenberg P, Glue P, Banfield CR et al. (1995b) Effects of felbamate on the pharmacokinetics of phenobarbital. Clin Pharmacol Ther 58:279–287

Rho JM, Donevan SD, Rogawski MA (1993) Mechanism of action of the anticonvulsant felbamate: opposing effects on NMDA and $GABA_A$ receptors. Ann Neurol 35:229–234

Rho JM, Donevan SD, Rogawski MA (1997) Barbiturate-like actions of the propanediol dicarbamates felbamate and meprobamate. J Pharmacol Exp Ther 280:1383–1391

Richens A, Banfield CR, Salfi M, Nomeir A, Lin CC, Jensen P, Affrime MB, Glue P (1997) Single and multiple dose pharmacokinetics of felbamate in the elderly. Br J Clin Pharmacol 44:129–134

Saano V, Glue P, Banfield CR et al. (1995) Effects of felbamate on the pharmacokinetics of a low-dose combination oral contraceptive. Clin Pharmacol Ther 58:523–531

Sachdeo R, Kramer LD, Rosenberg A, Sachdeo S (1992) Felbamate monotherapy: controlled trial in patients with partial onset seizures. Ann Neurol 32:386–392

Serra M, Cuccu R, Ghiani CA, Pisu MG, Murgia A, Biggio G (1997) Antagonism of convulsions but failure to enhance GABA(A) receptor function by felbamate in mice tolerant to diazepam. Neurochem Res 22:693–697

Shuaib A, Waqaar T, Ijaz MS, Kanthan R, Wishart T, Howlett W (1996) Neuroprotection with felbamate: a 7- and 28-day study in transient forebrain ischemia in gerbils. Brain Res 727:65–70

Srinivasan J, Richens A, Davies JA (1996) Effects of felbamate on veratridine- and K(+)-stimulated release of glutamate from mouse cortex. Eur J Pharmacol 315:285–288

Stefani A, Calabresi P, Pisani A, Mercuri NB, Siniscalchi A, Bernardi G (1996) Felbamate inhibits dihydropyridine-sensitive calcium channels in central neurons. J Pharmacol Exp Ther 277:121–127

Subramaniam S, Rho JM, Penix L, Donevan SD, Fielding RP, Rogawski MA (1995) Felbamate block of the N-methyl-D-aspartate receptor. J Pharmacol Exp Ther 273:878–886

Swinyard EA, Woodhead JH, Franklin MR, Sofia RD, Kupferberg HJ (1987) The effect of chronic felbamate administration on anticonvulsant activity and hepatic drug metabolizing enzymes in mice and rats. Epilepsia 28:295–300

Taglialatela M, Ongini E, Brown AM, Di Renzo G, Annunziato L (1996) Felbamate inhibits cloned voltage-dependent Na^+ channels from human and rat brain. Eur J Pharmacol 316:373–377

Taylor LA, McQuade RD, Tice MA (1995) Felbamate, a novel antiepileptic drug, reverses N-methyl-D-aspartate/glycine-stimulated increases in intracellular Ca^{2+} concentration. Eur J Pharmacol 289:229–233

Theodore WH, Raubertas R, Porter RJ et al. (1991) Felbamate: a clinical trial for complex partial seizures. Epilepsia 32:392–397

Theodore WH, Jensen P, Kwan RM (1995a) Felbamate: clinical use. In: Levy RH, Mattson RH, Meldrum BS (eds) Antiepileptic drugs, 4th edn. Raven Press, New York, pp. 817–822

Theodore WH, Albert P, Stertz B et al. (1995b) Felbamate monotherapy: implications for antiepileptic drug development. Epilepsia 36:1105–1110

Thompson CD, Kinter MT, Macdonald TL (1996) Synthesis and in vitro reactivity of 3-carbamoyl-2-phenylpropionaldehyde and 2-phenylpropenal: putative reactive metabolites of felbamate. Chem Res Toxicol 9:1225–1229

Ticku MK, Kamatchi GL, Sofia RD (1991) Effect of anticonvulsant felbamate on $GABA_A$ receptor system. Epilepsia 32:389–391

Travaglini MT, Morrison RC, Ackerman BH, Haith LR Jr, Patton ML (1995) Toxic epidermal necrolysis after initiation of felbamate therapy. Pharmacotherapy 15:260–264

Wagner ML, Graves NM, Marienau K, Holmes GB, Remmel RP, Leppik IE (1991) Discontinuation of phenytoin and carbamazepine in patients receiving felbamate. Epilepsia 32:398–406

Wagner ML, Remmel RP, Graves NM, Leppik IE (1993) Effect of felbamate on carbamazepine and its major metabolites. Clin Pharmacol Ther 53:536–543

Wagner ML, Graves NM, Leppik IE, Remmel RP, Shumaker RC, Ward DL, Perhach JL (1994) The effect of felbamate on valproic acid disposition. Clin Pharmacol Ther 56:494–502

Wallis RA, Panizzon KL (1995) Felbamate neuroprotection against CA1 traumatic neuronal injury. Eur J Pharmacol 294:475–482

Wamsley JK, Sofia RD, Faull RL, Narang N, Ary T, McCabe RT (1994) Interaction of felbamate with [^{3}H]DCKA-labeled strychnine-insensitive glycine receptors in human postmortem brain. Exp Neurol 129:244–250

Wasterlain CG, Adams LM, Wichmann JK, Sofia RD (1996) Felbamate protects CA1 neurons from apoptosis in a gerbil model of global ischemia. Stroke 27:1236–1240

White HS, Wolf HH, Swinyard EA, Skeen GA, Sofia RD (1992) A neuropharmacological evaluation of felbamate as a novel anticonvulsant. Epilepsia 33:564–572
White HS, Harmsworth WL, Sofia RD, Wolf HH (1995) Felbamate modulates the strychnine-insensitive glycine receptor. Epilepsy Res 20:41–48
Wilensky AJ, Friel PN, Ojemann LM, Kupferberg HJ, Levy RH (1985) Pharmacokinetics of W-554 (ADD 03055) in epileptic patients. Epilepsia 26:602–606

CHAPTER 21

Drugs Under Clinical Trial

E. Perucca

A. Introduction

Over the last decade, the introduction of novel antiepileptic drugs brought new hope to the multitude of patients whose seizures are not completely controlled by established anticonvulsants. However, while it has to be acknowledged that recently licensed drugs represent a valuable addition to the therapeutic armamentarium, it is a fact that these drugs produce freedom from seizures in no more than 10%–15% of patients refractory to older agents (Perucca 1996). Moreover, none of the new agents is ideal in terms of its pharmacokinetic properties, interaction potential, spectrum of activity and side effect profile. Therefore the search for newer drugs with improved efficacy and safety goes on.

Although important advances have been made in elucidating the pathogenesis of epilepsy, our knowledge is still insufficient to allow a fully rational design of new drugs. This is especially true for drugs targeted at solving the problem of refractory epilepsies, whose pathophysiological basis remains poorly understood. This situation, however, may change in the future as a result of ongoing progress in developing new epilepsy models and systems for assessing modes of drug action at biochemical, electrophysiological and molecular levels.

While the need for better antiepileptic drugs remains unchanged, the interest of the pharmaceutical industry towards the development of new agents has sadly been declining. This is due to a combination of factors, such as skyrocketing development costs, the crowded and competitive nature of the epilepsy drug market, and disillusion (born out from experience with recently developed drugs) about the probability that an excellent activity profile in preclinical models will translate into a major therapeutic breakthrough. Despite these limitations, a number of pharmaceutical companies are still actively pursuing the discovery of new drugs, and some of these agents are progressing through the various stages of development.

Drug development is a risky venture involving continuous re-evaluation based on new scientific information and financial considerations. This is exemplified by the fact that out of 14 drugs in clinical development listed in a recent review (Porter 1990), the vast majority (denzimol, eterobarb, flumazenil, flupirtine, milacemide, MK-801, nafimidone, Org-6370 and ralitoline) are no longer being actively developed for the treatment of epilepsy, at least to the author's knowledge. Only four compounds (felbamate, gabapentin, topiramate and zonisamide) progressed to the marketing stage, and one (stiripentol) is still under evaluation. With the realization that part of the following information may similarly become outdated in the next few years, this chapter will attempt to review antiepileptic drugs which are undergoing clinical testing at the time of writing. Since data become obsolete more rapidly for agents at early stages of development, attention will focus mainly on those compounds for which substantial clinical experience is already available. Drugs which may have potential value in the management of epilepsy but are licensed for other indications (e.g. allopurinol, flunarizine, nimodipine, flumazenil) and are not being actively developed as antiepileptic agents will not be considered further in this chapter.

B. Levetiracetam

Levetiracetam (ucb LO59) is a piracetam derivative originally developed as a cognition-enhancing agent. An interesting point about this compound is that its anticonvulsant activity was not apparent in routine maximal electroshock (MES) and pentylenetetrazole (PTZ) tests, but could be demonstrated in other epilepsy models. Levetiracetam is currently under evaluation for use in epilepsy and anxiety.

I. Chemistry

Levetiracetam (Fig. 1), the (S)-enantiomer of alpha-ethyl-2-oxo-pyrrolidine acetamide, is a soluble ethyl derivative of the nootropic drug piracetam.

II. Pharmacodynamics

1. Anticonvulsant Activity in Animal Models

Levetiracetam has been reported to possess broad-spectrum seizure protective activity in a variety of animal models, including tonic and clonic audiogenic seizures in mice, tonic audiogenic seizures in rats, tonic and clonic seizures induced by bicuculline in mice, and tonic seizures induced by bicuculline or intracerebral ventricular *N*-methyl-D-aspartate (NMDA) in mice,

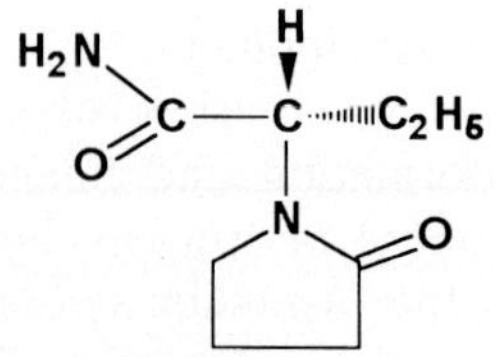

Fig. 1. Molecular structure of levetiracetam

and spontaneous EEG spike-wave activity in rats. In these models, ED_{50} values were generally in the 5–30 mg/kg range (GOWER et al. 1992, 1995; KAPETANOVIC and KUPFERBERG 1997). In rodents, levetiracetam is remarkably potent (ED_{50} 7 mg/kg) against seizures induced by pilocarpine, but it is only weakly active (ED_{50} 97 mg/kg) against DMCM-induced convulsions and it is inactive (>170 mg/kg) against seizures induced by systemically administered NMDA, kainate and AMPA (GOWER et al. 1992; KLITGAARD et al. 1996a,b). The drug's anticonvulsant effects remain generally undiminished after repeated administration.

The activity of levetiracetam is especially evident with submaximal convulsant stimuli. For example, the drug is inactive or only weakly active in the classical subcutaneous (s.c.) pentylenetetrazole (PTZ) test, but it potently inhibits seizures induced by submaximal pentylenetetrazole doses in mice as well as spike-and-wave EEG discharges after low-dose pentylenetetrazole in rats. Although there is controversy about potency in the maximum electroshock seizure test (GOWERS et al. 1992; LÖSCHER and HÖNACK 1993; KAPETANOVIC and KUPFERBERG 1997), in one study levetiracetam was ineffective at doses up to 500 mg/kg in mice and rats, but activity became evident under threshold conditions or when supramaximal currents were lowered (LÖSCHER and HÖNACK 1993). Based on the above findings, the activity profile in animal models has been considered as virtually unique (KLITGAARD et al. 1996a; KAPETANOVIC and KUPFERBERG 1997).

In separate experiments, levetiracetam was effective against amygdala-kindled seizures in rats (GOWER et al. 1992; LÖSCHER and HÖNACK 1993) and corneally kindled seizures in mice (MATAGNE and KLITGAARD 1996), results predictive of efficacy in partial seizures. In the pentylenetetrazole kindling model in mice, levetiracetam shows antiepileptogenic in addition to anticonvulsant activity (GOWER et al. 1992).

2. Mechanism of Action

The mechanism of action of levetiracetam is unknown. The drug has no significant affinity for known GABA, benzodiazepine, glycine, adenosine and various excitatory amino acid-related receptors, or Ca^{2+}, K^{+} and Cl^{-} channels. However, it does bind stereoselectively to a synaptic site in rat brain from which it can be displaced by ethosuximide, pentylenetetrazole and piracetam, but not by other conventional anticonvulsants (NOYER et al. 1995; HARIA and BALFOUR 1997). A stereoselective mode of action is confirmed by the fact that the R-enantiomer is inactive in seizure models (GOWER et al. 1992; GOWER and MATAGNE 1994). In vivo, levetiracetam reduces bicuculline-induced neuronal hyperexcitability in rat hippocampal CA_3 cells through an action which does not appear to be mediated by a GABAergic mechanism (MARGINEANU and WULFERT 1995). Although levetiracetam does not affect the GABA synthesizing and degrading enzymes glutamic acid decarboxylase (GAD) and GABA-transaminase (GABA-T) in vitro, it does affect the activity of these enzymes in vivo, possibly as a consequence of postsynaptic changes in transmitter function (LÖSCHER et al. 1996). In particular, levetiracetam has been found to increase GABA-T activity and to decrease GAD activity in the striatum, and to modify GABA turnover in various brain regions, including the striatum and the substantia nigra. Levetiracetam also decreases spontaneous neuronal firing in the substantia nigra, an action which has been considered as potentially important in mediating its anticonvulsant effects (LÖSCHER et al. 1996). Levetiracetam has also been found to inhibit bicuculline- and haloperidol-induced release of dopamine from cerebral ventricular perfusates in rats (ZHANG et al. 1993), but the relevance of this effect to antiepileptic activity is unclear.

3. Other Pharmacological Effects and Toxicology Data

In rodent models, levetiracetam has been found to possess anxiolytic effects in a broad range of tests, and to reduce the cognitive impairment associated with seizures, scopolamine or cerebral ischaemia. Levetiracetam also protects against mortality due to anoxia, and it reduces cerebral oedema associated with ischaemia (UCB S.A., data on file).

A remarkable feature of levetiracetam is its low neurotoxicity (GOWER et al. 1992; LÖSCHER and HÖNACK 1993; KLITGAARD et al, 1997). In the rotarod test, open field exploration and an Irwin-type observation test, only mild sedation and a slight increase in locomotor activity were observed at doses 50–100 times higher than the anticonvulsant doses (GOWER et al. 1992). After intraperitoneal administration, the TD_{50} value in the chimney test is about 1700 mg/kg in rats and 1170 mg/kg in mice. In both species, the TD_{50} value in the rotarod test is >1700 mg/kg.

III. Pharmacokinetics

Levetiracetam is absorbed rapidly from the gastrointestinal tract, peak plasma concentrations usually being observed within 1–2 h (EDELBROECK et al. 1993; PATSALOS et al. 1995; STABLES et al. 1995). The absolute oral bioavailability of the drug is close to 100%. Concomitant intake of food produces a slight delay in absorption (T_{max} 2.25 h), but the extent of absorption is unaffected (UCB S.A., data on file). Levetiracetam is not bound to plasma proteins and has an apparent volume of distribution of 0.5–0.7 l/kg. The half-life is about 6–8 h in young healthy subjects, 4–8 h in epileptic patients and about 10–11 h in elderly subjects. The plasma clearance is in the order of 1.0–1.2 ml/min/kg in young healthy subjects and 0.6 ml/min/kg in elderly subjects. In patients with impaired kidney function, the rate of elimination is reduced in proportion to the creatinine clearance. Levetiracetam is eliminated mainly by renal excretion, with about 50%–70% of the dose being recovered unchanged in urine. An inactive acidic metabolite obtained by hydrolysis of the acetamide group (ucb LO57) accounts for about one-quarter of the dose. Two minor metabolites related to hydroxylation and opening of the 2-oxo-pyrrolidinine ring have also been detected in urine. The drug's pharmacokinetics are reportedly linear after single oral doses of up to 5000 mg and multiple doses ranging from 1000 to 3000 mg/day (HARIA and BALFOUR 1997; UCB S.A., data on file).

IV. Drug Interactions

In vitro, levetiracetam does not inhibit various human isoforms of cytochrome P450 (CYP2A6, CYP2C8/9/10, CYP2D6 and CYP3A4), various glucuronotransferases, and epoxide hydrolase (UCB S.A., data on file). Preliminary data suggest that levetiracetam does not affect the concentration of concomitant anticonvulsants such as carbamazepine, phenobarbitone, primidone, valproic acid, clobazam and desmethylclobazem (BIALER et al. 1996; PATSALOS et al. 1996; MARIA and BALFOUR 1997). An increase in serum concentration of phenytoin by 27%–52% has been described in four patients (SHARIEF et al 1996), but more data are required to confirm this interaction. Levetiracetam (500 mg b.i.d. for one contraceptive cycle) did not influence significantly the kinetics of ethinyloestradiol and levonorgestrel in 18 healthy females (GIULIANO et al. 1996).

V. Antiepileptic Efficacy and Adverse Effects

An early study showed that levetiracetam is effective in abolishing the photoparoxysmal EEG response in patients with photosensitive epilepsy, the effect being detected at 1 h after a single 750–1000 mg dose and lasting for up to 6–30 h (KASTELEIJN-NOLSTE-TRENITE et al. 1996). A significant reduction in the frequency of refractory partial onset seizures has been demonstrated in two separate multicentre parallel-group placebo-controlled add-on trials in Europe and the United States (SHORVON 1997). In the European trial, the proportions of patients achieving a greater than 50% seizure reduction during treatment with levetiracetam 1000 and 2000 mg/day were 23% ($n = 101$) and 31% ($n = 98$) respectively, compared with 11% ($n = 107$) among patients given placebo (WIESHMANN et al, 1997). In the United States trial, a 50% reduction in seizure frequency occurred in 39% of 101 patients given 3000 mg daily, in 32% of 98 patients given 1000 mg daily and in 10% of 95 patients given placebo (DREIFUSS et al, 1996). Remarkably, 8% of patients assigned to the 3000 mg group were completely free from seizures over the entire 14-week evaluation period, while none of the patients taking placebo was seizure-free.

Levetiracetam is generally well tolerated, the most common dose-related adverse effects being drowsiness, tiredness, asthenia and headache. Other possible effects may include depression, diplopia, dizziness, unsteadiness, nausea, memory impairment, and mood or behavioural changes (DE DEYN et al. 1992; SINGH et al. 1992; ABOU-KHALIL et al. 1996; KASTELEIJN-NOLSTE-TRENITE et al. 1996; HARIA and BALFOUR 1997), although in the controlled trials reported to date the incidence of these events was generally no greater than in patients receiving placebo (WIESHMANN et al, 1997). No significant changes in cognitive function have been detected in ten patients with epilepsy treated with add-on levetiracetam at dosages up to 1500 mg/day for 1 week (NEYENS et al 1995).

C. Losigamone

Identification of losigamone (AO-33, ADD 137022) resulted from the pharmacological screening of derivatives of natural 5- and 6-membered lactones occurring in various plants of the *Piper* species (STEIN et al. 1991). In this program several tetronic acid derivatives were found to possess anticonvulsant activity, and losigamone was selected for further development based on results of additional tests performed by the Willmar Schwabe Arzneimittel Company in Germany in cooperation with the Epilepsy Branch of the National Institutes of Health in Bethesda, Maryland.

I. Chemistry

Losigamone or (+/–)5(R,S), alpha(S,R)-5-[(2-chlorophenyl) hydroxymethyl)]-4-methoxy(5H)-furanone (Fig. 2) is a white crystalline powder with a slight metallic taste, a melting point of 148 °C and a molecular weight of 254.67. The drug has no acidic or basic properties and is poorly soluble in water (0.04%). Losigamone contains two asymmetrical carbon atoms in a racemate having a threo configuration. While the (+)-isomer (AO-242) is more potent than the (–)-isomer (AO-294) in most pharmacological tests (ZHANG et al. 1992), the reverse is true in other models (DIMPFEL et al. 1995).

II. Pharmacodynamics

1. Anticonvulsant Activity in Animal Models

In rodents, losigamone causes dose-dependent inhibition of the tonic hind leg extension produced by electric shock, pentylenetetrazole, bicuculline, nicotine and 4-aminopyridine (STEIN 1995). Losigamone also inhibits clonic seizures induced by pentylenetetrazole, bicuculline and picrotoxin, whereas it has no effect on the hind leg extension caused by strychnine and picrotoxin or the

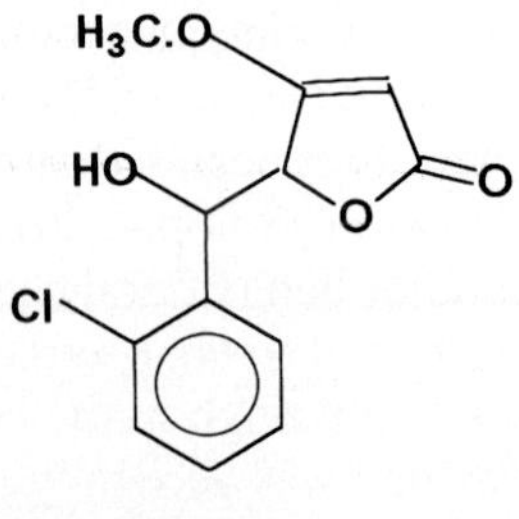

Fig. 2. Molecular structure of losigamone

clonic seizures induced by NMDA (STEIN 1995). The degree and duration of protection varies with the species, the route of administration and the type of convulsive stimulus. In the maximum electroshock seizure test in rats and mice, orally administered losigamone shows comparable potency to phenytoin and is more potent than valproate and ethosuximide. In the pentylenetetrazole test, losigamone is more potent than ethosuximide, valproate and phenytoin in mice, but it is inactive in rats (Table 1). This species-specific difference resides primarily in the (+)-enantiomer. In fact, while both enantiomers are active in the maximum electroshock seizure test, with the (+)-form being more potent than the (–)-form, activity in the pentylenetetrazole test in mice is observed only with the (+)-isomer (CHATTERJEE, personal communication). After oral administration, the protective index compares favourably with that of valproate and ethosuximide in the maximum electroshock seizure test in mice and rats, and with that of valproate, phenytoin and ethosuximide in the pentylenetetrazole test in mice. Administration of losigamone for five to seven daily doses (7 mg/kg) in rats showed no evidence of tolerance to anticonvulsant activity (STEIN 1995).

Other models in which losigamone has been found to be active include audiogenic seizures in rats and gerbils, and pentylenetetrazole-induced kindling in mice (CHATTERJEE, personal communication). Dose-dependent effects in these models are observed at oral doses between 20 and 80 mg/kg. In the GEARS model of absence epilepsy, losigamone, unlike carbamazepine and phenytoin, does not aggravate seizures but suppresses them at high doses (>80 mg/kg).

2. Mechanism of Action

Experiments in rat hippocampal slices have shown that losigamone, at micromolar concentrations, reduces the frequency of spontaneous and stimulus-induced epileptiform discharges in the presence of picrotoxin (KOHR and HEINEMANN 1990a) or low Ca^{2+} or low Mg^{2+} artificial cerebrospinal fluid (KOHR and HEINEMANN 1990b). Seizure-like events produced by perfusion with high K^+, low Mg^{2+} and low Ca^{2+} fluid in the same model are similarly inhibited (LECHLINGER et al. 1998). In the low Mg^{2+} model, losigamone also inhibits epileptiform discharges in the CA_1 and CA_3 regions of the hippocampus and in the entorhinal cortex (ZHANG et al. 1992). At the latter site, late recurrent discharges are suppressed by losigamone but not by ethosuximide, trimethadione, phenytoin, carbamazepine, phenobarbitone and midazolam, even when the latter were tested at concentrations far above the usual therapeutic ranges. Other experiments in the entorhinal cortex indicated that losigamone reduced repetitive spike firing elicited by depolarizing current and depressed moderately stimulus-induced excitatory postsynaptic potentials, while monosynaptic fast and slow inhibitory postsynaptic potentials were unaffected (SCHMITZ et al. 1995). In separate experiments, losigamone has been found to decrease 4-aminopyridine-induced epileptiform activity in rat hippocampal slices

Table 1. Comparative anticonvulsant activity (ED_{50}) and neurotoxicity (TD_{50}, rotarod test) of losigamone and reference antiepileptic drugs following oral administration in mice and rats. Data derived from Stein (1995) and Chatterjee (1997 personal communication). Time of test ranged from 0.25 to 4 h, depending on substance and model

Substance	TD_{50}[a]		ED_{50} (MES)[a]		ED_{50} (scPTZ)[a]	
	Mouse	Rat	Mouse	Rat	Mouse	Rat
Losigamone	149 (114–184)	384 (254–500)	19.9 (18–21) PI = 7.5	6.7 (4.6–9.8) PI = 57	34 (27–43) PI = 4.3	>400 PI = <1
Carbamazepine	96 (86–109)	361 (319–402)	12 (8–15) PI = 8.0	3.6 (2.4–25) PI = 100	41 (31–60) PI = 2.3	>250 PI < 1.4
Phenytoin	87 (80–96)	>300	9.0 (7–11) PI = 9.6	30 (22–39) PI = NA	>300 PI < 0.3	>300 PI = NA
Phenobarbitone	97 (80–115)	61 (44–96)	20 (15–32) PI = 4.8	9 (8–12) PI = 6.7	13 (8–19) PI = 7.5	12 (8–15) PI = 5.1
Ethosuximide	879 (840–934)	1012 (902–1109)	>2000 PI = <0.4	>1200 PI = <0.8	193 (159–218) PI = 4.5	54 (46–60) PI = 19
Valproate	1264 (800–2250)	280 (191–353)	655 (605–718) PI = 1.9	490 (351–728) PI = 0.6	388 (349–439) PI = 3.3	180 (147–210) PI = 1.6

[a] mg/kg, means and 95% confidence interval. PI, protective index (TD_{50}/ED_{50}).
MES, maximum electroshock seizures; PTZ, pentylenetetrazole.

(YONEKAWA et al 1995). Overall, analysis of electrophysiological effects in the above studies suggested that reduction in cellular excitability by losigamone may involve a non-synaptic or direct membrane action, possibly involving inhibition of Na^+ or Ca^{2+} currents or activation of K^+ currents (KOHR and HEINEMANN 1990b; SCHMITZ et al. 1995). An inhibiting action of losigamone on voltage-dependent Ca^{2+} currents has been demonstrated in rat dorsal root ganglion neurons (STEIN 1995), though Ca^{2+} entry was unaffected when presynaptic transmission was blocked (KOHR and HEINEMANN 1990b). A primarily presynaptic mode of action dependent on functional Na^+ channels was suggested by recent experiments in cultured rat hippocampal neurons (JUNGCLAUS et al. 1997).

In contrast to the findings discussed above, other lines of evidence indicate that a contribution of postsynaptic actions cannot be fully excluded in explaining losigamone's effects. Although losigamone does not bind to GABA, picrotoxin or benzodiazepine receptors, an action on Cl^- currents is suggested by the observation that losigamone enhanced the Cl^- uptake in mouse spinal cord neurons in the absence of GABA, and potentiated the effects of GABA in this model (DIMPFEL et al. 1995). Both actions were antagonized by tetrodotoxin and bicuculline, and it was suggested that at least part of the antiepileptic activity of losigamone may be mediated by stimulation of $GABA_A$ receptor-gated Cl^- channels. Additional actions which might contribute to antiepileptic activity but have been observed only at high concentrations of losigamone (>100 μM) include inhibition of glutamate and aspartate release from mouse cortex (SRINIVASAN et al. 1995) and partial blockade of adenosine uptake into mouse brain synaptosomes (STEIN 1995).

3. Other Pharmacological Effects and Toxicology Data

At non-toxic doses, losigamone has been found to possess anxiolytic, antidepressant and memory enhancing effects in animal models (WILLMAR-SCHWABE, data on file). At dosages up to 25 or 50 mg/kg, losigamone does not affect cardiovascular function, body temperature and motility in rodents adversely. A change in motility pattern and slight sedation may be observed at 100 mg/kg (STEIN 1995). In toxicity studies, the no-effect dosages were 15–20 mg/kg and <5 mg/kg with 4-week and 26-week dosing respectively in rats, and 200–100 mg/kg and 30 mg/kg with 4-week and 26-week dosing respectively in dogs (STEIN 1995). Mutagenicity tests were negative. Teratogenicity tests showed no evidence of altered foetal development, apart from reduced body weight and minor retardation of ossification at the highest dose (400 mg/kg) in rats and occasional, possibly non-drug-related, skeletal variations at 60 and 100 mg/kg in rabbits (STEIN 1995).

III. Pharmacokinetics

Unless specified otherwise, pharmacokinetic studies were conducted by using non-enantioselective assays. In healthy volunteers, losigamone displays linear kinetics after single oral doses ranging from 100 to 700 mg, and after multiple doses up to 600 mg t.i.d. for 28 days (STEIN et al. 1995; BIBER and DIENEL 1996). Absorption from the gastrointestinal tract is rapid, with peak plasma concentrations usually being observed after 2–3 h. Losigamone is approximately 60% bound to plasma proteins (STEIN et al. 1991) and has an apparent volume of distribution (Vd/F) of about 1.5 l/kg (STEIN et al. 1995). In patients who took losigamone for up to 5–14 h before undergoing epilepsy surgery, the concentration of the drug in the brain has been found to be on average 30% higher than in plasma, and more than 3 times higher than in the CSF (WILLMAR-SCHWABE, data on file).

The mean apparent oral clearance (CL/F) of losigamone after single doses in healthy volunteers is about 300–400 ml/min, while the half-life and mean residence time average around 4 and 7 h respectively. There are, however, important differences between the enantiomers. After a single 100 mg oral dose of the individual isomers, the apparent oral clearance of the (–)-enantiomer is more than 10 times greater than that of the (+)-enantiomer (1863 vs. 171 ml/min), and the half-life of the (–)-enantiomer is also shorter (2.2 vs. 4.8 h) (BIBER, personal communication). A slight increase in clearance of the racemate without change in its half-life has been described after multiple doses (BIBER and DIENEL 1996). Pharmacodynamic studies in healthy volunteers based on the recording of auditory evoked potentials suggest that the duration of effect may be longer than anticipated from the drug's kinetics in plasma (SCHAFFLER et al. 1996).

Less than 1% of an administered dose of losigamone is excreted unchanged in the urine, and about 15% is excreted as a glucuronide conjugate. A conjugate also accounts for 11%–32% of the total concentration of the drug in serum (WAD and KRAER 1997). Losigamone is eliminated primarily by oxidative biotransformation, and the (–)-enantiomer undergoes more extensive first-pass metabolism than the other isomer. Of five biotransformation products obtained from studies with human liver microsomes, metabolites M_1 and M_5 were identified as phenolic analogues, with M_5 probably corresponding to 5'-hydroxy-(±)-losigamone (TORCHIN et al. 1995). Metabolites M_3 and M_4 were considered to be precursors of M_5, whereas M_2 was probably a non-phenolic substance. These studies confirmed that the drug's metabolism is stereoselective, with M_1 being primarily produced from the (+)-isomer and M_3, M_4 and M_5 being formed preferentially from the (–)-isomer. Interestingly, the formation of M_1 from the (+)-losigamone in vitro is markedly inhibited by (–)-losigamone. Cytochrome CYP2A6 appears to be the main isoenzyme involved in the metabolism of both isomers.

IV. Drug Interactions

The pharmacokinetics of losigamone are affected by concomitant anticonvulsants. In particular, carbamazepine and phenytoin accelerate the elimination of losigamone, resulting in mean CL/F values slightly in excess of

500–600 ml/min and mean half-lives of the order of 3.8 h (Kramer et al. 1995a, 1996; Dienel and Biber 1996). Compared to non-induced volunteers, plasma losigamone levels in phenytoin or carbamazepine-comedicated patients are reduced by about one-third. Other inducing agents such as the barbiturates are also likely to accelerate losigamone elimination. On the other hand, valproic acid (Kramer et al. 1995b) and lamotrigine (Dienel and Biber 1996) have been reported not to affect losigamone pharmacokinetics.

At dosages up to 1800 mg/day for up to 28 days in healthy volunteers, losigamone does not stimulate the metabolism of antipyrine and caffeine (Biber and Dienel 1996). However, losigamone (1000 mg daily) may reduce the plasma concentration of valproic acid slightly, possibly by inducing its metabolism (Kramer et al. 1995b, 1996). In studies conducted in healthy volunteers and epileptic patients, losigamone did not affect the serum concentration of phenytoin, carbamazepine, carbamazepine-10,11-epoxide and lamotrigine (Kramer et al. 1995a; Stein 1995; Runge et al. 1996a,b).

V. Antiepileptic Efficacy and Adverse Effects

In 2 small pilot open add-on studies in patients with refractory partial epilepsy, 5 out of 9 (Stein 1995) and 6 out of 20 patients (Runge et al. 1996) reported a >50% reduction in seizure frequency after treatment for 6 and 24 months respectively. The optimal dosage based on these preliminary data was about 1500 mg/day in three divided doses, and there was evidence that tolerability decreased at higher dosages (Stein 1995). A multicenter placebo-controlled add-on randomized trial at a dosage of 500 mg t.i.d. in 203 patients with partial epilepsy has been completed (Elger et al. 1996). Evidence of superiority over placebo was obtained, with a median seizure reduction of 15% in the losigamone group compared with 7% in the placebo group ($p < 0.005$).

The most common adverse events recorded during losigamone treatment are dizziness and fatigue. Other possible side effects include headache, sedation, diplopia, ataxia, dysarthria, restlessness, nausea, vomiting and palpitations (Stein 1995; Biber and Dienel 1996; Runge et al. 1996). In healthy volunteers, transient increases in SGOT and SGPT values have been recorded. Although there are also reports of elevated liver enzyme levels in chronically treated patients (Morris and Wenger 1996), none of over 400 patients taking losigamone dosages up to 500 mg t.i.d. in add-on studies has dropped out because of hepatic toxicity (Biber and Dienel 1996).

D. Remacemide

Remacemide hydrochloride (AR-R 12924AA, remacemide, formerly FPL 12924) was discovered from a screening of potential new anticonvulsants and neuroprotectants conducted by Fisons (currently Astra Charnwood) in conjunction with the Antiepileptic Drug Development Program of the National

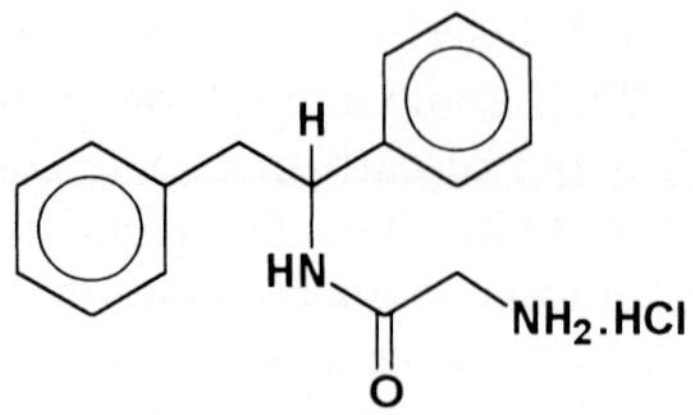

Fig. 3. Molecular structure of remacemide hydrochloride

Institutes of Health in Bethesda (Clark et al. 1995). Remacemide has undergone extensive preclinical testing and is currently in late phase 2 development.

I. Chemistry

Remacemide or (±)2-amino-*N*-(l-methyl-1,2-diphenylethyl)-acetamide monohydrochloride (Fig. 3), the anhydrous salt of a base with a pK_a of 8.0, is a white crystalline powder, readily soluble in water (40 g/l). It has a molecular weight of 304.82 and a melting point of 260 °C. Both the clinically used drug and its desglycinyl-metabolite AR-R 12495 are racemic mixtures of two enantiomers. Remacemide and AR-R 12495 can be measured in body fluids by HPLC with UV detection at 210 nm (Flynn et al. 1992; Wilson et al. 1992).

II. Pharmacodynamics

1. Anticonvulsant Activity in Animal Models

Remacemide and its desglycinyl metabolite exhibit anticonvulsant potency in a number of pharmacological models, including the maximum electroshock seizure test, audiogenic seizures, seizures induced by NMDA, kainic acid and 4-aminopyridine in mice (Stagnitto et al. 1990; Garske et al. 1991; Palmer et al. 1991, 1992a,b; 1993; Clark et al. 1995), and experimental status epilepticus induced by injection of homocysteine thiolactone in rats with a cortical cobalt focus (Walton et al. 1996). The drug shows no significant protective activity against a variety of other chemical convulsants, including pentylenetetrazole, picrotoxin, bicuculline and strychnine. Although remacemide failed to prevent kindled seizures induced by subthreshold bicorneal stimulation in rats (Garske et al. 1991; Palmer et al. 1992a), more recent work indicated suppressive activity against kindled seizures following rapid hippocampal stimulation in the same species (Clark et al. 1995). In the maximum electroshock seizure test, no evidence of tolerance could be demonstrated after repeated daily dosing in rats (Garske et al. 1991). In mice, however, some attenuation of the anticonvulsant effect developed over time.

Since both remacemide and the desglycinyl metabolite are racemic mixtures, the pharmacological properties of the individual enantiomers have been investigated (Garske et al. 1991; Palmer et al. 1991). Some differences have

Table 2. Potency of remacemide (RMC) and its desglycinyl metabolite (D-RMC) in various models for anticonvulsant activity. Unless specified otherwise, all tests were performed in mice. (Data derived from CLARK et al 1995)

Model	RMC		D-RMC	
	ED_{50} (mg/kg)		ED_{50} (mg/kg)	
	p.o.	i.p.	p.o.	i.p.
MES test (mouse)	48	21.5	40	17.1
MES test (rat)	21.5	12.2	9.8	4.0
NMDA-induced convulsions	–	57	–	32
NMDA-induced mortality	–	32	–	17
Kainate-induced convulsions	–	60	–	Inactive
Kainate-induced mortality	–	28	–	Inactive
4-Aminopyridine-induced seizures	–	18.3	–	17.8
Audiogenic seizures	–	19.6	–	11.9

been detected, with the S-enantiomers being slightly more potent than the R-enantiomers, or the racemates, both in protecting against maximum electroshock seizures and in producing neurotoxic impairment (PALMER et al. 1991). These differences, however, were considered insignificant in biological terms.

The desglycinyl metabolite is more potent than the parent drug in some models but less active in others (Table 2), suggesting that its mechanisms of action do not overlap fully with those of the unchanged compound. Although in most tests the desglycinyl metabolite is more potent than remacemide, it is also more toxic. In particular, after oral administration in mice the protective index (TD_{50} for neurotoxicity in the inverted screen test/ED_{50} in the maximum electroshock seizure test) was 2.4 for the desglycinyl metabolite and 7.7 for remacemide (PALMER et al. 1991). In rats, the protective index (TD_{50} for neurotoxicity in the gangplank escape test/ED_{50} in the maximum electroshock seizure test) by the oral route was 15.5 for the desglycinyl metabolite and 39.6 for remacemide (GARSKE et al. 1991). These findings justified selection of the parent drug rather than its desglycinyl metabolite for clinical development.

2. Mechanism of Action

The primary mechanisms of action of remacemide appear to involve blockade of voltage-dependent Na^+ channels and non-competitive antagonism of NMDA receptors. An action on Na^+ channels is suggested by remacemide-induced inhibition of sustained repetitive firing in cultured neurons (CHEUNG et al. 1992; WAMIL et al. 1996). In this model, the desglycinyl metabolite shows an IC_{50} value of 0.8–1.2 μM, and is 10 times more potent than the parent drug (IC_{50} 8 μM). However, it is of interest that in cell cultures the activity of the parent drug, unlike that of the metabolite, increases with time (WAMIL et al. 1996). An action on Na^+ channels is also suggested by a moderate affinity of both compounds for the batrachotoxin binding site, with K_d values of 15.6 μM for remacemide and 7.9 μM for the desglycinyl metabolite.

The desglycinyl metabolite is also more potent than remacemide as an antagonist at the NMDA subtype of the glutamate receptor (PALMER et al. 1993; CLARK et al. 1995; WAMIL et al. 1996). The IC_{50} value for inhibition of MK-801 binding is 0.48 μM for the desglycinyl metabolite, compared with 68 μM for the parent drug. In line with these observations, the isomers of the desglycinyl metabolite inhibited NMDA-induced currents in cultured neurones with an IC_{50} of 0.6–4.0 μM, whereas IC_{50} values for the remacemide isomers were in the range of 67–75 μM. In vivo, the difference in potency between remacemide and the desglycinyl metabolite in inhibiting NMDA-induced seizures and mortality are less marked (Table 2), presumably because in vitro the metabolite contributes to the effects of the parent drug.

In a neurochemical study in rats, 5-day treatment with remacemide (up to 75 mg/kg intraperitoneally) was associated with increased brain GABA transaminase activity and decreased glutamate decarboxylase activity (LEACH et al. 1996a; SILLS et al. 1996). The brain GABA content was not affected, but glutamate levels were reduced to 75% of control values. Whether the above effects are related to Na^+ channel blockade, NMDA antagonism or some other mechanism is unclear, but the reduction in glutamate levels may contribute to anticonvulsant activity. Apart from the desglycinyl metabolite, minor biotransformation products of remacemide retain some degree of activity (PALMER et al. 1992a, 1993; CLARK et al. 1995). These include a *p*-hydroxy-desglycinyl metabolite (AR-R 14331), which has affinity for the NMDA receptor, and an *N*-hydroxy-desglycinyl metabolite, which shows anticonvulsant potency comparable to the parent drug. Most of the other identified metabolism show no appreciable pharmacological activity (PALMER et al. 1992a).

3. Other Pharmacological Effects and Toxicology Data

Remacemide prolonged the survival time in mice exposed to an hypoxia environment (PALMER et al. 1991) and protected against neuronal damage in rodents, cats and dogs subjected to global or focal cerebral ischaemia (PALMER et al. 1991; BANNAN et al. 1994; JAMIESON 1995). These effects are likely to be mediated by NMDA receptor antagonism and inhibition of excitotoxicity.

In two animal models of Parkinson's disease (the monoamine-depleted rat and the MPTP-lesioned rhesus monkey), remacemide provided adjunctive benefit with L-DOPA in alleviating Parkinsonian signs (GREENAMYRE et al. 1994). Based on these data, exploratory trials in patients with Parkinson's disease are going on.

In animal models, remacemide differs from other more potent non-competitive NMDA receptor antagonists in that it has less potential for inducing adverse behavioural effects. In particular, remacemide given to rats at oral doses up to 30 times the ED_{50} in the maximum electroshock seizure test failed to produce a phencyclidine-like behaviour in an open-field test (PALMER et al.

1993). Moreover, remacemide did not substitute for phencyclidine in rats trained to discriminate phencyclidine in a lever-pressing task. Unlike phencyclidine and MK-801, remacemide failed to facilitate reward self-stimulation in rats with chronic electrode implants in the median forebrain bundle (Clark et al. 1995).

In toxicological studies in rodents, high doses of remacemide (>400 mg/kg) produce excitatory central nervous system effects such as tremors, ataxia and seizures. Dogs are more sensitive to such effects, possibly because they show much higher plasma levels of the desglycinyl metabolite than other species (Clark et al. 1995). In rats, large acute doses of remacemide (>160 mg subcutaneously) cause neuronal vacuolation in various brain regions, an effect known with other NMDA antagonists (Olney et al. 1989). Such an effect, however, has been considered an acute and transient phenomenon unlikely to be relevant to human safety, being related particularly to desglycinyl metabolite concentrations which are much higher than those observed clinically (Clark et al. 1995).

Remacemide causes vomiting in dogs and monkeys, and minor gastritis has been seen in rats dosed with 200–350 mg/kg per day. The drug showed no evidence of genotoxicity in a variety of tests, and teratogenicity studies in rats and rabbits were also negative (Clark et al. 1995).

III. Pharmacokinetics

Although remacemide and its desglycinyl metabolite are racemic mixtures, pharmacokinetic parameters have been reported only for the racemates. Preliminary evidence, however, indicates that pharmacokinetic differences between the enantiomers are less than twofold (Palmer et al. 1992a; Jamieson 1995). The lack of major pharmacodynamic differences between the enantiomers means that kinetic parameters calculated for the racemate are biologically relevant.

After single oral doses up to 500 mg in healthy volunteers, remacemide shows linear kinetics (Palmer et al. 1993; Clark et al. 1995). Its absorption from the gastrointestinal tract is rapid and peak plasma concentrations are observed within 1–2 h for the parent drug and 4–6 h for the desglycinyl metabolite (Clark et al. 1995). Concomitant ingestion of food does not affect the extent of absorption, but it may delay the time to peak concentration (Palmer et al. 1993).

In healthy subjects who received a single intravenous dose, remacemide shows a volume of distribution of 5–6 l/kg (Clark et al. 1995), which indicates extensive penetration into tissues. Remacemide is about 75% bound to plasma proteins, while the desglycinyl metabolite is about 90% protein-bound. Remacemide concentrations in the CSF are similar to its unbound plasma concentrations (Lindstrom et al. 1996).

In healthy volunteers, remacemide is eliminated from plasma with a half-life of 3–4 h, whereas the half-life of the desglycinyl metabolite is about

12–18h. After intravenous dosing, the plasma clearance of remacemide is about 13ml/min/kg (PALMER et al. 1992a; CLARK et al. 1995). In healthy subjects treated with doses up to 400mg twice daily for up to 28days, the steady-state pharmacokinetics are linear and predictable from the single-dose data. In subjects given 300mg twice daily, peak and trough levels of the desglycinyl metabolite averaged 143ng/ml and 89ng/ml respectively, compared with 1069ng/ml and 124ng/ml respectively for the parent drug (CLARK et al. 1995). In a multiple ascending dose study (up to 150mg q.i.d) in 12 volunteers aged 60–71 years, remacemide kinetics were similar to those seen in younger subjects. The half-life of the desglycinyl metabolite was slightly longer than that recorded in young volunteers (19–21h vs. 13–17h), but peak steady-state concentrations of this metabolite were similar (ASTRA CHARNWOOD, data on file).

Only negligible amounts (<1%) of orally administered remacemide are excreted unchanged in urine. As discussed above, an important metabolic pathway involves the drug's conversion to the active desglycinyl metabolite, a reaction catalysed by aminopeptidases in hepatic and extrahepatic tissues. Additional biotransformation routes include oxidation by cytochrome P450 mixed function oxidases in the liver, and glucuronidation to a carbamoyl glucuronide (CLARK et al. 1995).

IV. Drug Interactions

Remacemide metabolism is enhanced by concurrent treatment with enzyme-inducing anticonvulsants such as carbamazepine and phenytoin. In patients receiving these drugs, the remacemide AUC in plasma is reduced by up to 50% compared with values recorded in healthy subjects (SCHEYER et al. 1992; CLARK et al. 1995; LEACH et al. 1995, 1996b). The metabolism of the desglycinyl metabolite is also probably stimulated by enzyme-inducing anticonvulsants, as indicated by the fact that its AUC and half-life are decreased by 70%–80%, and by 40% respectively compared with values in healthy volunteers. On the other hand, concomitant treatment with valproate has no major effects on the kinetics of remacemide and its desglycinyl metabolite (ASTRA CHARNWOOD, data on file).

When remacemide is added to pre-existing carbamazepine therapy, plasma carbamazepine concentrations may increase. In one study in which add-on remacemide was given at a dosage of 300mg q.i.d., carbamazepine plasma concentrations increased by 28% on the average (range –27% to 98%), while the levels of carbamazepine-10,11-epoxide showed no consistent change (LEACH et al. 1995, 1996b; RILEY et al, 1996). In some cases, an increase in plasma phenytoin levels has also been observed (CLARK et al. 1995; RILEY et al, 1996), while plasma valproic acid levels are generally unaffected by remacemide. These interactions are likely to be explained by the ability of remacemide to inhibit to some extent the activity of cytochromes CYP3A4 and CYP2C9, which are known to be involved in the metabolism of carbamazepine and phenytoin respectively (RILEY et al. 1996). Compared with remacemide, the desglycinyl metabolite is a weaker inhibitor of CYP3A4 and

CYP2C9, but a more potent inhibitor of CYP2D6 ($K_i = 4\,\mu M$), an observation whose clinical significance remains to be determined (RILEY et al. 1996). In a single-dose double-blind study in 30 healthy subjects, coadministration of remacemide 300 mg did not aggravate the psychomotor impairment caused by 0.7 g/kg alcohol (LOCKTON et al. 1996).

V. Antiepileptic Efficacy and Adverse Effects

In a double-blind add-on cross-over trial in 28 patients with refractory epilepsy, mostly with partial seizures (CRAWFORD et al. 1992), the median seizure frequency in the 22 patients completing the trial was 6/month on remacemide (150 mg q.i.d) and 9/month on placebo ($p < 0.05$). Compared with the baseline value, a >50% reduction in seizure frequency was observed in 32% of patients on remacemide compared with 9% of those on placebo, but interpretation of these findings is complicated by a modest rise in plasma carbamazepine levels in the active treatment period. Two other double-blind placebo-controlled add-on trials, using a parallel-group design, have assessed the efficacy and safety of 3-months treatment with remacemide in patients with refractory partial seizures (BIALER et al. 1996; JONES et al. 1996). In one study, patients received doses of 300, 600 and 1200 mg daily in a q.i.d. regimen, while the other study tested doses of 300, 600 and 800 mg daily in a b.i.d. regimen. Changes in plasma levels of concomitantly administered carbamazepine and phenytoin were minimized by adjusting the dosage of any comedication. In the q.i.d. study, a significant ($p = 0.038$) difference in responder rate (proportion of patients who experienced at least a 50% reduction in seizure frequency) was observed between remacemide 1200 mg daily (23%) and placebo (7%). In the other study, there was a trend towards a greater responder rate with remacemide 400 mg b.i.d. (31%), as compared with placebo (15%). Although this difference failed to reach statistical significance when the treatment groups were compared overall, remacemide 400 mg b.i.d. was superior to placebo in a pairwise comparison ($p = 0.043$).

The most common adverse effects encountered with remacemide used alone included dizziness, ataxia, somnolence, abdominal pain, dyspepsia, nausea, vomiting and fatigue. Common adverse events in patients receiving a combination of remacemide and carbamazepine or phenytoin also included visual disturbances (diplopia, vision abnormal), amnesia, confusion, nervousness, irritability, impaired concentration and emotional lability. These unwanted effects were generally mild to moderate in severity (ASTRA CHARNWOOD, data on file).

E. Rufinamide

Rufinamide (CGP 33101) or 1-(2,6-difluorobenzyl)-1*H*-1,2,3-triazole-4-carboxamide is a novel anticonvulsant discovered by Novartis and is currently in phase III development.

I. Pharmacodynamics

In rodent models of epilepsy, rufinamide is particularly effective in inhibiting maximum electroshock-induced tonic-clonic seizures (oral ED_{50}, 5–17 mg/kg), while its potency in antagonizing clonic seizures induced by pentylenetetrazole, bicuculline or picrotoxin is lower. Rufinamide has also been found effective in delaying kindling development and suppressing afterdischarges in amygdala-kindled cats, and in reducing seizure frequency in rhesus monkeys with chronic alumina foci in the motor cortex. Hippocampal and cortical afterdischarges induced by electrical stimulation in non-kindled cats are also inhibited by rufinamide. The protective index is generally higher than that of most common anticonvulsants (SCHMUTZ et al. 1993; NOVARTIS, data on file).

The primary mode of action of rufinamide is likely to involve inhibition of spread of seizure activity through blockade of voltage-dependent Na^+ channels (SCHMUTZ et al. 1993). In binding studies, rufinamide does not interact directly with a variety of neurotransmitter systems, including those involving GABA, acetylcholine, monoamines, NMDA and other excitatory amino acids (NOVARTIS, data on file).

II. Pharmacokinetics and Drug Interactions

When rufinamide is administered in tablet form, its peak plasma levels are usually achieved within 1.5–3 h at doses up to 150 mg and within 5–6 h at higher doses (CHEUNG et al. 1995; BIALER et al. 1996; NOVARTIS, data on file). The extent of the drug's absorption is about 50% when it is taken on an empty stomach but increases to about 70% when it is ingested with food (WALDMEIER et al. 1996). Plasma rufinamide concentrations increase less than proportionally with increasing dosages, probably due to capacity-limited absorption (BIALER et al. 1996). Using 400 mg b.i.d as a reference, doubling the dose to 800 mg b.i.d. increased the amount of systemically available drug by only 73% instead of 100% as expected from dose-proportionality considerations (NOVARTIS, data on file). Rufinamide is about 34% bound to plasma proteins, mainly albumin. Less than 2% of an orally administered dose is excreted unchanged in urine. Rufinamide is extensively metabolized, primarily through hydrolysis of the carboxylamide group, and the main product found in urine is the inactive carboxylic acid derivative CGP 47292 (WALDMEIER et al. 1996). Although a few other minor metabolites are produced, cytochrome P450 (CYP450) isoenzymes do not appear to play an important role in rufinamide biotransformation (BIALER et al. 1996). The half-life of rufinamide is about 8–12 h (mean 9.5 h) in healthy volunteers, but it may be shortened to an average of about 6 and 7 h in patients comedicated with phenytoin or carbamazepine, and slightly prolonged to an average of 10.5 h in patients comedicated with valproic acid; NOVARTIS, data on file). In a study which assessed its population kinetics, rufinamide clearance was found to be increased by about 20% in patients receiving phenytoin and primidone, reduced by about 20% in patients taking valproic acid, and unaffected in patients comedicated with phenobarbitone, carbamazepine, oxcarbazepine and vigabatrin (NOVARTIS, data on file). Rufinamide is devoid of inhibitory effects on a variety of CYP450 drug metabolizing enzymes (KAPEGHIAN et al. 1996). Preliminary observations suggest that plasma levels of associated anticonvulsants are not modified by rufinamide (BIALER et al. 1996).

III. Antiepileptic Efficacy and Adverse Effects

A parallel-group double-blind placebo-controlled add-on trial compared rufinamide dosages of 200, 400, 800 and 1600 mg/day in patients with refractory partial epilepsy (BIALER et al. 1996). The mean seizure frequency on the combined active doses (400, 800 and 1600 mg/day) was approximately 15% lower than when the patients received placebo.

Single doses of the drug up to 1200 mg and multiple doses up to 2400 mg/day appear to be well tolerated in patients with epilepsy. In the double-blind trial discussed above, the most common adverse events in patients who received rufinamide included headache (26%), fatigue (19%), dizziness (14%), viral infection (11%), nausea (8%) and diplopia (7%). Patients receiving placebo, however, exhibited a similar side effect profile, except for slightly lower frequencies of dizziness (10%), somnolence (4%) and diplopia (3%).

F. Stiripentol

Stiripentol is an allylic alcohol selected for development from related compounds because of its anticonvulsant properties. The drug has been used clinically for about 20 years, but demonstration of its antiepileptic effects in the clinical setting has been hampered by prominent pharmacokinetic interactions with concomitantly administered anticonvulsants (BEBIN et al. 1994).

I. Chemistry

Stiripentol is 4,4-dimethyl-1-[(3,4 methylenedioxy)phenyl]-1-penten-3-ol (Fig. 4). It exists in two enantiomeric forms and has a molecular weight of 234. Stiripentol is soluble in ethanol and acetone, virtually insoluble in water, and its concentration in body fluids can be determined by HPLC with UV detection at 254 nm (LIN and LEVY 1983).

II. Pharmacodynamics

1. Anticonvulsant Activity in Animal Models

Stiripentol exhibits broad spectrum anticonvulsant activity in animal models. In rodents, the drug is effective against seizures induced by electrical stimula-

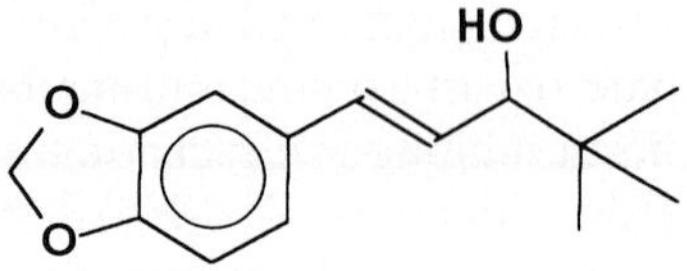

Fig. 4. Molecular structure of stiripentol

tion (maximum electroshock seizures) and chemical convulsants such as pentylenetetrazole and bicuculline, though it is only weakly active against convulsions induced by strychnine (ASTOIN et al. 1978; POISSON et al. 1984; LOISEAU and DUCHE 1995). After intraperitoneal dosing, the ED_{50} is approximately 240 mg/kg in the maximum electroshock seizure test in rats and 200 mg/kg in the pentylenetetrazole test in mice (POISSON et al. 1984). In protecting against pentylenetetnazole-induced seizures, the (+)-enantiomer is 2.4 times more potent than the (–)-enantiomer (SHEN et al. 1992). During repeated dosing, some tolerance to the anticonvulsant activity develops but the animals also become more resistant to neurotoxicity and the protective index remains substantially unchanged (LOISEAU and DUCHE 1995). At intraperitoneal dosages ranging between 125 and 500 mg/kg, stiripentol suppressed spike-and-wave discharges in a genetic model of petit mal epilepsy in Wistar rats (MICHELETTI et al. 1988). In an alumina-gel rhesus monkey model of focal epilepsy, stiripentol reduced the frequency of interictal EEG spike discharges and showed an activity similar to valproate in delaying seizures activated by a 4-deoxypiridine challenge (LOCKARD et al. 1985; LOISEAU and DUCHE 1995).

2. Mechanism of Action

Stiripentol has no affinity for $GABA_A$, $GABA_B$, glycinergic or benzodiazepine receptors, but it inhibits the synaptosomal uptake of glycine and GABA at concentrations compatible with its pharmacological activity (POISSON et al. 1984; LOISEAU and DUCHE 1995). In addition, stiripentol may enhance the activity of β-hydroxybutyrate dehydrogenase and inhibit GABA-transaminase in rat brain (WEGMAN et al. 1978), which may explain the increased brain GABA levels observed at 30 min after intraperitoneal administration of a 300 mg/kg dose (LOISEAU and DUCHE 1995). A GABA-mediated mode of action is also suggested by the finding that ^{3}H-stiripentol shows a distribution similar to that of endogenous GABA in rat brain (WEGMAN et al. 1979). Studies of the action of stiripentol on excitatory neurotransmission and ion channel conductance do not appear to have been performed, and therefore alternative or additional modes of action cannot be excluded.

3. Other Pharmacological Effects and Toxicology Data

In standard animal models, stiripentol showed no significant pharmacological actions outside the central nervous system, and results of acute and chronic toxicity studies were unremarkable (LOISEAU and DUCHE 1995). Stiripentol is devoid of mutagenic activity in the Ames test using *Salmonella typhimurium* and in the micronucleus test in the mouse. No evidence of teratogenicity was observed at doses up to 800 mg/kg/day in mice and rabbits.

III. Pharmacokinetics

Virtually all pharmacokinetic information for the drug in humans was obtained using non-enantioselective assays. This represents an important limitation in view of the evidence that in a rat model the two enantiomers differ both in anticonvulsant potency and in kinetic behaviour (SHEN et al. 1992).

After single 300–1200 mg oral doses in healthy subjects, stiripentol is absorbed rapidly from the gastrointestinal tract, peak plasma concentrations being usually achieved within 2 h (LEVY et al. 1983). The drug's absorption may be critically dependent on the formulation used, as indicated by the fact that intake of a single dose as a solution resulted in a bioavailability of only 21 ± 9%, as compared with the powder form. This was tentatively ascribed to precipitation of drug crystals in the aqueous environment of the gastrointestinal tract.

Stiripentol is 99% bound to plasma proteins (LEVY et al. 1983). After intravenous injection of the ^{3}H-labelled drug in rats, the highest radioactivity at 30 min was found in liver and kidneys (PIERI et al. 1982). In the central nervous system, the maximal radioactivity was detected in the cerebellum. Elimination after single oral doses in healthy volunteers appears to be multiphasic and non-linear, with a mean residence time of 4 h and an oral clearance of 1.3–1.8 l/h/kg (LEVY et al. 1983). In healthy subjects given a single 300 mg dose followed by 1200 mg/day in four divided doses for 1 week, the drug's clearance decreased eightfold during the multiple dosing, suggesting that its elimination is capacity limited (LEVY et al. 1983). Studies in healthy subjects at dosages up to 1800 mg/day and in epileptic patients at dosages up to 2400 mg/day confirmed that the elimination of stiripentol follows Michaelis-Menten kinetics (LEVY et al. 1984a,b). In agreement with this kinetic behaviour, steady–state serum concentrations of the drug increase non-linearly with increasing dosage (LEVY et al. 1984a, 1987a). In one study in epileptic patients receiving concomitant anticonvulsants, the steady-state concentration of stiripentol increased by 253% following a dosage increment from 600 to 1200 mg/day, and further doubling of the dose to 2400 mg/day caused an almost 400% rise in serum concentration (LEVY et al. 1984b). The apparent oral clearance decreased from 1.7 l/h/kg at 600 mg/day to 0.35 l/h/kg at 2400 mg/day; these values, in any case, are much higher than those observed in healthy subjects, due to stimulation of stiripentol elimination by enzyme-inducing anticonvulsants (see below). In a group of paediatric patients, the oral clearance of stiripentol was on the average lower than that observed in a group of adult patients on polytherapy receiving equivalent dosages, (FARWELL et al. 1993).

The non-linear kinetics of stiripentol appears to be due to saturation of the enzyme systems responsible for its metabolism. In fact, only trace amounts of the drug are excreted unchanged in urine. Five distinct metabolic pathways have been identified, those most important quantitatively being conjugation with glucuronic acid (20%–30% of the dose), opening of the methylenedioxy ring with formation of a dihydroxy derivative (11%–14%), and O-methylation of catechol metabolites at positions 3 and 4 (17%–24%) (MORELAND et al. 1986; LOISEAU et al. 1995). The rate of formation of metabolites resulting from conjugation and from ring opening in the methylendioxy moiety (*p*-hydroxy and *m*-hydroxy-metabolites) varies with dosage, indicating that these pathways contribute to the capacity-dependent nature of stiripentol elimination. Many phase I metabolites are also excreted as conjugates. Overall, renally excreted metabolites account for 73% of the dose, with an additional 18% of the dose being recovered in the faeces (MORELAND et al. 1986).

IV. Drug Interactions

The metabolism of stiripentol is accelerated by concomitant treatment with enzyme-inducing anticonvulsants. In patients comedicated with carbamazepine, phenytoin or barbiturates, stiripentol clearance at a dosage of 1200 mg/day was three-fold higher than in healthy subjects given the same dosage, although interindividual variability was considerable (LEVY et al. 1984b). Stiripentol is a potent inhibitor of oxidative drug metabolism and by this mechanism may increase the serum concentration of phenytoin (LEVY et al. 1984b; LOISEAU et al. 1995; MATHER et al. 1995), carbamazepine (LEVY et al. 1987a,b; LOISEAU et al. 1987; KERR et al. 1991; MATHER et al. 1995), phenobarbitone (LEVY et al. 1984b; LOISEAU et al. 1988, 1995), primidone (BEBIN et al. 1994; LOISEAU et al. 1995) and valproic acid (LEVY et al. 1987a, 1988, 1990). Most of these interactions are clinically important and may require adjustments in the dosage of associated drugs.

V. Efficacy and Adverse Effects

Evaluation of the efficacy of stiripentol has been hampered by drug interactions, which makes blind assessment difficult. In add-on open studies, an appreciable proportion of patients with difficult-to-treat epilepsy has been reported to benefit from stiripentol (LOISEAU et al. 1995), but the data are difficult to interpret because of their uncontrolled nature and the possibility that improvement was related to a rise in the serum levels of concomitant medication. Both partial seizures and a variety of generalized seizures, especially typical and atypical absences, are said to be improved by stiripentol, usually at maintenance dosages of 1000–3000 mg/day in adults and 20–70 mg/kg/day in children (LOISEAU et al. 1989, 1995; FARWELL et al. 1993).

In some studies, seizures were suppressed even when serum levels of concomitant drugs were kept unchanged, suggesting that stiripentol itself was responsible for the clinical improvement (LOISEAU et al. 1988). One double-blind placebo-controlled trial which attempted to maintain unaltered serum levels of comedication in 201 patients with partial seizures has been performed (LOISEAU et al. 1990). Although a >50% reduction in seizure rate was observed in 47% of patients treated with stiripentol (2000 mg/day) compared with 19% in placebo-treated patients, the results were considered non-conclusive because despite dosage adjustments serum carbamazepine levels increased in the stiripentol group (LOISEAU et al. 1995). To circumvent the problem of drug interactions, in some studies an attempt has been made to discontinue comedication and stabilize patients on stiripentol monotherapy. However, the efficacy of stiripentol under these conditions was not impressive, as most patients showed a deterioration in seizure control (LOISEAU et al. 1995).

As for clinical improvement, side effects may be related to the stiripentol itself or to interactions with other drugs. Adverse effects most commonly encountered in clinical trials include gastrointestinal disturbances (nausea, vomiting, gastric or abdominal discomfort, anorexia), insomnia and drowsiness. Acute psychotic reactions have been described occasionally (LOISEAU et al. 1995).

G. Drugs in Early Clinical Development

I. 534U87

534U87 or 4-amino-1-(2,6-difluorobenzyl)-1*H*-1,2,3-triazolo (4,5-c)-pyridine hydrochloride is a novel compound which is especially potent against maximum electroshock-induced seizures, with an oral ED_{50} of 2–4 mg/kg in rats, while it is inactive or far less active in chemical convulsant tests (GLAXO-WELLCOME, data on file). Its mode of action is unknown. Following administration of single 450 mg oral doses in healthy volunteers, 534U87 was absorbed with a median T_{max} of 4 h and eliminated with a half-life of about 19 h (YAU et al. 1995). In healthy subjects, single doses up to 800 mg and multiple doses up to 300 mg b.i.d. for 10 days were tolerated without serious side effects. The adverse events most commonly encountered in these studies were headache, nausea, dyspepsia and dizziness or lightheadedness. Pilot studies in epileptic patients are progress.

II. Abecarnil

Abercanil is a β-carboline endowed with partial agonist activity at benzodiazepine receptor sites. Abecarnil shows seizure-protecting activity in various models of epilepsy and, unlike conventional benzodiazepines, its repeated administration is associated with little or no tolerance to its anticonvulsant effects (SERRA et al 1996). In early clinical studies, abecarnil has been found effective in suppressing the photoparoxysmal EEG response in patients with photosensitive epilepsy (KASTELEIJN et al. 1996).

III. Anti-epilepsirine

Anti-epilepsirine is a new drug under clinical development in China. At dosages of 150–500 mg/kg per day in rats, it produces dose-dependent protection against pentylenetetrazole-induced seizures, whereas even at the highest dosage it has no effect in amygdaloid-kindled seizures (WANG et al, 1997). Promising results have been reported in preliminary controlled trials in children with primary generalized seizures.

IV. AWD-140-190

AWD 140-190 [4-(*p*-bromophenyl)-3-morpholino-1*H*-pyrrole-2-carboxylic acid methyl ester] is active against maximum electroshock seizures, audiogenic seizures in DBA/2 mice and corneally and amygdala-kindled seizures in rats, with an overall high protective index in these models (ROSTOCK et al. 1996a, 1997; TOBER 1996). The compound shows no protective activity against seizures induced chemically by pentylenetetrazole, bicuculline and strychnine. The mode of action probably involves blockade of use-dependent Na^+ channels (ROSTOCK et al. 1995, 1996a).

V. D-2916 (Soretolide)

D-2916, *N*-(5-methyl-3-isoxazolyl)-2,6-dimethyl benzamide, currently known as sore to lide, shows in animal models an anticonvulsant profile similar to that of carbamazepine, being particularly potent in protecting against maximum electroshock-induced seizures (LEPAGE et al. 1992; GILLARDIN et al. 1993). Its precise mode of action is unknown. In healthy volunteers, D-2916 is absorbed rapidly from the gastrointestinal tract (BIOCODEX, data on file). The drug is about 75% bound to plasma proteins and undergoes extensive and rapid conversion by cytochromes CYPlA2 and CYP2Cl9 to the hydroxylated active metabolite D-3187 (LEPAGE et al. 1995; HARR et al. 1996), which is found in plasma at concentrations much higher than those of the parent drug. In healthy volunteers, the half-life of D-2916 is 3–9 h, while the half-life of D3187 is of the order of 5–14 h (BIOCODEX, data on file). In vitro, D-2916 and D-3187 has been found to cause inhibition of the activity of cytochrome CYP2Cl9. Clinical trials are in progress.

VI. D-23129 (Retigabine)

D-23129, or *N*-[2-amino-4-(4-fluorobenzylamino)-phenyl] carbamic acid ethyl ester, currently known as retigabine is a flupirtine derivative which is effective against seizures induced by maximum electroshock, pentylenetetrazole, picrotoxin, penicillin, kainate and intracerebroventricular NMDA, and seizures occurring in genetic models such as DBA/2 mice, GEPR-3 and GEPR-9 rats (KAPETANOVIC and RUNDFELDT 1996; ROSTOCK et al 1996b). D-23129 also shows remarkable potency in delaying epileptogenesis and in protecting against seizures in the amygdala-kindled model (KAPETANOVIC and RUNDFELDT 1996; TOBER et al. 1996). In 4-aminopyridine-treated rat hippocampal slices, D-23129 fully suppresses spontaneous bursts in CA_1 and CA_3 areas, and eliminates afterdischarge-like trains of population spikes induced by a single electrical stimulation pulse without interfering with the normal evoked potential (YONEKAWA et al. 1995). Finally, D-23129 has been found to improve learning and memory in rat models of cerebral ischaemia and electroshock-induced amnesia (ROSTOCK et al. 1996b,c). Its primary modes of action are thought to involve increase in K^+ conductance and enhancement of GABAergic transmission through stimulation of GABA synthesis and amplification of GABA-induced currents (KAPETANOVIC 1995, 1996; BIALER et al. 1996; KAPETANOVIC and RUNDFELDT 1996; ROSTOCK et al. 1996b). Additional possible actions may include inhibition of glutamergic transmission and blockade of Na^+ and Ca^{2+} channels. After single oral doses ranging from 25 to 600 mg in healthy subjects, D-23129 follows linear pharmacokinetics. Peak plasma concentrations occur within 2 h and the elimination half-life is about 9.5 h (ARZNEIMITTELWERK DRESDEN GMBH, data on file). Studies with human liver microsomes demonstrated the existence of *N*-glucuronide conjugates with minimal oxidative metabolism (BIALER et al. 1996). Clinical development is ongoing.

VII. Dezinamide

Dezinamide [ADD 94057, AHR-11748, 3-(trifluoromethyl) phenoxy)-l-azetidinecarboxamide] is the demethylated metabolite of fluzinamide, a potential anticonvulsant whose development was discontinued because of toxicity problems not observed with the metabolite. In animal models, dezinamide is active against seizures induced by maximum electroshock, pentylenetetrazole, bicuculline, picrotoxin and amygdaloid kindling (ALBERTSON and WALBY 1987; JOHNSON et al. 1990). Its mode of action has not been fully characterized, but there is unconfirmed evidence that blockade of voltage-dependent Na^+ channels may be involved (VICTOR 1997).

Dezinamide is absorbed rapidly from the gastrointestinal tract, is about 85% bound to plasma proteins and shows a volume of distribution of about 1 l/kg. It is eliminated primarily by metabolism. After single dose administration to epileptic patients, the half-life is 2–5 h in smokers and 5–11 h in non-smokers (PLEDGER et al. 1992; PRIVITERA et al 1994; VICTOR 1997). At steady-state, plasma dezinamide levels are greater than predicted from single-dose kinetics and may increase disproportionately with increasing dosage, due to the presence of Michaelis-Menten kinetics. In a preliminary double-blind placebo-controlled add-on cross-over trial, 7 of 15 patients with refractory partial epilepsy showed a greater than 50% reduction in seizure frequency, but interpretation of results was complicated by a modest increase in the plasma levels of phenytoin (PRIVITERA et al. 1994). Adverse events encountered in early clinical studies include headache, fatigue, ataxia, blurred vision, diplopia, dizziness, mild confusion and nausea. In addition to the interaction with phenytoin, there is a possibility of dezinamide increasing the serum levels of carbamazepine-10,11-epoxide through inhibition of epoxide hydrolase (VICTOR 1997).

VIII. Ganaxolone

Ganaxolone (CCD 1042), the 36-methyl-substituted analogue of the endogenous neuroactive steroid 3 A-hydroxy-5 A-pregnan-20-one, is a stereoselective high-affinity positive modulator of the $GABA_A$ receptor. In animal models, ganaxolone shows potent activity against seizures induced by pentylenetetrazole, bicuculline, aminophylline and corneal kindling, while it is less potent against maximum electroshock-induced seizures (KOKATE et al. 1996; CARTER et al. 1997). When ganaxolone is administered after a high-fat meal in healthy volunteers, plasma drug concentrations reach a peak within 1–3 h and thereafter decline biexponentially, with a terminal half-life of 37–70 h (MONAGHAM et al. 1997). In healthy volunteers given doses up to 500 mg t.i.d. for up to 14 days, the most commonly observed adverse events were sedation, dizziness, headache, gastrointestinal disturbances, fatigue, unsteady gait and impaired concentration (MONAGHAM et al. 1996, 1997). Interestingly, side effects were twice as common in females as in males despite similar plasma drug levels in the two genders. In a small preliminary trial in paediatric patients given dosages up to 12 mg/kg t.i.d., adverse events included somnolence, sleep disturbances, nervousness, constipation and, in one case, disturbed behaviour and cognition. No apparent changes in the plasma levels of concurrent anticonvulsants were seen in this preliminary study (LECHTENBERG et al. 1996).

IX. Isobutyl-GABA (Pregabalin)

S-(+)-3-Isobutyl-GABA or pregabalin, or (S)-3-(aminomethyl)-5-methylhexanoic acid (PD144723, CI-1008) is an orally active structural analogue of both GABA and gabapentin. In animal models, S-(+)-3-isobutyl-GABA is more potent than gabapentin in protecting against electrically induced seizures (TAYLOR et al. 1993). Since the R-(–)-isomer is much less active in seizure models, its mode of action must involve a stereoselective mechanism, possibly related to its ability to displace gabapentin from a high-affinity binding site in the brain which has been recently associated with the subunit of a voltage-dependent L-type Ca^{2+} channel (GEE et al 1996). Isobutyl-GABA has also been found to activate L-glutamic acid decarboxylase, but this effects occurs at concentrations greater than those required to produce anticonvulsant effects in vivo (YUEN et al. 1994). The drug is currently in phase I clinical development.

X. LY300164

LY300164 [GIKY 53773; (R)-7-acetyl-5-(4-aminophenyl)-8,9-dihydro-8-methyl-7*H*-1,3-dioxolo(4,5-h) (2,3) benzodiazepine] is an orally active non-competitive antagonist at AMPA receptor sites. Since the opposite isomer (LY300165) is devoid of antagonistic activity, interaction with the AMPA receptor is enantioselective. Although LY300164 does possess a benzodiazepine structure, its affinity for benzodiazepine receptors is very weak and is not considered important in mediating its pharmacological effects. In experiments in vitro, LY300164 attenuates excitatory neurotransmission in rat cortex and hippocampus, and protects hippocampal neurons from degeneration induced by excessive AMPA receptor activation. In vivo, LY300164 inhibits firing rates induced by AMPA (but not NMDA) in rat spinal cord neurons, and protects rodents against seizures induced by maximum electroshock, pentylenetetrazole and other chemoconvulsants (ELI LILLY Co., data on file).

After single oral doses, peak plasma concentrations of LY300164 are achieved within 2.5 h. About 75% of the drug in plasma is protein bound. Non-linear kinetics, with a more than proportional increase in AUC and C_{max} with increasing dosages, have been observed after single and multiple doses in healthy volunteers (ELI LILLY Co., data on file). Pharmacokinetic evaluation indicated that LY300164 is most likely to be eliminated according to a combination of a first-order and a capacity-limited process, with the latter becoming saturated at plasma levels of about 200 ng/ml. At dosing regimens resulting in levels higher than these (single doses above 50 mg and multiple doses above 20 mg t.i.d.), the half-life is about 8 h and plasma concentrations of the drug are expected to increase linearly with dose. LY300164 is extensively metabolized. Although its metabolic pathways in man have not been fully characterized, acetylation appears to be an important route. At steady-state, the apparent oral clearance of LY300164 in slow-acetylators is on the average about 50% lower than in fast acetylators, though there is considerable variability and some overlapping between the two groups. Preliminary in vitro studies suggest that LY300164 may act as a suicidal inhibitor of cytochrome CYP3 A (ELI LILLY Co., data on file), so that one might predict that the drug would interfere with the metabolism of CYP3 A substrates such as carbamazepine and ethosuximide. In phase I studies in healthy volunteers, doses up to 20 mg 8 hourly were well tolerated, but sedation, postural dizziness, paraesthesias, euphoria and psychomotor impairment were noted at higher doses. Efficacy trials in patients with epilepsy are in progress.

XI. Monohydroxycarbazepine

Monohydroxycarbazepine [10,11-dihydro-10-hydroxy-5*H*-dibenz(b,f) azepine-5-carboxamide; CGP47779] is the active metabolite of oxcarbazepine, a drug which is available commercially in many countries (GRANT and FAULDS 1991). Since oxcarbazepine is considered to act as a prodrug for monohydroxycarbazepine, the metabolite has been studied extensively. Chemically, it is a racemic mixture of a (R)- and a (S)-enantiomer, known as CGP13698 and CGP13751 respectively, which show comparable anticonvulsant activities in animal models. The mode of action is considered to involve blockade of Na^+ channels but other mechanisms, including an effect on K^+ channels and inhibition of voltage-dependent Ca^{2+} channels, may contribute (McLEAN et al 1994; STEFANI et al 1997). The half-life of metabolically derived monohydroxycarbazepine averages 8–20h (GRANT and FAULDS 1992; TARTARA et al 1993). The compound is eliminated primarily by conjugation with glucuronic acid, with a small amount being converted to the inactive di-hydroxy-derivative (GRANT and FAULDS 1992). Since monohydroxycarbazepine is more water soluble than oxcarbazepine, it is undergoing clinical development as an injectable formulation for intravenous and, possibly, intramuscular use. Following intravenous administration of racemic monohydroxycarbazepine in healthy subjects, the half-life is about 11h for the (S)-enantiomer and 9h for the (R)-enantiomer. The clearance is also higher for the (R)-enantiomer (4.3 l/h vs. 3.1 l/h for the (S)-enantiomer – NOVARTIS, data on file). Clinical trials are in progress to assess the efficacy and safety of monohydroxycarbazepine in patients with refractory partial seizures who are undergoing evaluation for epilepsy surgery.

XII. PNU-151774

PNU-151774 or (S)-(+)-2-[4-(3-fluorobenzyloxy)benzylamino] propanamide methanesulphonate is a potent Na^+ and Ca^{2+} channel blocker which also shows MAO-B inhibiting properties in rat and human tissues and an affinity for the sigma-1 receptor in receptor ligand assays (PHARMACIA-UPJOHN, data on file). PNU-151774 is endowed with broad spectrum activity in various seizure models, including kindling and kainate-induced status epilepticus in rats. It is also effective in preventing neuronal cell loss induced by kainic acid in rats and cerebral ischaemia in the gerbil. Its neuroprotective effects may be related to its ability to inhibit excitatory neurotransmitter release. Because of its high potency and excellent therapeutic index in preclinical models, PNU-151774 has been selected for clinical development.

XIII. *N*-Valproyl-glycinamide

N-Valproyl-glycinamide (TV 1901) was selected for development from a series of N-valproyl derivatives of GABA and glycine (BIALER et al. 1996). It shows protective activity against maximum electroshock- and pentylenetetrazole-induced seizures, and against seizures induced by corneal kindling in rodents. In these models, the anticonvulsant profile differs from that of valproic acid, and the protective index (ratio of minimal neurotoxic dose to effective anticonvulsant dose) is also greater than that for valproate. After single oral doses of 1 and 4g given to healthy volunteers, *N*-valproyl-glycinamide is absorbed rapidly and is eliminated with a mean half-life of 7–8 h and a CL/F value of about 6.5 l/h (Bialer et al. 1996; Teva Pharm. Ind. Ltd., data on file). After a 4 g dose, about 20% of the dose is excreted unchanged and 39% is excreted as valproyl glycine. Clinical development is in progress.

XIV. SB-204269

SB-204269 [*trans*-(+)-6-acetyl-4*S*-(4-fluoro-benzoyl amino)-3,4-dihydro-2,2-dimethyl-2*H*-benzo(b)pyran-3*R*-ol hemihydrate] is a compound structurally unrelated to other anticonvulsants, and is effective in protecting against seizures in both the maximum electroshock and the maximum electroshock seizure threshold tests, in inhibiting tonic limb extensor seizures produced by pentylenetetrazole infusion (without affecting myoclonic seizures induced by this agent), and in blocking epileptiform activity induced by electrical stimulation and ionic manipulation in hippocampal brain slices (Chan et al. 1996; Upton et al. 1997). Overall, its pharmacological profile is predictive of activity against partial seizures and generalized tonic-clonic seizures. Because of its virtual lack of neurotoxicity in animal models, its protective index is extremely high compared to those reported for existing anticonvulsants. Its mode of action involves inhibition of seizure spread and does not appear to be related to blockade of Na^+ channels, inhibition of glutamate release or modulation of GABA transmission (Upton et al. 1997). Evidence has been provided that its anticonvulsant action may be mediated by a stereoselective interaction with a novel binding site in the brain, which is distinct from that related to the sites of action of other known anticonvulsants, including gabapentin and levetiracetam (Herdon et al. 1997).

H. Conclusion

A number of new antiepileptic drugs are progressing steadily through clinical development. For some of these compounds, such as levetiracetam, losigamone, remacemide and stiripentol, a relatively large number of patients have been exposed and appreciable efficacy and safety data are already available. For other compounds, clinical experience is as yet too limited to allow meaningful evaluation of their therapeutic potential. Even for compounds which eventually will make their way to licensing and marketing, acquisition of new information is a never ending process and their roles in the management in epilepsy can only be defined through further studies and general clinical experience.

References

Abou-Khalil B, Nasreddine W, Fakhoury T, Atkinson D, Beydoun A (1996) Efficacy and safety of ucb LO59 as an adjunctive treatment in refractory partial epilepsy: results of open-label treatment at two centres. Epilepsia 37 [Suppl 5]:169

Albertson TE, Walby WF (1987) The anticonvulsant action of AHR-11748 on kindled amygdaloid seizures in rats. Epilepsy Res 1:126–133
Astoin J, Marivain A, Riveron A, Crucifix M, Lapotre M, Torrens Y (1978) Action de nouveaux alcools alpha-ethyleniques sur le systeme nerveux central. Eur J Med Chem Chim Ther 13:41–47
Bannan PE, Graham DI, Lees KR, McCulloch LJ (1994) Neuroprotective effect of remacemide hydrochloride in focal ischaemia in the cat. Brain Res 664:271–275
Bebin M, Black TP (1994) New anticonvulsant drugs. Focus on flunarizine, fosphenytoin, midazolam and stiripentol. Drugs 48:153–171
Bialer M, Johannessen SI, Kupferberg HJ, Levy RH, Loiseau P, Perucca E (1996) Progress report on new antiepileptic drugs: a summary of the Third Eilat Conference. Epilepsy Res 25:299–319
Biber A, Dienel A (1996) Pharmacokinetic of losigamone, a new antiepileptic drug, in healthy male volunteers. Int J Clin Pharmacol Ther 34:6–11
Carter RB, Wood PL, Wieland S et al. (1997) Characterization of the anticonvulsant properties of ganaxolone (CCD 1042, 3 A-hydroxy-3β-methyl-5 A-pregnan-20-one), a selective high-affinity steroid modulator of the $GABA_A$ receptor. J Pharmacol Exp Ther 280:1284–1295
Chan WN, Evans JM, Hadley MS et al. (1996) Synthesis of novel trans-4-(substituted-benzamido)-3,4-dihydro-2H-benso(b)-pyran-3-ol derivatives as potential anticonvulsant agents with a distinctive binding profile. J Med Chem 39:4357–4359
Cheung H, Wamil AW, Harris EW, McLean MJ (1992) Effects of remacemide hydrochloride, its desglycinated metabolite and isomers on sustained repetitive firing in mouse spinal cord cultured neurones. FASEB J 6:A1879
Cheung WK, Kianifard F, Wong A et al. (1995) Intra- and inter- subject variabilities of CGP 33101 after replicate single oral doses of two 200-mg tablets and 400-mg suspension. Pharm Res 12:1878–1882
Clark B, Hutchison JB, Jamieson V, Jones T, Palmer GC, Scheyer RD (1995) Potential antiepileptic drugs: Remacemide. In: Levy RH, Mattson RH, Meldrum BS (eds) Antiepileptic drugs. Raven Press, New York, pp. 1035–1044
Cower AJ, Noyer M, Verloes R, Cobert J, Wulfert E (1992) ucb LO59, a novel anticonvulsant drug: pharmacological profile in animals. Eur J Pharmacol 222:193–203
Crawford P, Richens A, Mawer G, Cooper P, Hutchinson JB (1992) A double-blind placebo-controlled crossover study of remacemide hydrochloride as adjunctive therapy in patients with refractory epilepsy. J Epilepsy 11 [Suppl A]:P7/13
De Deyn PP, Bielen E, Saxena V, et al. (1992) Assessment of the safety of orally administered ucb LO59 as add-on therapy in patients treated with antiepileptic drugs. Seizure 1 [Suppl A]:P7/15
Dienel A, Biber A (1996) Losigamone: comprehensive summary of safety and tolerability in volunteers. Epilepsia 37 [Suppl 4]:63–64
Dimpfel W, Chatterjee SS, Noldner M, Ticku MK (1995) Effects of the anticonvulsant losigamone and its isomers on the $GABA_A$ receptor system. Epilepsia 36:983–989
Dreifuss F, Cereghino J, Debrabandere L, Johnscher J (1996) Multicentre, double-blind placebo-controlled trial of ucb LO59 (500 mg b.i.d. and 1500 mg b.i.d.) as add-on therapy in patients with refractory partial epilepsy. Platform presentation at the Annual Meeting of the American Epilepsy Society, San Francisco, December 7–10
Edelbroeck PM, de Wilde-Ockeleon JM, Kasteleijn-Nolste-Trenite DGA, Alpherts WCJ, Meijer JWA (1993) Evaluation of the pharmacokinetics and neuropsychometrics parameters in chronic comedicated epileptic patients of three increasing dosages of a novel antiepileptic drug, ucb LO59 250 mg capsules per each dose for one week followed by two weeks of placebo. Epilepsia 34 [Suppl 2]:7
Elger CE, Stefan H, Runge U, Dienel A and the Losigamone Study Group (1996) Losigamone, double-blind study of 1,500 mg/day versus placebo in patients with focal epilepsy. Epilepsia 37 [Suppl 4]:64
Farwell JR, Anderson GD, Kerr B, et al. (1993) Stiripentol in atypical absence seizures in children: an open trial. Epilepsia 34:305–311

Flynn JW, O'Brien JE (1992) High-performance liquid chromatographic method for the simultaneous measuremenmt of remacemide hydrochloride (a novel anticonvulsant and cerebroprotectant) and an active metabolite in human plasma. J Chromatogr 583:91–97

Garske GE, Palmer GC, Napier JJ et al. (1991) Preclinical profile of the anticonvulsant remacemide and its enantiomers in the rat. Epilepsy Res 9:161–174

Gee N, Brown JP, Dissanayake VUK, Offord J, Thurlow R, Woodruff GN (1996) The novel anticonvulsant drug, gabapentin (Neurontin), binds to the alpha2delta subunit of a calcium channel. J Biol Chem 271:6768–5776

Gillardin JM, Verleye M, Ralambosoa C, Lepage F, Levy RH (1993) Anticonvulsant profile and plasma-brain concentrations of a new 2,6-dimethylbenzamide-N-(5-methyl-3-isoxazolyl)(D2916) in rats. Epilepsia 34 [Suppl 6]:38

Giuliano RA, Hiersemensel R, Baltes E, Johnscher G, Janik F, Weber W (1996) Influence of a new antiepileptic drug (levetiracetam, uab LO59) on the pharmacokinetics and pharmacodynamics of oral contraceptives. Epilepsia 37 [Suppl 4]:90

Gower AJ, Matagne A (1994) Levetiracetam (UCB LO59]: anticonvulsant effects are mediated by the parent compound. Epilepsia 35 [Suppl 7]:75

Gower AJ, Noyer M, Verloes R, Gobert J, Wulfert E (1992) Ucb LO59, a novel anticonvulsant: pharmacological profile in animals. Eur J Pharmacol 222:193–203

Gower AJ, Hirsch E, Boehrer A, Noyer M, Marescaux C (1995) Effects of levetiracetam, a novel antiepileptic drug, on convulsant activity in two genetic rat models of epilepsy. Epilepsy Res 22:207–213

Grant SM, Faulds D (1992) Oxcarbazepine. A review of its pharmacology and therapeutic potential in epilepsy, trigeminal neuralgia and affective disorders. Drugs 43:873–888

Greenamyre JT, Eller RV, Zhang Z, Ovadia A, Kurlan R, Gash DM (1994) Antiparkinsonian effects of remacemide hydrochloride, a glutamate antagonist, in rodent and primate models of Parkinson's disease. Ann Neurol 35:655–661

Haria M, Balfour JA (1997) Levetiracetam. CNS Drugs 7:159–164

Harr JE, Maher GG, Kunze KL, Lepage F, Levy RH (1996) Predictions of drug interactions based on identification of CYP450 isoforms which metabolize and are inhibited by D2916, a novel anticonvulsant. Meeting of the American Association of Pharmaceutical Scientists, Seattle, October 28–31 (abstract)

Herdon HJ, Jerman JC, Stean TO et al. (1997) Characterization of the binding of (^{3}H)-SB-204269, a radioactive form of the new anticonvulsant SB-204269, to a novel binding site in rat brain membranes. Brit J Pharmacol 121:1687–1691

Jamieson V (1995) Preclinical and early clinical experience. In: Remacemide hydrochloride – Anticonvulsant and neuroprotectant? Satellite Symposium to the 21st International Epilepsy Symposium, Sydney, 2 September 1995

Johnson DN, Osman MA, Cheng LK, Swinyard EA (1990) Pharmacodynamics and pharmacokinetics of AHR-11748, a new antiepileptic agent, in rodents. Epilepsy Res 5:185–191

Jones MW, Blume W, Guberman A, Lee M, Pillay N, Weaver D, Veloso F (1996) Remacemide hydrochloride (300 mg, 600 mg, 800 mg/day) efficacy and safety versus placebo in patients with refractory epilepsy. Epilepsia 37 [Suppl 5]:166

Jungclaus M, Sokolowa S, Heinemann U, Draguhn A (1997) Losigamone decreases the spontaneous synaptic activity in cultured hippocampal neurons. Eur. J. Pharmacol. 325:245–251

Kapeghian JC, Madan A, Parkinson A, Tripp SL, Probst A (1996) Evaluation of rufinamide (CGP33101), a novel anticonvulsant, for potential drug interactions in vitro. Epilepsia 37 [Suppl 5]:26

Kapetanovic IM, Kupferberg HJ (1997). Preclinical profile of levetiracetam (ucb LO59]: Lack of effect against MES and s.c. PTZ seizures contrasted by a potent broad spectrum protection in animal models of epilepsy. Poster presented at 8th International Bethel-Cleveland Epilepsy Symposium, Bielefeld, Germany, 24–27 April 1997

Kapetanovic IM, Rundfeldt C (1996) D-23129: anticonvulsant compound. CNS Drug Rev 2:308–321
Kapetanovic IM, Yonekawa WD, Kupferberg HJ (1995) The effect of anticonvulsant compounds on 4-aminopyridine-induced de novo synthesis of neurotransmitter amino acids in rat hippocampus in vitro. Epilepsy Res 20:113–120
Kapetanovic IM, Yonekawa WD, Kupferberg HJ (1996) D-23129 stimulated de novo synthesis of GABA in rat hippocampal slices is blocked by an inhibitor of the Na+/K+ antiporter. Epilepsia 37 [Suppl 5]:81
Kastelejin-Nolste-Trenite DGA, Marescaux C, Stodieck S, Edelbroek PM, Oosting J (1996a) Photosensitive epilepsy: a model to study the effects of antiepileptic drugs. Evaluation of the piracetam analogue, levetiracetam. Epilepsy Res 25:225–230
Kastelejin-Nolste-Trenite DGA, Voskuyl RA, Spekreijse S et al. (1996b) Effect of abecarnil, a partial benzodiazepine receptor agonist, in human and animal models. Epilepsia 37 [Suppl 4]:153
Kerr BM, Martinez-Lage JM, Viteri C et al. (1991) Carbamazepine dose requirements during stiripentol therapy: influence of cytochrome P450 inhibition by stiripentol. Epilepsia 32:267–274
Klitgaard H, Matagne A, Gobert J, Wulfert E (1996a) Anticonvulsant properties of levetiracetam (ucb L059) in mice: comparison with currently prescribed and newly developed antiepileptic drugs. Epilepsia 37 [Suppl 4]:132
Klitgaard H, Matagne A, Gobert J, Wulfert E (1996b) Levetiracetam (ucb L059) prevents limbic seizures induced by pilocarpine and kainic acid in rats. Epilepsia 37 [Suppl 4]:118
Klitgaard H, Matagne A, Gobert J, Wulfert E (1997) Levetiracetam (ucb L059) displays an unusually high margin between protective and neurotoxic doses in kindling models of partial epilepsy. Epilepsia 38 [Suppl 3]:177
Kohr G, Heinemann U (1990a) Anticonvulsant effects of tetronic acid derivatives on picrotoxin-induced epileptiform activity in rat hippocampal slices. Neurosci Lett 112:43–47
Kohr G, Heinemann U (1990b) Effects of tetronic acid derivatives AO-33 (losigamone) and AO-78 on epileptiform activity and on stimulus-induced calcium concentration changes in rat hippocampal slices. Epilepsy Res 7:49–55
Kokate TG, Yamaguchi S, Fazilat S, Rogawski MA (1996) Anticonvulsant activity of the neuroactive steroid ganaxolone (CCD 1042) in mice. Epilepsia 37 [Suppl 5]:81
Kramer G, Wad N, Bredel-Geissler A, Biber A, Dienel A (1995a) Losigamone-phenytoin interaction: a placebo-controlled, double-blind study in healthy volunteers. Epilepsia 36 [Suppl 3]:S163
Kramer G, Wad N, Bredel-Geissler, Biber A, Dienel A (1995b) Losigamone-valproate interaction: a placebo-controlled, double-blind study in healthy volunteers. Epilepsia 36 [Suppl 4]:53
Kramer G, Wad N, Bredel-Geissler A, Dienel A, Biber A (1996) Losigamone interactions with antiepileptic drugs in healthy volunteers. Epilepsia 37 [Suppl 4]:89
Leach JP, Blacklaw J, Stewart M et al. (1995) Mutual pharmacokinetic interactions between remacemide hydrochloride and carbamazepine. Epilepsia 36 [Suppl 3]:163
Leach JP, Sills GJ, Butler E, Forrest G, Thompson GG, Brodie MJ (1996a) Neurochemical actions of remacemide in mouse brain. Epilepsia 37 [Suppl 4]:69
Leach JP, Blacklaw J, Jamieson V, Jones T, Richens A, Brodie MJ (1996b) Mutual interaction between remacemide hydrochloride and carbamazepine: two drugs with active metabolites. Epilepsia 37:1100–1106
Lechlinger A, Stabel J, Igelmund P, Heinemann U (1998) Pharmacological and electrographic properties of epileptiform activity induced by elevated K^+ and lowered Ca^{2+} and Mg^{2+} concentrations in rat hippocampal slices. Brain Res (in press)
Lechtenberg R, Villeneuve N, Monaghan EP, Densel MB, Rey E, Dulac O (1996) An open-label dose-escalation study to evaluate the safety and tolerability of ganaxolone in the treatment of refractory epilepsy in pediatric patients. Epilepsia 37 [Suppl 5]:204

Lepage F, Tombret F, Cuvier G, Marivain A, Gillardin JM (1992) New N-aryl isoxazolecarboxamides and N-isoxazolylbenzamides as anticonvulsant agents. Eur J Med Chem 27:581–593

Lepage F, Gillardin JM, Tombret F, Girard P, Descombe JJ, Tang C, Mather G, Levy RH, Baillie A (1995) Human and rat metabolism of D2916 and anticonvulsant properties of its metabolites. Epilepsia 36 [Suppl 4]:49

Levy RH, Lin HS, Blehaut H, Tor JA (1983) Pharmacokinetics of stiripentol in normal man: evidence of nonlinearity. J Clin Pharmacol 23:523–533

Levy RH, Loiseau P, Guyot M, Blehaut HM, Tor J, Moreland TA (1984a) Michaelis-Menten kinetics of stiripentol in normal humans. Epilepsia 25:486–491

Levy RH, Loiseau P, Guyot M, Blehaut HM, Tor J, Moreland TA (1984b) Stiripentol kinetics in epilepsy: nonlinearity and interactions. Clin Pharmacol Ther 36:661–669

Levy RH, Loiseau P, Guyot M, Acheacampong A, Tor J, Rettenmeier AW (1987a) Effects of stiripentol on valproate plasma level and metabolism. Epilepsia 28:605

Levy RH, Martinez-Lage M, Kerr BM (1987b) Effect of stiripentol on the formation and elimination of carbamazepine epoxide. 17th International Epilepsy Congress, Jerusalem, Israel, 6–11 September 1987, abstract 71

Levy RH, Loiseau P, Guyot M, Acheacampong A, Tor J (1988) Effect of stiripentol dose on valproate metabolism. Epilepsia 29:709

Levy RH, Rettenmeier AW, Anderson GD, et al. (1990) Effects of polytherapy with phenytoin, carbamazepine and stiripentol on formation of 4-ene-valproate, a hepatotoxic metabolite of valproic acid. Clin Pharmacol Ther 48:225–235

Lin HS, Levy RH (1983) Pharmacokinetic profile of a new anticonvulsant, stiripentol, in the rhesus monkey. Epilepsia 24:692–702

Lindstrom P, Ben Menachem E, Soderfeldt B (1996) CSF concentrations of remacemide and its desglycinyl metabolite in a double-blind placebo controlled study of 3 doses (300, 600, 1200 mg) remacemide hydrochloride as add-on therapy in patients with refractory epilepsy. Epilepsia 37 [Suppl 5]:166

Lockard JS, Levy RH, Rhodes PH, Moore DF (1985) Stiripentol in acute/chronic efficacy tests in monkeys model. Epilepsia 26:704–712

Lockton JA, Wesnes K, Rolan P, Stephenson N (1996) Volunteer study of the potential interaction between remacemide hydrochloride 300 mg and alcohol 0.7 g/kg. Epilepsia 37 [Suppl 4]:35

Loiseau P, Duche B (1995) Potential antiepileptic drugs: stiripentol. In: Levy RH, Mattson RH, Meldrum BS (eds) Antiepileptic drugs. Raven Press, New York, pp. 1045–1056

Loiseau P, Tor J (1987) Stiripentol in absence seizures. Epilepsia 28:579

Loiseau P, Duche B, Tor J (1989) Stiripentol in absence seizures. An open study updated. Epilepsia 30:639

Loiseau P, Strube E, Tor J, Levy RH, Dodrill C (1988a) Evaluation neuropsychologique et therapeutique du stiripentol dans l'epilepsie. Resultats preliminaires. Rev Neurol 144:165–172

Loiseau P, Strube E, Tor J et al. (1988b) Evaluation neuropsychologique et therapeutique du stiripentol dans l'epilepsie. Resultats preliminaires. Rev Neurol 144:165–172

Loiseau P, Levy RH, Houin G, Rascol O, Dordain G (1990) Randomized, double-blind parallel multicenter trial of stiripentol added to carbamazepine in the treatment of carbamazepine-resistant epilepsies. An interim analysis. Epilepsia 31:618–619

Löscher W, Hönack D (1993) Profile of ucb LO59, a novel anticonvulsant drug, in models of partial and generalized epilepsy in mice and rats. Eur J Pharmacol 232:147–158

Löscher W, Hönack D, Bloms-Funke, P (1996). The novel antiepileptic drug levetiracetam (ucb LO59) induces alteration in GABA metabolism and turnover in discrete areas of rat brain and reduces neuronal activity in substantia nigra pars reticulata. Brain Res 735:208–216

Margineanu D, Wulfert E (1995) ucb LO59, a novel anticonvulsant, reduces bicuculline-induced neuronal hyperexcitability in rat hippocampal CA3 in vivo. Eur J Pharmacol 286:321–325
Matagne A, Klitgaard H (1996) Corneally kindled seizures in mice: anticonvulsant action of levetiracetam (ucb LO59) in a new screening model with relevance for partial epilepsy. Epilepsia 37 [Suppl 4]:140
Mather GG, Bishop FE, Trager WF, Kunze KK, Thummel KE, Shen DD, Roskos LK, Lepage F, Guilardin JM, Levy RH (1995) Mechanisms of stiripentol interactions with carbamazepine and phenytoin. Epilepsia 36 [Suppl 3]:162
McLean MJ, Schmutz M, Wamil AW, Olpe HR, Portet C, Feldmann KF (1994) Oxcarbazepine: mechanisms of action. Epilepsia 35 [Suppl 3]:5–9
Micheletti G, Vergnes M, Lannes B, Tor J, Marescaux C, Depaulis A, Warter JM (1988) Effect of stiripentol on petit-mal like epilepsy in Wistar rats. Epilepsia 29:709
Monaghan EP, Densel MB, Lechtenberg R (1996) Gender differences in sensitivity to ganaxolone, a neuroactive steroid under investigation as an antiepileptic drug. Epilepsia 37 [Suppl 5]:171
Monagham EP, Navalta LA, Shum L, Ashbrook DW, Lee DA (1997) Initial human experience with ganaxolone, a neuroactive steroid with antiepileptic activity. Epilepsia 38:1026–1031
Moreland TA, Astoin J, Lepage F (1986) The metabolic fate of stiripentol in man. Drug Metab Dispos 14:654–662
Morris GL, Wenger B (1996) Losigamone in the long-term treatment of partial seizures. Epilepsia 37 [Suppl 4]:71
Neyens LGJ, Alpherts WCJ, Aldenkamp AP (1995) Cognitive effects of a new pyrrolidine derivative (levetiracetam) in patients with epilepsy. Progr Neuropsych Biol Psychiatr 19:411–419
Noyer A, Gillard M, Matagne A, Henichart J-P, Wulfert (1995) The novel antiepileptic drug levetiracetam (LO59) appears to act via a specific binding site in CNS membranes. Eur J Pharmacol 286:137–146
Olney JW, Labruyere J, Price MT (1989) Pathological changes induced in cerebrocortical neurones by phencyclidine and related drugs. Science 244:1360–1362
Palmer GC, Stagnitto ML, Ordy JM et al. (1991) Preclinical profile of stereoisomers of the anticonvulsant remacemide in mice. Epilepsy Res 8:36–48
Palmer GC, Murray RJ, Wilson TCM et al. (1992a) Biological profile of the metabolites and potential metabolites of the anticonvulsant remacemide. Epilepsy Res 12:9–20
Palmer GC, Harris EW, Ray R, Stagnitto ML, Schmiesing RJ (1992b) Classification of compounds for prevention of NMDLA-induced seizures/mortality or maximal electroshock and pentylentetrazol seizures in mice and antagonism of MK-801 binding in vitro. Arch Int Pharmacodyn Ther 317:16–34
Palmer GC, Clark B, Hutchison JB (1993) Antiepileptic and neuroprotective potential of remacemide hydrochloride. Drugs of the Future 18:1021–1042
Patsalos PN, Walker MC, Ratnaraj N, Sander JWAS, Shorvon SD (1995) The pharmacokinetics of levetiracetam (UCB LO59) in patients with intractable epilepsy. Epilepsia 36 [Suppl 4]:52
Perucca E (1996) The new generation of antiepileptic drugs: Advantages and disadvantages. Brit J Clin Pharmacol 42:531–543
Pieri F, Wegman R, Astoin J (1982) Etude pharmacocinetique du ^{3}H–stiripentol chez le rat. Eur J Drug Metab Pharmacokinet 7:5–10
Pledger GW, Laxer KD, Sahlroot JT et al. (1992) Pharmacokinetics and dose-tolerability study of ADD 94057 in comedicated patients with partial seizures. Epilepsia 33:112–118
Poisson M, Huguet F, Savatier A, Bakri-Logeais F, Narcisse G (1984) A new type of anticonvulsant, stiripentol. Arznm Forsch 34:199–204
Porter RJ (1990) Substances in clinical development. In: Dam M, Gram L (eds) Comprehensive epileptology. Raven Press, New York, pp. 671–682

Privitera MD, Treiman DM, Pledger GW et al. (1994) Dezinamide for partial seizures: results of a e-of-1 design trial. Neurology 44:1453–1458
Riley RJ, Slee D, Martin CA, Webborn PJH, Wattam DG, Jones T, Logan CJ (1996) In vitro evaluation of pharmacokinetic interactions between remacemide hydrochloride and established anticonvulsants. Brit J Clin Pharmacol 41:461P
Rostock A, Rundfeldt C, Tober C, Bartsch R (1995) AWD 140–190: a new anticonvulsant with a very good margin of safety. Arch Pharmacol 351 [Suppl R]:159
Rostock A, Tober G, Rundfeldt C, Bartsch R, Stark B, Kronbach T (1996a) High brain and plasma levels of AWD 140-190 in vivo are consistent with anticonvulsant activity and with use dependent sodium channel blockade. Epilepsia 37 [Suppl 5]:63
Rostock A, Tober G, Rundfeldt C et al. (1996b) D-23129: a new anticonvulsant with a broad spectrum of activity in animal models of epileptic seizures. Epilepsy Res 23:211–223
Rostock A, Bartsch R, Engel J (1996c) D-23129, a new anticonvulsant improves learning and memory in rat models of cerebral deficiency. Epilepsia 37 [Suppl 4]:140
Rostock A, Tober C, Rundfeldt C et al. (1997) AWD 140-190: a new anticonvulsant with a very good margin of safety. Epilepsy Res 28:17–28
Runge U, Rabending G, Dienel A (1996a) Losigamone: preliminary efficacy with 1,500 mg fixed daily dose for >6 months in patients with focal epilepsy. Epilepsia 37 [Suppl 4]:75
Schaffler K, Wauschkuhn CH, Dienel A, Biber A (1996) Losigamone has a longer CNS bioavailability in volunteers than is expected from pharmacokinetics. Epilepsia 37 [Suppl 4]:159
Scheyer RD, Cramer JA, Leppik IE et al. (1992) Remacemide elimination after initial and chronic dosing. Clin Pharmacol Ther 51:189
Schmitz D, Gloveli T, Heinemann U (1995) Effects of losigamone on synaptic potentials and spike frequency habituation in rat entorhinal cortex and hippocampal CA1 neurons. Neuroscience Lett 200:141–143
Schmutz M, Allgeier H, Jeker A et al. (1993) Anticonvulsant profile of CGP 33101 in animals. Epilepsia 34 [Suppl 2]:122
Serra M, Ghiani CA, Maciovcco E, Pisu MG, Tuligi G, Porceddu ML, Biggio G (1996) Failure of chronic treatment with abecarnil to induce contingent and noncontingent tolerance in pentylenetetrazol-kindled rats. Epilepsia 37:332–335
Sharief MK, Singh P, Sander JWAS (1996) Efficacy and tolerability study of ucb LO59 in patients with refractory epilepsy. J Epilepsy 9:106–112
Shen DD, Levy RH, Savitch JL, Boddy AV, Tombret F, Lepage F (1992) Comparative anticonvulsant potency and pharmacokinetics of (+) and (–)-enantiomers of stiripentol. Epilepsy Res 12:29–36
Shorvon SD (1997) Comparative evidence on efficacy and safety of different dosages of levetiracetam in add-on treatment of partial epilepsy. Epilepsia 38 [Suppl 3]:78
Sills GJJ, Leach JP, Patsalos PN, Brodie MJ (1996) Effects of new antiepileptic drugs on enzymes of the GABA Shunt. Epilepsia 37 [Suppl 5]:24
Singh P, Sharief MK, Sander JWAS, Patsalos PN, Shorvon SD (1992) A pilot study of the efficacy and tolerability of LO59 in patients with refractory epilepsy. Seizure 1 [Suppl A]:P7/46
Stables J, Bialer M, Johannessen SI, Kupferberg HJ, Levy RH, Loiseau P, Perucca E (1995) Progress report on new antiepileptic drugs. A summary of the Second Eilat Conference. Epilepsy Res 22:235–246
Srivanasan J, Richens A, Davies JA (1995) Losigamone reduces glutamate and aspartate release from mouse cortex. Brit J Pharmacol (Brighton BPS 1995) Sigra Canale Farmacia 507395
Stagnitto ML, Palmer GC, Ordy JM et al. (1990) Preclinical profile of remacemide: a novel anticonvulsant effective against maximal electroshock seizures in mice. Epilepsy Res 7:11–28
Stefani A, Spadoni F, Bernardi G (1997) Voltage-activated calcium channels: targets of antiepileptic drug therapy? Epilepsia 38:959–965

Stein U (1995) Potential antiepileptic drugs: Losigamone. In: Levy RH, Mattson RH, Meldrum BS (eds) Antiepileptic drugs. Raven Press, New York, pp. 1025–1034
Stein U, Klessing K, Chatterjee SS (1991) Losigamone. In: Pisani F, Perucca E, Avanzini G, Richens A (eds) New antiepileptic drugs. Elsevier, Amsterdam, pp. 129–133
Tartara A, Galimberti CA, Manni R et al. (1993) The pharmacokinetics of oxcarbazepine and its active metabolite 10-hydroxy-carbazepine in healthy subjects and in epileptic patients treated with phenobarbitone or valproic acid. Brit J Clin Pharmacol 36:366–368
Taylor CP, Vartanian MG, Yuen P-W, Bigge C, Suman, Chauhan N, Hill DR (1993) Potent and stereospecific anticonvulsant activity of 3-isobutyl GABA relates to in vitro binding at a novel site labeled by titriated gabapentin. Epilepsy Res 14:11–15
Tober C (1996) Effects of AWD 140-190 on the kindling development in the amygdala kindling model in rats. Epilepsia 37 [Suppl 4]:161
Tober C, Rostock A, Rundfeldt, Bartsch R (1996) D-23129: a potent anticonvulsant in the amygdala kindling model of complex partial seizures. Eur J Pharmacol 303:163–169
Torchin CD, McNeilly PJ, Kapetanovic IM, Strong JM, Kupferberg HJ (1996) Stereoselective metabolism of a new anticonvulsant drug candidate, losigamone, by human liver microsomes. Drug Metab Disp 24:1002–1008
Upton N, Blackburn TP, Cooper D et al. (1997) Profile of SB-2-4269, a novel anticonvulsant drug, in rat models of focal and generalized epileptic seizures. Brit J Pharmacol 121:1679–1686
Victor SJ (1997) Dezinamide. In: Engel J, Pedley TA (eds) Epilepsy – a comprehensive textbook. Lippincott-Raven, New York, 1655–1658
Wad N, Kramer G (1997) Losigamone: detection of its glucuronide in serum. Epilepsia 38 [Suppl 3]:148
Waldmeier F, Gschwind HP, Rouan MC, Sioufi A, Czendlik C (1996) Metabolism of the new anticonvulsive trial drug rufinamide (CGP 33101) in healthy male volunteers. Epilepsia 37 [Suppl 5]:167
Walton NY, Treiman DM (1996) Remacemide versus phenytoin for treatment of experimental status epilepticus. Epilepsia 37 [Suppl 5]:212
Wamil AW, Cheung H, Harris EW, McLean MJ (1996) Remacemide HC1 and its metabolite, AR-C 12495AA, limit action potential firing frequency and block NMDA responses of mouse spinal cord neurons in cell culture. Epilepsy Res 23:1–14
Wang L, Walson PD, Zuo CH (1997) Clinical and experimental evaluation of antiepilepsirine. Epilepsia 38 [Suppl 3]:101
Wegman R, Llies A, Aurousseau M (1979a) Enzymologie pharmacocellulaire du mode d' action du stiripentol au cours de l'epilepsie cardiazolique. III. Les metabolismes protidique, nucleoprotidique, lipidique et des proteoglycanes. Cell Mol Biol 24:51–60
Wegman R, Llies A, Aurousseau M (1979b) Enzymologie pharmacocellulaire du mode d'action du stiripentol au cours de l'epilepsie cardiazolique. IV. Repartition cellulaire et tissulaire du ^{3}H-stiripentol. Cell Mol Biol 24:51–60
Wieshmann U, Janz D, Loewenthal A, Shorvon S, Bielen E, Hiersemenzel R, Johnscher G and the European Epilepsy Study of Levetiracetam (1997) Efficacy and tolerability of levetiracetam (ucb LO59) add-on treatment in refractory patients with partial onset epileptic seizures. Poster presented at 8th International Bethel-Cleveland Epilepsy Symposium, Bielefeld, Germany, 24–27 April 1997
Wilson TC, Eismen MS, Machulskis GE (1992) Quantitation of the novel anticonvulsant remacemide hydrochloride in rat and dog plasma and urine: Application of the plasma methodology to measure the plasma protein binding of remacemide hydrochloride. J Chromatogr 582:195–202
Yau MK, Rudd GD, DellaMaestra WE (1995) Acute dose tolerance and pharmacokinetics of 534U87 in healthy male volunteers. Epilepsia 36 [Suppl 4]:53

Yonekawa WD, Kapetanovic IM, Kupferberg HJ (1995) The effects of anticonvulsant agents on 4-aminopyridine induced epileptiform activity in rat hippocampus in vitro. Epilepsy Res 20:137–150

Yuen P-W, Kanter GD, Taylor CP, Vartanian MG (1994) Enantioselective synthesis of PD144723: a potent stereospecific anticonvulsant. Bioorgan Med Chem Lett 4:823–826

Zhang CL, Chatterjee SS, Stein U, Heinemann U (1992) Comparison of the effects of losigamone and its isomers on maximal electroshock-induced convulsions in mice and on three different patterns of low magnesium induced epileptiform activity in slices of the rat temporal cortex. Naunyn Schmiedbergs Arch Pharmacol 345:85–92

Zhang X, Wulfert E, Hanin I (1993). Effects of ucb LO59, a potential anticonvulsant agent, on release of dopamine (DA) and its metabolites from cerebral ventricular perfusate induced by bicuculline (BIC) and haloperidol (HAL) in rats. Pharmacologist 35:187

CHAPTER 22

Anticonvulsant Combinations and Interactions

P.N. Patsalos

A. Introduction

Combination anticonvulsant therapy (the use of two or more drugs) is common in patients with chronic active epilepsy and in patients with multiple seizure types for whom different drugs may be prescribed for each seizure type. These patients represent approximately 30% of patients with epilepsy and because of the long-term nature of epilepsy and its treatment, the possibility of anticonvolsant drug interactions at some time during treatment is high. Furthermore, polytherapy is often prescribed for brief periods, either during optimization of therapy in newly diagnosed patients, or during seizure exacerbations, in patients who eventually experience good seizure control with a single drug.

In this chapter, the various anticonvulsant drug interactions that are considered clinically significant, in that they may cause complications in the management of the patient, are reviewed. Interactions that are likely to be experienced frequently, or whose outcome is potentially hazardous, are particularly emphasized. The drugs are reviewed in the chronological order in which they have become available for general use (Table 1).

B. Extent of the Problem

The more drugs a patient takes, including over-the-counter drugs, the greater the likelihood that a drug interaction will occur. At greatest risk of suffering clinically serious adverse interactions are the elderly and those who are severely ill, since they are more likely to be treated with several drugs, including drugs used for the treatment of unrelated medical conditions, and also because their drug dosage requirements may be reduced due to renal or hepatic disease or to changes in tissue responsiveness.

Many interactions involving anticonvulsant drugs have been documented over the years, but fortunately in most situations their clinical importance is probably small. However, the significance of an interaction can vary greatly from patient to patient, depending on the relative dosage of the interacting drugs, the previous drug exposure and the genetic constitution. Thus, an interaction resulting in a marked or even modest elevation of a low anticonvulsant concentration may result in improved seizure control, whilst a small elevation

Table 1. Anticonvulsant drugs marketed in (a) the United Kingdom and (b) various countries around the world, but not in the United Kingdom

Drug	Year introduced
(a)	
Phenobarbitone	1912
Phenytoin	1938
Primidone	1952
Ethosuximide	1960
Carbamazepine	1963
Diazepam	1973
Clonazepam	1974
Valproate	1974
Clobazam	1982
Vigabatrin	1989
Lamotrigine	1991
Gabapentin	1993
Topiramate	1995
Tiagabine	1998
(b)	
Felbamate	
Oxcarbazepine	
Zonisamide	

of a nearly toxic concentration may precipitate toxicity. It is therefore important to consider the end result in the individual patient. A marked deviation in the plasma anticonvulsant drug concentration in an unusually susceptible individual receiving drug polytherapy that causes little change in the majority of patients, is equally significant.

C. Pharmacokinetic Interactions

Pharmacokinetic interactions are those in which the processes by which drugs are absorbed, distributed, metabolized and excreted are affected. The key mechanism of interaction of the anticonvulsant drugs relates to the inhibition or induction of drug metabolism. Inhibition results from competition between drugs for the same active site on the enzyme which is involved in their metabolism; circulating concentrations of the inhibited drug increase to reach a new steady state between 4 and 6 half-lives after the interaction. Consequently, pharmacological potentiation will occur quickly if the drug has a short half-life and more slowly if it has a long half-life (Table 2). Toxicity or undesirable effects are likely to occur if dosage reduction is not undertaken.

In contrast, induction involves the synthesis of new enzyme and requires time for protein synthesis so that many days may pass before it is complete. The consequent enhancement of metabolism usually results in decreased

Table 2. Minimum elapsed-time required for a new steady state plasma concentration to be achieved, and consequently for complete pharmacological potentiation after inhibition of hepatic metabolism

Anticonvulsant drug	Time (days)
Phenobarbitone	20
Phenytoin	14
Primidone (phenobarbitone metabolite)	20
Ethosuximide	12
Carbamazepine	5
Valproic acid	3
Lamotrigine	5

efficacy of standard doses of the affected drug. Generally, increasing the drug dose can restore the pharmacological response of a drug whose plasma concentration has been reduced by enzyme induction. The process goes in reverse when the inducer is withdrawn, with an increase in plasma concentrations of the target drug and hence an increased potential for toxic side effects. However, such toxicity can be avoided by appropriate dosage readjustment.

Enzyme induction can be associated with a paradoxical potentiation of a drug's therapeutic and/or toxic effects if pharmacologically active metabolites are present. The most important example of this is carbamazepine, which is metabolized to carbamazepine-epoxide, but the same applies to diazepam and clobazam which are metabolized, respectively, to the active metabolites *N*-desmethyldiazepam and *N*-desmethylclobazam.

I. Cytochrome P450

Cytochrome P450, a group of monooxygenases, is by far the most important drug-metabolizing enzyme system. Of the nine first line, generally available, anticonvulsant drugs, four are hepatic enzyme inducers (phenobarbitone, primidone, phenytoin and carbamazepine). Not only is the magnitude of the induction dose-dependent, but in addition there is evidence to suggest that the different anticonvulsant drugs stimulate different cytochrome P450 isoenzymes (Table 3). Thus their inducing spectra may not be identical. This may explain in part the poorly predictable nature of induction interactions and the fact that phenobarbitone can increase the metabolic clearances of other concomitant enzyme-inducing anticonvulsant drugs.

Most pharmacokinetic drug interactions have been discovered as a result of an unexpected change in the clinical status of a patient after a drug is added to, or withdrawn from, existing medication. However, in recent years it has been recognized that the drug interaction potential of a drug can substantially affect the ease with which this drug is used. Consequently, interaction studies

Table 3. Human cytochrome P450 isoenzymes involved in drug metabolism

Isoenzyme	Drug substrate	Examples of	
		Isoenzyme inducers	Isoenzyme inhibitors
CYP1A1	Benzo-pyrene	Cigarette smoke	Ciprofloxacin Enoxacin
CYP1A2	Caffeine Carbamazepine Lidocaine Oestradiol Procarbazine Propafenone Theobromine Theophylline Tamoxifen Verapamil	Charcoal-broiled foods Cigarette smoke Omeprazole Oxfendazole Phenobarbitone	Ciprofloxacin Norfloxacin
CYP2A6	Cocaine	Clofibrate	Coumarin
CYP2B	Coumarin Cyclophosphamide Diazepam Ethosuximide Ethylmorphine Ifosphamide Trimethadone Warfarin	Dexamethasone Phenobarbitone Phenytoin Testosterone	Chloramphenicol Orphenadrine Secobarbitone
CYP2C8	Carbamazepine Phenytoin	Dexamethasone Phenobarbitone	Amiodarone Cimetidine Methylpyriline
CYP2C9	Fluconazole Ibuprofen Phenytoin Tolbutamide Warfarin	Dexamethasone Phenobarbitone	Amiodarone Cimetidine Fluconazole Methylpyriline Miconazole
CYP2C19	Cimetidine Diazepam Fluoxetine Omeprazole Phenytoin	Dexamethasone Phenobarbitone	Amiodarone Cimetidine Ketoconazole Methylpyriline
CYP2D6	Amitriptyline Chlomipramine Clozapine Codeine Haloperidol Imipramine Lidocaine Omeprazole Propranolol Timolol	None identified	Chlomipramine Cimetidine Fluoxetine Propafenone Quinidine Thioridazine

Table 3. *Continued*

Isoenzyme	Drug substrate	Examples of	
		Isoenzyme inducers	Isoenzyme inhibitors
CYP2E1	Diethyl ether Enflurane Ethanol Ethosuximide Halothane Isoflurane Paracetamol Theophylline	Ethanol Isoniazid	Disulfiram
CYP3A4	Amiodarone Carbamazepine Cyclosporin Diazepam Erythromycin Ethosuximide Felodipine Imipramine Midazolam Nifedipine Quinidine Tamoxifen Warfarin	Carbamazepine Cortisol Dexamethasone Phenobarbitone Phenytoin Rifampicin	Erythromycin Ethinyloesradiol Ketoconazole Fluconazole Miconazole Verapamil

are an integral part of phase I and II development for all new putative anticonvulsant drugs.

Cytochrome P450 enzymes are located in almost every tissue but the liver has by far the highest concentrations. In human liver, more than 25 different isoenzymes of cytochrome P450 have been identified, which, based on their amino acid sequence homology, have been categorized into 4 families (Table 3). It is now recognized that members of the CYP3A subfamily (particularly CYP3A4) are among the most important of all human drug-metabolizing enzymes, whilst, in contrast, CYP4 plays only a small role (Spatzenegger and Jaeger 1995). Presently, it is considered that only CYP2C9, CYP2C19 and CYP3A4 are important in terms of understanding anticonvulsant drug interactions. CYP3A appears to be particularly susceptible to induction and inhibition by many compounds. Consequently drug-drug interactions involving CYP3A are common and are often of clinical significance. Interactions can be expected and are more likely to occur between two drugs if both are specifically metabolized by the same form of P450 or if one of them is a specific inducer or a specific inhibitor of the form of P450 responsible for the metabolism of the other. Even though drug interactions can be anticipated, based on knowledge of the substrates of the isoenzyme concerned, and whether the drug involved is an inducer or an inhibitor, the magnitude of the interaction cannot be predicted and must be determined in clinical studies.

A marked interindividual variability in metabolizing ability which can be as large as 5- to 20-fold, even in the absence of liver dysfunction, is the hallmark of CYP3A metabolism. This is not due to genetic polymorphism but is the consequence of a combination of genetic and environmental factors and also the isoenzyme's particular susceptibility to induction and inhibition by many compounds.

D. Pharmacodynamic Interactions

Pharmacodynamic interactions are those where the effects of one drug are changed by the presence of another drug at its site of action. Drugs may compete directly for a receptor (leading to additive, synergistic or antagonistic effects) but often the interaction may be more indirect, involving interference with physiological mechanisms. These interactions are more difficult to identify and are usually delineated only after an unexpected change in the clinical status of a patient cannot be ascribed definitively to a pharmacokinetic interaction.

E. Interactions of the Generally Available Anticonvulsant Drugs

I. Pharmacokinetic Interactions

1. Phenobarbitone

Both hepatic metabolism and renal excretion eliminate phenobarbitone. The main aromatic hydroxylation pathway of the drug is catalysed by various CYP isoenzymes. Phenobarbitone is the prototype drug which induces CYP2C and CYP3A isoenzymes (Table 3).

a) Interactions Affecting Phenobarbitone

Plasma phenobarbitone concentrations are affected by a variety of drugs (Table 4). Most changes are modest (10%–20%) and in most settings these interactions probably are not clinically significant.

α) Valproic Acid

Valproic acid inhibits the metabolism of phenobarbitone, resulting in a 50% increase in phenobarbitone's half-life and a concurrent increase in its plasma concentrations (Table 5). This interaction occurs in most patients and can lead to sedation and drowsiness necessitating a reduction in phenobarbitone dosage in up to 80% of patients (YUKAWA et al. 1989).

Table 4. Miscellaneous interactions affecting phenobarbitone

Drug	Phenobarbitone	Mechanism
Acetazolamide	↑	INH
Activated charcoal	↓	DA
Ammonium chloride	↓	Reduction in tubular reabsorption
Antacids	↓	DA
Chloramphenicol	↑	INH
Dextropropoxyphene	↑	INH
Dicoumarol	↓	IND
Folic acid	↓	IND
Frusemide (furosemide)	↑	INH
Methsuximide	↑	INH
Methylphenidate	↑	INH
Pheneturide	↑	INH
Pyridoxine	↓	IND?
Thioridazine	↑	INH/IND
Valproic acid*	↓	Decreased plasma protein binding

INH, hepatic inhibition; IND, hepatic induction; DA, decreased absorption.
* Free non-protein-bound concentration; however, the major effect of valproate is to inhibit phenobarbitone metabolism (see text for further details).

β) Phenytoin

Plasma phenobarbitone concentrations increase upon introduction of phenytoin comedication. The most probable mechanism of this interaction is competitive inhibition of phenobarbitone hydroxylation by phenytoin. A recent prospective controlled study of the effects of the reduction and discontinuation of phenytoin therapy on concomitant phenobarbitone concentrations in ten patients with intractable epilepsy observed that phenobarbitone concentrations decreased by a mean of 30%, with new steady-state concentrations being achieved by 4 weeks after the discontinuation of phenytoin intake (Duncan et al. 1991). The protracted time course reflects the long half-life of phenobarbitone.

γ) Miscellaneous Interactions

The interaction of phenobarbitone with activated charcoal (Table 4) is exploited clinically to hasten the elimination of phenobarbitone in overdosed patients. Activated charcoal interacts by impairing phenobarbitone absorption and accelerating its elimination by absorbing any of the drug secreted into the intestine. Patients overdosed with other anticonvulsant drugs including phenytoin and carbamazepine can be treated similarly (Mauro et al. 1987). Another useful interaction that can be exploited for the treatment of patients who have taken an overdose of phenobarbitone is one that occurs with ammonium chloride or other urine-alkalinizing drugs (Powell et al. 1981). These drugs

Table 5. Expected changes in plasma concentrations when a generally available anticonvulsant drug (ACD) is added to an existing ACD regimen

Added ACD	Existing ACD								
	PB	PHT	PRM	ESM	CBZ	DZP	CZP	VPA	CLB
PB	AI?	PHT⇑⇓	NCCP	ESM↓	CBZ⇓	DZP↓	CZP↓	VPA⇓	CLB↓ NDMC↑
PHT	PB⇑	AI	PRM↑↓ PB↑	ESM↓	CBZ⇓	DZP↓	CZP↓	VPA⇓	CLB↓ NDMC↑
PRM	NCCP	PHT⇑⇓	AI?	ESM↓	CBZ⇓	DZP↓	CZP↓	VPA⇓	CLB↓ NDMC↑
ESM	NA	PHT↑	NA	–	NA	NA	NA	VPA⇓	NA
CBZ	NA	PHT⇑⇓	PRM↓ PB↑	ESM↓	AI	DZP↓	CZP↓	VPA⇓	CLB↑ NDMC↑
DZP	NA	PHT↑↓	NA	NA	NA	–	NA	NA	NA
CZP	NA	PHT↑↓	NA	NA	CBZ↓	NA	–	NA	NA
VPA	PB⇑	PHT⇑⇓	PRM↑ PB⇑	ESM↑↓	CBZ-E⇑	DZP⇑*	NA	–	NA
CLB	PB↑	PHT↑↓	PRM↑ PB↑	NA	CBZ↓	NA	NA	VPA↑	–

CBZ, carbamazepine; CBZ-E, carbamazepine-epoxide; CLB, clobazam; CZP, clonazepam; DZP, diazepam; ESM, ethosuximide; NDMC, *N*-desmethylclobazam; PB, phenobarbitone; PHT, phenytoin; PRM, primidone; VPA, valproic acid; NA, none anticipated; AI, autoinduction; NCCP, not commonly coprescribed; ↓ an infrequently observed decrease in plasma concentration; ⇓ a frequently observed decrease in plasma concentration; ↑ an infrequently observed increase in plasma concentration; ⇑ a frequently observed increase in plasma concentration.

* Free pharmacologically active concentration.

Table 6. Miscellaneous interactions where phenobarbitone reduces plasma concentrations of other drugs

Drug affected	Mechanism
Acetaminophen (paracetamol)	IND
Antipyrine (phenazole)	IND
Cimetidine	IND/DA
Chloramphenicol	IND
Chlorpromazine	IND
Cyclosporin	IND/DA
Desipramine	IND
Dicoumarol	IND/DA
Digitoxin	IND
Griseofulvin	IND/DA
Haloperidol	IND
Lignocaine (lidocaine)	IND/PROT
Meperidine (pethidine)	IND
Mesoridazine	IND
Methadone	IND
Methsuximide	IND
Misonidazole	IND
Nortryptyline	IND
Phenylbutazone	IND
Theophylline	IND
Warfarin	IND

IND, hepatic induction; DA, decreased absorption; PROT, protein binding.

increase urinary elimination of phenobarbitone by reducing its reabsorption from the renal tubules.

b) Interactions Where Phenobarbitone Affects Other Drugs

Table 6 shows the various drugs whose plasma concentrations have been reported to be lowered by phenobarbitone. For some drugs, the interaction may be very significant.

α) Anticoagulants

Enzyme induction by phenobarbitone can reduce the plasma concentration of the anticoagulants bishydroxycourmarin (dicoumanol) and warfarin, and consequently their anticoagulant effect. This is a potentially dangerous interaction requiring an increased anticoagulant dosage, guided by prothrombin time determinations; the increase may be as much as tenfold (Breckenridge 1974). Upon withdrawal of phenobarbitone (and indeed withdrawal of any other inducing drugs) it is necessary reduce to the anticoagulant dose if a serious risk of haemorrhage is to be avoided.

β) Calcium Antagonists

The bioavailabilities of felodipine and nimodipine, calcium antagonists used in the treatment of hypertension and heart failure, are substantially reduced in patients coprescribed phenobarbitone. The mechanism of these interactions is induction of first-pass metabolism and they can be associated with plasma concentrations for felodipine and nimodipine which are below 7% and 15% respectively of those in normal uninduced subjects (TARTARA et al. 1991).

γ) Oral Contraceptives

During phenobarbitone comedication, women taking oral contraceptives can experience breakthrough bleeding and be at an increased risk of pregnancy (BACK et al. 1988). Data from the Committee on Safety of Medicines for the period 1973 to 1984 showed that, of a total of 43 cases of contraceptive failure reported, phenobarbitone accounted for 20 and phenytoin for 25 (BACK et al. 1988). Two modes of interaction are thought to be responsible for the contraceptive failure. Firstly, because of induction of the metabolism of synthetic oral steroids (oestrogen and/or progesterone), insufficient hormone concentrations are available to block ovulation. Secondly, by enhancing the synthesis of sex hormone-binding globulin, which is involved in the binding of sex steroids, a decrease in the pharmacologically active free concentration of circulating hormones occurs, and this too contributes to failure to block ovulation.

δ) Paracetamol

Patients receiving phenobarbitone do badly after a paracetamol overdose as they are particularly susceptible to acute hepatic necrosis. This can be attributed to the formation of a hepatotoxic highly reactive metabolite of paracetamol consequent on induction of paracetamol metabolism by phenobarbitone (or by other anticonvulsant drug inducers).

ε) Valproic Acid

Patients, particularly children, are more likely to develop valproic acid-associated hyperammonaemia and liver toxicity when taking phenobarbitone comedication, compared with those taking valproic acid monotherapy. This effect may be due to enhanced production of toxic metabolites.

ζ) Miscellaneous Interactions

Other clinical disorders which may be exacerbated by the enzyme-inducing properties of phenobarbitone include steroid-treated adrenal insufficiency, asthma, rheumatoid arthritis and pemphigus vulgaris (SEHGAL and JRIVASTAVA 1988). In steroid-dependent patients, phenobarbitone can precipitate acute asthma attacks. A vicious cycle may develop subsequently, as hypoxaemia provoked by worsening asthma may lead to further enzyme induction.

Although the decrease in plasma concentrations of drugs such as cyclosporin, cimetidine and griseofulvin is primarily due to induction, there is evidence to suggest that reduced gastrointestinal absorption may also be in part responsible (BEUREY et al. 1982; CARTENSEN et al. 1986).

2. Phenytoin

Of all the anticonvulsants, phenytoin is the one most commonly reported as associated with clinically significant interactions (Table 5). Although this can be attributed in part to its duration and frequency of use, a greater contributing factor is phenytoin's unique pharmacokinetic and physiological properties. Thus, because phenytoin is both extensively bound to plasma proteins and also very loosely bound to hepatic cytochrome P450 enzymes, it is particularly susceptible to competitive displacement and metabolic inhibitory interactions. Furthermore, phenytoin is a potent inducer of hepatic drug metabolizing enzymes. Also, its metabolism is saturable at therapeutic concentrations. Thus, it is necessary only to inhibit its metabolism slightly to produce a disproportionate increase in circulating phenytoin concentration and an enhanced risk of toxicity. Phenytoin is almost completely eliminated by hepatic metabolism (less than 5% being excreted unchanged) with most metabolism occurring via CYP2C9, although some is metabolized by CYP2C19.

a) Interactions Affecting Phenytoin

Table 7 shows the various drugs that have been reported to affect phenytoin plasma concentrations. The clinical significance of the different interactions is variable but may be particularly significant in patients already taking maximum tolerable phenytoin doses.

α) Alcohol

Overall, mild to moderate alcohol consumption does not affect phenytoin metabolism significantly. However, acute alcohol ingestion can be associated with elevated plasma phenytoin concentrations whilst long term exposure to large amounts of alcohol results in hepatic enzyme induction, enhanced phenytoin metabolism, and reduced plasma phenytoin concentrations with possible loss of seizure control. In addition, seizure control can be lost because alcohol may itself be epileptogenic and also because alcohol related memory impairment may result in poor compliance with treatment.

β) Amiodarone

Amiodarone inhibits the metabolism of phenytoin and also displaces phenytoin from its plasma protein binding sites. This dual interaction can result in a twofold increase in plasma phenytoin concentrations within 2–4 weeks after initiation of amiodarone therapy. A further complication is that amiodarone itself can cause similar neurological toxicity to that observed with phenytoin.

Table 7. Miscellaneous interactions affecting phenytoin

Drug	Phenytoin plasma concentration	Mechanism
Activated charcoal	↓	DA
Allopurinol	↑	INH
Acyclovir	↓	DA
Azopropazone	↑↓	PROT
Bromfenac	↓	IND
Ceftriaxone	↑*	PROT
Chloramphenicol	↑	INH
Cisplatin	↓	DA
Clobazam	↑	INH
Cyclosporin	↑	INH
Diazoxide	↑↓	PROT
Disulfiram	↑	INH
Fluconazole	↑	INH
Fluoxetine	↑	INH
Folic acid	↓	IND
Methotrexate	↓	DA
Miconazole	↑	?
Nafcillin	↑*	PROT
Nisoldipine	↓	IND
Nitrofurantoin	↓	?
Nutrient formulae	↓	DA
Omeprazol	↑	INH
Oxacillin	↓	DA
Phenylbutazone	↑↓	INH/PROT
Rifampicin	↓	IND
Salicylate	↑↓	PROT
Sulfamethoxazole	↑*	PROT
Sulfonamides (sulphaphenazole, sulphadiazine)	↑	INH
Sulphafurazole	↑↓	PROT
Sulphanethoxypyrine	↑↓	PROT
Tamoxifen	↑	INH
Theophylline	↓	DA
Ticlopidine	↑	INH
Tolbutamine	↑↓	INH/PROT
Vinblastine	↑	DA

INH, hepatic inhibition; IND, hepatic induction; DA, decreased absorption; PROT, protein binding.
* Free (non-protein-bound) concentration.

Thus, there is a need to be cautious about interpreting the clinical signs of toxicity during comedication with phenytoin and amiodarone (SHACKLEFORD and WATSON 1987).

γ) Antiulcer Agents

Phenytoin absorption can be significantly reduced by high dose (15–45 ml) antacids (aluminium and magnesium hydroxide and calcium carbonate) and by the gastric protective agent sucralfate (D'ARCY and MCELNAY 1987). However, small doses of antacids (<10 ml) generally have little effect on phenytoin bioavailability. In order to avoid this interaction, ingestion of antacids and phenytoin should be separated by 1–2 h.

Cimetidine, a H_2 receptor antagonist, dose dependently inhibits the metabolism of phenytoin. The resultant 20%–30% elevation in plasma phenytoin concentrations can trigger toxicity, necessitating a reduction in phenytoin dosage (LEVINE et al. 1985). Furthermore, during neurosurgical procedures there is an increased risk of severe thrombocytopenia when cimetidine and phenytoin combination therapy is used (YUE et al. 1987). Thus, during such procedures, cimetidine and phenytoin in combination should be avoided.

δ) Carbamazepine

The interaction between phenytoin and carbamazepine is controversial, with reports that plasma phenytoin concentrations are both elevated and reduced (LAI et al. 1992). These differences can be explained on the basis of carbamazepine acting both as an inhibitor and an inducer of phenytoin metabolism. The mechanism that determines whether induction or inhibition prevails is not known but probably relates to the relative doses and plasma concentrations of the two drugs.

ε) Isoniazid

Isoniazid inhibits the metabolism of phenytoin. Thus, patients receiving chronic phenytoin therapy who are administered isoniazid commonly experience drowsiness and intoxication (KAY et al. 1985). Approximately 10%–15% of patients experience intoxication and the risk of intoxication is greater in those individuals who are slow acetylators of isoniazid because they are more likely to achieve sufficiently high isoniazid plasma concentrations to inhibit phenytoin metabolism. This interaction can occur rapidly and the phenytoin dose should be adjusted accordingly, based on plasma phenytoin concentrations.

ζ) Phenobarbitone

Phenobarbitone is both a strong inducer of phenytoin metabolism and an inhibitor. Thus when phenytoin and phenobarbitone are coingested, plasma phenytoin concentrations may be lowered, elevated or unaffected. The mechanism which determines whether induction or inhibition will prevail is not known but it has been pointed out that induction prevails if the dose of phenytoin is relatively high and inhibition prevails when the phenobarbitone dose is high. Thus, if a patient's enzymes are highly induced as a result of the administration either of a low dose of phenobarbitone on a long-term basis or a high dose on a short-term basis, and the patient is then given phenytoin, any further increase of the phenobarbitone dosage might provoke inhibition of phenytoin metabolism. The inhibition will result in elevated plasma phenytoin concentrations, since maximum induction by phenobarbitone would have already taken place. This bidirectional interaction can be significant in some patients.

η) Valproic Acid

Valproic acid both displaces phenytoin from its plasma protein binding sites and inhibits phenytoin metabolism. This dual interaction between valproic acid and phenytoin is transient and unpredictable and plasma phenytoin concentration values can be potentially misleading in these circumstances. These two effects can be opposite in nature, and the clinical significance of the interaction depends on whether or not phenytoin metabolism is close to saturation. Displacement of phenytoin from its protein binding sites results in an increase in the free phenytoin concentration. However, in patients where phenytoin metabolism is not saturated, the increase is transient because a rapid redistribution of phenytoin throughout body tissues occurs and in addition there is a compensatory rise in metabolism so that the free phenytoin concentration returns to its value before valproic acid was introduced. Even though plasma total phenytoin concentrations decrease, dosage of the drug should not be increased. If phenytoin dosage adjustment is considered necessary, changes should be made based on its free drug concentration. In contrast, phenytoin dosage reduction would be necessary in patients whose phenytoin metabolism is close to saturation, since the displacement coupled with metabolic inhibition by valproic acid can increase phenytoin total concentrations substantially and precipitate neurological toxicity.

θ) Miscellaneous Interactions

The intestinal absorption of phenytoin is significantly reduced by nutritional formulae administered by nasogastric tube. Plasma phenytoin concentration can be reduced by as much as 75% (Pearce 1988). It is suggested that patients receiving phenytoin orally should be monitored carefully when feeding with a nutritional formula is commenced or stopped. Furthermore, caution should be exercised if changes are made in the type of formula used, since while"Isocal" and "Osmolite" formulae interact with phenytoin, the formula "Ensure" does not.

Like valproic acid, numerous other drugs (azapropazone, ceftriaxone, diazoxide, nafcillin, phenylbutazone, salicylate, sulfamethoxazole, sulphafurazole, sulphamethoxypyridine and tolbutamide) have been reported to interact with phenytoin by displacing it from its plasma protein binding sites (Dasgupta et al. 1991). However, as in the case of valproic acid, an adjustment to phenytoin dosage will be necessary only if phenytoin metabolism is close to saturation and in particular if the displacement interaction is associated with simultaneous inhibition of phenytoin metabolism, as may occur with tolbutamide and phenylbutazone (McGovern et al. 1984; Tassaneeyakul et al. 1992).

b) Interactions Where Phenytoin Affects Other Drugs

Phenytoin, like phenobarbitone, is a potent inducer of hepatic enzymes. Consequently phenytoin comedication can be associated with decreases in the plasma concentrations of target drugs by as much as 50%. Therefore appropriate dosage adjustments need to be made and if, subsequently, phenytoin is withdrawn, toxicity may result if readjustment of the dosage of the concomitant drug is not undertaken.

α) Anticoagulant Drugs

Phenytoin interacts with the anticoagulants dicoumarol and warfarin in a contradictory manner. Thus, whilst phenytoin induces the metabolism of dicoumarol, it inhibits the metabolism of warfarin, resulting in increased plasma warfarin concentrations and possible haemorrhage.

β) Dexamethasone

Dexamethasone clearance is enhanced by phenytoin. As a consequence, patients without Cushing's syndrome but taking phenytoin medication have less than normal suppression of urinary 17-hydroxycorticosteroid secretion after a "low dose" dexamethasone test, but normal suppression after a "high dose" test, which is suggestive of Cushing's disease. Thus, the dexamethasone suppression test needs to be interpreted with caution in patients receiving phenytoin or other hepatic enzyme-inducing anticonvulsant drugs.

Dexamethasone is useful in the control of raised intracranial pressure and consequently is frequently prescribed in conjunction with phenytoin in patients undergoing craniotomy. However in these patients dexamethasone doses several times larger than normal are required, and this too can be attributed to enzyme-induction.

γ) Theophylline

Theophylline, a widely used bronchodilator with a narrow therapeutic index, requires careful dose titration, particularly in the elderly. Phenytoin can increase theophylline clearance by as much as 35%–75% (CROWLEY et al. 1987) and, in contrast to other inducers in the elderly (e.g. dichlorphenazone and rifampacin), this induction effect of phenytoin is maintained in old age. As well, cigarette smoking further enhances the clearance of theophylline, since smoking and phenytoin have an additive inducing effect on theophylline metabolism.

δ) Miscellaneous Interactions

There are many other drugs whose metabolism is enhanced by phenytoin (Table 8), the most important being carbamazepine, chloramphenicol, dicoumarol, digoxin, folic acid, methadone, midazolam, pethidine, oral contraceptives, and valproic acid.

Table 8. Drugs/compounds whose metabolism may be induced by concurrent treatment with carbamazepine

Acetaminophen (paracetamol)	Methsuximide
Amitriptyline	Methylprednisolone
Busulphan	Metronidazole
Chloramphenicol	Metyrapone
Chlorpromazine	Mexilitine
Chlopropamide	Midazolam
Cimetidine	Misonidazole
Clobazam	Nimodipine
Clonazepam	Nisoldipine
Clopenthixol	Nitroglycerine (glyceryl trinitrate)
Clozapine	Nomifensine
Codeine	Nortriptyline
Cyclophosphamide	Oral contraceptives (ethinyloestradiol and levonorgestrel)
Cyclosporin	Paroxetine
Desipramine	Pethidine (meperidine)
Desmethylchlomipramine	Phenacetin
Dexamethasone	Phenazone (antipyrine)
Dicoumarol	Phenylbutazone
Digitoxin	Phenobarbitone
Disopyrimide	Phenytoin
Doxycycline	Praziquantal
Etopside	Prednisolone
Ethosuximide	Prednisone
Felodipine	Primidone
Fenoprofen	Propoxyphene (dextropropoxyphene)
Fentanyl	Propranolol (plus other β-blockers)
Flunarizine	Protriptyline
Flupenthixol	Psoralens
Griseofulvin	Quinine
Haloperidol	Quinidine
Imipramine	Theophylline
Itraconazole	Thyroxine
Ketoconazole	Tiralazad
Lidocaine (lignocaine)	Trazodone
Mainserin	Valproic acid
Mesoridazine	Vitamin D derivatives
Methadone	Warfarin
Methoxsalen (8-methoxypsoralen)	

These interactions can also be expected to occur with the other enzyme-inducing anticonvulsant drugs.

Phenytoin impairs the absorption of cyclosporin, frusemide and praziquantal and thus their bioavailabilities can be reduced by as much as 75%, 50% and 75% respectively (BITTENCOURT et al. 1992). The interaction with cyclosporin is rather controversial since when cyclosporin is administered intravenously, phenytoin comedication results in a 50% reduction in the cyclosporin AUC, suggestive of hepatic enzyme induction (KEOWN et al. 1984). In approximately 50% of patients receiving phenytoin, plasma folate concentrations tend to be lower; this reduction may be attributed in part to impaired folate absorption (CARL and SMITH 1992).

3. Primidone

Because primidone is metabolized to two pharmacologically active metabolites, phenobarbitone and phenylethylmalonamide, the interpretation of interactions between primidone and other drugs is not straightforward.

a) Interactions Affecting Primidone

All the known interactions of phenobarbitone (see above) should also be expected to occur in patients taking primidone. In addition, acetazolamide impairs the absorption of primidone whilst nicotinamide and isoniazid inhibit its metabolism, resulting in a lower plasma phenobarbitone to primidone ratio. Conversely, a higher plasma phenobarbitone to primidone ratio is observed in patients taking primidone and another enzyme-inducing drug, e.g. phenytoin or carbamazepine (SATO et al. 1992).

b) Interactions Where Primidone Affects Other Drugs

As the primary metabolite of primidone, phenobarbitone, is a potent hepatic enzyme-inducer, it might be expected to induce the metabolism of a variety of drugs, thus requiring dosage adjustment of concomitant drugs (see Table 6).

4. Ethosuximide

Most of an ethosuximide dose is eliminated via hepatic metabolism (60%–70%), but approximately 20% is excreted unchanged via the kidneys. A wide spectrum of CYP isoenzymes (CYP3A4, CYP2E1, CYP2B and CYP2 C) is involved in its metabolic hydroxylation and this may explain why only potent enzyme-inducers alter the clearance of ethosuximide. Ethosuximide is not an enzyme-inducer, is not bound to plasma proteins and has a low capacity to alter the pharmacokinetics of other drugs. Thus, there are few interactions involving ethosuximide and in most cases they are of little clinical significance (Table 5).

a) Interactions Affecting Ethosuximide

Ethosuximide metabolism is enhanced by enzyme-inducing anticonvulsant drugs, resulting in lower plasma ethosuximide concentrations (DUNCAN et al. 1991), and is inhibited by isoniazid, resulting in higher plasma ethosuximide concentrations. The effect of valproic acid on plasma ethosuximide concentration is variable: an increase, a decrease, or no effect can occur.

b) Interactions Where Ethosuximide Affects Other Drugs

During ethosuximide and valproic acid comedication, the plasma valproic acid concentration can be reduced by approximately 30% (SALKE-KELLERMANN et al. 1997). The mechanism of this interaction is not clear.

5. Carbamazepine

Carbamazepine has numerous characteristics which make it particularly susceptible to drug interactions. Firstly, it is a potent hepatic enzyme-inducer; secondly, it exhibits autoinduction (i.e. it induces its own metabolism); thirdly, it is metabolized to an epoxide metabolite (carbamazepine-10,11-epoxide) which is pharmacologically active. Interactions affecting the epoxide metabolite are being increasingly seen as clinically important since the epoxide metabolite contributes not only to the efficacy of carbamazepine but also to its toxicity. Furthermore, interactions affecting the epoxide metabolite can precipitate neurological toxicity and may pass undetected since therapeutic monitoring of the epoxide is not commonly undertaken and carbamazepine plasma concentrations may not change.

The hepatic isoenzymes responsible for the metabolism of carbamazepine are CYP3A4, CYP2C8 and CYP1A2, with CYP3A4 being the main enzyme system responsible for the conversion of carbamazepine to its epoxide, as it accounts for 30%–50% of the carbamazepine clearance (KERR et al. 1994). Consequently, drugs that inhibit (e.g. ketoconazole, danazol, cimetidine and macrolide antibiotics) or induce CYP3A4 (e.g. barbiturates and phenytoin) can be expected to elevate and lower, respectively, carbamazepine plasma concentrations.

a) Interactions Affecting Carbamazepine

α) Antibiotics

Carbamazepine toxicity (confusion, somnolence, ataxia, vertigo, nausea and vomiting) can present soon after starting erythromycin therapy, and is usually associated with an up to threefold increase in plasma carbamazepine concentrations. The severity of the interaction depends on the duration of antibiotic therapy. The interaction is reversed rapidly upon withdrawal of the antibiotic. Carbamazepine metabolism is inhibited by erythromycin. This inhibition can also occur with other macrolide antibiotics including clarithromycin, flurithromycin, josamycin, ponsinomycin and triacelyloleandomycin (WROBLEWSKI et al. 1988; COUET et al. 1990). Plasma carbamazepine concentrations should be monitored whenever macrolide therapy is contemplated.

β) Antidepressants

While tricyclic antidepressants have not been reported to affect the kinetics of carbamazepine, there is evidence to suggest that the selective serotonin reuptake inhibitors fluoxitine, fluvoxamine and sertraline (but not paroxetine) may increase plasma carbamazepine concentrations, possibly by inhibiting carbamazepine metabolism (GRIMSLEY et al. 1991). However, these interactions have not been confirmed in all studies.

γ) Anticonvulsant Drugs (Enzyme-Inducing)

Carbamazepine metabolism is highly inducible by other enzyme-inducing anticonvulsant drugs. Thus the addition of primidone, phenobarbitone or phenytoin (all hepatic enzyme inducers) to carbamazepine therapy is commonly associated with a significant reduction in the carbamazepine plasma concentration. Concurrent increases in carbamazepine-epoxide concentrations have been reported but more often these remain unchanged. Of particular clinical significance may be the diurnal fluctuations (50%–90%) and concurrent intermittent side effects of carbamazepine that occur during polytherapy with enzyme-inducing drugs. In monotherapy, plasma carbamazepine concentrations vary by only 23%–45%.

δ) Calcium Channel Blockers

Calcium channel blockers have variable effects on carbamazepine metabolism. Verapamil and diltiazem can almost double carbamazepine plasma concentrations, resulting in toxic side effects. In contrast, nifedipine does not exhibit any significant interaction with carbamazepine (BAHLS et al. 1991).

ε) Cimetidine

Cimetidine inhibits the metabolism of carbamazepine and thus, during comedication with cimetidine, a 20%–30% increase in plasma carbamazepine concentrations can be expected (DALTON et al. 1988). In some patients with peptic ulcers, the intake of cimetidine may continue for a long time and thus the clinical significance of this interaction may increase with time as carbamazepine accumulates. Thus, an H_2-antagonist that is devoid of hepatic enzyme inhibitory effects (e.g. ranitidine or famotidine) should be considered for patients taking carbamazepine.

ζ) Imidazole Drugs

Carbamazepine intoxication has been reported to occur during coingestion of a variety of imidazole drugs (e.g. isoniazid, nafimidone, stiripentol and denzimol). These drugs appear to be potent inhibitors of carbamazepine metabolism and result in plasma carbamazepine concentrations increasing as much as twofold.

η) Valproic Acid

Valproic acid coadministration can quadruple plasma carbamazepine-epoxide concentrations in some patients. This can occur in the absence of any marked changes in the plasma carbamazepine concentration and can be associated with significant neurotoxicity. The mechanism of this interaction is primarily by inhibition of epoxide hydrolase, the enzyme that is responsible for the metabolism of carbamazepine-epoxide, but inhibition of the glucuronidation of the *trans*-diol metabolite of carbamazepine may also occur (BERNUS et al. 1997)

An even greater interaction involving carbamazepine-epoxide occurs with valpromide, an amide derivative of valproic acid. During comedication with valpromide an up to eightfold increase in carbamazepine-epoxide concentrations can occur (PISANI et al. 1988). It is therefore not advisable to use valpromide and valproic acid interchangeably. More recently, valnoctamide, a mild tranquilizer available over the counter and an isomer of valpromide, has similarly been observed to increase plasma carbamazepine-epoxide concentrations fivefold (PISANI et al. 1993).

θ) Miscellaneous Interactions

Carbamazepine metabolism is inhibited by a variety of drugs including danazol, haloperidol, omeprazole and propoxyphene (HAYDEN and BUCHANAN 1991; NAIDU et al. 1994; IWAHASHI et al. 1995). In particular the analgesic propoxyphene has been associated with increases in carbamazepine plasma concentrations of 30%–60%. Thus patients taking carbamazepine should avoid analgesic preparations containing propoxyphene and instead use codeine or ibuprofen for analgesia.

b) Interactions Where Carbamazepine Affects Other Drugs

Carbamazepine induces the metabolism of a wide variety of concurrently administered drugs (Table 8). However, in many studies the patients investigated were receiving a combination of carbamazepine and other enzyme-inducing drugs such as phenytoin and phenobarbitone. Consequently, the specific contribution of carbamazepine to the observed effects has not been determined in all cases.

The spectrum of enzymes whose activity is stimulated by carbamazepine has not been clearly defined but almost certainly includes CYP3A4 because the metabolism of drugs that are substrates for this isoenzyme (e.g. cyclosporin and steroidal oral contraceptives) is enhanced in patients treated with carbamazepine. However, it is very likely that carbamazepine induces other oxidative isoenzymes as well as non-oxidative enzymes such as glucuronyl-transferases.

Drugs whose clinical effects may be significantly affected include antidepressants, β-blockers, haloperidol, felodipine, oral anticoagulants, steroidal oral contraceptives, theophylline and trazodone (CRAWFORD et al. 1990; BROSEN and KRAGH-SORENSEN 1993; OTANI et al. 1996). Carbamazepine also induces the metabolism of the anaesthetic fentanyl so that it is required in higher doses during craniotomies (Tempelhoff et al. 1990). Midazolam, used as an oral hypnotic, is affected similarly (Beckman et al. 1996).

Plasma concentrations of clonazepam, ethosuximide, phenytoin, primidone and valproic acid tend to be lower during comedication with carbamazepine (Table 5). The clinical significance of these interactions is variable, but dosage adjustments may become necessary in some patients (Duncan et al. 1991).

Carbamazepine impairs the absorption of praziquantal so that during comedication its bioavailability is reduced by more than 90% (Bittencourt et al. 1992). Cyclosporin bioavailability is also reduced during comedication with carbamazepine. However, as with phenytoin, this effect may in part be due to hepatic enzyme induction. Finally, in patients with normal adrenopituitary function, a depressed response to the low-dose dexamethasone suppression test and to the oral metyrapone test can occur during carbamazepine therapy. These positively misleading results can be attributed to hepatic enzyme induction by carbamazepine.

6. Diazepam

a) Interactions Affecting Diazepam

Diazepam is involved in few interactions (Table 5). Enzyme-inducing anticonvulsant drugs have been shown to increase the clearance of diazepam. Valproic acid interacts with diazepam in two ways. Firstly, it displaces diazepam from its plasma protein binding sites and increases its free (pharmacologically active) concentration; secondly, it inhibits diazepam metabolism (Dhillon and Richens 1982). Thus during combination therapy an enhanced CNS-depressant effect of diazepam is commonly observed. Cimetidine, ciprofloxacin, disulfiram, erythromycin, omeprazole and venlafaxine may inhibit the metabolism of diazepam. The interaction mechanism in these cases may be competition for the CYP2C19 catabolic pathway; however, the clinical significance of these effects is unknown.

b) Interactions Where Diazepam Affects Other Drugs

The effect of diazepam on phenytoin is controversial, with phenytoin metabolism being enhanced or inhibited in different patients.

7. Clonazepam

a) Interactions Affecting Clonazepam

In contrast to the primary metabolites of clobazam and diazepam, the primary metabolite of clonazepam (a 7-amino derivative) is not pharmacologically active. The efficacy of clonazepam is attenuated during comedication with hepatic enzyme-inducing anticonvulsant drugs. Plasma clonazepam concentrations can be expected to be lower in these patients.

b) Interactions Where Clonazepam Affects Other Drugs

The interaction with phenytoin is controversial (Table 5). Plasma phenytoin concentrations may rise, fall or stay the same.

8. Valproic Acid

Valproic acid is almost completely eliminated by metabolism, with less than 4% of a dose being excreted unchanged in the urine. About 40% of valproic acid's clearance takes place by direct conjugation, 30% by mitochondrial β-oxidation and approximately 10% by CYP-dependent oxidation. Valproic acid does not induce hepatic enzymes but does inhibit hepatic metabolism. Some of the many metabolites of valproic acid are pharmacologically active and may contribute to its efficacy and its hepatotoxicity. Because valproic acid is highly bound to plasma proteins, it readily displaces other bound anticonvulsant drugs.

a) Interactions Affecting Valproic Acid

Interactions affecting valproic acid are few and rarely of clinical significance. Lower valproic acid plasma concentrations are achieved during comedication with antacids, adriamycin and cisplatin, due to reduced gastrointestinal absorption. In addition plasma protein binding displacement interactions with naproxen, phenylbutazone and salicylic acid can also result in lower valproic acid plasma concentrations. However, these interactions may on occasion be associated with an elevation in plasma total concentrations of valproic acid, since valproic acid exhibits saturable binding to plasma proteins. Hyperactivity and acute toxic psychosis can occur when salicylic acid is coingested with valproic acid (ABBOTT et al. 1986; GOULDEN et al. 1987).

Lower (50%) valproic acid plasma concentrations are also observed during comedication with carbamazepine, phenobarbitone, phenytoin and primidone and are due to hepatic enzyme induction and resultant increased valproic acid and clearance (Table 5). The clinical consequence of these interactions can be a reduction of seizure control necessitating an increase in valproic acid dosage. However, a more adverse consequence is the increased incidence of valproic acid-associated hepatotoxicity which may be the result of the increased production of the metabolites 4-en- and 2-4-dien-valproic acid. Chlorpromazine may increase plasma valproic acid concentrations. Acyclovir may reduce valproic acid bioavailability by reducing its gastrointestinal absorption (PARMEGGIANI et al. 1995).

b) Interactions Where Valproic Acid Affects Other Drugs

Valproic acid is a potent metabolic inhibitor, affecting both oxidative pathways and glucuronide conjugation pathways. The inhibitory interactions with carbamazepine, diazepam, ethosuximide, lamotrigine, phenobarbitone and phenytoin are discussed elsewhere. Valproic acid also inhibits the metabolism of amitriptyline, clomipramine, nimodipine and nortiptyline and increases their bioavailabilities by 50%–86% (Tartara et al. 1991).

9. Clobazam

a) Interactions Affecting Clobazam

Carbamazepine, phenobarbitone, phenytoin and primidone lower plasma clobazam concentrations and elevate desmethyl-clobazam concentrations (Table 5). The mechanism of this interaction is induction of metabolism, but other mechanisms may also be involved. Since the desmethyl-clobazam metabolite of the drug is not only pharmacologically active but may have even greater anticonvulsant efficacy than clobazam itself, these interactions may be of benefit therapeutically.

Alcohol and cimetidine may also significantly increase plasma clobazam concentrations

b) Interactions Where Clobazam Affects Other Drugs

Clobazam can raise plasma phenobarbitone, phenytoin and valproic acid concentrations and precipitate toxicity (Table 5). Also, during comedication with carbamazepine, clobazam can enhance carbamazepine metabolism by as much as 50%, probably by inducing its epoxidation (Munoz et al. 1990).

II. Pharmacodynamic Interactions

Although pharmacodynamic interactions involving anticonvulsant drugs have been well documented in animal studies (Bourgeois and Wad 1988), there are little data on the occurrence and magnitude of such interactions in man. This can be attributed to the difficulty in identifying such interactions and also, in part, to the fact that in many situations simultaneous pharmacokinetic changes may contribute to the overall effect.

1. Interactions Between Anticonvulsant Drugs

It is well documented that in 10%–15% of patients who are refractory to single anticonvulsant drug therapy, duo therapy often provides better seizure control. Indeed, numerous anticonvulsant drug combinations are widely used because they are considered to be more effective in controlling various seizure types than either drug used alone. Such combinations include valproic acid plus ethosuximide, carbamazepine plus valproic acid and clonazepam plus valproic acid (Mireles and Leppik 1985; Ketter et al. 1992). The use of these synergistic combinations is not based on scientific evidence from clinical trials but is instead based on clinical experience. However, undesirable potentiation of side effects may also occur, consequent to pharmacodynamic interactions. For example, valproic acid-associated stupor and coma is observed in patients receiving other anticonvulsant drugs, particularly phenobarbitone.

Furthermore, anticonvulsant drug polytherapy has been associated with enhanced cognitive side effects. What is not clear, however, is whether the more severe seizure disorder that may be associated with these patients taking polytherapy regimens may be contributing to the impaired cognition.

2. Interactions Between Anticonvulsant Drugs and Other Drugs

During chronic polytherapy with anticonvulsant drugs, agents such as atracurium, frusemide, metocurine, pancuronium and vecuronium appear to be less effective at conventional doses (ORNSTEIN et al. 1985; ROTH and EBRAHIM 1987; TEMPELHOFF et al. 1990). It has been suggested that anticonvulsant-treated patients have a reduced sensitivity to these drugs, but the exact mechanism is not clear.

Furthermore, alcohol, phenothiazine and various antihistamines exhibit enhanced CNS depression and some neuroleptic drugs and antidepressants have the potential to lower the seizure threshold and to exacerbate seizures if taken with anticonvulsant drugs. During combination therapy with lithium and carbamazepine or phenytoin, some patients have presented with neurotoxicity, e.g. confusion, disorientation, drowsiness, ataxia and occasionally course tremor, hyperreflexia and cerebellar signs (SHUKLA et al. 1984). These side effects were not considered to be the result of pharmacokinetic interactions, since the plasma concentrations of carbamazepine, phenytoin and lithium were unaffected.

F. Interactions of the Recently Licensed Anticonvulsant Drugs

I. Pharmacokinetic Interactions

1. Vigabatrin

Vigabatrin is not protein bound, is minimally metabolized and is primarily (70%) excreted as unchanged drug in urine with a clearance similar to the value of the glomerular filtration rate. Therefore, theoretically, pharmacokinetic interactions involving vigabatrin should be minimal (PATSALOS 1999).

a) Interactions Affecting Vigabatrin

Even though vigabatrin is minimally metabolized, half-life values of 4–6h (compared with 5–7h in healthy volunteers) can be expected in patients with epilepsy who are also taking hepatic enzyme-inducing anticonvulsant drugs. These interactions are not of clinical relevance and to the present there have been no reports in relation to any other drug affecting the pharmacokinetics of vigabatrin.

b) Interactions Where Vigabatrin Affects Other Drugs

Interactions whereby vigabatrin affects the pharmacokinetics of other drugs would not be expected to occur. Its use, however, has been associated with a 7% reduction in plasma phenobarbitone concentrations and an 11% reduction in plasma primidone concentrations. Although these interactions are not considered clinically significant, a more significant interaction occurs between vigabatrin and phenytoin (Tables 9, 10). When vigabatrin is coadministered with phenytoin, a 20%–30% reduction in plasma phenytoin concentrations is seen after approximately 1 month. The mechanism of this interaction is unknown (protein binding displacement, induction of hepatic enzymes or an effect on absorption have been excluded) but the interaction can be clinically significant in some patients and may require an increase in phenytoin dosage to maintain seizure control (Browne et al. 1987; Rimmer and Richens 1989). The withdrawal of vigabatrin may on occasion precipitate phenytoin toxicity and a need to decrease phenytoin dosage.

2. Lamotrigine

Lamotrigine is primarily metabolized by hepatic *N*-glucuronidation (65% of the dose) with some (10%) being excreted unchanged in the urine. Only 60% is bound to plasma proteins.

a) Interactions Affecting Lamotrigine

The N-glucuronidation of lamotrigine is particularly susceptible to inhibition and induction. Thus, whilst in healthy volunteers the mean elimination half-life of lamotrigine is approximately 24h, its half-life is reduced to a mean of 15h in patients with epilepsy already receiving enzyme-inducing drugs such as carbamazepine, phenobarbitone and phenytoin. In contrast, valproic acid inhibits the metabolism of lamotrigine so that, typically, half-life values of the order of 60h are observed (Yuen et al. 1992). Interestingly, in patients treated with a combination of valproic acid and enzyme-inducing drugs, mean half-life values of 30h have been reported for lamotrigine. Thus, in prescribing lamotrigine a different dosing strategy for the drug needs to be used depending on what comedication is prescribed (Tables 9, 10).

b) Interactions Where Lamotrigine Affects Other Drugs

The lack of any induction effects on hepatic drug metabolizing enzymes by lamotrigine and its relatively low binding to plasma proteins (60%) suggest that interactions with concomitant drugs will be minimal. Nevertheless, lamotrigine has been associated with a 25% reduction in steady-state plasma valproic acid concentrations (Anderson et al. 1996). Also, during comedication with carbamazepine, plasma carbamazepine-epoxide concentrations have been observed to increase by as much as 45%, resulting in significant neuro-

Table 9. Effect of generally available anticonvulsant drugs (ACDs) on plasma concentration of newly licensed ACDs

Added ACD	Existing ACD							
	VGT	LTG	GBP	TPM	FBM	OXC	TGB	ZNS
PB	VGT↓	LTG⇓	NA	TPM⇓	FBM⇓	OXC⇓ 10-OH-OXC⇓	TGB⇓	ZNS⇓
PHT	VGT↓	LTG⇓	NA	TPM⇓	FBM⇓	OXC⇓ 10-OH-OXC⇓	TGB⇓	ZNS⇓
PRM	VGT↓	LTG⇓	NA	TPM⇓	FBM⇓	?	TGB⇓	ZNS⇓
ESM	NA	NA	NA	NA	?	?	?	?
CBZ	VGT↓	LTG⇓	NA	TPM⇓	FBM⇓	OXC⇓ 10-OH-OXC⇓	TGB⇓	ZNS⇓
VPA	NA	LTG⇑	NA	NA	NA	NA	NA	NA

For an explanation of abbreviations, see Table 10.

Table 10. Effect of newly licensed anticonvulsant drugs (ACDs) on plasma concentration of generally available ACDs

Added ACD	Existing ACD					
	PB	PHT	PRM	ESM	CBZ	VPA
VGT	PB↓	PHT⇓	PRM↓ PB↓	NA	NA	NA
LTG	NA	NA	NA	NA	CBZ-E↑	NA
GBP	NA	NA	NA	NA	NA	NA
TPM	NA	PHT⇑	NA	NA	NA	VPA⇓
FBM	PB⇑	PHT⇑	?	?	CBZ⇓ CBZ-E⇑	VPA⇑
OXC	NA	NA	NA	NA	NA	NA
TGB	NA	NA	NA	?	NA	VPA↓
ZNS	NA	PHT⇑	NA	?	CBZ⇑	NA

CBZ, carbamazepine; CBZ-E, carbamazepine-epoxide; ESM, ethosuximide; FBM, felbamate; GBP, gabapentin; LTG, lamotrigine; OXC, oxcarbazepine; 10-OH-OXC, 10,11-dihydroxycarbazepine; PB, phenobarbitone; PHT, phenytoin; PRM, primidone; TGB, tiagabine; TPM, topiramate; VPA, valproic acid; VGT, vigabatrin; ZNS, zonisamide; NA, none anticipated; ? indicates an unknown effect; ↓ an infrequently observed decrease in plasma concentration; ⇓ a frequently observed decrease in plasma concentration; ↑ an infrequently observed increase in plasma concentration; ⇓ a frequently observed increase in plasma concentration.

logical side effects (WARNER et al. 1992). However, the relevance and mechanism of these interactions are unknown.

Paracetamol (acetaminophen), like lamotrigine, is primarily metabolized by glucuronidation. During comedication its metabolism is enhanced (20%) by lamotrigine (DEPOT et al. 1990). The clinical significance of this interaction is at present uncertain.

3. Gabapentin

Gabapentin is not bound to plasma proteins and is not metabolized, the whole ingested dose being excreted unchanged in urine. Theoretically, therefore, gabapentin should not be a target for drug interactions and indeed no significant interactions have been reported to the present (Tables 9, 10).

a) Interactions Affecting Gabapentin

Gabapentin absorption can be affected by antacids containing magnesium or aluminium hydroxides and the interactions can reduce gabapentin plasma concentrations by up to 24% (BUSCH et al 1992).

b) Interactions Where Gabapentin Affects Other Drugs

With the exception of a single case of phenytoin toxicity in a patient comedicated with gabapentin, carbamazepine and clobazam, there is little evidence of gabapentin affecting the pharmacokinetics of other drugs (TYNDEL 1994).

4. Topiramate

Whilst more than 60% of a topiramate dose is excreted unchanged in the urine of uninduced patients, only 30% is excreted unchanged in patient taking enzyme-inducing anticonvulsant drugs. Thus, in patients taking inducing drugs, metabolic elimination is a major determinant of topiramate disposition. Topiramate appears to inhibit the activity of CYP2C19 and induce that of CYP3A.

a) Interactions Affecting Topiramate

Hepatic enzyme-inducing anticonvulsant drugs such as carbamazepine, phenobarbitone and phenytoin induce the metabolism of topiramate, so that topiramate plasma concentrations can be expected to decrease by approximately 50% (Tables 9, 10; SACHDEO et al. 1996).

b) Interactions Where Topiramate Affects Other Drugs

In addition to phenytoin inducing the metabolism of topiramate, topiramate can increase phenytoin plasma concentrations (probably by inhibition of CYP2C19) by as much as 25% in those patients whose phenytoin metabolism is at or near saturation. Interestingly, topiramate dose-dependently decreases plasma valproic acid concentrations; the significance of this is unknown (ROSENFELD et al. 1997b). In addition, topiramate enhances the metabolism of digoxin and oral contraceptives. Consequently plasma digoxin concentrations should be monitored when topiramate is added to or withdrawn from a patient's therapy. Also, an approximate 30% increase in the clearance of the oestrogen component of oral contraceptive preparations makes it advisable to prescribe an oral contraceptive containing at least 25 g oestrogen for women taking topiramate (ROSENFELD et al. 1997a).

5. Felbamate

Approximately 50% of a felbamate dose is eliminated by hepatic metabolism, with about 15% being eliminated via reactions catalysed by CYP3A4 and CYP2E1 isoenzymes. At clinically relevant plasma concentrations, felbamate is thought to induce CYP3A4 and to inhibit CYP2C19 and β-oxidation.

a) Interactions Affecting Felbamate

Carbamazepine and phenytoin induce the metabolism of felbamate, resulting in lower than expected steady-state plasma felbamate concentrations (WAGNER et al. 1993). In contrast, vigabatrin and lamotrigine have no effect.

b) Interactions Where Felbamate Affects Other Drugs

Felbamate exhibits significant pharmacokinetic interactions with phenytoin, phenobarbitone, valproic acid and carbamazepine, but not with lamotrigine or oxcarbazepine (GRAVES et al. 1989; WAGNER et al. 1993; REIDENBERG et al. 1995; HOOPER et al. 1996). Plasma phenytoin, phenobarbitone and valproic acid concentrations have been reported to rise by 20%, 24% and 50% respectively in some patients, upon the introduction of felbamate. The increase in plasma valproic acid concentrations can be attributed to inhibition of the β-oxidation pathway for valproic acid. During comedication with carbamazepine, plasma concentrations of the latter decrease by 20%. This reduction is associated with a concurrent increase in the plasma concentration of carbamazepine-epoxide, the pharmacologically active metabolite of carbamazepine.

Felbamate has been observed to interact with oral contraceptives in that gestodene and ethinyloestradiol plasma concentration are reduced; however, the effect on ethinyloestradiol is probably of little clinical significance (SAANO et al. 1995).

6. Oxcarbazepine

Oxcarbazepine, a keto derivative of carbamazepine, can be considered a prodrug since it is rapidly biotransformed to two metabolites of which the primary one 10,11-dihydro-10-hydroxycarbazepine is pharmacologically active. Because ketone reductase and glucuronyl-transferase enzymes are primarily responsible for the metabolism of oxcarbazepine, and unlike cytochrome P450-dependent enzymes are less prone to induction and inhibitory effects, oxcarbazepine exhibits no, or only a weak, enzyme induction potential in man (PATSALOS et al. 1990). Oxcarbazepine seems to alter significantly the pharmacokinetics of some compounds that are primarily metabolized by CYP3A3 and CYP3A4.

a) Interactions Affecting Oxcarbazepine

Carbamazepine, phenytoin and phenobarbitone, but not valproic acid, induce the metabolism of the hydroxycarbazepine metabolite of oxcarbazepine (TARTARA et al. 1993; MCKEE et al. 1994). Whether the magnitude of these interactions is clinically significant needs to be ascertained. However, crossover studies of carbamazepine to oxcarbazepine therapy have been associated with an elevation in plasma concentrations of concomitant anticonvulsant drugs (e.g. phenytoin and valproic acid). Therefore if patients are to be switched from carbamazepine to oxcarbazepine, reduction of concomitant drug dosage regimens will be necessary if the precipitation of toxicity is to be avoided.

A small but statistically significant decrease in plasma hydroxycarbazepine concentrations is observed when oxcarbazepine is coadministered with viloxazine (11%) and verapamil (20%) (KRAMER et al. 1991; PISANI et al. 1994).

b) Interactions Where Oxcarbazepine Affects Other Drugs

A significant decrease in the bioavailability of an oral contraceptive pill (containing the hormones ethinyloestradiol and levonorgestrel) secondary to oxcarbazepine comedication has been observed (KLOSTERKOV JENSEN et al. 1992). Repeated coadministration of oxcarbazepine, but not single doses of the drug, decreases the bioavailability of the calcium antagonist felodipine (ZACARA et al. 1993). These effects may reflect the induction of a cytochrome P450 isoenzyme.

7. Tiagabine

Tiagabine is substantially bound to plasma proteins (96%) and extensively metabolized by the liver (CYP3A), with only a small proportion of the dose being excreted unchanged in the urine.

a) Interactions Affecting Tiagabine

During comedication with enzyme-inducing anticonvulsants (carbamazepine, phenobarbitone and phenytoin) the metabolism of tiagabine is accelerated so that its elimination half-life is decreased from 5–8h to 2–3h. Naproxen, salicylates and valproic acid displace tiagabine from its protein binding sites in vitro, but the in vivo clinical relevance of this is unknown (So et al. 1995).

b) Interactions Where Tiagabine Affects Other Drugs

Even though tiagabine is extensively metabolized by CYP3A it does not appear to induce or inhibit this isoenzyme's activity. Thus, with the exception of an occasional small decline in plasma valproic acid concentrations, tiagabine comedication has had no effect on the pharmacokinetics of other drugs.

8. Zonisamide

The metabolism of zonisamide is saturable, resulting in a non-linear relationship between its plasma concentrations and its dose. Numerous hepatic metabolic pathways are involved in its metabolism and it appears that the drug induces the activity of CYP3A and inhibits that of CYP2C19.

a) Interactions Affecting Zonisamide

The metabolism of zonisamide is inducible by enzyme-inducing anticonvulsant drugs (Ojemann et al. 1986). Thus in patients prescribed carbamazepine and phenytoin, zonisamide half-lives of 27–36h can be expected, which are approximately 50% shorter than those in individuals not receiving these drugs.

b) Interactions Where Zonisamide Affects Other Drugs

Plasma concentrations of concurrently administered carbamazepine and phenytoin may be elevated during comedication with zonisamide, so that it is advisable to monitor plasma concentrations of these drugs when zonisamide is added to therapy or its use is discontinued (Kaneko et al. 1993). To the present no other interactions have been reported.

II. Pharmacodynamic Interactions

1. Interactions Between Anticonvulsant Drugs

It has recently been reported that lamotrigine in combination with valproic acid is more efficacious than either drug administered alone (Brodie et al. 1997). However, undesirable potentiation of side effects may also occur and valproic acid-associated tremor during the comedication has been reported (Reutens et al. 1993). A similar anticonvulsant synergism has been reported for tiagabine and vigabatrin in combination (Leach and Brodie 1994).

2. Interactions Between Anticonvulsant Drugs and Other Drugs

To the present, none has been reported.

G. Conclusions

Anticonvulsant drugs are widely used, with at least 4 million patients worldwide taking polytherapy regimens. Also, because of the long-term nature of epilepsy it is not unusual for drugs used to treat conditions other than epilepsy to be prescribed as well. Consequently, the possibility of pharmacokinetic interactions is high. The large number of such interactions that have been described in recent years relates in part to the widespread availability of therapeutic drug monitoring in the management of epilepsy. However, the more recent understanding of which specific cytochrome P450 isoenzymes are responsible for anticonvulsant drug metabolism has also contributed significantly, particularly in relation to the newly licensed drugs.

Although there are long lists of potentially interacting drugs, it is impractical for the clinician to memorize these. The best approach to the prevention of potentially harmful effects of anticonvulsant drug interactions is to remember those that are most likely to be encountered and which are clinically relevant, to understand their underlying mechanisms and to measure plasma anticonvulsant drug concentrations whenever a drug combination is in use. Knowledge of the mechanism of an interaction may allow anticipation of its observed effect.

Although in general drug interactions, particularly those encountered with the widely available anticonvulsant drugs, are considered problematic and to be avoided where possible, it should be remembered that they may not always be detrimental, and can be used to improve seizure control. Furthermore, interactions involving the newly licensed and expensive anticonvulsant drugs may actually allow more patients to have access to these drugs. Thus, deliberate coprescribing of drugs which allow the dosage of a new anticonvulsant drug to be reduced, while maintaining its blood concentration within its target range, may not only be therapeutically sound but may prove economically efficient.

Finally, even though possible pharmacokinetic interactions of the new anticonvulsant drugs have been investigated extensively, pharmacodynamic interactions, which are at least as important, are largely unknown and need careful investigation. It is possible that through extensive clinical experience with these new drugs still more interactions may be identified.

References

Abbott FS, Kassam J, Orr MJ, Farrell K (1986) The effect of aspirin on valproic acid metabolism. Clin Pharmacol Therap 40:94–100

Anderson GD, Yau MK, Gidal BE, Harris SJ, Levy RH, Lai AA, Wolf KB, Wargin WA, Dren AT (1996) Bidirectional interaction of valproate and lamotrigine in healthy subjects. Clin Pharmacol Ther 60:145–156

Back DJ, Grimmer SFM, Orme MLE, Proudlove C, Mann RD, Breckenridge AM (1988) Evaluation of Committee on Safety of Medicines yellow card reports on oral contraceptive-drug interactions with anti-convulsants and antibiotics. Br J Clin Pharmacol 25:527–532

Bahls FH, Ozuna J, Ritchie DE (1991) Interaction between calcium channel blockers and the antiepileptic drugs carbamazepine and phenytoin. Neurology 41:740–742

Beckman JT, Olkkola KT, Ojala M, Laaksovirta H, Neuvonen PJ (1996) Concentrations and effects of oral midazolam are greatly reduced in patients treated with carbamazepine or phenytoin. Epilepsia 37:253–257

Bernus I, Dickinson RG, Hooper WD, Eadie MJ (1997) The mechanism of the carbamazepine-valproate interaction in humans. Br J Clin Pharmacol 44:21–27
Beurey J, Weber M, Vignaud JM (1982) Treatment of tinea capitis: metabolic interference of griseofulvin with phenobarbital. Annals Dermatol Venerol 109:567–570
Bittencourt PRM, Cracia CM, Martins R, Fernandes AG, Diekmann HW, Jung W (1992) Phenytoin and carbamazepine decrease oral bioavailability of praziquantel. Neurology 42:492–496
Bourgeois BFD, Wad N (1988) Combined administration of carbamazepine and phenobarbital: effect on anticonvulsant activity and neurotoxicity. Epilepsia 29:482–487
Breckenridge A (1974) Drug interactions with oral anticoagulants. Br Med J 2:397–400
Brodie MJ, Yuen AWC, 105 Study Group (1997) Lamotrigine substitution study: evidence for synergism with sodium valproate. Epilepsy Res 26:423–432
Brosen K, Kragh-Sorensen P (1993) Concomitant intake of nortriptyline and carbamazepine. Ther Drug Monit 15:258–260
Browne TR, Mattson RH, Penry JK et al. (1987) Vigabatrin for refractory complex partial seizures: multi-centre single-blind study with long term follow up. Neurology 37:184–189
Busch JA, Radulovic LL, Bockbrader HN (1992) Effect of maalox TC on single-dose pharmacokinetics of gabapentin capsules in healthy subjects. Pharm Res 9 [Suppl 2]:S315
Carl GF, Smith ML (1992) Phenytoin-folate interaction: differing effects of the sodium salt and the free acid of phenytoin. Epilepsia 33:372–375
Cartensen H, Jacobsen N, Dieperink H (1986) Interaction between cyclosporin A and phenobarbitone. Br J Clin Pharmacol 21:550–551
Couet W, Istin B, Ingrand I, Girault J, Fourtillan JB (1990) Effect of ponsinomycin on single-dose kinetics and metabolism of carbamazepine. Ther Drug Monit 12:144–149
Crawford P, Chadwick DJ, Martin C, Tjia J, Back DJ, Orme M (1990) The interaction of phenytoin and carbamazepine with combined oral contraceptive steroids. Br J Clin Pharmacol 30:892–896
Crowley JJ, Cusack BJ, Jue SG, Koup JR, Vestal RE (1987) Cigarette smoking and theophylline metabolism: effect of phenytoin. Clin Pharmacol Ther 42:334–340
Dalton MJ, Powell JR, Messenheimer JA, Clark J (1986) Cimetidine and carbamazepine: a complex drug interaction. Epilepsia 27:553–558
D'Arcy PF, McElnay JC (1987) Drug-antacid interactions of clinical importance. Drug Intel Clin Pharm 21:607–617
Dasgupta A, Dennen DA, Dean R, McLawhon RW (1991) Displacement of phenytoin from serum protein carriers by antibiotics: Studies with ceftriaxone, nafcillin and sulfamethoxazole. Clin Chem 37:98–100
Depot M, Powell JR, Messenheimer JA, Cloutier G, Dalton MJ (1990) Kinetic effects of multiple oral doses of acetaminophen on a single oral dose of lamotrigine. Clin Pharmacol Ther 48:346–355
Dhillon S, Richens A (1982) Valproic acid and diazepam interaction in vivo. Br J Clin Pharmacol 13:553–560
Duncan JS, Patsalos PN, Shorvon SD (1991) Effects of discontinuation of phenytoin, carbamazepine, and valproate on concomitant antiepileptic medication. Epilepsia 32:101–115
Goulden KJ, Dooley JM, Camfield PR, Fraser AD (1987) Clinical vaproate toxicity induced by acetylsalicylic acid. Neurology 37:1392–1394
Graves NM, Holmes GB, Fuerst RH, Leppik IE (1989) Effect of felbamate on phenytoin and carbamazepine serum concentrations. Epilepsia 30:225–229
Grimsley SR, Jann MW, Carter JG, D'Mello AP, D'Souza MJ (1991) Increased carbamazepine plasma concentrations after fluoxetine coadministration. Clin Pharmacol Ther 50:10–15

Hayden M, Buchanan NH (1991) Danazol: carbamazepine interaction. Med J Aust 155:851
Hooper WD, Franklin ME, Glue P et al. (1996) Effect of felbamate on valproic acid disposition in healthy volunteers: Inhibition of β-oxidation. Epilepsia 37:91–97
Iwahashi K, Miyatake R, Suwaki H, Hosokawa K, Ichikawa Y (1995) The drug-drug interaction effects of haloperidol on plasma carbamazepine levels. Clin Neuropharmacol 18:233–236
Kaneko S, Hayashimoto A, Niwayama H, Fukushima Y (1993) Effects of zonisamide on serum levels of phenytoin and carbamazepine. J Jpn Epilepsy Soc 11:31–35
Kay L, Kampmann JP, Svendsen TL, Vergman B, Hansen JEM, Skovsted L, Kristensen M (1985) Influence of rifampicin and isoniazid on the kinetics of phenytoin. Br J Clin Pharmacol 20:323–326
Kerr BM, Thummel KE, Wurden CJ, Klein SM, Kroetz DL, Gonzalez FJ, Levy RH (1994) Human liver carbamazepine metabolism: role of CYP3A4 and CYP2C8 in 10,11-epoxide formation. Biochem Pharmacol 47:1969–1979
Ketter TA, Pazzaglia PJ, Post RM (1992) Synergy of carbamazepine and valproic acid in affective illness: case report and review of the literature. J Clin Psychopharmacol 12:276–281
Klosterskov Jensen P, Saano V, Haring P, Svenstrup B, Menge GP (1992) Possible interaction between oxcarbazepine and an oral contraceptive. Epilepsia 33:1149–1152
Kramer G, Tettenborn B, Flesch G (1991) Oxcarbazepine-verapamil drug interaction in healthy volunteers. Epilepsia 32 [Suppl 1]:70–71
Leach JP, Brodie MJ (1994) Synergism with GABAergic drugs in refractory epilepsy. Lancet 343:1650
Levine M, Jones MW, Sheppard I (1985) Differential effects of cimetidine on serum concentrations of carbamazepine and phenytoin. Neurology 35:562–565
Mauro LS, Mauro VF, Brown DL, Somani P (1987) Enhancement of phenytoin elimination by multiple-dose activated charcoal. Annals Emerg Med 16:1132–1135
McGovern B, Geer VR, La Ruia PJ, Garan H, Ruskin JN (1984) Possible interaction between amiodarone and phenytoin. Ann Intern Med 101:650–651
McKee PJW, Blacklaw J, Forrest G, Gillham RA, Walker SM, Conelly D, Brodie MJ (1994) A double-blind, placebo-controlled interaction study between oxcarbazepine and carbamazepine, sodium valproate and phenytoin in epileptic patients. Br J Clin Pharmacol 37:27–32
Munoz JJ, De Salamanca RE, Diaz-Obregon C, Timoneda FL (1990) The effect of clobazam on steady state plasma concentrations of carbamazepine and its metabolites. Br J Clin Pharmacol 29:763–765
Naidu MUR, Shobha JC, Dixit VK, Kumar A, Kumar TR, Sekhar KR, Sekhar EC (1994) Effect of multiple dose omeprazole on the pharmacokinetics of carbamazepine. Drug Invest 7:8–12
Ojemann LM, Shastri RA, Wilensky AJ, Friel PN, Levy RH, McLean JR, Buchanan RA (1986) Comparative pharmacokinetics of zonisamide (CI-912) in epileptic patients on carbamazepine or phenytoin monotherapy. Ther Drug Monit 8:293–296
Ornstein E, Matteo RS, Young WL, Diaz J (1985) Resistance to metocurine-induced neuromuscular blockade in patients receiving phenytoin. Anesthesiology 63:294–298
Otani K, Ishida M, Kaneko S, Mihara K, Ohkubo T, Osanai T, Sugawara K (1996) Effects of carbamazepine coadministration on plasma concentrations of trazodone and its active metabolite, m-chlorphenylpiperazine. Ther Drug Monit 18:164–167
Parmeggiani A, Riva R, Posar A, Rossi PG (1995) Possible interaction between acyclovir and antiepileptic treatment. Ther Drug Monit 17:312–315
Patsalos PN (1999) New antiepileptic drugs. Ann Clin Biochem 36:10–19
Patsalos PN, Zakrzewska JM, Elyas AA (1990) Dose dependent enzyme induction by oxcarbazepine? Eur J Clin Pharmacol 39:187–188

Pearce GA (1988) Apparent inhibition of phenytoin absorption by an enteral nutrient formula. Aust J Hosp Pharm 18:289–292

Pisani F, Fazio A, Oteri G, Artesi C, Xiao B, Perucca E, DiPerri R (1994) Effects of the antidepressant drug viloxazine on oxcarbazepine and its hydroxylated metabolites in patients with epilepsy. Acta Neurol Scand 90:130–132

Pisani F, Fazio A, Oteri G, Spira E, Perucca E, Bertilsson L (1988) Effect of valpromide on the pharmacokinetics of carbamazepine-10, 11-epoxide. Br J Clin Pharmacol 25:611–613

Pisani F, Haj-Yehia A, Fazio A et al. (1993) Carbamazepine-valnoctamide interaction in epileptic patients: In vitro/in vivo correlation. Epilepsia 34:954–959

Powell JR, Nelson E, Conrad KA, Likes K, Byers J (1981) Phenobarbital clearance, elimination with alkaline diuresis, and bioavailability in adults. Clin Pharmacol Ther 29:273–274

Reidenberg P, Glue P, Banfield CR et al. (1995) Effects of felbamate on the pharmacokinetics of phenobarbital. Clin Pharmacol Ther 58:279–287

Reutens DC, Duncan JS, Patsalos PN (1993) Disabling tremor after lamotrigine with sodium valproate. Lancet 342:185–186

Rimmer EM, Richens A (1989) Interaction between vigabatrin and phenytoin. Br J Clin Pharmacol 27 [Suppl 1]:S27–S33

Rosenfeld WE, Doose DR, Walker SA, Nayak RK (1997a) Effect of topiramate on the pharmacokinetics of an oral contraceptive containing norethindrone and ethinyl estradiol in patients with epilepsy. Epilepsia 38:317–323

Rosenfeld WE, Liao S, Kramer LD, Anderson G, Palmer M, Levy RH, Nayak RK (1997b) Comparison of the steady-state pharmacokinetics of topiramate and valproate in patients with epilepsy during monotherapy and concomitant therapy. Epilepsia 38:324–333

Roth S, Ebrahim ZY (1987) Resistance to pancuronium in patients receiving carbamazepine. Anesthesiology 66:691–693

Saano V, Glue P, Banfield CR et al. (1995) Effects of felbamate on the pharmacokinetics of a low-dose combination oral contraceptive. Clin Pharmacol Ther 58:523–531

Sachdeo RC, Sachdeo SK, Walker SA, Kramer LD, Nayak RK, Doose DR (1996) Steady-state pharmacokinetics of topiramate and carbamazepine in patients with epilepsy during monotherapy and concomitant therapy. Epilepsia 37:774–780

Salke-Kellermann RA, May T, Boenigt HE (1997) Influence of ethosuximide on valproic acid serum concentrations. Epilepsy Res 26:345–349

Sato J, Sekizawa Y, Yoshida A et al. (1992) Single-dose kinetics of primidone in human subjects: effect of phenytoin on formulation and elimination of active metabolites of primidone, phenobarbital and phenylethylmalonamide. J Pharmacobiol-Dyn 15:467–472

Sehgal VN, Jrivastava G (1988) Corticosteroid – irresponsive pemphigus vulgaris following antiepileptic therapy. Internat J Dermatol 27:258

Shackleford EJ, Watson FT (1987) Amiodarone-phenytoin interaction. Drug Intel Clin Pharm 21:921

Shukla S, Goodwin CD, Long LEG, Miller MG (1984) Lithium-carbamazepine neurotoxicity and risk factors. Amer J Psychiat 141:1604–1606

So EL, Wolff D, Graves NM, Leppik IE, Cascino GD, Pixton GC, Gustavson LE (1995) Pharmacokinetics of tiagabine as add-on therapy in patients taking enzyme-inducing antiepilepsy drugs. Epilepsy Res 22:221–226

Spatzenegger M, Jaeger W (1995) Clinical importance of cytochrome P450 in drug metabolism. Drug Metab Rev 27:397–417

Tartara A, Galimberti CA, Manni R et al. (1991) Differential effects of valproic acid and enzyme-inducing anticonvulsants on nimodipine pharmacokinetics in epileptic patients. Br J Clin Pharmacol 32:335–340

Tartara A, Galimberti CA, Manni R et al. (1993) The pharmacokinetics of oxcarbazepine and its active metabolite 10-hydroxy-carbazepine in healthy subjects and

in epileptic patients treated with phenobarbitone and valproic acid. Br J Clin Pharmacol 36:366–368
Tassaneeyakul W, Veronese ME, Birkett DJ, Doecke CJ, McManus ME, Sansom LN, Miners JO (1992) Co-regulation of phenytoin and tolbutamide metabolism in humans. Br J Clin Pharmacol 34:494–498
Tempelhoff R, Modica PA, Spitznayel EC (1990) Antiepileptic therapy increases fentanyl requirements during anaesthesia for craniotomy. Can J Anaesth 37:327–332
Tyndal F (1994) Interaction of gabapentin with other antiepileptics. Lancet 343:1363–1364
Wagner ML, Remmel RP, Graves NM, Leppik IE (1993) Effect of felbamate on carbamazepine and its major metabolites. Clin Pharmacol Ther 53:536–543
Warner T, Patsalos PN, Prevett M, Elyas AA, Duncan JS (1992) Lamotrigine-induced carbamazepine toxicity: an interaction with carbamazepine-10, 11-epoxide. Epilepsy Res 11:147–150
Wroblewski BA, Singer WD, Whyte J (1986) Carbamazepine-erythromycin interaction. Case studies and clinical significance. J Amer Med Assoc 255:1165–1167
Yue CP, Mann KS, Chan KH (1987) Severe thrombocytopenia due to combined cimetidine and phentoin therapy. Neurosurgery 20:963–965
Yuen AWC, Land G, Weatherley BC, Peck AW (1992) Sodium valproate acutely inhibits lamotrigine metabolism. Br J Clin Pharmacol 33:511–513
Yukawa E, Higuchi S, Aoyama T (1989) The effect of concurrent administration of sodium valproate on serum concentrations of primidone and its metabolite phenobarbital. J Clin Pharm Ther 14:387–392
Zaccara G, Gangemi PF, Bendoni L, Menge GP, Schwabe S, Monza GC (1993) Influence of single and repeated doses of oxcarbazepine on the pharmacokinetic profile of felodipine. Ther Drug Monit 15:39–42

CHAPTER 23

The Use of Antiepileptic Drugs in Clinical Practice

M.J. EADIE

A. Introduction

The first reasonably effective drug therapy for epilepsy became available in 1857 (LOCOCK 1857). Over the subsequent years, the number of available efficacious antiepileptic drugs has increased and their pattern of clinical use has evolved progressively. Since the previous version of the present book appeared in 1985 there has been continuing gradual, rationally based development in the practice of antiepileptic drug therapy. As well, the use of what are customarily regarded as antiepileptic drugs for indications other than epilepsy has grown.

B. Changes in Antiepileptic Drug Use for Epilepsy

The changes in the ways in which antiepileptic drugs have been used to treat epilepsy in recent years appear to depend on several factors, particularly those discussed below.

I. Increased Knowledge of the Natural History of Epilepsy

In the past decade a considerable amount has been published concerning the natural history of epilepsy, though nearly all of it necessarily deals with treated epilepsy. Much of this work has emanated from careful community-based investigations, instead of being drawn mainly from patients referred to specialized epilepsy services, which were the sources of most earlier data. It has become clear that such previous referral patterns led to patients with difficult-to-control epilepsy, with its less favourable outlook for cure, tending to be over-represented in many earlier studies on the prognosis of the disorder. The widely accepted and long-standing view that epilepsy, once established in a patient, would persist for that patient's lifetime (GOWERS 1881), is no longer sustainable. In at least two out of three persons with epilepsy (or seven in ten) treated with antiepileptic drugs, the disorder will become inactive after a few years (ANNEGERS et al. 1979a; SANDER 1993; COCKERELL et al. 1995). Recently, indications have become available that a similar relatively favourable outlook also probably applies for the untreated disorder (O'DONOGHUE and SANDER 1996). Drug therapy may prevent the occurrence of epileptic seizures, but whether it influences the ultimate outcome for the average patient with epilepsy has now become rather less certain (O'Donoghue and Sander 1996; Shinnar and Berg 1996). This uncertainty, of course, is not necessarily an argument against treating epilepsy with antiepileptic drugs: as stated above, epileptic seizures may be prevented by such treatment, and seizures can have very deleterious consequences for the sufferer's physical health, psychological and social life, and career prospects. They also involve an increased risk of sudden, otherwise unexplained death (Cockerell 1996), though this sometimes appears to be associated with evidence of non-compliance with prescribed therapy (Lund and Gormsen 1985). The probable failure of antiepileptic drug therapy to influence the long-term remission rate in epilepsy may be an argument against giving an excessive priority to achieving early, complete control of seizures, as was sometimes suggested to be desirable in the recent past (Reynolds 1987, 1988; Oller-Daurella and Oller 1991). Avoidance of even the first seizure in those at increased risk of such an event, e.g. after head injury (Temkin et al. 1990), no longer seems as important as it did a few years ago.

Data such as those above, and accumulating information about prognostic factors for particular epileptic seizure syndromes, are having an increasing influence on clinical practice. However, it should be kept in mind that those who manage most patients with epilepsy will probably also continue to be responsible for the care of an atypically severe population of epilepsy sufferers. They will therefore need to interpret information derived from general community-based studies in the light of this realization.

II. A More Critical Application of Pharmacokinetic Concepts

In the 1970s, with the increasingly widespread availability of facilities for monitoring plasma anticonvulsant concentrations, it became clear that the monitoring often led to improved seizure control and to fewer adverse effects of antiepileptic therapy. The monitoring was no doubt sometimes used uncritically (Beardsley et al. 1983: Schoenenberger et al. 1995), and the expectation developed that achieving a "therapeutic" range plasma concentration of an antiepileptic drug represented the optimal possible management of a given patient's epilepsy with that drug. This view probably arose because the plasma concentration of an exogenous foreign substance was interpreted in a way that was more appropriate to the evaluation of the plasma concentration of an endogenous physiological material, e.g. glucose, urea. Accumulating experience has increasingly revealed the fallacies inherent in such a pattern of interpretation of plasma drug concentration data and the limited benefits that may emanate from it. As a result, over the past decade plasma antiepileptic drug concentration monitoring has increasingly been used with a more critical appreciation of its merits. The monitoring is thus perceived as an extremely valuable aid to clinical judgement in achieving seizure control, but not as the ultimate tool for this purpose. This more critical attitude to monitoring has been reinforced by the marketing of new antiepileptic drugs (see below) for which therapeutic range plasma concentrations have not yet been defined. Dosages of these newer drugs have to be adjusted on a basis of clinical judgement assisted by insight into pharmacokinetic principles, unaided (or unhampered) by plasma drug concentration data. Doing this has again brought home the realization that antiepileptic drugs can be used successfully without the need for plasma drug concentration monitoring.

Over the past quarter of a century, monitoring of plasma antiepileptic drug concentrations has provided valuable insights into the management of the drug therapy of epilepsy. Monitoring is now probably being used less than it was as an almost unthinking routine and increasingly in a more discriminating way (Mattson 1995), as a better balanced and more realistic perspective develops regarding its virtues and its limitations.

III. The Availability of New Antiepileptic Drugs

Over the past 5 years several new antiepileptic drugs have been marketed in various countries (vigabatrin, lamotrigine, gabapentin, topiramate, tiagabine, zonisamide, oxcarbazepine, felbamate). The number of agents available for treating epilepsy has more than doubled over this comparatively short period, and additional drugs are being developed (Chaps. 6 and 21, this volume). There has not yet been time for these newly introduced drugs to find their definitive places in the epileptologist's therapeutic armamentarium. They have so far been studied mainly as add-on therapy in patients whose seizure disorders have proved resistant to longer-established therapies, and in contemporary medical practice they are used mainly in this clinical situation. However, data are beginning to appear comparing their efficacies and adverse effect profiles with those of the older drugs when used as monotherapy at the outset of the treatment of epilepsy (Brodie et al. 1995; Tanganelli and Regesta 1996; Christe et al. 1997).

IV. A Better Understanding of the Mechanisms of Action of Antiepileptic Drugs

A reasonably satisfactory understanding of the biochemical mechanisms of action of nearly all the marketed antiepileptic drugs has become available over the past decade (Macdonald and Kelly 1994). This knowledge has opened the way to using rational combinations of antiepileptic drugs which might be expected to yield more successful control of epilepsy by interfering with the molecular mechanisms involved in epileptogenesis at more than one separate stage of the process. At present, antiepileptic drug combinations are nearly always used only after therapy with single agents has failed. However, with experience, the use of rational drug combinations from the outset of therapy may prove beneficial in certain epilepsies for which the chances of control by antiepileptic drug monotherapy are not particularly favourable.

V. The Maturing of the Surgical Therapy of Epilepsy

The surgery of epilepsy has developed to a stage at which, in many centres, it represents a realistic alternative to further trials of antiepileptic drug combinations, in particular when a seizure disorder is present which is likely to benefit from operation and several attempts at antiepileptic drug monotherapy have failed. This additional therapeutic option will often shorten the time available to the prescriber for trying the numerous possible permutations and combinations of the older and newer antiepileptic drugs, before the patient requests what may be perceived as a definitive cure. This has made it even more desirable to select the potentially most appropriate antiepileptic drugs and drug combinations for each patient as early as possible in the course of therapy.

C. The Decision to Prescribe Antiepileptic Drug Therapy

The decision to use antiepileptic drugs will probably be made in one of three main sets of circumstances, viz.

1. When the patient is considered to be at a high enough risk of developing seizures, though no seizure has yet occurred
2. When no more than a solitary seizure has occurred, and
3. When the patient has already experienced more than one seizure, i.e. when the patient has epilepsy (in the conventional sense of that term).

I. Prevention of Anticipated (Usually Situation-Related) Seizures

After head injuries, particularly ones which penetrate the substance of the brain, or after neurosurgical operations involving the cerebral cortex (Deutschman and Haines 1985), the risk of seizures is often considered high enough for prophylactic anticonvulsant therapy to be used without waiting for the first seizure to occur. The antiepileptic drugs used for partial (localization-relation) epilepsies are usually employed (see below) and decrease the short and medium term risk of seizures occurring (Shinnar and Berg 1996). However, antiepileptic drug therapy in these circumstances is now known to make little difference to the risk of later continuing epilepsy developing (Shinnar and Berg 1996). Knowledge of this lack of long term dividend is likely to reduce enthusiasm for the use of such antiepileptic drug prophylaxis, unless significant advantage to the patient would accrue from preventing seizures in the first few months after the cerebral insult.

The risk of eclamptic seizures around the time of labour in hypertensive pregnant epileptic women is also high enough to warrant attempts at seizure prevention. In this situation magnesium sulphate is probably the preferred therapy, having proven at the least more effective than phenytoin (Lucas et al. 1995).

II. After a Solitary Seizure

Patients who present after a solitary seizure are unlikely to be fully representative of the epileptic population in the community. Solitary seizure sufferers are more likely to have had tonic-clonic seizures, whereas those with simple partial seizures, absences and myoclonic attacks will tend to be underrepresented because patients with these relatively less severe epilepsies usually have experienced multiple episodes before they first present clinically. A decade ago it was thought that the solitary seizure usually represented the beginning of an ongoing seizure disorder, i.e. epilepsy (REYNOLDS 1987; HART et al. 1990). Therefore it was argued that the occurrence of a solitary seizure usually warranted the prescription of antiepileptic drug therapy unless the attack was precipitated by circumstances which were unlikely to occur again, e.g. heavy alcohol intake, a very recent head injury, aseptic meningitis. The main exception to this early treatment policy was the first simple febrile convulsion in infancy. In this syndrome, even though further febrile illnesses and seizures might occur, it was already believed that continuous prophylactic antiepileptic therapy was unnecessary. Phenobarbitone (FAERO et al. 1972) and valproate (CAVAZUTTI 1975) were known to prevent further attacks, but this prevention did not influence the (low) risk of subsequent non-febrile epilepsy (ANNEGERS et al. 1979b). Antiepileptic therapy taken at times of heightened seizure risk was considered a preferable course (ROSMAN 1997).

It is known that appropriate antiepileptic drug prophylaxis will halve the risk of recurrence of an initial single non-situation-related seizure (FIRST SEIZURE TRIAL GROUP 1993). Published figures for the chance of further seizures after a single fit vary, but the meta-analysis of BERG and SHINNAR (1991) indicates that the best estimate of the risk is in the range 40%–52%. Not all solitary seizures come to medical attention at or near their time of occurrence. For solitary seizures which present to medical practitioners at or soon after their occurrence, the 78% risk of recurrence within 3 years found in the National General Practice Study of Epilepsy (HART et al. 1990) probably provides the best available estimate of the risk. Risk factors for further attacks after a single seizure are known (EADIE 1996). They include the presence of abnormal neurological signs, the seizures being partial ones, and the age of the patient being below 16 years or the patient being elderly. The risk diminishes the longer the patient goes without a further seizure. The presence of epileptiform abnormalities in the routine EEG increases the risk of recurrence (VAN DONSELAAR et al. 1992). Antiepileptic drug therapy probably appears indicated if one or more of the risk factors applies after a solitary seizure has occurred. Otherwise, and particularly if more than 6 months have elapsed between the seizure and the time of presentation (since most solitary seizures which go on to epilepsy have done so by this time), the risk of a further episode appears too low to warrant therapy unless another attack would hold unusually severe disadvantages for the patient.

Because of the types of epilepsy likely to present as a solitary seizure, if an antiepileptic drug is to be used carbamazepine will probably be the preferred agent at the present time. Phenytoin, phenobarbitone and valproate are the main alternatives in contemporary practice, but this situation may change as the newer antiepileptic drugs increasingly find their places in therapeutics.

III. Definite Epilepsy

Most patients for whom antiepileptic drugs are prescribed will have already experienced two or more epileptic events before their initial clinical presentation. Unless a definite and avoidable circumstance has precipitated all the patient's seizures, antiepileptic drug therapy will nearly always be indicated. Rarely the advantages of treatment may be outweighed by the disadvantages, e.g. in a severely intellectually retarded, unemployable individual who over a long period has had only occasional minor seizures which have caused minimal interference with his or her life, and who may have developed severely disturbed behaviour when given various sedatives in the past. In such instances antiepileptic drug therapy may be considered undesirable.

In some epilepsies, e.g. the Lennox-Gastaut syndrome (Yagi 1996), it will be accepted from the outset that antiepileptic therapy will probably be required for many years and perhaps for the remainder of the patient's life. However, in the majority of patients who have experienced no more than a few epileptic seizures by their time of presentation, antiepileptic treatment is likely to be necessary for only a few years.

The choice of appropriate drug therapy for such epilepsy is discussed below.

D. The Choice of an Antiepileptic Drug

Some antiepileptic drugs appear to be more satisfactory for certain epilepsies than for others, as discussed in Chap. 1. Correlations between the drugs and the epileptic syndromes for which they appear most useful are set out in Table 1, though there is not as much statistical evidence available for the correlations as might have been expected (Chadwick and Turnbull 1985). When the matter has been investigated in controlled clinical trials, the differences between the drugs have tended to relate as much to the incidences and severities of adverse effects as to the drug's actual abilities to prevent seizures in the different epilepsies (Heller et al. 1995; de Silva et al. 1996). In the large scale study of Mattson et al. (1985) carbamazepine, phenytoin, phenobarbitone and primidone did not differ significantly in their abilities to control generalized tonic-clonic seizures in those who could tolerate the agent used, but phenobarbitone, and even more so primidone, had to be ceased more frequently than the other drugs because of unwanted effects. In that study, carbamazepine and phenytoin were more effective than the other drugs in pre-

Table 1. Correlation between epilepsies (ILAE Classification 1989, condensed) and effective antiepileptic drugs for each syndrome

Epileptic syndrome	Effective drugs
1. Localization-related epilepsies (whether or not they become secondarily generalized)	Carbamazepine; phenytoin; phenobarbitone[a]; valproate; vigabatrin; lamotrigine; gabapentin; felbamate; topiramate; tiagabine
2. Generalized epilepsies	
Absences	Valproate; ethosuximide[b]; clonazepam
Myoclonic epilepsies	
In infancy (West's syndrome)	ACTH: vigabatrin; valproate; ? clonazepam
Lennox-Gastaut syndrome	Felbamate[c]; valproate
Juvenile myoclonic epilepsy	Valproate; phenobarbitone[a]; clonazepam; lamotrigine
Tonic, clonic, tonic-clonic seizures	Valproate; phenobarbitone[a]; carbamazepine; phenytoin; lamotrigine
3. Indeterminate types of epilepsy	Carbamazepine; valproate; phenytoin; phenobarbitone[a]; lamotrigine; vigabatrin; topiramate
4. Situation-related epilepsies	
Febrile convulsions of infancy	Valproate; phenobarbitone[a]; diazepam

[a] Also methylphenobarbitone or primidone.
[b] An agent effective against bilateral tonic-clonic seizures may also be necessary.
[c] Felbamate's availability is limited by its toxicity.

venting partial seizures. Later, the study of MATTSON et al. (1992) showed that, whilst carbamazepine and valproate were equi-effective in controlling secondarily generalized tonic-clonic seizures in adults, the former was superior in preventing complex partial seizures. In some of the above studies it was not clear whether all varieties of seizure were suppressed in patients, or only the more severe, and more readily remembered, ones.

Considering the known frequencies of the different epileptic syndromes in the community, and the largely equal overall efficacies of carbamazepine and valproate in adult onset epilepsy (RICHENS et al. 1994), the data of Table 1 would suggest that one or other of these two agents should suffice to manage most patients with epilepsy. This would be so if it were not that an appreciable number of patients experience unacceptable adverse effects from these drugs, so that therapeutic alternatives are desirable. Rarely, some of the adverse effects of these two drugs may be lethal, e.g. valproate-associated hepatotoxicity (ZIMMERMAN and ISHAK 1982). As well, carbamazepine and particularly valproate, taken during pregnancy, can occasionally be associated with spina bifida in the offspring (ROSA 1991; OMTZIGT et al. 1992). This latter contingency can make valproate an unwise choice of therapy in young females with juvenile myoclonic epilepsy, a relatively common syndrome for which the drug usually is a very satisfactory agent from the point of view of controlling seizures without producing adverse effects. Unfortunately, valproate often needs to be taken over many years, during which unanticipated pregnancy may occur. Access to a wider range of antiepileptic agents than valproate and carbamazepine is desirable even for the physician who manages only a few patients with epilepsy, whilst for the 25%–30% of patients with epilepsy whose seizure disorders are not controlled with the older established drugs, the availability of as many additional potentially effective agents as possible offers advantages.

As experience with the antiepileptic drugs introduced in the past 5 years grows, and some of the antiepileptic drugs now under development come into use, the relative positions in the order of preference of the agents listed in Table 1, when used for various major epileptic syndromes, may alter, reflecting knowledge of a changed balance between efficacy, safety and cost. A contemporary meta-analysis has failed to detect conclusive differences in efficacy and tolerability between gabapentin, lamotrigine, tiagabine, topiramate, vigabatrin and zonisamide in refractory partial epilepsy (Marson et al. 1996). However, at the time of writing vigabatrin is emerging as a possible drug of first choice in West's syndrome (Appleton 1995: Aicardi et al. 1996) and it may have a useful role in managing the Lennox-Gastaut syndrome (Feucht and Branter-Inthaler 1994).

E. Initiating Drug Therapy

In recent years there has been widespread acceptance of the dictum that a single antiepileptic drug should be used whenever possible in treating epilepsy (Reynolds and Shorvon 1981). The short and medium term aim of antiepileptic drug therapy is to prevent all further epileptic seizures occurring in the patient, employing an agent which produces no adverse effects. Success in achieving these goals must, in the final analysis, be assessed clinically. However, at least for the longer-established antiepileptic drugs, ranges of plasma drug concentrations are known which correlate in most patients with seizure control in the absence of adverse effects. Such "therapeutic" ranges can be used to provide a short term indication of the potential adequacy of antiepileptic drug therapy until enough time has elapsed for clinical data to make clear whether or not seizures really are controlled. Use of the therapeutic ranges should not be substituted for clinical judgement in the recognition of adverse effects arising from the prescribed drug treatment. However, the development of otherwise obscure symptoms and signs in the presence of supratherapeutic plasma drug concentrations does suggest that overdosage probably exists. In patients who have an epilepsy in which seizures have already occurred frequently, or in which frequent seizures can be expected, e.g. absence epilepsy, the clinical response of the seizure disorder will nearly always be obvious fairly quickly. Here plasma antiepileptic drug concentration monitoring is nearly always not needed to determine the adequacy of therapy. In contrast, in the more common situation of managing patients who have varieties of epilepsy in which seizures are unlikely to occur frequently, or patients in whom the

Table 2. Therapeutic ranges of plasma concentration for the established antiepileptic drugs, and the average drug dose required to achieve a mid-therapeutic range plasma concentration at steady state. (After EADIE and TYRER 1989)

Drug	Therapeutic range		Dose (mg/kg/day)	
	(mg/l)	(μmol/l)		
Carbamazepine	6–12	25–50	Approx.	30
Ethosuximide	40–100	300–700		30
Methylphenobarbitone	See phenobarbitone		>40 years	4
			15–40 years	6.5
			<15 years	7.5
Phenobarbitone	10–30	45–130	>40 years	2
			15–40 years	2.5
			5–<15 years	3
			<5 years	4.5
Phenytoin	10–20	40–80	Adults	6
			<13 years	11
Primidone	See phenobarbitone		Adults	11
Valproate	50–100	300–600	–	–

natural history of the disorder is unknown at the stage when treatment is commenced, the plasma antiepileptic drug concentrations do provide a useful preliminary guide to the adequacy of therapy before enough time has elapsed for the clinical response to be clear. Generally accepted therapeutic ranges of plasma concentrations of the antiepileptic drugs are listed in Table 2. In making use of these ranges several points should be remembered, viz.:

1. The range is not some intrinsic property of the drug itself, but is the result of the interaction between drug and the seizure disorder for which it is prescribed in numbers of individual patients. The range for a given drug may differ for different types of epileptic seizure. Thus SCHMIDT et al. (1986) found a mean plasma phenytoin concentration of 14 mg/l was associated with prevention of bilateral tonic-clonic seizures, whereas a mean concentration of 23 mg/l was needed for prevention of partial seizures.
2. The range is a population statistic, and will not necessarily be valid for every treated individual. Sometimes seizures in a patient will be fully controlled only at plasma antiepileptic drug concentrations which are above the therapeutic range for the population, yet no adverse effects may be present in the patient who is being treated. Conversely, subtherapeutic plasma concentrations may suffice for full seizure prevention in some patients, whilst in other patients such concentrations may be associated with troublesome or even unacceptable adverse effects.

At the start of antiepileptic drug therapy in a patient, purely pharmacokinetic (and simplistic) considerations would suggest that the dose chosen

Table 3. Antiepileptic drug half-lives and times to achieve steady-state conditions after a dosage change

Drug	Half-life (h)	Time for steady state (days)
Carbamazepine	25–50[a]	6
Clonazepam	24–36	5–8
Ethosuximide	30–70	6–14
Gabapentin	8	2
Lamotrigine	30	6
Phenobarbitone	70–120	14–21
Phenytoin	15–20[b]	3–5
Tiagabine	5–13	1–3
Topiramate	18–23	4–5
Valproate	8–12	2–3
Vigabatrin	4–8	2

[a] Shortens on continuing exposure to the drug.
[b] Is concentration dependent.

should yield a steady-state therapeutic range plasma concentration of the drug throughout the whole of the dosage interval, and that the dosage interval should be approximately the duration of the half-life of the drug. Once there has been time for a steady state to be present (Table 3), and the patient remains clinically free from adverse effects, the plasma drug concentration should be measured and the drug dose altered if the concentration is not reasonably close to its target value, unless it is already clear that the patient's seizures are controlled. Clinical experience suggests that some modification of such a theoretically derived treatment policy may sometimes be desirable. Except for phenytoin and valproate (in most instances), antiepileptic drugs given in their full anticipated dosage from the outset of therapy may cause many patients to experience troublesome, and sometimes unacceptable, sedation. Carbamazepine metabolism undergoes antoinduction over the first few days and weeks of exposure to the drug (EICHELBAUM et al. 1975), and there is some evidence for lesser degrees of such a phenomenon in relation to phenytoin (DICKINSON et al. 1985) and valproate (personal unpublished data). Autoinduction will reduce the plasma concentration of the drug over some days or weeks and consequently may lessen the degree of initial sedation from the antiepileptic drug. It also appears likely that true pharmacological tolerance to this sedation may occur, though this is difficult to prove in humans. To allow time for these various adaptive phenomena to take effect, it is often prudent to prescribe one-fourth or one-third of the expected daily dose of the antiepileptic drug initially, and to increase the dose in stages at weekly or fortnightly intervals till the definitive dose is reached, assuming that no significant adverse effects have appeared before this time. Such a progressive introduction of therapy may delay seizure control in those with frequently occurring attacks, though in such epilepsy it may also avoid unnecessarily high antiepileptic drug dosage should seizures be suppressed at a lower dose and lower plasma drug concentration than anticipated. When it is feasible, antiepileptic drugs are probably best taken twice a day, even if half-life considerations would allow less frequent drug intake. Twice daily dosage appears to offer the best chance of long term compliance with a dosage regimen. It also minimizes the consequences of omitting a single dose of a drug which is slowly enough eliminated to permit once daily dosage. Omission of a single daily dose of a drug with a 24 h half-life (which results in no drug intake for 48 h) could lead to an appreciable fall in plasma and tissue antiepileptic drug concentrations by the time the next dose is taken, and this might allow previously controlled seizures to break through.

As mentioned above, once there has been time for a steady state to be reached at the anticipated appropriate antiepileptic drug dosage, the plasma drug (or drug metabolite in the cases of methylphenobarbitone and primidone) concentration should be measured, if feasible. Should possible adverse effects have occurred already, the drug concentration considered in relation to the therapeutic range for the drug may help decide whether the patient is overdosed and merely needs less of the drug, or whether the patient is sensitive to, or intolerant of, the drug. In the latter case it would be best to substitute another agent. If no adverse effects are present and it is clear that a satisfactory dosage is already being prescribed, i.e. previously frequent seizures have ceased, the drug concentration that then applies will serve as a baseline for future interpretation of the clinical situation should subsequent treatment difficulties arise. That concentration is a therapeutic one for the patient concerned, whatever its numerical value. If there are no adverse effects but it is uncertain whether enough drug is being taken to prevent the patient's seizures (usually because the natural history of the patient's epilepsy is unknown at that stage), the dosage should not be altered if the plasma antiepileptic drug concentration is within or above the therapeutic range. If the concentration is subtherapeutic, and the patient is known to be compliant with the prescribed dosage, the dose should be increased by an amount calculated sufficient to maintain a plasma drug concentration within the therapeutic range (providing no adverse effects then develop).

Empirical data show that, at least for phenytoin, phenobarbitone and ethosuximide, steady-state plasma drug concentrations in individual patients rise more than proportionately in relation to the size of the dosage increments prescribed (Eadie 1976). In the case of phenytoin this non-linearity is due to increasing saturation of the body's capacity to *para*-hydroxylate the drug as the dose is increased (Eadie et al. 1976). In contrast, steady-state plasma carbamazepine concentrations rise less than expected relative to dosage increase in the individual, due to ongoing dose-dependent autoinduction of metabolism of the drug given in monotherapy (Bernus et al. 1996). These nonlinearities need to be kept in mind when adjusting dosages of these particular drugs. Plasma phenobarbitone concentrations rise very much in proportion to the size of methylphenobarbitone dosage increments. The relationships between dosage and steady-state plasma concentrations of the other marketed antiepileptic drugs in the individual patient do not yet appear to have been defined adequately.

F. Continuing Drug Therapy

Once the patient with epilepsy is established on apparently satisfactory drug therapy a number of management situations may arise. Below, they are considered individually, though in practice two or more may at times coexist.

I. No Further Seizures and No Adverse Effects Occur

This is the ideal therapeutic situation. It is attained within 2 or 3 years of the onset of epilepsy in some 75% of patients (REYNOLDS et al. 1983). In these circumstances, all that needs to be done is to continue the successful therapy in unaltered dosage, to put in place measures intended to help ensure long term compliance with the therapy (PETERSON et al. 1984), and to review the patient at intervals to ensure that all remains well. Although it is not strictly necessary, plasma antiepileptic drug concentrations may be measured at intervals, partly to provide an ongoing baseline against which to interpret any therapeutic difficulty which may happen to arise later, and partly as a way of checking on, and thus helping to maintain, compliance with the treatment. If the plasma antiepileptic drug concentration declines at some stage, and continues to remain low, but seizures not recur, there is reason to hope that the underlying epileptic process has become inactive. If so, withdrawal of therapy (see below) can be considered at that time in the hope that the epileptic process in the patient is in lasting remission.

II. Adverse Effects Occur

The type and severity of adverse effects will determine the appropriate therapeutic action. If the adverse effect that occurs appears to involve hypersensitivity mechanisms it will usually be necessary to withdraw the culprit drug and to substitute another appropriate agent. In this case the situation then becomes that of antiepileptic drug therapy begun anew. If the adverse effect is one whose severity is probably dose-proportional, the appropriate course of action is to reduce the dose of the antiepileptic drug. This may remedy the adverse effect, though possibly at the price of decreased seizure control. This latter situation is discussed immediately below.

III. Seizures Continue Despite Therapy

In this situation there are two likely explanations, viz. (a) the patient is not taking a sufficient dose of the antiepileptic drug that is being used, or (b) the epilepsy is not responsive to the drug used, either because the diagnosis of the epileptic syndrome present is incorrect so that an inappropriate drug has been prescribed, or the diagnosis is correct but for some reason the underlying epileptic process is resistant to the drug prescribed.

If the plasma antiepileptic drug concentration is below the therapeutic range, underdosage is likely to explain the continuing seizures so that a higher drug dose should be used to try to obtain seizure control. If the concentration is within the therapeutic range, the diagnosis of the type of epilepsy present should be reconsidered, and the presence of hitherto undetected progressive brain pathology should be excluded as far as it can be. If the diagnosis of the epileptic syndrome appears correct, the appropriate course is to increase the antiepileptic drug dose cautiously, and to continue to do this whenever steady-state conditions apply but seizures continue to occur, until adverse effects of the therapy preclude any further dose increase. If seizures come under control with increasing antiepileptic drug dosage, and adverse effects remain absent, the patient has moved into the desirable situation of being free both of seizures and of adverse effects, and is managed accordingly. If dosage incrementation produces adverse effects before seizure control occurs, it will be necessary to exchange the drug in use for another potentially appropriate agent. The changeover is best made in stages over some days or weeks.

IV. Antiepileptic Drug Monotherapy Fails

Should all the longer established antiepileptic drugs appropriate for a patient's type of epilepsy fail to control the disorder when used as monotherapy in doses which leave the patient free from adverse effects, there remain three main treatment possibilities, viz. (a) to try one or other of the new anticonvulsants in monotherapy, though marketing approval indications may deter such a course in some countries, (b) to use antiepileptic drug combinations, or (c) to examine the possibility of epilepsy surgery (which will not be considered further in the present text).

At the time of writing, there is not a great deal of information available regarding the use of the newer antiepileptic drugs as monotherapy in refractory epilepsy. They have usually been studied by being added to existing (inadequate) therapy, and have shown efficacy in these circumstances. Antiepileptic drug combinations involving the longer marketed agents may be effective in some patients in whom the drugs which are to be combined have already failed when used in monotherapy. While Schmidt (1982) found adding a second antiepileptic drug led to significantly improved seizure control in only 13% of patients with monotherapy-refractory partial seizures, Mattson (1994) stated that antiepileptic drug combinations produced improved seizure control in half the patients in whom monotherapy had failed.

1. Antiepileptic Drug Combinations

If two antiepileptic drugs are to be used in combination, it is sensible to prescribe agents which are known to interfere with different aspects of the molecular mechanisms of epileptogenesis to try to obtain enhanced

Table 4. Known biochemical actions of the antiepileptic drugs

Group	Action	Drugs
I	Blocking voltage-dependent Na^+ channels	Phenytoin; carbamazepine; valproate; lamotrigine; topiramate
II	Increasing postsynaptic Cl^- entry at $GABA_A$ receptors	
	Directly	Phenobarbitone; topiramate
	By facilitating GABA effects	Benzodiazepines
	By increasing synaptic GABA concentrations[a]	Vigabatrin; valproate; tiagabine
III	Interfering with glutaminergic neurotransmission	Lamotrigine; ? gabapentin; ? topiramate
IV	Blocking "T" type thalamic Ca^{2+} channels	Ethosuximide; valproate

[a] May also have effects at $GABA_B$ receptors.

therapeutic efficacy. However, combinations of agents with the same molecular mechanism of action are neither contraindicated nor illogical if the mechanisms responsible for the toxicities of the two substances differ. The known biochemical mechanisms of action of the marketed antiepileptic drugs are summarized in Table 4. An agent from group I and one from group II of the table, or one each from groups I and III, or from groups II and III, might comprise suitable combinations, so long as the epileptic syndrome that is present is known to respond to both of the agents chosen. As yet, there is not a great deal of evidence that such theoretically based expectations are borne out in practice. For absence seizures, where only the agents in group IV are useful, the combination of ethosuximide and valproate has been reported to be successful when each drug, used alone, had failed to prevent the attacks (PERUCCA 1995).

With the use of antiepileptic drug combinations, there is an increased possibility of adverse effects occurring. These must be watched for carefully, and appropriate action taken should they develop.

2. Pharmacokinetic Interactions Between Anticonvulsants

When two or more antiepileptic drugs are used together, pharmacodynamic interactions may occur. As mentioned above, some such interactions may be beneficial to the patient. Others may result in adverse effects, e.g. sedation. Pharmacokinetic interactions may also occur between two antiepileptic agents used in combination. Many such interactions are known (Table 5, Chap. 22, this volume). When these interactions affect the drug originally used they can be detected by measuring its plasma concentration before and 1–3 weeks after the second agent is added. The interpretation is simpler if the dose of the first agent has not been changed. Interactions affecting the added agent are harder to detect in a given patient, but can be suspected if the plasma concentrations

Table 5. Pharmacokinetic interactions between antiepileptic drugs. (After PATSALOS and DUNCAN 1993)

Drug	Clearance	
	Increased by	Decreased by
Carbamazepine	Phenobarbitone; phenytoin; primidone	[a]
Ethosuximide	Carbamazepine; primidone; valproate (inconstant)	Methylphenobarbitone; valproate (inconstant)
Gabapentin	–	–
Lamotrigine	Carbamazepine; phenobarbitone; phenytoin	Valproate
Phenobarbitone		Phenytoin; valproate
Phenytoin	Carbamazepine (inconstant); clonazepam (inconstant); valproate (inconsistent); vigabatrin	Carbamazepine (inconstant); clonazepam (inconstant); ethosuximide; sulthiame; valproate (at high phenytoin concentrations)
Tiagabine	?	?
Topiramate	Carbamazepine; phenytoin	–
Valproate	Carbamazepine; phenobarbitone; phenytoin	–
Vigabatrin	–	–

[a] Carbamazepine-10,11-epoxide clearance is decreased by lamotrigine and valproate.

of the added drug proves to be unusually high or unusually low relative to its dose. If plasma concentrations of the initially prescribed drug fall after a second agent is added, and seizures continue, the more appropriate course of action may be to increase the dose of the first drug rather than to increase that of the second.

One pharmacokinetic interaction which may not be detected readily, but which is often responsible for adverse effects, is that which follows the addition of phenytoin or phenobarbitone to existing carbamazepine therapy. In this interaction plasma carbamazepine concentration may fall to some extent, yet the patient may experience increased sedation or ataxia because the plasma carbamazepine-10,11-epoxide concentration tends to rise (MCKAUGE et al. 1981). The plasma concentrations of this carbamazepine metabolite are not measured routinely, though it is both an antiepileptic agent and a sedative. Reduction in carbamazepine dose is more appropriate than reduction in the dose of the added drug in this circumstance.

V. The Patient's Physiological Status Alters

1. Age

Although many patients with epilepsy receive antiepileptic drugs for only a few years before their treatment can be withdrawn successfully, some persons need the therapy over most of the course of their lives. Age-related alterations in drug clearance may then produce the need for dosage adjustments at times. The clearances of those antiepileptic drugs which are eliminated mainly or exclusively by being metabolized, expressed relative to body weight, tend to be lower in the neonate, to increase in the first year of life, remain high throughout childhood, and begin to decline gradually at or after puberty, the decline continuing into old age. This type of behaviour is likely to apply to all the currently available antiepileptic drugs except vigabatrin and gabapentin, though phenytoin clearance relative to body weight decreases fairly abruptly around the time of puberty. Vigabatrin and gabapentin are cleared mainly by renal excretion in unmetabolized form. Their clearances diminish from middle age onwards, as renal function declines (as it normally does). This knowledge of the age-related behaviour of antiepileptic drug clearance may help in determining appropriate initial antiepileptic drug dosage, and in anticipating the dosage alterations which may be required during a prolonged course of antiepileptic drug therapy which could encompass much of a patient's lifespan.

2. Menstrual Cycle

Plasma concentrations of phenytoin, carbamazepine and phenobarbitone tend to fall in the premenstrual week in at least some women with epilepsy. This fall may contribute to a tendency for their epileptic seizures to occur mainly or exclusively around the time of menstruation (Herkes et al. 1993). Some women with such catamenial epilepsy also tend to have more seizures at mid-cycle, if ovulation occurs. In women with catamenial epilepsy it has been suggested that higher antiepileptic drug doses should be taken in the premenstrual week, though it may sometimes be difficult for the patient to know exactly when to commence the higher dosage in each menstrual cycle because of unpredictability of the lengths of individual cycles. So long as the patient does not develop overdosage manifestations it may be better for higher antiepileptic drug doses to be taken throughout the whole cycle in the hope that the premenstrual drug concentrations will then suffice to prevent seizures.

3. Pregnancy

The optimal use of antiepileptic drugs during pregnancy involves reconciling what is best for the mother with what is best for her baby. Intake of antiepileptic drugs during pregnancy is associated with an increased risk of teratogenesis. To minimize this risk it has been advised that only one antiepileptic drug should be taken whenever feasible, and that its dose should be the lowest one which will control seizures in the mother (Lindhout and Omtzigt 1994). In earlier studies (Knight and Rhind 1975), epileptic seizures were reported to become more frequent during pregnancy. However, more recent work has failed to confirm this (Tomson et al. 1994), perhaps because over the intervening years the widening use of plasma antiepileptic drug concentration monitoring may have made therapeutic practice more efficient. Clearances of phenytoin (Dam et al. 1976), phenobarbitone (Lander et al. 1977) and probably valproate (Philbert and Dam 1982), but not carbamazepine, unless it is used in combination with phenytoin or phenobarbitone (Bernus et al. 1995), increase as pregnancy progresses, and return progressively to pre-pregnancy values over a few weeks or months after childbirth. Information is not yet available for the dispositions of the newer antiepileptic drugs in pregnancy. Ideally the plasma antiepileptic drug concentrations which were present before pregnancy should have been associated with as complete and adverse effect-free control of seizures as was possible in the patient. It would then be sensible to monitor the plasma drug concentration every few weeks during pregnancy, and to adjust the antiepileptic drug dosage as necessary to maintain the plasma drug concentrations close to their pre-pregnancy value throughout the pregnancy. The maternal plasma drug concentrations should also be monitored fortnightly in the postnatal period, and the drug dosage reduced when the plasma drug concentration begins to rise, thus avoiding the appearance of overdosage manifestations. In interpreting the drug concentration values, some allowance may need to be made for the fact that the plasma protein binding capacity, at least for phenytoin, is reduced in the last trimester of pregnancy (Dean et al. 1980). Therefore a 10%–15% fall in whole plasma phenytoin concentration may not necessarily be associated with compromised seizure control in later pregnancy. Ideally, plasma water drug concentrations rather than whole plasma drug concentrations would be monitored during pregnancy. Fortunately, salivary concentrations of phenytoin, carbamazepine and ethosuximide correlate closely with the plasma water concentrations of these substances (McAuliffe et al. 1977), as do salivary phenobarbitone concentrations if a correction is first made to allow for the effect that the measured pH difference between plasma and saliva has on the phenobarbitone ionized fractions in the two fluids.

In practice, if the above policy is followed, phenytoin doses will usually need to be increased in pregnancy, as will carbamazepine doses if the drug is used in combination with phenytoin or phenobarbitone. Phenobarbitone or drugs metabolized to it are now not often used in Western societies and valproate intake in pregnancy is undesirable because of the risk of spina bifida in the offspring. Unless the mother experiences troublesome overdosage symptoms in the postpartum period, breast feeding is very unlikely to provide enough antiepileptic drug in milk to produce adverse effects in a baby previously exposed to the drug in utero.

There is a 1.2-fold to 3-fold increase in perinatal mortality in the infants of epileptic mothers (Hiilesmaa 1992), but there is no increase in the incidence of other obstetric problems except for the hazard of teratogenesis and the chance of a neonatal bleeding diathesis which can be prevented by giving the mother an injection of vitamin K during labour. If a foetus has been exposed to antiepileptic drugs, particularly valproate or carbamazepine, in the first trimester of pregnancy, a high resolution ultrasound scan and measurement of plasma α-fetoprotein concentration should be offered, to enable the mother to take an informed decision about continuing the pregnancy in the unlikely event that spina bifida is present.

4. Intercurrent Illness

Intercurrent illness which impairs the function of the organs involved in eliminating the antiepileptic drugs is likely to necessitate a decrease in drug dosage. If renal insufficiency develops, doses of vigabatrin and gabapentin, the only marketed antiepileptic drugs which are eliminated mainly by renal excretion in largely unmetabolized form, will probably need to be lowered. Hepatic insufficiency is likely to reduce the body's capacity to tolerate previously satisfactory dosages of any of the remaining antiepileptic drugs, all of which are cleared predominantly by being metabolized in the liver. Diseases which reduce plasma albumin concentrations will alter the relationship between the whole plasma drug concentration and the biological effects of the drug. When such diseases are present it is desirable to monitor drug concentrations in plasma water (or drug concentrations in saliva, if these are known to reflect plasma water drug concentrations), as a guide to antiepileptic drug dosage. Plasma water drug concentration monitoring is unnecessary for drugs which exhibit little or no binding to plasma proteins, e.g. ethosuximide, gabapentin.

Drugs prescribed to treat an intercurrent illness may alter the dispositions of any antiepileptic drug or drugs which are being taken by the patient. Such pharmacokinetic interactions are too numerous to be mentioned individually at this point, but are described in Chap. 22 and other chapters of this book. They can be detected by measuring the plasma antiepileptic drug concentration just before the other agent is added to the patient's therapy, and again 1 or 2 weeks later. The information from these paired measurements can be used to guide any antiepileptic drug dosage adjustment that then appears desirable.

VI. Status Epilepticus Occurs

Status epilepticus may complicate the ongoing management of epilepsy, in which case it often proves due to omission of prescribed antiepileptic therapy. Alternatively, it may be the presenting manifestation of epilepsy. The factors responsible for the occurrence of the status should be diagnosed quickly and, as far as possible, corrected. Appropriate supportive care, e.g. maintenance of the airway, of blood oxygenation and of fluid balance, is essential. Various antiepileptic drug regimens are used in different centres to control the status, though there are no comparative studies to determine which regimen is the best (WALKER et al. 1995). Unless the sufferer can swallow with safety at the time when treatment of status epilepticus is commenced, the antiepileptic drug therapy must be given parenterally, and preferably intravenously. The doses used depend on whether or not the sufferer has already been taking antiepileptic drugs before the status develops.

1. Generalized Convulsive Status Epilepticus

At the time of writing, the commonly used agents for convulsive status epilepticus are phenytoin and diazepam (or another benzodiazepine) whilst phenobarbitone, pentobarbitone, thiopentone or inhalational anaesthetics may be employed in resistant cases (WALKER et al. 1995).

In previously untreated instances of convulsive status epilepticus, an initial intravenous dose of 10–15 mg/kg phenytoin might be infused over a period of 1–2 h. If the phenytoin pro-drug phosphenytoin is available, it may be given intravenously more conveniently, and rather more rapidly, than phenytoin, and in similar molar dosage. As alternatives, diazepam 0.1 mg/kg or clonazepam 0.03–0.05 mg/kg might be given intravenously over 5 min, initially. If the benzodiazepines are used, another antiepileptic drug better suited to long term intake will need to be prescribed for subsequent maintenance therapy. Parenteral drug administration is continued at appropriate intervals until seizures cease or evidence of beginning cardiorespiratory depression appears. If the patient had already been receiving therapy with the antiepileptic drug chosen for intravenous administration, a similar regimen, though with a perhaps 30%–50% lower dose, might be employed unless there was evidence that treatment had been omitted recently, in which case a fuller dosage could be used. It would appear sensible to use more of the antiepileptic drug the patient was already taking, particularly if that drug had been effective in treating the patient's seizures previously, in preference to trying a different agent. This would avoid hypersensitivity type adverse effects which might follow the administration of a drug to which the patient had not been exposed previously. Unfortunately, many anticonvulsants are not marketed in a dosage form suitable for parenteral use. Therefore the choice of parenteral antiepileptic drug is somewhat limited (being restricted to phenytoin, phenobarbitone, diazepam, clonazepam and certain other benzodiazepines including midazolam, and in some countries valproate). However, certain drugs with seizure-suppressing effects, which are too sedating or otherwise unsuitable for regular use in the long term treatment of epilepsy, e.g. amylobarbitone, chlormethiazole, paraldehyde, can be given intravenously to control convulsive status epilepticus.

When convulsive status epilepticus is controlled, parenteral antiepileptic drug therapy is continued until the patient is again able to take drugs by mouth safely. Oral maintenance therapy is then organized, or reinstituted, as the case may be, along the lines described earlier in this chapter.

2. Non-convulsive Status Epilepticus

In partial or absence seizure status, if the patient can swallow with safety, oral therapy may be used from the outset. Clonazepam or valproate, orally or parenterally, is probably the preferred agent in these situations, though the other drugs employed for convulsive status are also useful in partial seizure status. Non-convulsive seizure status does not usually constitute the emergency that convulsive status does. As a consequence, antiepileptic drug therapy can be adjusted in less haste to control the episode.

G. Duration of Therapy

Evidence has emerged that antiepileptic drug therapy suppresses seizures but probably does not cure epilepsy, which itself often goes into remission while the drug therapy continues to be taken. As a result, the argument for achieving prompt, prolonged and complete control of all epileptic seizures in the patient may not appear as pressing as it seemed to be a decade ago.

The meta-analysis of Berg and Shinnar (1994) showed that, if a patient had been completely free from seizures for 2 or more years, there were 29 in 100 chances that the disorder would relapse within 2 years of commencing any withdrawal of therapy. Some other published figures for the relapse rate have been 36% (Shinnar et al. 1994), 20% (Bouma et al. 1987: Eadie 1994) and 14% (Matricardi et al. 1989). The MRC Antiepileptic Drug Withdrawal Study Group (1993) found that the following factors increased the risk of relapse after antiepileptic drug withdrawal: age above 16 years, taking more than one antiepileptic drug, seizures continuing after antiepileptic drug therapy commenced, having bilateral tonic-clonic seizures or myoclonic seizures, and there being a relative short seizure-free period before drug withdrawal was begun. Eadie (1994) found that a patient's reaching the point of withdrawing antiepileptic drug therapy was favoured by an earlier age of onset of epilepsy, a history of birth difficulty, having had only a solitary seizure before treatment began, and having no abnormal neurological signs on examination. Epilepsy beginning after the age of 12 years, and epilepsy needing two or more antiepileptic drugs to achieve seizure control, decreased the chances of a successful withdrawal of therapy. Oller-Daurella and Oller (1991) showed that delay in treating epilepsy decreased the prospect of successfully withdrawing therapy. In essence, the nature of the epileptic syndrome that is present, and whether or not structural brain pathology underlies the epilepsy, appear the main determinants of the success or otherwise of ceasing therapy. On the whole, generalized epilepsies beginning after the first decade of life, including juvenile myoclonic epilepsy, respond well to appropriate antiepileptic drugs but, with the exception of absence seizures (Sato et al. 1983), tend to relapse at some stage after therapy is withdrawn.

It is uncertain whether persisting paroxysmal activity in the routine surface lead EEG at the time of withdrawal of therapy provides a useful prognostic guide (Galimberti et al. 1993; Tinuper et al. 1996), though paroxysmal EEG abnormalities developing during the course of the withdrawal have unfavourable connotations. For fully controlled epilepsies with a good outlook for continuing freedom from seizures after withdrawal of antiepileptic drug therapy, one recent study showed that as little as 12 months without seizures may be sufficient to allow successful phasing out of drug intake (Braathen and THEORELL 1995). However, it is often difficult to know exactly when the period of epilepsy control has begun in a patient who has had only occasional seizures. Therefore in practice a 2 or 3 year period without seizures is usually considered necessary before withdrawal of antiepileptic drug therapy is considered. The extensive data of OLLER-DAURELLA et al. (1976) showed that the risk of epilepsy relapse after withdrawal of antiepileptic drug therapy decreased with increasing duration of seizure control over a period of at least 20 years. However, beyond 5 years of seizure control there was relatively little further reduction in the risk of relapse. In practice, even when the time and circumstances seem propitious for a withdrawal of antiepileptic drug therapy, and the patient knows there are four in five chances that his or her seizures will not recur, some epilepsy sufferers will elect to continue therapy because of the fear of further attacks and their consequences. Practical guidelines for withdrawing antiepileptic drug therapy have been discussed by CHADWICK (1994).

In some 20% of patients with epilepsy (SHORVON 1996) it will prove impossible to control the seizures with all currently available therapy. There is then little alternative to using what experience in the patient has shown is the most effective and least toxic drug or drug combination for an indefinite period. Adverse effects must be watched for carefully, particularly delayed onset ones, e.g. folate depletion and its consequences, and osteomalacia. If these begin to emerge, appropriate remedial action should be taken.

H. Withdrawal of Therapy

Although there appears to be no proof that rapid withdrawal of antiepileptic drug therapy leads to a worse outcome than gradual withdrawal, antiepileptic drug dosage is usually phased down in stages over several months. Thus the daily drug dose might be reduced in 25% steps at monthly or even second monthly intervals till drug intake is ceased. If two antiepileptic drugs are used, the drug thought less important for control of the patient's epilepsy is withdrawn first, and then the more important drug. The risk of relapse is greatest during the withdrawal process, and over the first few months afterwards. Some 70% of the risk of relapse has been consumed by the time a year has passed following the commencement of the withdrawal of therapy (EADIE 1994).

I. Use of Antiepileptic Drugs for Indications Other than Epilepsy

For many years, the agents customarily regarded as antiepileptic drugs have also been used to treat disorders other than epilepsy. Most antiepileptic drugs have tranquillizing properties, and these probably account for some of the beneficial actions attributed to the drugs. Over the years, phenytoin has achieved a rather wide array of uses (EADIE and TYRER 1989), and is still sometimes employed in managing myotonia, occasional forms of migraine, trigeminal neuralgia, cardiac arrhythmias and, in recent times, cocaine abuse (Crosby et al. 1996). Carbamazepine is the treatment of choice for trigeminal neuralgia, and may be useful in various painful peripheral neuropathies. It is now being increasingly employed in the management of bipolar affective disorders (Bowden 1996). Valproate is also used in trigeminal and other neuralgias (Peiris et al. 1980) and in mania (Fenn et al. 1996), and appears to be a migraine prophylactic (Mathew et al. 1995; Lenaerts et al. 1996). Primidone is employed to suppress essential tremor (Findley et al. 1985). Clonazepam is used for some types of non-epileptic myoclonus (Goldberg and Dorman 1976) and for trigeminal neuralgia. There are suggestions that vigabatrin and gabapentin may have "neuroprotective" actions that may prove useful in neurological disorders where the pathogenic mechanism is thought to involve glutamate-mediated excitotoxicity (Gurney et al. 1996). Uses of antiepileptic drugs apart from epilepsy may be regarded as outside the terms of reference of the present book, but some of them are mentioned above to illustrate additional ways in which these agents are coming to be employed in contemporary medicine.

References

Aicardi J, Mumford JP, Dumas C, Wood S (1996) Vigabatrin as initial therapy for infantile spasms: a European retrospective survey. Sabril IS Investigator and Peer Review Group. Epilepsia 37:638–642

Annegers JF, Hauser WA, Elveback LR (1979a) Remission of seizures and relapse in patients with epilepsy. Epilepsia 20:729–737

Annegers JF, Hauser WA, Elveback LR, Kurland LT (1979b) The risk of epilepsy following febrile convulsions. Neurology 29:297–303

Appleton RE (1995) Vigabatrin in the management of generalized seizures in children. Seizure 4:45–48

Beardsley RS, Freeman JM, Appel FA (1983) Anticonvulsant serum levels are useful only if the physician appropriately uses them: an assessment of the impact of providing serum level data to physicians. Epilepsia 24:330–335

Berg AT, Shinnar S (1991) The risk of seizure recurrence following a first unprovoked seizure: a quantitative review. Neurology 41:965–972

Berg AT, Shinnar S (1994) Relapse following discontinuation of antiepileptic drugs: a meta-analysis. Neurology 44:601–608

Bernus I, Hooper WD, Dickinson RG, Eadie MJ (1995) Metabolism of carbamazepine and co-administered anticonvulsants during pregnancy. Epilepsy Res 21:65–75

Bernus I, Dickinson RG, Hooper WD, Eadie MJ (1996) Dose-dependent metabolism of carbamazepine in humans. Epilepsy Res 24:163–172

Bouma PAD, Peters ACB, Arts RJHM, Stinjen T, Van Rossum J (1987) Discontinuation of antiepileptic therapy: a prospective study in children. J Neurol Neurosurg Psychiat 50:1579–1583

Bowden CL (1996) Role of newer medications for bipolar disorder. J Clin Psychopharmacol 16:48S–55 S

Braathen G, Theorell K (1995) Is one year treatment enough in uncomplicated epilepsy? Epilepsia 36 [Suppl 3]:S163

Brodie MJ, Richens A, Yuen AWC (1995) Double-blind comparison of lamotrigine and carbamazepine in newly diagnosed epilepsy. Lancet 345:476–479

Cavazutti GB (1975) Prevention of febrile convulsions with dipropylacetate (Depakine). Epilepsia 16:647–648
Chadwick D (1994) A practical guide to discontinuing antiepileptic drugs. CNS Drugs 2:423–428
Chadwick D, Turnbull DM (1985) The comparative efficacy of antiepileptic drugs for partial and tonic-clonic seizures. J Neurol Neurosurg Psychiat 48:1073–1077
Christe W, Krämer G, Vigonius U, Pohlmann H, Steinhoff BJ, Brodie MJ, Moore A (1997) A double-blind controlled clinical trial: oxcarbazepine versus sodium valproate in adults with newly diagnosed epilepsy. Epilepsy Res 26:451–460
Cockerell OC (1996) The mortality of epilepsy. Current Opin Neurol 9:93–96
Cockerell OC, Johnson AL, Sander JW, Hart YM, Shorvon SD (1995) Remission of epilepsy: results from the National General Practice Study of epilepsy. Lancet 346:140–144
Commission on Classification and Terminology of the International League Against Epilepsy (1989) Proposal for revised classification of epilepsies and epileptic syndromes. Epilepsia 30:389–399
Crosby RD, Pearson VL, Eller C, Winegarden T, Graves NL (1996) Phenytoin in the treatment of cocaine abuse: a double-blind study. Clin Pharmacol Ther 59:458–468
Dam M, Mygind KI, Christiansen J (1976) Antiepileptic drugs: plasma clearance during pregnancy. In: Janz D (ed) Epileptology. Thieme, Stuttgart, pp 179–183
de Silva M, MacArdle B, McGowan M et al. (1996) Randomized comparative monotherapy trial of phenobarbitone, phenytoin, carbamazepine, or sodium valproate for newly diagnosed childhood epilepsy. Lancet 347:709–713
Dean M, Stock B, Patterson RJ, Levy R (1980) Serum protein binding and after pregnancy in humans. Clin Pharmacol Ther 28:253–261
Deutschman CS, Haines SJ (1985) Anticonvulsant prophylaxis in neurological surgery. Neurosurgery 17:510–517
Dickinson RG, Hooper WD, Patterson M, Eadie MJ, Maguire B (1985) Extent of urinary excretion of p-hydroxyphenytoin in healthy subjects given phenytoin. Ther Drug Monit 7:283–289
Eadie MJ (1976) Plasma level monitoring of anticonvulsants. Clin Pharmacokinet 1:52–66
Eadie MJ (1994) Epileptic seizures in 1902 patients: a perspective from a consultant neurological practice (1961–1991). Epilepsy Res 17:55–79
Eadie MJ (1996) The single seizure: to treat or not to treat. CNS Drugs 5:83–86
Eadie MJ, Tyrer JH (1989) Anticonvulsant therapy: pharmacological basis and practice. 3rd edn. Churchill-Livingstone, Edinburgh
Eadie MJ, Tyrer JH, Bochner F, Hooper WD (1976) The elimination of phenytoin in man. Clin Exptl Pharmacol Physiol 3:217–224
Eichelbaum M, Ekbom K, Bertilsson L, Ringberger VA, Rane A (1975) Plasma kinetics of carbamazepine and its epoxide metabolite in man after single and multiple doses. Europ J Clin Pharmacol 8:337–341
Faero O, Kastrup KW, Lykkegaard Nielsen E, Melchior JC, Thorn I (1972) Successful prophylaxis of febrile convulsions with phenobarbital. Epilepsia 13:279–285
Fenn HH, Robinson D, Luby D, Dangel C, Buxton E, Beattie M, Kraemer H, Yesavage JA (1996) Trends in pharmacotherapy of schizoaffective and bipolar affective disorders: a 5-year naturalistic study. Am J Psychiatry 153:711–713
Feucht M, Brantner-Inthaler S (1994) Gamma-vinyl-GABA (vigabatrin) in the therapy of Lennox-Gastaut syndrome: an open study. Epilepsia 35:993–998
Findley LJ, Cleeves L, Calzetti S (1985) Primidone in essential tremor of the hands and head: a double blind controlled study. J Neurol Neurosurg Psychiat 48:911–915
First Seizure Trial Group (1993) Randomized clinical trial on the efficacy of antiepileptic drugs in reducing the risk of relapse after a first unprovoked tonic-clonic seizure. Neurology 43:478–483
Galimberti CA, Manni R, Parietti L, Marchioni E, Tartara A (1993) Drug withdrawal in patients with epilepsy: prognostic value of the EEG. Seizure 2:213–220

Goldberg MA, Dorman JD (1976) Intention myoclonus: successful treatment with clonazepam. Neurology 26:24–26
Gowers WR (1881) Epilepsy and other chronic convulsive disorders. J and A Churchill, London
Gurney ME, Cutting FB, Zhai P, Doble A, Taylor CP, Andrus PK, Hall ED (1996) Benefit of vitamin E, riluzole, and gabapentin in a transgenic model of familial amyotrophic lateral sclerosis. Ann Neurol 39:147–157
Hart YM, Sander JWAS, Johnson AL, Shorvon SD (1990) National General Practice Study of epilepsy: recurrence after a first seizure. Lancet 336:1271–1274
Heller AJ, Chesterman P, Elwes RD, Crawford P, Chadwick D, Johnson AL, Reynolds EH (1995) Phenobarbitone, phenytoin, carbamazepine, or sodium valproate for newly diagnosed adult epilepsy: a randomised comparative monotherapy trial. J Neurol Neurosurg Psychiat 58:44–50
Herkes GK, Eadie MJ, Sharbrough F, Moyer T (1993) Patterns of seizure occurrence in catamenial epilepsy. Epilepsy Res 15:47–52
Hiilesmaa VK (1992) Pregnancy and birth in women with epilepsy. Neurology 42 [Suppl 5]:8–11
Knight AH, Rhind EG (1975) Epilepsy and pregnancy: a study of 153 pregnancies in 59 patients. Epilepsia 16:99–110
Lander CM, Edwards VE, Eadie MJ, Tyrer JH (1977) Plasma anticonvulsant concentrations during pregnancy. Neurology 27:128–131
Lenaerts M, Bastings E, Sianard J, Schoenen J (1996) Sodium valproate in severe migraine and tension-type headache: an open study of long-term efficacy and correlation with blood levels. Acta Neurol Belg 96:126–129
Lindhout D, Omtzigt JGC (1994) Teratogenic effects of antiepileptic drugs: implications for the management of epilepsy in women of childbearing age. Epilepsia 35 [Suppl 4]:S19–S28
Locock C (1857) Discussion of paper by E.H.Sieveking. Analysis of fifty-two cases of epilepsy observed by the author. Lancet 1:527–528
Lucas MJ, Leveno KJ, Cunningham FG (1995) A comparison of magnesium sulphate with phenytoin for the prevention of eclampsia. New Eng J Med 333:201–205
Lund A, Gormsen H (1985) The role of antiepileptics in sudden death. Acta Neurol Scand 72:444–446
Macdonald RL, Kelly KM (1994) Mechanism of action of currently prescribed and newly developed antiepileptic drugs. Epilepsia 36 [Suppl 4]:S41–S50
Marson AG, Kadir ZA, Chadwick DW (1996) New antiepileptic drugs: a systematic review of their efficacy and tolerability. Brit Med J 313:1169–1174
Mathew NT, Saper JR, Silberstein SD, Rankin L, Markley HG, Solomon S, Rapoport AM, Silber CJ, Deaton RL (1995) Migraine prophylaxis with divalproex. Arch Neurol 52:281–286
Matricardi M, Brincotti M, Benedetti P (1989) Outcome after discontinuation of antiepileptic drug therapy in children with epilepsy. Epilepsia 30:582–589
Mattson RH (1994) Current challenges in the treatment of epilepsy. Neurology 44 [Suppl 5]:S4–S9
Mattson RH (1995) Antiepileptic drug monitoring: a reappraisal. Epilepsia 36 [Suppl 5]:S22–S29
Mattson RH, Cramer JA, Collins JF et al. (1985) Comparison of carbamazepine, phenobarbital, phenytoin, and primidone in partial and secondarily generalized tonic-clonic seizures. New Eng J Med 313:145–151
Mattson RH, Cramer JA, Collins JF and Department of Veterans Affairs Epilepsy Cooperative Study No 264 Group (1992) A comparison of valproate with carbamazepine for the treatment of complex partial seizures and secondarily generalised tonic-clonic seizures in adults. New Engl J Med 327:765–771
McAuliffe JJ, Sherwin AL, Leppik IE, Fayle SA, Pippenger CE (1977) Salivary levels of anticonvulsants: a practical approach to drug monitoring. Neurology 27:409–413

McKauge L, Tyrer JH, Eadie MJ (1981) Factors influencing simultaneous concentrations of carbamazepine and its epoxide in plasma. Ther Drug Monit 3:63–70
Medical Research Council Antiepileptic Drug Withdrawal Study Group (1993) Prognostic index for recurrence of seizures after remission of epilepsy. Brit Med J 306:1374–1378
O'Donoghue M, Sander JWAS (1996) Does early anti-epileptic drug treatment alter the prognosis for remission of the epilepsies? J Roy Soc Med 89:245–258
Oller-Daurella L, Oller LF-V (1991) Influence of "lost time" on the outcome of epilepsy. Eur Neurol 31:175–177
Oller-Daurella L, Pamies R, Oller L (1976) Reduction or discontinuance of antiepileptic drugs in patients seizure-free for more than 5 years. In: Janz D (ed) Epileptology. Thieme, Stuttgart, pp. 218–227
Omtzigt JGC, Los FJ, Grobbee DE et al. (1992) The risk of spina bifida aperta after first-trimester exposure to valproate in a prenatal cohort. Neurology 42 [Suppl 5]:119–125
Patsalos PN, Duncan JS (1993) Antiepileptic drugs. A review of clinically significant drug interactions. Drug Safety 9:156–184
Peiris JB, Perera GLS, Devendra SV, Lionel NWD (1980) Sodium valproate in trigeminal neuralgia. M J Australia 2:278
Perucca E (1995) Pharmacological principles as a basis for polytherapy. Acta Neurol Scand [Suppl 162]:31–34
Peterson GM, McLean S, Millingen KS (1984) A randomised trial of strategies to improve patient compliance with anticonvulsant therapy. Epilepsia 25:412–417
Philbert A, Dam M (1982) The epileptic mother and her child. Epilepsia 23:85–99
Reynolds EH (1987) Early treatment and prognosis of epilepsy. Epilepsia 28:97–106
Reynolds EH (1988) The prevention of chronic epilepsy. Epilepsia 29 [Suppl 1]:S25–S28
Reynolds EH, Shorvon SD (1981) Monotherapy or polytherapy for epilepsy. Epilepsia 22:1–10
Reynolds EH, Elwes RDC, Shorvon SD (1983) Why does epilepsy become intractable? Prevention of chronic epilepsy. Lancet:582–584
Richens A, Davidson DLW, Cartlidge NEF, Easter DJ (1994) A multicentre comparative trial of sodium valproate and carbamazepine in adult onset epilepsy. J Neurol Neurosurg Psychiat 57:682–687
Rosa FW (1991) Spina bifida in infants of women treated with carbamazepine during pregnancy. New Eng J Med 324:674–677
Rosman NP (1997) Therapeutic options in the management of febrile seizures. CNS Drugs 7:26–36
Sander JW (1993) Some aspects of the prognosis in the epilepsies: a review. Epilepsia 34:1007–1016
Sato S, Dreifuss FE, Penry JK, Kirby DD, Palesch Y (1983) Long-term follow-up of absence seizures. Neurology 33:1590–1595
Schmidt D (1982) Two antiepileptic drugs for intractable epilepsy with complex-partial seizures. J Neurol Neurosurg Psychiat 45:1119–1124
Schmidt D, Einicke I, Haenel F (1986) The influence of seizure type on the efficacy of plasma concentrations of phenytoin, phenobarbital, and carbamazepine. Arch Neurol 43:263–265
Schoenenberger RA, Tanasijevic MJ, Jha A, Bates DW (1995) Appropriateness of antiepileptic drug level monitoring. J Amer Med Assoc 274:1622–1626
Shinnar S, Berg AT (1996) Does antiepileptic drug therapy prevent the development of "chronic" epilepsy? Epilepsia 37:701–708
Shinnar S, Berg AT, Moshe SL, Kang H, O'Dell C, Alemany M, Goldennsohn ES, Hauser AW (1994) Discontinuing antiepileptic drugs in children with epilepsy: a prospective study. Ann Neurol 35:534–545
Shorvon SD (1996) The epidemiology and treatment of chronic and refractory epilepsy. Epilepsia 37 [Suppl 2]:S1–S3

Tanganelli P, Regesta G (1996) Vigabatrin vs. carbamazepine monotherapy in newly diagnosed focal epilepsy: a randomized response conditional cross-over study. Epilepsy Res 25:257–262

Temkin NR, Dikmen SS, Wilensky A, Keihm J, Chabal S, Winn HR (1990) A randomized double-blind study of phenytoin for the prevention of post-traumatic seizures. New Eng J Med 323:497–502

Tinuper P, Avoni P, Riva R, Provini F, Lugaresi E, Baruzzi A (1996) The prognostic value of the electroencephalogram in antiepileptic drug withdrawal in partial epilepsies. Neurology 47:76–78

Tomson T, Lindbom U, Ekqvist B, Sundqvist A (1994) Epilepsy and pregnancy: a prospective study of seizure control in relation to free and total plasma concentrations of carbamazepine and phenytoin. Epilepsia 35:122–130

van Donselaar CAQ, Schimsheimer R-J, Geerts AT, Declerck AC (1992) Value of the electroencephalogram in adult patients with untreated idiopathic first seizures. Arch Neurol 49:231–237

Walker MC, Smith SJ, Shorvon SD (1995) The intensive care treatment of convulsive status epilepticus in the UK. Results of a national survey and recommendations. Anaesthesia 50:130–135

Yagi K (1996) Evolution of Lennox-Gastaut syndrome: a long-term longitudinal study. Epilepsia 37 [Suppl 3]:48–51

Zimmerman HJ, Ishak KG (1982) Valproate-induced hepatic injury. Analysis of 23 fatal cases. Hepatology 2:591–597

Subject Index

Printing: Saladruck, Berlin
Binding: Buchbinderei Lüderitz & Bauer, Berlin